CLINICAL OPTICS

CLINICAL OPTICS

SECOND EDITION

Troy E. Fannin, O.D.
Professor Emeritus of Optometry
University of Houston
College of Optometry
Houston

Theodore Grosvenor, O.D., Ph.D.
Professor of Optometry
Indiana University
School of Optometry
Bloomington

Butterworth-Heinemann
Boston   Oxford   Johannesburg   Melbourne   New Delhi   Singapore

Copyright © 1996 by Butterworth-Heinemann

⟨R A member of the Reed Elsevier group

Every effort has been made to ensure that the drug dosage schedules within this text are accurate and conform to standards accepted at time of publication. However, as treatment recommendations vary in the light of continuing research and clinical experience, the reader is advised to verify drug dosage schedules herein with information found on product information sheets. This is especially true in cases of new or infrequently used drugs.

Recognizing the importance of preserving what has been written, ∞ Butterworth-Heinemann prints its books on acid-free paper whenever possible.

Library of Congress Cataloging-in-Publication Data
Fannin, Troy E.
    Clinical optics / Troy E. Fannin, Theodore P. Grosvenor. — 2nd
ed.
        p.   cm.
    Includes bibliographical references and index.
    ISBN 0-7506-9670-2 (alk. paper)
    1. Optometry.   2. Physiological optics.   I. Grosvenor, Theodore
P. II. Title.
    [DNLM: 1. Refraction, Ocular. 2. Lenses. 3. Optics.   WW 300
F213c 1996]
RE951.F36   1996
617.7´5—dc20
DNLM/DLC
for Library of Congress   96–191
                                                                            CIP

British Library Cataloguing-in-Publication Data
A catalogue record for this book is available from the British Library.

The publisher offers discounts on bulk orders of this book.
For information, please write:
Manager of Special Sales
Butterworth-Heinemann
225 Wildwood Avenue
Woburn, MA 01801-2041
Tel: 781-904-2500
Fax: 781-904-2620

For more information on all B-H publications available, contact our World Wide Web home page at: http://www.bh.com/

10 9 8 7 6 5 4

Printed in the United States of America

Contents

Preface

During the period of almost a decade since the publication of the first edition of *Clinical Optics*, many advances have occurred in the development of ophthalmic lens materials and lens designs.

Chapter 1, Ophthalmic Lens Materials, presents the physical and optical properties of the many recently introduced high-index glass and plastic lens materials, and the discussion of protective lenses has been expanded. Chapter 6, Aberrations and Ophthalmic Lens Design, describes the newly-available aspheric lens designs—for minus lenses as well as plus lenses.

The most extensive revisions are found in Chapter 7, Absorptive Lenses and Lens Coatings, and in Chapter 8, Multifocal Lenses. Chapter 7 describes recent research on the harmful effects of ultraviolet and short-wavelength visible radiation, as well as lens materials that are available to absorb the harmful radiation. The chapter also describes recent developments in both glass and plastic photochromic lens materials.

Chapter 8 emphasizes the many recently introduced occupational lenses—particularly lenses designed to be used with video display terminals—and the ever-increasing variety of progressive addition lenses, particularly multi-design lenses, which are designed to provide optimum performance regardless of the required addition.

Less extensive revisions have been made in the other chapters. The usefulness of the book has also been enhanced by the inclusion of many additional tables, illustrations, and study questions.

We want to thank Dean Jerald Strickland, of the University of Houston College of Optometry for his encouragement and support. We appreciate the efforts of Ms. Enita Torres, Director of the Audio-Visual Department of the University of Houston College of Optometry, and her staff for conscientiously completing the additional illustrations. We also wish to acknowledge the assistance of several individuals who made valuable suggestions concerning the textbook revision—Dr. Gregory Stephens, Dr. Clifford Brooks, and Mr. John Ross.

Preface to the First Edition

This textbook is intended primarily for use by optometry students, but should prove useful also in programs for the training of optometric technicians and dispensing opticians.

In optometric educational programs, the subject of clinical optics (or ophthalmic optics, as it is sometimes called) is normally presented subsequent to courses in geometrical and physical optics. It is assumed, therefore, that the student taking up the subject of clinical optics will have an understanding of the following topics: the laws of reflection and refraction; the optical principles both of thin lenses and of thick lens systems; the optical principles of cylindrical and toric lenses; the optical principles of prisms; and the principles of chromatic dispersion, lens aberrations, interference, diffraction, and polarization.

In the past, a number of different "sign conventions" have been used by authors of optics textbooks. Nomenclature and notation (or symbols) have also varied from one textbook to another. Fortunately, in recent years most optometric textbooks in the English-speaking world have adopted the sign convention and nomenclature used by British authors including Emsley, Fincham and Freeman, and Bennett.

The introductory chapter will present the sign convention, nomenclature, and notation to be used throughout this textbook. For any terminology not included in the introductory chapter, the reader may wish to refer to W. A. H. Fincham and M. H. Freeman's *Optics*, 9th edition, London: Butterworth–Heinemann, 1980.

INTRODUCTION

Sign Convention, Nomenclature, and Notation

Sign convention, nomenclature, and notation establish the ground rules, or *standard of reference*, for all labeling and measurements. On the basis of this standard of reference, equations are developed that express the fundamental relationships of image formation by optical systems.

0.1. Sign Convention

Throughout this textbook, the English system, as employed by Fincham and Freeman,[1] is used. As illustrated in Figure 0–1, the elements of this sign convention are as follows:

1. Incident light is considered as traveling from *left to right*. An arrowhead on a ray indicates the direction in which the light is traveling.
2. All distances (object distances, image distances, focal lengths, etc.) are measured *from the optical system.*
    a. If measured in the direction in which light is traveling (from left to right), distances are considered as *positive.*
    b. If measured in the direction opposite to that in which light is traveling (from right to left), distances are considered as *negative.*
3. Vertical distances measured from the optic axis to a point above the optic axis are *positive,* whereas vertical distances measured to a point below the optic axis are *negative.*
4. The angle between a ray and the optic axis is measured from the ray to the optic axis.
5. Angles of incidence, refraction, and reflection are measured from the normal to the ray.
6. Angles measured in a counterclockwise direction are considered as *positive;* angles measured in a clockwise direction are considered as *negative.*
7. An arrowhead on a line or a curve, fixing the limit of a given distance or angle, indicates the *direction* in which the distance or the angle is measured.
8. *Vergence* is defined as the curvature of a wavefront at a specific distance from the origin, or focus. As shown in Figure 0–2, if a wavefront is moving toward its focus (converging rays), the vergence is *positive* (A); if a wavefront is emanating from its origin (diverging rays), the vergence is *negative* (B). The unit used for specification of vergence is the *diopter.* For a given wavefront, the vergence, in diopters, is given by the reciprocal of the distance (expressed in meters) from the wavefront to its center of curvature. Thus, the vergence of the converging wavefront shown in Figure 0–2A is +0.50 D; the vergence of the diverging wavefront shown in Figure 0–2B is –0.25 D.

Important Note. Plus and minus signs are assigned to actual *values.* They are not assigned to symbols (i.e., letters) used in mathematical expressions, but to the numbers substituted for these symbols in solving problems.

0.2. Nomenclature

A *ray* is a hypothetical line extending from the origin or focus of a wavefront and is perpendicular to all wavefronts emanating from the origin or moving toward the focus of the wavefront. A ray represents the direction of propagation of the wavefront. Rays are considered to emanate from point sources or from any of an infinite number of points comprising an extended object, or a source of finite size.

A *pencil* is a bundle of rays emanating from a point source after passing through a limiting aperture. The *chief ray* is the ray passing through the center of a limiting aperture.

A *beam* of light is a collection of pencils arising from an extended source, or source of finite size.

An *object* is the physical source of light (or of no light) that exists in object space. Objects, also called sources, may be either point sources or sources of finite size.

Objects may be either *real* or *virtual* (Figure 0–3). Real objects are those from which light actually radiates or from which it is reflected (A). The object presented to the first source of an optical system is always real. Virtual objects are those toward which light is converging before interruption by a subsequent surface of an optical system (B).

An *image*, produced by an optical system, is the optical counterpart of an object. It is formed by the light traveling from the object, in image space, after the optical system has acted on it. Images may be either *real* or *virtual* (Figure 0–4).

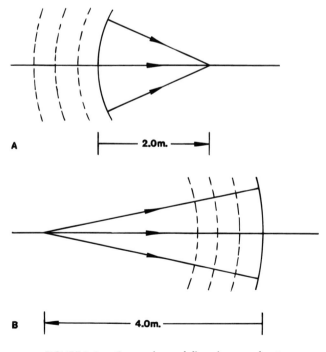

FIGURE 0–2.   **Converging and diverging wavefronts.**

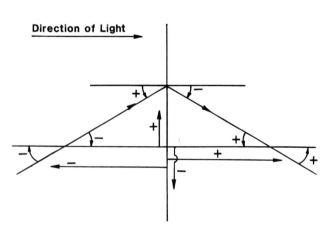

FIGURE 0–1.   **Elements of the sign convention.**

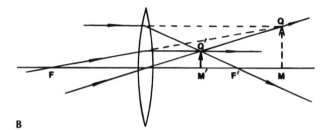

FIGURE 0–3.   Real and virtual objects. A, MQ is a real object; B, MQ is a virtual object.

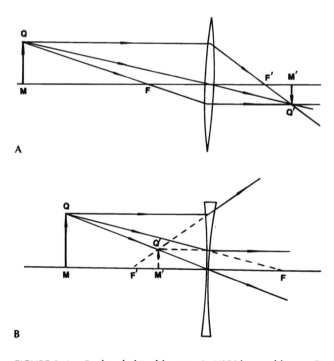

FIGURE 0–4.   Real and virtual images. A, M'Q' is a real image; B, M'Q' is a virtual image.

A real image is one that is actually reached (and formed) by *converging* light rays (A). A real image will be formed on a screen if the screen is placed in the image plane. A virtual image is formed by light that appears to be *diverging* from points in an optical system after treatment by the system (B). Such an image will not be found on a screen placed in the image plane, but may be found by placing a convex lens in the optical system with the result that a real image will be formed. Because the human eye is a converging optical

system, a virtual image may be seen by an observer looking through the optical system.

Object space is the space in which light travels before encountering an optical system. Object space also encompasses the space beyond the optical system, in which light would have traveled had the optical system not interrupted it.

Image space is that space in which light travels after being acted on by the optical system. Like object space, it encompasses the space on both sides of the system: the side on which it is actually traveling and the side from which it appears to have come.

The word *primary*, when used in conjunction with focal points, principal points, and nodal points, applies to points in object space; the word *secondary* applies to points in image space.

0.3. Notation

The following general notation is used in the text:

1. Lowercase letters are used to designate distances, angles, and constants such as an index of refraction.
2. Capital letters are used to denote points, reciprocals of distances, and complicated quantities involving a number of terms and variables.
3. Corresponding object and image quantities are differentiated by following the image quantity by a "prime" ('). For example, f and f' denote the primary and secondary focal lengths, respectively.
4. Subscript numerals are used to designate the order in which the surfaces of a lens or an element of a system are encountered by incident light. For example, F_1 and F_2 denote the front and back surfaces of a lens, respectively.

Commonly used notations include the following:

Indices of Refraction

n, n'	Refractive indices of object and image space.
$n_1, n_2, \ldots$	Index of refraction of the first medium, second medium, etc.

Object and Image Distances and Sizes

l, l'	Distance of object and image from the optical system.
h, h'	Sizes of object and image.

Focal Lengths and Extra-Focal Distances

f, f'	The primary and secondary focal lengths, measured from the optical system.
x, x'	The extra-focal distances, or distances of the object and image from the primary and secondary focal points.

Radii and Curvatures of Surfaces

$r_1, r_2, \ldots$	Radius of the first surface, second surface, etc.
$C_1, C_2, \ldots$	Center of curvature of the first surface, second surface, etc.
$R_1, R_2, \ldots$	Curvature of the first surface, second surface, etc.

Angles

i, i'	Angle of incidence and angle of refraction, respectively.
α, α'	Angular size of object and image, respectively.

Vergence

L	Vergence in object space (n/l).
L'	Vergence in image space (n'/l').

Refracting Power

F	Power of an optical system; ability to change vergence of light.
F_1, F_2	Refracting power of front and back lens surfaces.
F_n	Front vertex power (neutralizing power).
F_v	Back vertex power.
F_e	Equivalent power.

Focal Points, Principal Points, Nodal Points

F, F'	Primary and secondary focal points (or focal planes).
P, P'	First and second principal points (or principal planes).
N, N'	First and second nodal points (or nodal planes).

Magnification

M	Lateral magnification of a lens (h'/h, or L/L').
M	Angular magnification of a lens ($\tan \alpha'/\tan \alpha$, or α'/α).

Prism Notation

β	Refracting angle of a prism.
ε	Refracting power of a prism; P may also be used.
Δ	The prism diopter.
d	Decentration.

Reference

1. Fincham, W. H. A., and Freeman, M. H. *Optics*, 9th edition. Butterworth–Heinemann, London, 1980.

Bibliography

The student may find the following textbooks, on the subject of clinical optics and related areas, to be helpful.

Jalie, M. *The Principles of Ophthalmic Lenses*, 3rd edition. Association of Dispensing Opticians, London, 1977.

Morgan, M. W. *The Optics of Ophthalmic Lenses*. Professional Press, Chicago, 1978.

Brooks, C. W., and Borish, I. M. *System of Ophthalmic Dispensing*. Professional Press, Chicago, 1979.

Stimson, R. L. *Ophthalmic Dispensing*, 3rd edition. Charles C Thomas, Springfield, IL, 1979.

Tunnacliffe, A. H., and Hirst, J. G. *Optics*. Association of Dispensing Opticians, London, 1981.

Sasieni, L. S. *Principles and Practice of Optical Dispensing and Fitting*, 3rd edition. Butterworths, Boston, 1975.

Drew, R. *Professional Ophthalmic Dispensing*. Professional Press, Chicago, 1970.

Keating, M. P. *Geometric, Physical, and Visual Optics*. Butterworths, Stoneham, MA, 1988.

Freeman, H. H. *Optics*, 10th edition. Butterworths, London, 1990.

CHAPTER ONE

Ophthalmic Lens Materials

Although lenses have been used as aids for vision in one form or another since ancient times, throughout most of the period of their use all such lenses were made of glass. Furthermore, from the eighteenth century until the period between World War I and World War II, virtually all single-vision lenses were made of a particular variety of glass known as *ophthalmic crown*.

Varieties of glass other than ophthalmic crown were first utilized for special purposes such as the reading segments of fused bifocal lenses, which were originally made of *flint* glass, having a higher index of refraction than crown glass. More recently, numerous high-index glasses have been developed, not only for bifocal segments but for higher powered single-vision lenses as well. World War II served as a stimulus for the development of plastic materials of optical quality, and the development of plastic ophthalmic lenses proceeded rapidly once the war was over. With the advent of large lens sizes during the 1970s, plastic lenses, only about half as heavy as glass lenses, have assumed an increasingly important role.

This chapter discusses both glass and plastic materials used for the manufacture of ophthalmic lenses in terms of development, their optical properties, and their impact resistance and other physical properties.

GLASS

1.1. History of Glassmaking

Although glass is one of the oldest and most commonplace materials known to man, many questions about the exact nature of glass are still unanswered. Glass may be defined as an amorphous solid material that is obtained by cooling, without crystallization, an inorganic mixture that has been found to fuse at high temperatures. Most liquids change from liquid to solid abruptly and at a definite temperature, but glass behaves in such a way that, on cooling, the viscosity increases continuously, and there is no fixed temperature at which the material solidifies. For this reason, glass is often called a "supercooled" liquid.

Innumerable varieties of glass are available today from the glass industry, formulated for specific and wide-ranging purposes. Although there is a large amount of information available today concerning the structure of glass, a generalized structural model of glass has yet to emerge. Because of the vast array of groups of materials capable of forming glass, a generally accepted structural model of glass is difficult to develop. ("Glass" is a generic term as is "metal"; when referring to different glass compositions it is appropriate to call them "glasses," just as one speaks of "metals.")

The raw materials used to make modern glasses usually include quartz sand, soda (as sodium carbonate), and lime (as carbon oxide). The quartz sand provides silica, which is the principal ingredient of glass. Since the melting temperature of quartz is high (above 1700°C), soda is added as a flux to assist melting. Lime is added to increase its chemical stability and to decrease the solubility of the glass in water.

The first glass used by man probably came from volcanoes. Natural glass formed by volcanic action can be found in many parts of the world; the most common form of natural glass is *obsidian*, a black, translucent material that can be chipped and flaked to make tools, weapons, and ornaments. Other glassy materials, known as *fulgurites*, are long slender tubes of fused sand formed by lightning.

It is not known when glass was first manufactured. As noted by Gasson,[1] Pliny the Elder, a Roman historian, gave one account of the possible origin of the manufacture of glass. He described how a ship laden with *natron*, soda blocks, was moved by Phoenician merchants on the banks of the river Belus near the Mediterranean Sea. The traders, while preparing a meal on the bank, used lumps of natron to support their pots. On being subjected to fire, the soda fused with the sand; to the Phoenicians' surprise, the natron melted and formed beneath the cooking pot a liquid that later cooled into a shining layer of what we now know as glass. According to Pliny, cited by Obrig,[2] production of *permanent* glass involved adding magnesium limestone to the mixture of sand and sodium carbonate, and the craft of glassmaking was imported from Syria into Egypt. At what stage *glassblowing* was invented is a matter of dispute. Although Obrig[2] stated that the art of glassblowing was known in Egypt as early as 2000 B.C., other writers, including Horne[3] and Gasson,[4] gave the Syrians credit for inventing the technique toward the end of the first century B.C.

Regardless of where or when glassmaking began, the craft first flourished in Egypt early in the Eighteenth Dynasty (1580–1358 B.C.). Sophisticated and beautifully made glass appeared abruptly during this dynasty, which suggests that the Egyptians may have imported the skill from elsewhere. In conquering Syria and Egypt during the first century of the Christian era, the Romans learned the glassmaking art and developed it into a large-scale industry. As the Roman Empire expanded, the art of glassmaking expanded to the boundaries of the empire; as the Roman Empire declined, the art of glassmaking also declined. With the fall of the Roman Empire, the centers of glassmaking returned to the Middle East, and remained there until the occurrence of the Renaissance in the West.

The manufacture of glass during the Renaissance period has been traced by Horne.[3] By the year 1000 A.D., glass was being made in Rhineland forest factories, wood was being used to fire the furnaces, and the ashes were being used for the potash flux needed for glassmaking. In the thirteenth century, glass furnaces were built in England (in Surrey and Sussex) by workers from Normandy, and the manufacture of windows and glass vessels was developed. By about 1550 A.D., a high-quality crystal glass had been developed in Venice and was exported to England. In an attempt to rival the Italian crystal, English glassmakers developed, in 1676, a form of crystal made of crushed flint stones (the first *flint* glass). By that time, glass was being produced in quantities in Italy, Germany, France, and England. As a result, a wide range of products made of glass was generally available.

1.2. The Development of Optical Glass

Glass has two properties that make it especially suitable for optical uses. It is transparent to the visible spectrum, and its surfaces may be worked so that they are also transparent and nonscattering.

One of the first references[4] to the use of the convex lens as a burning glass was made by the Greek playwright Aristophanes (450–388 B.C.) in his *Comedy of the Clouds*, written in 423 B.C.:

STREPSIADES: You have seen at the druggist's that fine transparent stone by which fires are kindled?
SOCRATES: You mean glass, do you not?
STREPSIADES: Just so.
SOCRATES: Well, what will you do with that?
STREPSIADES: When a summons is sent to me, I will take this stone, and placing myself between it and the sun, I will, though at a distance, melt all the writing on the summons. (Strepsiades was referring to the wax tablets used for writing at that time.)

The invention of spectacles (if we define *spectacles* as two lenses mounted in a frame and used for the correction of ametropia) apparently occurred late in the thirteenth century. As noted by Hofstetter,[5] possible inventors of spectacles were the Chinese (as reported by Marco Polo in 1270), Roger Bacon, and Salvino degli Armati and Alesandro di Spina, both of Italy. The early lenses were apparently used only for the correction of *presbyopia*. However, during this time, good-quality homogeneous optical glass was not available. The invention of the movable-type printing press by Johannes Gutenberg in Germany in 1440 greatly popularized reading and gave impetus to the craft of spectacle making, but the need for high-quality optical glass became obvious only with the invention of the telescope by Galileo, in 1608.

The experiments of Fraunhofer on the analysis of the sun's spectrum, his specification of the refraction and dispersion of glass in terms of certain lines of the spectrum, and his interest in the color correction of telescope lenses all served to provide the stimulus for the Englishman John Dolland to construct in 1757 an *achromatic lens*, made of crown and flint glass components. Unfortunately, the varieties of optical glass available were not of sufficient homogeneity for use in telescope lenses.

Early optical glasses were known as either crown or flint glass. These terms originated in interesting ways. The adjective "crown" was originally applied to window glass used for seventeenth- and eighteenth-century houses in England. This glass was blown and whirled into a disk with a knot left in the center by the working rod. Before the development of optical glasses especially made for lenses, pieces of crown glass were used for ophthalmic lenses and the lenses were known as crown lenses. Today, *crown* refers to glass whose primary ingredients are silica, soda or potash, and lime.

In 1676 George Ravenscroft, an Englishman, used ground flints as a source of silica and incorporated a relatively large quantity of lead as one of the basic constituents of glass. The glass became known as flint glass. It was softer, heavier, clearer, and more brilliant than any other glass then available and was used for drinking vessels, bowls, and quality crystalware. Today, *flint* glasses are those that contain lead oxide.

One of the earliest makers of optical glass was P. L. Guinand of Switzerland, who discovered around 1814 that the homogeneity of glass could be greatly increased by *stirring* the glass while it was in the crucible in the molten state. In 1827 Michael Faraday began studies to improve the quality of optical glass in England. He developed methods of purifying the substances and constructed a *platinum* crucible that was remarkably resistant to attack by molten glass. However, this event went rather unnoticed and platinum did not come into use for nearly a century after Faraday's work. In 1839 the Chance brothers of England began the manufacture of a large range of optical glasses.

Beginning in 1876, Ernst Abbe and Otto Schott, of Jena, Germany, collaborated in experimenting with a large number of chemical oxides in the manufacture of glass and developed a wide range of new glasses for optical purposes. Before 1880, the only types of glasses of optical quality were crown and flint. The addition of lead oxide to flint glass increased both the refractive index and the dispersive power compared with that of crown glass. The invention of barium crown glass by Abbe in 1880 introduced a glass of high refractive index without an appreciable increase in dispersive power. As a result of the researches of Abbe and Schott, the firm of Carl Zeiss soon gained preeminence in the manufacture of optical glass.

In the United States, glassmaking was one of the first industries started in the Colony of Virginia, near Jamestown, in 1607. The Colony is said to have produced colored glass beads for use in trading with Indians. The first American attempt at producing optical glass was made by George Macbeth of the Macbeth-Evans Glass Company in 1889 at Elwood, Indiana, but was soon abandoned. The next attempt was made by Bausch & Lomb Optical Company in 1912, and by 1915 Bausch & Lomb was producing substantial amounts of optical glass of good quality. In the early months of 1917, when the imminence of the entry of the United States into World War I was apparent, the supply of optical glass was extremely critical. Imported stocks from Germany, Great Britain, and France were eliminated or were severely curtailed. In this emergency, the United States government set out to speed up the production of optical glass. With this stimulus, over 600,000 pounds of optical glass were produced during the remaining months of the war. Today, Corning, Inc., Pittsburgh Plate Glass Company, and Schott Glass Technologies, Inc., comprise the major glass manufacturers in the United States.

1.3. The Manufacture of Optical Glass

The process of optical glassmaking has been described in some detail by Obrig,[2] and his description serves as a basis for this discussion. The art of glassmaking consists of melting together the necessary ingredients at a temperature high enough to produce a liquid mass sufficiently fluid to permit any bubbles to escape, of mixing the molten mass thoroughly by stirring so that the composition is the same throughout, and of pouring and rolling the glass into a large sheet that is cooled slowly or is cooled by letting the pot and the glass cool together at room temperature.

The ingredients are put into a *melting pot* 36 inches in diameter and 32 inches high, sufficient to make about 1000 pounds of glass. The ingredients making up the batch depend, of course, on the type of glass being made, but are principally oxides or salts of metals including silica, sodium and potassium, calcium, and aluminum. An additional ingredient, called *cullet*, is waste glass from previous melts. It is added to save valuable raw materials and to form a *glaze* on the surface of the pot, which reduces the corrosive action of the pot by the melting of the raw materials.

Before furnace operations are begun, the pot is gradually raised to a temperature of 800° to 1000°C and kept there for 3 to 5 days, after which the pot is glazed by the use of small pieces of cullet. The ingredients are then added at intervals until the temperature of the pot is raised to about 1400°C. During the melting process, the batch is full of bubbles of escaping gas. The escaping of the gas is known as *fining;* toward the end of the melting and fining process (which requires several hours) scum, stones, and other materials rise to the top of the batch and are skimmed off. The melt is then stirred constantly with long clay rods, which may be moved either mechanically or by hand.

After the melting, fining, and stirring processes are completed, the molten glass has the consistency of heavy syrup. When cooled to a temperature of 1200°C, it is poured and rolled into sheets of various thicknesses, and each sheet of glass is placed in a heated annealing oven where it is gradually cooled to room temperature. After annealing, the glass is cut into small pieces, is reheated, and is then either pressed or molded into *rough blanks*. After inspection, the rough blanks are blocked on grinding shells and the first surface is ground and polished to the desired curvature. The blanks are then reblocked, and ground and polished on the second side.

This process, called the *batch process*, was formerly used for the manufacture of all optical glass. Now, it is used only for the production of relatively small quantities of glass, for example, special types of glass such as high-index glass and many varieties of colored glass. An automated method known as the *continuous-flow process* is now used for making large quantities of a particular type of glass. The process differs from the batch process in that the molten glass is not poured into sheets but is extruded, by means of a continuous process, and pressed into molds to make the rough blanks.

1.4. Varieties of Optical Glass

The critical properties of optical glass are the *refractive index*, n, the *dispersion*, expressed by the Abbe number, V, and the *specific gravity*. Since refractive index and dispersion vary for different wavelengths of light, it is necessary to measure them at some known wavelength standard. In the United States the convention is that the wavelength standard is the Fraunhofer d line, which is the yellow helium line of wavelength 587.56 nm. Therefore, the index is labeled n_d and the Abbe number, also called constringence, is labeled V_d. The index of refraction for the d line, n_d, is defined as

$$n_d = \frac{\text{velocity of helium light in a vacuum}}{\text{velocity of helium light in an optical medium}} \quad (1.1)$$

Two other indices are of interest because they define the Abbe number for dispersion. The first, n_F, is the refractive index of the Fraunhofer F line at the blue end of the spectrum, with a wavelength of 486.13 nm; the other, n_C, is the refractive index for the Fraunhofer C line at the red end of the spectrum, with a wavelength of 656.27 nm. The Abbe number is defined as

$$V_d = \frac{n_d - 1}{n_F - n_C} \quad (1.2)$$

The Abbe number is the reciprocal of the relative dispersion expression,

$$\frac{n_F - n_C}{n_d - 1}$$

Because the V value is the reciprocal of relative dispersion, the optical medium having a high V value has a low dispersion, and vice versa. Furthermore, as shown in Chapter 6, Section 6.3, the longitudinal chromatic aberration of a lens is defined as

$$C.A. = \frac{F_d}{V_d}$$

and the chromatic aberration of a prism is defined as

$$C.A. = \frac{\varepsilon_d}{V_d}$$

Every material has its unique weight per unit volume, known as *density*. *Specific gravity* is the ratio of the weight of a substance to the weight of water with the same volume. For example, 1 cubic foot of glass weighs 158.6 lb, and water weighs 62.5 lb per cubic foot. The specific gravity of glass is therefore given by the expression

$$\text{Specific gravity} = \frac{158.6}{62.5} = 2.54.$$

When the volume is measured in cubic centimeters (cm^3), the density and specific gravity have the same numerical value because the density of water is 1.00 g/cm.^{3}

As discussed earlier, the terms "crown" and "flint" applied to optical glass have lost their original meanings. Now, arbitrarily, glasses with Abbe numbers greater than 50 are called crown glasses, and glasses having Abbe numbers less than 50 are called flint glasses.

Not all glasses are classified by this system. Many glasses are designated by descriptive names, for example, High-Lite (made by Schott), or abbreviations such as LHI. The most meaningful classification is a six-digit designation whose first three digits are the decimal of the index of refraction and whose remaining three digits are the Abbe value. Thus, ophthalmic crown glass is designated "523590."

The three main varieties of optical glass are ophthalmic crown glass, flint glasses, and barium crown glasses. *Ophthalmic crown* derives its name, as already discussed, from the sheets of glass originally blown for window glass. However, "crown" now is used to refer to the composition of the glass rather than to its method of manufacture. The ingredients of ophthalmic crown glass are silica (sand) (70%); sodium oxide (soda) (14–16%); calcium oxide (lime) (11–13%); and small percentages of potassium, borax, antimony, and arsenic. Ophthalmic crown glass is used for the great majority of single-vision glass lenses, and for the distance portion of most glass bifocal and trifocal lenses. As already noted, its index of refraction is 1.523 and its Abbe value is 59.

Flint glasses contain from 45% to 65% lead oxide, from 25% to 45% silica, and about 10% mixture of soda and potassium oxide. As compared with crown glass, flint glasses have a higher index of refraction (from 1.580 for light flint to 1.690 for dense flint) and a higher chromatic dispersion (an Abbe value of 30 to 40). They are used for bifocal segments for some *fused* bifocals (in which the segment must have a higher index of refraction than does the major lens) and, until recently, for single-vision lenses of high power, because the high index of refraction allows a *thinner* (although heavier) lens to be produced. Other high-index glasses have largely supplanted flint for this purpose.

Barium crown glasses contain from 25% to 40% barium oxide, which has the same effect as lead oxide in increasing the index of refraction, but without as great an increase in chromatic dispersion. These glasses have indices of refraction from 1.541 to 1.616, and Abbe values from 55 to 59 (comparable to that of crown glass). Their main use is for segments of Nokrome's series of fused bifocals. The optical properties of high-index glasses developed for fused bifocal segments, as compared with those of ophthalmic crown glass, are shown in Table 1–1.

In recent years, many specific varieties of glass, having special properties, have been developed. These include high-index glasses with refractive indices of 1.60, 1.70, and 1.80. These glasses have a high content of titanium oxide and are useful for reducing the thickness of high-powered lenses. Characteristics of some of these glasses are shown in Table 1–2.

Glass for *absorptive lenses* is made by the addition of metallic oxides to the raw materials in the batch. For example, the addition of cobalt results in a *blue* lens, chromium oxide in a *green* lens, magnesium in a *violet* lens, and uranium in a *yellow* lens. These and other metallic oxides may be used in combination to achieve the desired effect. In addition, cerium oxide and other materials have the property of absorbing *ultraviolet* radiation, and iron oxide has the property of absorbing *infrared* radiation.

Photochromic glass contains silver halide crystals, which under the influence of ultraviolet radiation separate into silver and halide ions. The silver and halide ions cluster together, and as the cluster becomes larger, it becomes opaque and causes the lenses to darken in the presence of ultraviolet light. In the absence of ultraviolet radiation, the silver and halide crystals recombine and cause the lenses to fade. The main types of photochromic glasses are *borosilicate* for Corning, Inc. lenses and *alumino-phosphate* for Chance-Pilkington Ltd. lenses.

Absorptive lenses (including photochromic lenses) are discussed in greater detail in Chapter 7.

TABLE 1–1
Optical Properties of Representative High-Index Glasses Developed for Multifocal Segment Compared with Ophthalmic Crown Glass

Glass	Refractive Index	Abbe No.	Specific Gravity	Use
Ophthalmic crown	1.523	58.9	2.54	Single vision, carrier of multifocals
Light barium crown	1.573	57.4	3.21	Intermediate segment of trifocal
Dense barium crown	1.616	55.1	3.36	Near segments of bifocals and trifocals
Dense flint	1.649	33.8	3.90	Segment of kryptok bifocals
Extra-dense flint	1.69	30.9	4.23	Segment of kryptok bifocals

TABLE 1–2
Optical Properties of Representative High-Index Glasses Compared with Ophthalmic Crown Glass

Manufacturer/Supplier	Glass	Refractive Index	Abbe No.	Specific Gravity
[Numerous]	Ophthalmic crown	1.52	58.9	2.54
Pilkington	Slimline 640	1.600	41.0	2.59
Hoya	LH-II	1.600	42.5	2.58
Corning	Photogray Extra 16*	1.600	42.2	2.73
Corning	Photobrown Extra 16*	1.600	42.2	2.73
Schott	S.1018	1.601	42.2	2.67
Rodenstock	High-Crown	1.604	41.8	2.67
Pilkington	Slimline 730	1.700	31.0	2.99
Pilkington	Slimline 750	1.700	51.0	3.38
Hoya	LHI	1.702	40.2	2.99
Schott	High-Lite	1.706	31.0	2.99
Rodenstock	Rodalent 1.7	1.706	39.3	3.20
Rodenstock	Rodalent 1.8	1.800	35.4	3.60
Ohara	Index 8	1.805	26.4	3.37
Pilkington	Slimline 825	1.805	25.0	3.35
Hoya	THI-II	1.806	33.3	3.47
Nikon	Pointal	1.830	32.0	3.59

* Photochromic glass.

1.5. Desirable Characteristics and Defects of Optical Glass

Desirable characteristics of optical glass, described by Obrig,[2] are:

1. Homogeneity in both chemical composition and physical state.
2. Correct index of refraction and chromatic dispersion values.
3. Freedom from color.
4. A high degree of transparency.
5. A high degree of chemical and physical stability.

Homogeneity

CHEMICAL COMPOSITION

Nonuniformity in the chemical composition of glass results in the following defects:

1. *Striae*—streaks or lines in the glass, caused by uneven mixing (also called *veins*), having a different index of refraction than the surrounding media.
2. *Bubbles*—usually formed during the melting and fining processes, occurring as a result of gaseous matter that fails to reach the surface before the glass cools (also referred to as seeds, air-bells, or boil).
3. *Inclusions*—consisting of stones and crystallites. Stones are undissolved particles of material in the finished glass. Crystallites are crystal bodies formed when the cooling process is too slow.
4. *Cloudiness*—caused by precipitated colloidal material (sulfates and chlorates) during the cooling period.

PHYSICAL STATE

Refractive index and structural characteristics of optical glass are strongly influenced by the thermal history of the material. Improper annealing procedures can produce (1) index differences throughout the bulk of the glass; (2) sufficient double refraction (birefringence) to cause image degradation; and (3) residual stress that may cause fracture or distortion when the glass is worked. Defects in the homogeneity of glass are found at final inspection of the glass or during the later stages of processing, either by a human inspector or by an optical inspection system.

Index of Refraction and Dispersion Values

Index of refraction is defined as the ratio of velocity of light in a vacuum to the velocity in a given medium *at a given wavelength*. For ophthalmic crown glass, the index of refraction with Fraunhofer d line (wavelength 587.56 nm)—but not for the C line (656.27 nm) or for the F line (486.13 nm)—is 1.523. Dispersive power is based on the change in index for different wavelengths (C and F, as compared with

d). If the index of refraction of a substance is the same for *all* wavelengths, there will be no chromatic dispersion. Therefore, not only must the refractive index for the d line be correct, but the indices for the C and F lines must also be controlled for the dispersive power (Abbe value) to be correct.

The index of refraction increases as the wavelength decreases. Dispersion usually increases in glasses of high refractive index. This is demonstrated in Table 1–2; for example, materials having refractive indices in excess of 1.80 have Abbe numbers between 32.0 and 35.4; patients may complain of seeing color fringes while wearing these lenses.

Table 1–2 also shows that specific gravity increases as index of refraction increases. This means that although a high-index lens may be thinner than a lens made of ophthalmic crown, one would expect the high-index lens to be heavier than the ophthalmic crown lens. However, this is not always true. As discussed in Chapter 11 and shown in Figure 11–18, a 1.70-index lens having a power of about ±8.00 D (and having a diameter of 50 mm and a minimum center thickness of 2.0 mm) is no heavier than an ophthalmic crown lens of the same power.

Color and Transparency

Clear optical glass must have the highest transparency and transmission possible for light in the spectral region for which it is designed. Clear optical glass transmits only 92% of the incident light as a result of loss of approximately 4% at each of the surfaces because of reflections. Surface reflections decrease with increasing wavelength; therefore, an optical glass with no absorption would have a spectral variation in transmission that would change the color of the light passing through it.

High-index glasses transmit less than 92% of the incident light because of increased surface reflectance. If a tint is specified, the glass must have the correct transmission properties. Transmission is specified in terms of a lens thickness of 2 mm; the thicker the lens, the lower the transmission. Unwanted color in a batch of glass is caused by the presence of impurities in the raw materials or is a result of material from the pot's walls entering into solution with the glass. Iron oxide is the most serious source of problems and causes an intense green or yellow discoloration.

Chemical and Physical Stability

Optical glass should be hard, durable, resistant to weather, and should not tarnish or stain. Flint and barium crown glasses are softer than ophthalmic crown glass, and are less chemically tolerant. Materials used for fused bifocals must be physically stable and the major lens and segment glasses must have equal expansion rates so that stress does not occur along the line of fusion.

PLASTIC MATERIALS

1.6. Characteristics

A plastic material is defined as "a polymeric material (usually organic) of large molecular weight which can be shaped by flow; usually refers to the final product with fillers, plasticizers, pigments and stabilizers included (versus the resin, the homogeneous starting material)."[6] Although terminology often changes with technology, the adjective "plastic" is still widely used to describe ophthalmic lenses made from one of these materials. In the early years of development, plastics had a reputation of being cheap substitutes for traditional materials, a reputation often abetted by improper processing or by incorrect use of materials. However, at the present time, if plastics are processed properly and tailored for appropriate applications, they may offer many advantages compared with the materials they replace.

Because of the negative connotation of the term "plastic," ophthalmic lens manufacturers have used other terms to describe lenses made of plastic materials, such as "organic" lenses (because the lenses are made by processes involving organic chemistry, as compared with the "mineral" nature of glass lenses, which are manufactured from mineral materials). Other adjectives used to describe plastic lenses are "resin" and "hard resin." No term has yet been universally adopted.

Most plastics are synthetic materials formed by combining various organic ingredients with inorganic materials such as carbon, hydrogen, oxygen, nitrogen, chlorine, and sulfur. Some raw materials, such as wood and cotton (cellulose) and milk (casein), may come directly from plant and animal sources. More commonly, the raw materials are derivatives of fossil-formed products such as oil, coal, and natural gas.

Although billions of pounds of plastics are produced each year, the amount used for optical purposes is only a very small fraction of the total. Most of the research efforts concerning the optical uses of plastic materials have been financed by private industry with the goal of developing new optical products with attractive properties and with desirable indices of refraction and dispersive powers. In many instances, the amount of information available is scanty because the material formulation and processing technology are proprietary secrets.

1.7. Manufacturing Processes

Plastic materials can be classified into two main groups, on the basis of the physical properties of the finished product: *thermoplastic* materials, which soften when heated and therefore can be remolded, and *thermosetting* materials, which once hardened cannot be softened, even at high temperatures.

Thermoplastic materials have their molecules arranged in long chains, and such materials are usually supplied in pellet, granular, or sheet form. The material softens when heated and can be stretched, pressed, or molded into complex shapes with no appreciable change in its chemical structure. When cooled, the material hardens and shrinks and has the same configuration as the mold in which it was heated. This process is known as *injection molding*. Since no chemical change transpires, the softening and hardening cycle may be repeated indefinitely. Thermoplastic materials are generally less dimensionally stable than thermosetting materials (described below) and they can withstand less heat without deformation. Examples of thermoplastic materials are acrylates (including the familiar trade names Plexiglas, Lucite, and polymethyl methacrylate used for the manufacture of "hard" contact lenses), cellulose acetate and cellulose nitrate (zylonite and celluloid, both of which are used for the manufacture of spectacle frames), polycarbonate, polystyrene, nylons, and vinyls.

Thermosetting materials are usually supplied in liquid monomer form and cast in molds. Plasticizers, filters, dyes, binding modifiers, other monomers, and catalysts may be added to the basic chemical compound. After the catalyst is added and the material is heated, *polymerization* occurs. This is the linking together of the molecules to form longer molecular chains, the molecules forming a three-dimensional, cross-linked, lattice pattern rather than the two-dimensional pattern of the thermoplastic material. This process transforms a liquid monomer first into a syrup, then into a gel, and finally into a solid. The relationship between the time and temperature required in the hardening process is known as the *curing cycle*. Once hardened, the material cannot be softened (even at high temperature). The process is irreversible, and it is this characteristic that distinguishes this material from the thermoplastic materials. If the thermosetting materials are subjected to a high temperature, the material decomposes without melting or substantially softening.

Thermosetting materials have good dimensional stability, are rigid, are relatively insensitive to heat, are flame resistant, can withstand solvents, and have relatively hard surfaces. Examples of thermosetting materials are allyl diglycol carbonate (Columbia Resin 39 [Pittsburgh Plate Glass], or CR-39, used for most plastic lenses), epoxies, phenolics (trade name, Bakelite), and melamine compounds (used for tableware).

When two monomers are mixed the resultant material, called a *copolymer*, possesses some of the characteristics of each of the constituent materials. The two monomers need not originate from the same group: One can be thermosetting and the other thermoplastic.

1.8. Development of Optical Plastics

Although plastic materials have been available for many years, plastic lenses are relatively new compared with glass lenses. They provided little competition to glass lenses until the decade of the 1970s. Because of Food and Drug Administration (FDA) requirements to test lenses for impact resistance, the increasing popularity of larger lens sizes, and the availability of an easily used dyeing system for creating "fashion tints," plastic lenses were suddenly in great demand.

Just as World War I served as the impetus for the development of the optical glass industry in the United States, World War II served as the impetus for the development of the plastics industry. One of the plastic materials developed during World War II was *polymethyl methacrylate* (PMMA), a synthetic thermoplastic resin developed for aircraft windshields. This material has been known in the United States by the trade names Lucite or Plexiglas, and in England by the trade name Perspex, and has been used for a variety of products from plumbing fixtures to the well-known PMMA contact lenses. This material was also used for the manufacture of spectacle lenses (such as the Igard lens, made in Great Britain), and although it had the advantage of being much more shatterproof than nontempered glass, it had the unfortunate disadvantage of scratching more easily. Another plastic material developed during World War II, also for use in military applications, was the material *allyl diglycol carbonate*, known as Columbia Resin 39, or CR-39. Just before 1940, the Columbia Southern Division of Pittsburgh Plate Glass Industries was asked to develop a lightweight transparent plastic material for use in military aircraft. Concentrating on thermosetting rather than on thermoplastic materials, a series of 170 clear allylic resins were compounded and tested. The 39 compound, designated as CR-39, was the allyl diglycol carbonate monomer, and it was selected as having the optimal properties for further development for use in military aircraft.

In 1947 Robert Graham, an optometrist, formed the Armorlite Lens Company in Pasadena, California, and later described[7] the first ophthalmic lenses made from CR-39 in the United States. The Armorlite Lens Company subsequently manufactured CR-39 lenses in commercial quantities for the optical professions. This material, although scratching more easily than glass, is much more scratch resistant than polymethyl methacrylate. The CR-39 lens, now over 45 years old, currently dominates the plastic lens market.

In 1957 General Electric developed a new plastic material, a *polycarbonate resin*, called Lexan. This material, of great mechanical strength and high service temperatures, was first produced in ophthalmic lenses in 1978 by Gentex Corporation.

In 1982 Corning Glass Works announced the development of a lens called Corlon, a two-layer ophthalmic composite material consisting of a glass lens backed by a very thin layer of polyurethane film, which is bonded to the back surface of the glass lens. Under a licensing agreement, the lens material is being made available to optical laboratories in stock single-vision lenses. Because delamination often occurred during surfacing and edging operations, Corning discontinued the manufacture of the Corlon lens.

1.9. Manufacture of Plastic Lenses

CR-39 Lenses

Ophthalmic lenses made of CR-39 are cast from allyl diglycol carbonate monomer. Currently, the only American source of allyl diglycol carbonate monomer is the Columbia Division of Pittsburgh Plate Glass Industries, which supplies it to qualified casters (ophthalmic and nonophthalmic) as a yellowish, viscous liquid that produces CR-39 in a variety of forms and sizes. Although the basic process of making CR-39 lenses is common to most manufacturers, some add a copolymer or other additives, such as antiyellowing agents, ultraviolet absorbers, and mold releasers. Although copolymers and additives may reduce lens shrinkage, make casting easier, and make lenses lighter and tougher, the lenses are usually impaired in other ways, such as being less scratch resistant.

After the catalyst and other ingredients are added, the liquid resin is poured into a mold. The mold consists of two glass surfaces, one concave and the other convex, assembled with a gasket of predetermined thickness to control center and edge thickness of the lens. The inside surfaces of the mold, which impart the curvature to the lens, are made with great precision and are highly polished to produce finished lens surfaces of high quality. The glass molds are chemically tempered to resist the flexing action caused by the shrinkage of the CR-39 material during polymerization. (Shrinkage is about 14%.) The entire mold is then placed in an oven and subjected to a controlled time/temperature relationship called the *cure cycle*. After completion of the cure cycle, the molds are removed from the oven, dismantled, and separated from the finished lenses.

The preparation of the monomer in combination with the cure cycle used determines the physical properties of the finished lens. Lower temperatures and longer curing times produce lenses that have superior rigidity, dimensional stability, impact resistance, and scratch resistance.

Polycarbonate Lenses

Polycarbonate is a thermoplastic material. It begins as a solid, is melted down, and is then injected into a mold at a temperature of about 320°C. In the injection process, the polycarbonate conforms, under pressure, to the highly polished metal surfaces of the injection mold. A device will squeeze the lens to prevent shrinkage and ensure optical accuracy of the surfaces. Each lens-forming cycle requires approximately 90 to 130 seconds. After removal from the molds, the lenses are inspected and processed through a coating machine. Because the surface hardness of polycarbonate is much softer than CR-39, *all* polycarbonate lenses receive a hard coating to increase scratch resistance and chemical protection. Once the coating process is completed, a heat-curing process produces polymerization and cross-linking of the coating. The coating solvents evaporate and leave behind a silica-based solid coating approximately 4 to 6 μm thick.

1.10. Optical and Physical Properties of Plastic Lenses

CR-39

This material has an index of refraction of 1.498, an Abbe value of 58, and a specific gravity of 1.32. Its desirable characteristics include the following:

1. *Lightness.* Because of its low specific gravity, a CR-39 plastic lens weighs approximately half ($1.32/2.54 = 0.52$) that of an ophthalmic crown glass lens of identical size and prescription. For a strong prescription requiring thick lenses or for use of a frame with a large eye size, the weight difference is significant.

2. *Impact Resistance.* Without the need for special treatment, CR-39 lenses are sufficiently impact resistant to pass the FDA impact-resistance tests.

3. *Chemical Inertness.* CR-39 lenses are resistant to virtually all solvents including acetone, benzene, and gasoline, and to most chemicals other than highly oxidizing acids.

4. *Resistance to Pitting.* CR-39 material is more resistant than glass to pitting from small hot particles such as welding spatter and particles thrown off grinding wheels.

5. *Resistance to Fogging.* CR-39 material has a much lower thermal conductivity than glass, and hence fogging and misting do not occur as readily from sudden temperature changes as they do with glass.

6. *Tintability.* Almost any tint or color can be applied to the surface of a CR-39 lens. A uniform tint over the entire surface or a gradient tint of varying intensity or color may be applied. If desired, the tint can be removed and the lens dyed with a different color.

7. *Versatility in Optical Design.* Repletion casting techniques permit optical designers more latitude in incorporating desirable optical features that traditionally have been prohibitive in cost and hence largely unavailable. Examples include aspheric surfaces for cataract lenses, magnifiers with aspheric surfaces, high-powered lenticular lenses, occupational trifocals, progressive addition multifocal lenses, and reverse slab-off construction—all of which are now available at a reasonable cost.

These lenses, however, are not without some disadvantages, which include:

1. *Surface Abrasion.* The resistance to surface abrasion is appreciably lower in CR-39 material than in ophthalmic crown glass. The surfaces must be worked carefully and patients must be instructed properly in their care. However, manufacturers have responded to this problem by developing durable, hard, coating systems that greatly improve scratch resistance. The coating should preferably be placed on *both* surfaces.

2. *Warpage upon Glazing.* Targrove et al.[8] reported after a 12-month evaluation that significant amounts of lens warpage were almost universally revealed by the use of a Geneva lens gauge. Such warping may go undetected on a lensometer if the front and back surface warpages are essentially equal. The base curves provided in a particular lens series for a given prescription are selected by the lens designer to minimize oblique astigmatism and mean power error. Warpage changes the initial form of the lens and affects its performance for these two aberrations, as well as the magnification and distortion properties of the lens. Smith and Wientzen[9] studied the theoretical performance changes caused by warpage and concluded that, if the manufacturer adheres to the 1-D tolerance for induced warpage as set forth in the American National Standards Institute

(ANSI) Z80.1-1995 *Prescription Ophthalmic Lenses—Recommendations,*[10] the changes were not likely to cause difficulties except for adaptation and annoying differences between one pair of glasses and another.

3. *Increased Thickness.* As a result of its relatively low index of refraction, a CR-39 lens of a given power has a greater thickness difference between the center and the edge than does a glass lens. The thickness difference is increased with large eye sizes, and may elicit patient complaints because of cosmetic appearance.

4. *Inferior Photochromic Properties.* No manufacturer has been successful in producing plastic photochromic lenses having permanent fading and darkening cycles. However, improvements have been made in such lenses (see Chapter 7).

5. *Index variability with temperature.* Although the refractive index homogeneity of optical plastics approaches that of standard optical glass, the change in refractive index as a function of temperature is about 50 times greater than that of optical glass.[11] This makes optical performance of optical plastics much less stable in thermally fluctuating environments.

Polycarbonate

The unique characteristic of polycarbonate is that it is vastly superior to both ophthalmic glass and CR-39 plastic in terms of impact resistance. Polycarbonate differs from CR-39 in having an index of refraction of 1.586, which is higher (rather than lower) than that of glass. Accordingly, the difference between center thickness and edge thickness is less than that for glass; for a minus lens having the same center thickness as a glass lens, this material produces a thinner edge. The specific gravity of polycarbonate material is less than that of CR-39 (1.20 compared with 1.32), resulting in a lens of lighter weight. For high-powered lenses, the decreased weight is enhanced by decreased edge thickness (minus lenses) or decreased center thickness (plus lenses).

The surface of a polycarbonate lens is inherently very soft and scratches easily. Therefore, all polycarbonate lenses are factory coated on both sides with a scratch-resistant coating. The coating produces a surface that is as scratch resistant as a coated CR-39 lens.

All polycarbonate lenses absorb ultraviolet radiation up to 380 nm without additional treatment. Tinting of polycarbonate lenses is accomplished with the dyes used for CR-39 lenses. Because polycarbonate does not accept dye, the color is absorbed by the lens coating.

Having a higher index of refraction, polycarbonate lenses may produce more reflections than ophthalmic crown glass or CR-39. The scratch-resistant coating may lower the intensity of the reflections; however, if reflections are a problem, an antireflection coating may also be applied to the lenses.

An optical disadvantage of polycarbonate, as compared with either CR-39 or spectacle crown glass, is its low Abbe number (constringence) and, therefore, its high dispersive power. This produces undesirable lateral chromatic aber-

TABLE 1–3
Optical Properties of Representative Newly-Introduced Plastic Lens Materials Compared with Ophthalmic Crown Glass, CR-39 Plastic, and Polycarbonate

Manufacturer/Supplier	Material	Refractive Index	Abbe No.	Specific Gravity
[Numerous]	Ophthalmic crown	1.523	58.9	2.54
Pittsburg Plate Glass	CR-39	1.498	58.0	1.32
[Numerous]	Polycarbonate	1.586	30.0	1.20
Transitions Optical	Transitions*	1.500	57.0	1.28
Sola	Spectralite	1.537	47.0	1.21
Signet Armorlite	RLX-Lite	1.537	36.0	1.21
Hoya	HiLux II	1.556	40.0	1.27
Pittsburg Plate Glass	HIP	1.556	37.7	1.221
Seiko	Diacoat Thin	1.556	40.0	1.27
Younger	Younger-Lite	1.556	37.7	1.216
Silor	Thin & Lite	1.595	36.0	1.37
Optima	Hyper-Index 1.60	1.597	37.0	1.34
Signet Armorlite	1.60 High Index	1.600	36.0	1.45
Hoya	Hi-Lux Excellence	1.600	36.0	1.34
Seiko	Super 1.6	1.600	34.0	1.38
Pentax	Superthin 1.6	1.600	36.0	1.34
Zeiss	Claret SL	1.600	36.0	1.34
Optima	Hyperindex 166	1.660	32.0	1.35
Nikon	NL IV HCC	1.660	32.0	1.35

* Photochromic plastic.

ration upon peripheral gaze, which the wearer perceives as color fringes on all contours. In combination with oblique astigmatism, this dispersion may produce a loss of image clarity when the wearer uses the peripheral portion of the lens. This chromatic aberration is a function of the Abbe number and the prismatic power at the peripheral point used by the eye. The prismatic effect, of course, depends on the power of the lens and the eccentricity of gaze according to Prentice's rule (see Chapter 4, Section 4.6).

The findings of two studies of the peripheral effects of chromatic dispersion on visual acuity are not in agreement. Meslin and Obrecht[12] concluded that aberrations linked to chromatic dispersion of lenses are less important than expected and that materials with lower constringences could be used for ophthalmic lenses. However, Hampton et al.[13] concluded that in certain combinations of prescription power and eccentricity of gaze, significant blurring of vision will occur because of the dispersion inherent in polycarbonate. Therefore, the prescriber should consider whether this disadvantage equals or exceeds its impact-resistant advantage.

Surfaces of polycarbonate lenses are difficult to mold in such a way that the lenses are free of surface waves or other noticeable blemishes. The material is also difficult to work with: Edging and beveling require special tools and techniques.

High-Index Plastic Lenses

With the increased interest in producing thinner, more cosmetically acceptable lenses, a profusion of high-index plastic materials has been developed with indices ranging from 1.54 to 1.66. The Abbe numbers are smaller than those of either ophthalmic crown glass or CR-39, but higher than that of polycarbonate. With the large variety of high-index materials available, it is difficult to make generalizations about their optical properties. Some lenses are made from known polymers such as polyurethane; others are made with polymers having undisclosed proprietary formulas. Although information concerning refractive index, Abbe number, and specific gravity is widely published, specific information such as lens design criteria, optical performance, ultraviolet protection, and impact resistance is not always available.

Understanding the individual requirements of the patient is the key to selecting appropriate lens design to match the patient's prescription, occupational demands, recreational activities, lifestyle, and budget. To make a valid comparison of high-index options, the prescriber must acquire an accurate knowledge of complex differences of high-index materials. Representative high-index plastic materials are listed in Table 1–3.

THE STRENGTH OF LENS MATERIALS

1.11. FDA Policies

Before 1971 whether a spectacle-wearer's lenses were rendered impact resistant was left to the discretion of the practitioner or the dispenser. However, on May 15, 1971, the FDA published in the *Federal Register* a statement of policy concerning impact-resistant lenses. The policy stated that all lenses had to be impact resistant by February 1972, unless the practitioner judged otherwise. The statement of policy began with the following paragraphs:

Examination of the data available on the frequency of eye injuries resulting from the shattering of ordinary crown glass lenses indicates that the use of these lenses constitutes an avoidable hazard to the eyes of the wearer.

The consensus of the ophthalmic community is that the number of eye injuries would be substantially reduced by the use of eyeglasses and sunglasses of either plastic lenses, heat-treated crown glass lenses, or lenses made impact resistant by other methods.

To protect the public more adequately from potential eye injury, eyeglasses and sunglasses must be fitted with impact resistant lenses, except in those cases where the physician or optometrist finds that such lenses will not fulfill the visual requirements of the particular patient, directs in writing the use of other lenses, and gives written notification to the patient.

The most recent edition of this ruling is provided in the *Federal Register*, 21 CFR 801.410, April, 1990.

Since impact-resistant lenses are available in both heat-tempered and chemically tempered crown glass, chemically tempered high-index glass, and both CR-39 and polycarbonate plastic materials (both of which are inherently impact resistant), it is unlikely that an occasion would arise in which a patient's visual requirements could *not* be met by the use of impact-resistant lenses. However, if such an occasion should arise, the practitioner must give the patient written notice that the lenses are not impact resistant. Unless such written notice is given, it is the *practitioner's* responsibility to make sure that the patient's prescription is filled with impact-resistant lenses.

The FDA policy gives the practitioner the option of ordering "heat-treated glass lenses, plastic lenses, laminated glass lenses, or glass lenses made impact resistant by other means," and states that all such lenses must be capable of withstanding an impact test in which "a 5/8-inch steel ball weighing approximately 0.56 ounce is dropped from a height of 50 inches upon the horizontal upper surface of the lens. The ball should strike within a 5/8-inch diameter circle located at the geometrical center of the lens." To pass the test, the lens must not fracture. *Fracture* means that the lens cracks, through its entire thickness and across an entire diameter, into two or more pieces, or that lens material visible to the naked eye becomes detached from the ocular surface.

Each lens must be submitted to the drop-ball test, with the exception of certain categories of lenses that the manufacturer must "subject to the impact test a statistically significant sampling of lenses from each production batch." These categories include (1) raised-edge multifocal lenses, such as "executive"-style bifocal or trifocal lenses; (2) laminated glass lenses, which are likely to crack as a result of drop-ball testing; (3) plastic lenses; and (4) nonprescription spectacle lenses ("over-the-counter lenses"). The manufacturer is responsible for deciding what constitutes a "batch," and what constitutes a statistically significant sample of a batch.

Lenses designed for special use, such as prism segment multifocals, eikonic lenses, custom laminates, and cemented assemblies, should be made impact resistant if possible; however, these lenses are exempt from impact testing.

The FDA policy does not specify a minimum thickness for a lens to be considered impact-resistant, and the ANSI Z80.1-1995 recommendations[10] contain no minimum-thickness requirement. However, the tolerance for thickness, when specified, is ±0.3 mm.

In describing to a patient lenses that meet the FDA requirements, the practitioner should make sure to use the term *impact-resistant*. Words such as "unbreakable" and "shatterproof" are misleading and should not be used.

1.12. The Strength of Glass

Glass has an extremely high theoretical tensile strength, in excess of 4,000,000 pounds per square inch.[14] However, annealed glass breaks at 2000 to 10,000 pounds per square inch, only a fraction of the theoretical strength, and is considered to be a weak material. Unlike metal, glass does not exhibit *ductility*; glass is so brittle that it displays virtually no plastic deformation before fracturing.

The difference between the theoretical and actual tensile strengths of glass is thought to be caused by *flaws* in glass materials. The flaws may be either intrinsic or acquired. Intrinsic flaws may result from slight material inhomogeneities at the time of manufacture or from residual stress during an improper annealing process; acquired flaws occur in the form of minute surface and edge imperfections, often known as *Griffith flaws*, and result from grinding, polishing, or edging operations or from handling during these processes. The surface and edge flaws are the primary contributors to reduced impact resistance of ophthalmic lens materials. Hence, surface and edge quality of ophthalmic lens materials largely control impact resistance.

When a stress field is applied to a lens, the flaws act as stress concentrators. The local stress is many times the nominal stress.[15] The flaws may widen under applied stress with the result that the strength of the lens is further reduced. Fracture propagation and failure occur when the stress at the flaw exceeds the intrinsic strength of the glass. A flaw or crack in a lens enlarges only as a result of the tensile stress on the lens surface—a crack has a tendency to close by compressive forces across the crack. If the surface is placed under compression, tensile stresses occur in the interior of the lens to compensate for the compressive stress. The compression makes the lens stronger because any applied tensile strength must overcome the built-in compression before the surfaces can be put under tension.

Brandt[16] lists four mechanisms by which a lens may fail under impact:

1. Fracture of front surface origin, caused by simple elastic denting of the surface only (Figure 1–1). This occurs primarily when the lens is hit by a small, lightweight, high-velocity missile.
2. Fracture of rear surface origin, caused by compound flexure of the lens (Figure 1–2). This fracture is usually caused by a missile of moderate mass and moderate velocity, striking a negative-powered lens whose center is thinner than the edge.
3. Edge fracture, caused by simple flexure or flattening of the lens (Figure 1–3). This usually occurs with a heavy,

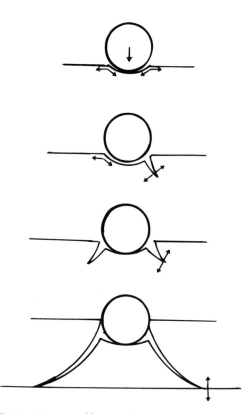

FIGURE 1-1.   **Fracture of front surface origin caused by simple elastic denting of the surface. (Reprinted with permission from N. M. Brandt, *Am. J. Optom. Physiol. Opt.*, Vol. 51, p. 985, © The American Academy of Optometry, 1974.)**

FIGURE 1-2.   **Fracture of rear surface origin caused by compound flexure of the lens. (Reprinted with permission from N. M. Brandt, *Am. J. Optom. Physiol. Opt.*, Vol. 51, p. 985, © The American Academy of Optometry, 1974.)**

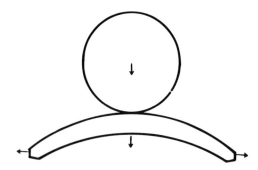

FIGURE 1-3.   **Edge fracture caused by simple flexure or flattening of lens. (Reprinted with permission from N. M. Brandt, *Am. J. Optom. Physiol. Opt.*, Vol. 51, p. 985, © The American Academy of Optometry, 1974.)**

low-velocity missile striking a positive lens whose edge is thinner than the center.

4. Edge fracture and failure, caused by elastic wave reflection (Figure 1-4). An elastic wave whose origin is the site of impact on the lens spreads to the edge that contains a flaw large enough to originate fracture.

1.13. Methods of Tempering Glass Lenses

Thermal tempering was the classic (and only) method of rendering ophthalmic lenses impact resistant until relatively recently, when the chemical tempering method was developed.

Thermal (Air) Tempering

The procedure for the toughening of glass by heating and cooling was developed during the seventeenth century concurrently with the development of similar procedures for the manufacture of steel armor plate. The early history of the toughening of glass, summarized below, has been discussed by Keeney.[17]

The *Prince Rupert drop*, named for Prince Rupert of Bavaria (1619–1682), is an interesting curiosity that demonstrates the strength of thermally tempered glass. The Prince Rupert drop is created by dropping a bit of molten glass into a container of cold water so that the drop is cooled with drastic suddenness. This action produces a pear-shaped drop of glass with a long tapering tail. The glass is extremely hard on its surface and the body of the drop will withstand a great impact; but if the tip of the tail is broken or scratched, the entire drop explodes into many fragments.

In 1874 Francis de la Bastie was issued a patent for a process of thermal tempering of glass by reheating the glass almost to its softening point and then quickly cooling it by immersing it in oil.[17] However, de la Bastie and other investigators of thermal tempering processes failed to understand the nature of the process; they believed they were *hardening* the surface of the glass. This misunderstanding—that thermally tempered glass is *hardened* glass, persists to the present day. Any treatment that places the surface of a lens under compression provides the lens with greater impact resistance than that possessed by ordinary annealed glass. Thermal (air) tempering is such a method.

FIGURE 1-4.   **Edge fracture and failure caused by elastic wave reflection. (Reprinted with permission from N. M. Brandt, *Am. J. Optom. Physiol. Opt.*, Vol. 51, p. 985, © The American Academy of Optometry, 1974.)**

In thermal tempering, the finished lens (without the frame) must be heated to a temperature near the softening point (about 650°C) and then rapidly cooled by a blast of air on both surfaces. The heating process causes the glass to expand, and the subsequent rapid cooling causes the surface to quickly become rigid while the interior mass of the lens is still slightly plastic. As the interior mass of the lens cools, it contracts and exerts tension on the resisting rigid surface volume. When reaching room temperature, the surface is under compression and the central portion of the lens (i.e., below the surface) is under tension. The layer of compression at the surface of the lens may be compared to the rim of a bicycle wheel.[18] Each of the spokes of the wheel has to be tightened, so as to place the spoke in just the right degree of tension. This tension exerts forces on the rim and keeps the rim in a state of compression.

Compression is not always uniform across the lens because the cooling rate varies with the volume of air reaching different parts of the lens surface and with the thickness of the lens. Careful control of heating time and temperature is required for air tempering. Proper heating produces a compression layer, which minimally distorts the lens surfaces. Overheating causes warping of the surfaces, and underheating leads to insufficient compression.

Compression of the surface with resulting tension of the internal portions produces *birefringence*, or double refraction, of the lens. If a heat-tempered lens is placed between two light-polarizing filters oriented at right angles to each other (in an instrument called a *polariscope*) the birefringence patterns are readily visible. The birefringence patterns are usually characterized as *Maltese cross* patterns, but an infinite number of patterns are possible. According to Wigglesworth,[19] lenses cannot reliably be assessed for impact resistance on the basis of their displayed birefringence patterns. Such a pattern indicates that the lens has been tempered, but unfortunately does not indicate whether the process was done satisfactorily.

Chemical Tempering

Although applied to ophthalmic lenses only relatively recently, techniques for chemical strengthening of glass are not new. In 1890 Tegetmeier[20] observed that large stresses could be generated in the surface of a glass by exposure to molten potassium or lithium salts. In 1965, 75 years after Tegetmeier's observation, Weber[21] was issued a patent for chemical strengthening of lenses by *ion-exchange injection*, in which large ions are exchanged for small ones below the strain temperature.

In 1971 Corning Glass Works adapted the ion-exchange process of chemical strengthening to ophthalmic lenses, and it was introduced to the ophthalmic community in 1972 when the FDA test requirements for impact resistance came into effect. In this process, the surface of the lens is put into compression, as with thermal tempering, but at a considerably lower temperature. The compression layer is created by exchanging small ions present in the glass with larger ions from a molten salt bath in which the lens is processed, as shown in Figure 1–5. The crowding of a large ion into a

FIGURE 1–5. **The ion exchange process used in chemical tempering. (Reprinted with the permission of Corning Glass Works, Corning, NY.)**

network site formerly occupied by a smaller ion causes a stress on the adjacent network if the network is stable. The "stuffing" action and resultant stress on the rigid network produces the compressive stress built into the surface of the glass. Since the exchange occurs at a temperature well below the strain point of the glass, the stresses are not relieved by network movement. Tensile stresses develop in the interior of the glass to compensate for the surface compression. By use of this process, a batch of finished lenses is "cooked" in a molten bath for a period of about 16 hours during which the large ions in the bath replace the smaller ions in the glass. The amount of ion exchange is proportional to the square root of the time and depends also on the temperature.

There are two ion-exchange systems used for ophthalmic lens tempering, and the composition of the glass determines the system used. For crown glass lenses, both clear and tinted, the bath consists of 100% KNO_3, and sodium ions in the lens are replaced by larger potassium ions present in the bath. However, for Corning photochromic lenses, the bath consists of 40% (by weight) $NaNO_3$ and 60% KNO_3, and the process involves two steps: (1) Lithium ions in the lens are first replaced by larger sodium ions present in the bath, and (2) sodium ions in the lens are then replaced by still larger potassium ions in the bath.

The required temperature varies, depending upon the variety of glass. For clear crown glass, the bath requires a temperature ±5 degrees of 470°C; for tinted crown glass the required temperature is ±5 degrees of 440°C. If clear and tinted crown glass are tempered in the same batch, a temperature ±5 degrees of 450°C is used. For photochromic lenses, the temperature is somewhat lower, ±5 degrees of 400°C.

Glass manufacturers have experimented with, and changed to some extent, the composition of ophthalmic crown glass to improve ion exchange. As a result, older lenses do not have the strength and compression levels of the newer formulations.

Because of the lower temperature (as compared with the temperature required for heat tempering), there is less chance of lens warpage, and irregularities do not occur as with heat tempering. Resurfacing and re-edging are possible with chemically tempered lenses, but not with heat-tempered lenses. After resurfacing and re-edging, however, the lenses should once again be submitted to the tempering process. Because the compressive stress developed in chemically strengthened lenses is much greater than that of heat-tempered lenses, these lenses are two to three times more impact resistant.

Some antireflective and tint *coatings* may be damaged or discolored at the temperature of the chemical bath; when chemically tempered lenses are to be coated, the coating operation should be done *after* the tempering operation. In addition, lenses that are to be coated should not be drop-ball tested until after the coating operation. Following this sequence will eliminate any lenses that may have been weakened by the coating process.

To visually identify a chemically tempered lens, the lens (removed from the frame) should be immersed in glycerin between crossed polarizing plates. When viewed through the surfaces, a narrow band is visible around the periphery of the lens. Commercial devices, such as Chem-Check (American Optical) and Tempr-A-Scope (Kirk Optical), are available for the visual identification of chemically tempered lenses.

One disadvantage of chemical tempering (chem-tempering) is that it requires a 16-hour (overnight) period, thus adding 1 day to the time required to receive the finished lens from the laboratory. However, the time delay is offset to some extent by the lenses being tempered in batches, in contrast to being thermal-tempered—a one-at-a-time process.

Equipment has been developed that ultrasonically stimulates the chem-tempering process.[22] The ultrasonic stimulation of a chem-tempering bath appears to result in higher strength lenses than conventional processing and requires a treatment time of only 2 1/2 to 4 hours. The ultrasonic stimulation appears to achieve this effect by improving the efficiency of transfer of potassium ions into the glass. Corning[23] has recently described a 2-hour chem-tempering process designed only for Corning photochromic glasses used for dress eyewear (trade names Photogray Extra, Photobrown Extra, Photogray II, and Photosun II).

1.14. Impact Resistance of Plastic Lenses

Both CR-39 and polycarbonate lenses, as already stated, are intrinsically impact resistant. However, their great advantage, as compared with lenses made of air-tempered or chemically tempered glass, is their *light weight.* Although CR-39 lenses are considerably lighter than glass lenses, for a lens of a given prescription and center thickness a polycarbonate lens (having an index of refraction of 1.586 and a specific gravity of 1.20) is lighter in weight than any other available lens. Both CR-39 and polycarbonate material have the disadvantage of being softer than glass and therefore being more easily scratched. The scratch resistance of CR-39 lenses can be increased by the use of a scratch-resistant coating, but polycarbonate material is so soft that such a coating is mandatory.

CR-39 Lenses

When the impact resistance of CR-39 lenses has been compared with that of air-tempered and chemically tempered glass lenses, conflicting (and interesting) results have been reported. Renaldo, Keeney, and Duerson,[24] using low-velocity drop-ball tests, found chemically tempered glass lenses to be 100% to 350% more impact resistant than air-tempered glass lenses. Wigglesworth[25] reported that 3-mm-thick, air-tempered glass lenses have a higher impact resistance than 3-mm CR-39 plastic lenses when tested with a 1-inch steel ball on the drop-ball test. However, with ballistic tests using a 1/8-inch steel ball, the positions were reversed—3-mm CR-39 lenses were more impact resistant than air-tempered lenses. Welsh et al.[26] tested untreated glass, air-tempered glass, chemically tempered glass, and CR-39 plastic lenses with a ballistic device using a 4.76-mm (3/8-inch) missile and found the CR-39 lens to have the greatest impact resistance and the untreated glass lens to have the least impact resistance. The differences between impact resistances of air-tempered and chemically tempered glass lenses were slight. Goldsmith and Gonden[27] applied strain to chemically tempered glass lenses and CR-39 plastic lenses with steel balls, aluminum cylinders, and pine boards at defined velocities. Fracture of chemically tempered glass lenses occurred in the range of 30,765 to 161,920 pounds per square inch; CR-39 plastic lenses survived in the range of 32,384 to 40,480 pounds per square inch but failed beyond that range.

Many other studies comparing impact resistance of CR-39 lenses to that of chemically tempered glass lenses have been reported. Analysis of the results of these studies indicates that chemically tempered glass lenses tend to be superior for large-mass, low-velocity objects (such as a large stone or a baseball), but CR-39 plastic lenses are likely to be superior for small, high-velocity, sharply pointed objects.

When plastic lenses fracture, they tend to break into a smaller number of pieces than do glass lenses, and the edges of the plastic fragments are not as sharp as the edges of glass fragments. Also, there are fewer small, fine particles originating at the line of fracture (i.e., flaking) of a plastic lens.

Surface scratching and pitting tend to reduce the survivability of all lenses. However, they compromise the strength of glass lenses more than that of plastic lenses because a glass lens depends for its strength on a compressive layer at the surface. Scratching the surface of a glass lens has the effect of reducing the surface compression and, therefore, reducing its impact resistance.

Polycarbonate Lenses

As stated earlier, polycarbonate is vastly superior to both ophthalmic crown glass and CR-39 plastic in terms of impact resistance. Polycarbonate is impact resistant because its molecules are extremely long chains of atoms that can slide back and forth on each other, with the result that the material can be flexed and even deformed permanently without breaking. The energy of an impact will flex or deform the lens rather than break it. Stephens and Davis[28] showed that polycarbonate has 21 times the impact resistance of CR-39 for 1/4-inch and 1/8-inch steel balls fired at high velocity.

Chou[29] emphasized that, although most eye injuries resulting from broken spectacle lenses are caused by large, slow-moving missiles, polycarbonate is the only available spectacle lens material that provides effective protection from fast-moving large or small missiles. Because of polycarbonate's high impact resistance, Chou recommends its use for industrial workers who are exposed to such objects, for others whose activities at work or play make them at risk for eye injury, and for amblyopic or monocular patients. When eye protection is the primary concern, polycarbonate is the lens of choice. Polycarbonate has experienced a slow but steady rise as a spectacle lens material and now claims about 13.3% of the market.[30]

A comparison of the mean fracture velocity of 3.0-mm-thick crown glass, CR-39, and polycarbonate lenses for a missile diameter of approximately 1/4 inch is shown in Table 1–4.[31-33]

Legal Ramifications

The question of the eyecare practitioner's legal responsibility in informing his or her patients about the impact resistance of lens materials has been raised in recent years. In lawsuits over eye injuries caused by spectacle lenses, lawyers have asked eyecare practitioners whether they were aware of the impact resistance of polycarbonate lenses, and why lenses made of this material had not been prescribed, offered, or provided.[29] The Optical Laboratories Association (OLA) has begun a campaign called *Duty to Warn*. In this campaign, eyecare professionals are advised to make sure that every patient ordering new eyewear is informed that polycarbonate exceeds all other materials in impact resistance. The OLA has also published a Duty-to-Warn kit that outlines a dispenser's responsibilities in warning patients about eye protection.[34]

As dispensers strive to create thinner lenses for patients, the drop-ball test required by the FDA and specified in the ANSI Z80.1-1995 recommendations becomes the critical factor in determining how far the thinness trend can evolve. Because the original lens manufacturers conduct batch impact testing of all plastic lenses (as permitted by the FDA), they extend to their purchasers a waiver eliminating the requirement for drop-ball testing. The waiver covers both finished stock lenses and semifinished blanks. The waiver is valid only if the purchaser processes or alters the lens in accordance with the disclaimer and its parameters printed on the package. Therefore, under the following conditions the waiver is void, and impact tests are required:

1. When a laboratory retailer applies a scratch-resistant coating to any material not normally requiring a scratch-resistant coating, such as CR-39 (polycarbonate and polyurethane lenses are normally given a scratch-resistant coating, and therefore remain covered by the waiver).
2. Any time an antireflective coating is applied by anyone other than the original manufacturer.
3. When laboratories process lenses to thicknesses smaller than those specified in the manufacturer's surfacing charts.

Any person who substantially alters the manufacturer's product shifts the responsibility. Thus, the professional who has an in-office finishing laboratory, for example, may now be regarded as the manufacturer/supplier for litigation purposes.

To help in the prevention of patient eye injury and resulting litigation, the practitioner should take the following steps[28]:

1. Be sure that the case history includes the patient's requirements for eye protection in industry, recreation, and hobbies. A patient questionnaire may prove useful.
2. Inform the patient of all lens materials available *before* frame selection and ordering the prescription.
3. Document the "Duty-to-Warn" discussion with the patient.
4. Make a record of your recommendations and the patient's choices, noting any rejections.
5. Stay up-to-date on new products and technology.
6. Be familiar with the current ANSI Z80.1 (dress eyewear) and ANSI Z87.1 (occupational) standards as well as the FDA impact-resistance regulations. Post copies or summaries of these standards in a conspicuous place.
7. Educate ancillary personnel concerning these standards and regulations.
8. When ordering eyewear for industrial safety purposes, never place industrial safety lenses in a frame not designed for industrial purposes; likewise, never place dress eyewear prescription lenses in a frame meeting the industrial safety standard.

TABLE 1–4
Mean Fracture Velocity of 3.0-mm-Thick Crown Glass, CR-39, and Polycarbonate Lenses for Missile Diameter Approximately 1/4 Inch

Lens Material	Thickness (mm)	Missile Diameter (mm)	Mean Fracture Velocity (m/s)	Source
Crown glass (untreated)	3.0	6.35	12.0	Wigglesworth[31]
Crown glass (thermal hardening)	3.0	6.35	18.0	Wigglesworth[31]
CR-39	3.0	6.35	49.0	Wigglesworth[31]
Crown glass (thermal hardening)	3.0	6.5	16.2	Oliver and Chou[32]
Crown glass (chemical hardening)	3.0	6.5	20.1	Oliver and Chou[32]
Polycarbonate (coated)	3.0	6.5	152.0	Greenberg et al.[33]
Polycarbonate (uncoated)	3.0	6.5	244.0	Greenberg et al.[33]

9. Always pass along to the patient any manufacturer's warning intended for the patient.
10. Never waive the impact-resistance requirement for dress eyewear.
11. Inform the patient that even though some lens materials are stronger than others, no lens is unbreakable or shatterproof. (Use "impact-resistant").
12. Always verify that all lens prescription parameters fall within established standards. This should be done *before* notifying the patient that the eyewear is available. Design a verification form that, minimally, includes the following:
    a. sphere, cylinder, and axis
    b. measurement of prism (lateral and vertical)
    c. quality of lens surfaces and bevel
    d. type of lens material
    e. center thickness
    f. base curve
    g. frame specifications
    h. impact resistance
    The form should become a permanent part of the patient's record.
13. Always carry sufficient malpractice insurance.

1.15. Lenses for Occupational and Educational Use

The standards for lenses and frames for occupational and educational use have been set forth by the American National Standards Institute, in ANSI Z87.1-1989, *Practice for Occupational and Educational Eye and Face Protection*.[35] The standard applies to all occupational and educational operations or processes except x-rays, gamma rays, high-energy particulate radiation, lasers, and masers.

Spectacles designed for industrial exposure must pass a more stringent drop-ball test than that required by the FDA for impact-resistant lenses. The lens must be removed from the frame and subjected to a test in which a 1-inch steel ball, weighing approximately 2.4 ounces, is dropped from a height of 50 inches onto the convex surface of the lens. The minimum thickness for a prescription lens is 3.0 mm, except lenses having plus power of 3.00 D or greater in the most plus meridian must have a minimum thickness no less than 2.5 mm.

All lenses must be marked in a permanent and legible manner with the manufacturer's monogram. If the lenses are general-purpose filter lenses, the shade number must follow the manufacturer's monogram. If photochromic lenses are provided, a "V" must accompany the manufacturer's monogram.

The optical performance standards for prescription lenses used in industrial eye protection devices are those specified in ANSI Z80.1. Although the ANSI Z80.1 tolerances are only recommendations for dress eyewear, they are mandatory for prescription industrial spectacles. A general-purpose filter is used for protection from excess optical radiation such as that occurring in welding. The shade number selected must meet the ANSI Z87.1 standards for minimum and maximum visible light transmittance (380–780 nm) and maximum for far ultraviolet (200–315 nm) and infrared (780–2000 nm) radiation transmittance. The near ultraviolet average transmittance (315–385) nm) must be less than one-tenth of the visible light transmittance. General-purpose filters must be supplied in pairs; for shade numbers 1.5 through 3.0, the luminous transmittance values must be within 10% of each other. For shade numbers 4.0 through 14.0, the luminous transmittance values must agree within 20%. All clear lenses must have luminous transmittance values greater than 85%.

Although the standard does not prohibit the general use of tints for industrial safety lenses, lenses having low-luminance transmittance, such as sunglasses, should not be worn indoors except when needed to filter excess optical radiation. Such lenses should not be worn for night driving. Because the fading process in photochromic lenses is not instantaneous, photochromic lenses should be used prudently in operations requiring critical acuity or fast reactions to the visual environment, particularly when the wearer moves from outdoors to indoors, as when a forklift operator passes from outdoors to indoors. Absorptive lenses, both for general wear and for occupational and educational use, are discussed in more detail in Chapter 7.

Frames used for prescription industrial eyewear must meet a number of performance standards such as impact resistance, flammability resistance, and corrosion resistance. All industrial spectacle frames must be marked with the A dimension (eye size), the distance between lenses (DBL), and the overall temple length. In addition, both the frame front and the temple must carry the manufacturer's monogram and "Z87" to indicate compliance with the standard. The use of frames not meeting the ANSI Z87.1 standard is definitely in violation of the standard, even though the lenses may be in compliance.

References

1. Gasson, W. The Early Story of Glass, Part I. *Optician*, Vol. 156, No. 4051, 1968.
2. Obrig, T. E. *Modern Ophthalmic Lenses and Optical Glass.* Chilton Co., Philadelphia, 1935.
3. Horne, D. F. *Spectacle Glass Technology.* Adam Hilger, Bristol, p. 1, 1978.
4. Gasson, W. The Early Story of Glass, Part II. *Optician*, Vol. 156, No. 4052, 1968.
5. Hofstetter, H. W. *Optometry: Professional, Economic and Legal Aspects.* C. V. Mosby Co., St. Louis, 1948.
6. *Dictionary of Scientific and Technical Terms*, 2nd edition. McGraw-Hill, New York, 1978.
7. Graham, R. A New, Light Weight and Unbreakable Plastic Ophthalmic Lens. *Am. J. Optom. Arch. Am. Acad. Optom.*, Vol. 24, pp. 495–497, 1947.
8. Targrove, B. D., Miller, J. W., Tredici, T. J., Kislin, B., Rahe, A. J., and Provines, W. F. Glass vs. Plastic Lenses—An Air Force Replacement and Durability Study. *Am. J. Optom. Arch. Am. Acad. Optom.*, Vol. 49, pp. 320–329, 1972.
9. Smith, F. D., and Wientzen, R. V. Prediction of Visual Effects from the Warpage of Spectacle Lenses. *Am. J. Optom. Arch. Am. Acad. Optom.*, Vol. 50, pp. 616–631, 1973.
10. *American National Standard for Ophthalmics: Prescription Ophthalmic Lenses—Recommendations.* ANSI Z80.1-1995. American National Standards Institute, New York, 1995.

11. Karow, H. H. *Fabrication Methods for Prescription Optics.* John Wesley and Sons, Inc., New York, 1993.

12. Meslin, D., and Obrecht, G. Effect of Chromatic Dispersion of a Lens on Visual Acuity. *Am. J. Optom. Physiol. Opt.* Vol. 65, pp. 25–28, 1988.

13. Hampton, L., Roth, N., Meyer-Arendt, T., and Shuman, D. Visual Acuity Degradation Resulting from Dispersion in Polycarbonate. *J. Am. Optom. Assoc.,* Vol. 62, pp. 760–765, 1991.

14. Chase, G. A., Kozlowski, T. P., and Krause, R. P. Chemical Strengthening of Ophthalmic Lenses. *Am. J. Optom. Arch. Am. Acad. Optom.,* Vol. 50, pp. 470–476, 1973.

15. Berger, R. E. Impact Testing of Ophthalmic Lenses: Stress Distribution and "Search" Theory. *J. Am. Optom. Assoc.,* Vol. 47, pp. 86–92, 1976.

16. Brandt, N. M. The Anatomy and Autopsy of an "Impact Resistant Lens." *Am. J. Optom. Physiol. Opt.,* Vol. 51, pp. 982–986, 1974.

17. Keeney, A. H. *Lens Materials in the Prevention of Eye Injuries.* Charles C Thomas, Springfield, IL, 1957.

18. Lueck, I. B. *Toughened Safety Lenses.* Scientific and Technical Publication No. 23. Bausch & Lomb, Inc., Rochester, NY, 1961.

19. Wigglesworth, E. C. The Birefringence Fallacy. *Am. J. Optom. Physiol. Opt.,* Vol. 52, pp. 320–327, 1975.

20. Tegetmeier, F. Electrical Conductivity of Glass and Rock Crystal. *Ann. Phys. Chem.,* Vol. 41, No. 18, p. 18, 1890.

21. Weber, N. U.S. Patent No. 3,218,220, 1965.

22. Duckworth, W. H., and Rosenfield, A. R. Strength of Glass Lenses Processed in Ultrasonically Stimulated Chemtempering Bath. *Am. J. Optom. Physiol. Opt.,* Vol. 61, pp. 48–53, 1984.

23. 2-Hour Chemtempering of Corning Photochromic Glasses. Corning Technical Bulletin, March, 1992.

24. Renaldo, D. P., Keeney, A. H., and Duerson, H. L., Jr. Ion Exchange Tempering of Glass Ophthalmic Lenses. *Am. J. Ophthalmol.,* Vol. 80, pp. 291–295, 1975.

25. Wigglesworth, E. C. The Comparative Performance of Eye Protection Materials. *Austr. J. Optom.,* Vol. 55, pp. 461–469, 1972.

26. Welsh, K. W., Miller, J. U., Kislin, B., Tredici, T. J., and Rahe, A. J. Ballistic Impact Testing of Scratched and Unscratched Ophthalmic Lenses. *Am. J. Optom. Physiol. Opt.,* Vol. 51, pp. 304–311, 1974.

27. Goldsmith, W., and Gonden, D. Fracture Resistance of Ophthalmic Lenses. *Am. J. Optom. Physiol. Opt.,* Vol. 60, pp. 914–919, 1983.

28. Stephens, G. L., and Davis, J. K. Spectacle Lenses. In W. Tasman and E. A. Yaeger, Eds., *Duane's Clinical Ophthalmology,* Lippincott, Philadelphia, 1993.

29. Chou, B. R. Choosing Candidates for Polycarbonate Lenses. *Optom. Today,* Vol. 2, No. 8, p. 25, 1994.

30. Bennett, I. Lab Survey Shows Growing Acceptance of New Technologies. *AOA News,* Vol. 33, No. 9, p. 17, 1994.

31. Wigglesworth, E. C. A Comparative Assessment of Eye Protection Devices and a Proposed System of Acceptance Testing and Grading. *Am. J. Optom. Arch. Am. Acad. Optom.,* Vol. 49, pp. 287–304, 1972.

32. Oliver, A. L., and Chou, B. R. A Ballistic Evaluation of Impact Resistance of Spectacle Lens Material. *Optom. Vis. Sci.,* Vol. 70, pp. 822–827, 1993.

33. Greenberg, I., Chase, G., and Lamarre, D. Statistical Protocol for Impact Testing Prescription Polycarbonate Safety Lenses. *Op. World,* Vol. 14, Mar/Apr pp. 7–8, 1985.

34. Bruneni, J. L. The Polycarbonate Handbook. *EyeQuest Magazine,* Vol. 5, No. 5 (Suppl.), pp. 28–30, 1995.

35. *American National Standard Practice for Occupational Eye and Face Protection,* Z87.1-1989. American National Standards Institute, Inc., New York, 1989.

Questions

1. Describe the "nature" of glass.

2. List the principal ingredients of ophthalmic glass.

3. Discuss the origin of the terms "crown" and "flint" used to describe glass.

4. Describe the batch process of ophthalmic glassmaking.

5. List the desirable characteristics of optical glass.

6. Describe the common defects found in the chemical composition of glass.

7. Distinguish between thermoplastic and thermosetting plastic materials.

8. Compare the characteristics of CR-39 and polycarbonate plastic lenses.

9. Describe the construction of the Corlon lens.

10. What is meant by the term "impact resistance"?

11. Describe how glass lenses are strengthened by thermal tempering.

12. Discuss the significance of birefringence patterns in thermally toughened lenses.

13. Describe the process of chemical tempering of glass lenses.

14. Discuss the relative impact resistance of CR-39 and chemically tempered lenses.

15. How are lenses designed for occupational use tested for resistance to breaking?

16. List the four mechanisms by which a lens may fail on impact.

17. Distinguish between the terms *density* and *specific gravity*.

18. Describe the thickness requirements for occupational lenses.

CHAPTER TWO

Characteristics of Ophthalmic Lenses

This chapter presents the fundamental characteristics of ophthalmic lenses in terms of both their physical and optical characteristics. Under the heading "Physical Characteristics," topics include the concept of curvature, surfaces of revolution, the relationship between curvature and refracting power, the lens measure (lens clock), lens form, lens blanks and base curves, specification of cylinder axes, prescription writing, and transposition. In the second part of the chapter, under the heading "Optical Characteristics," topics include basic terminology, image formation by spherical lenses, image formation by cylindrical and toric lenses, the concept of the conoid of Sturm, the power in an oblique meridian of a cylindrical or toric lens, obliquely crossed cylinders, astigmatism due to lens tilt, and the optical principles of the Maddox rod. (The discussion of optical characteristics of ophthalmic lenses continues in Chapters 3 and 4, which consider power specification and measurement as well as ophthalmic prisms and decentration.)

_____PHYSICAL CHARACTERISTICS_____

2.1. Curvature

The curvature of a surface is defined as the angle through which the surface turns in a unit length of arc. Referring to Figure 2–1, an object traveling in a circular arc, AB, at point A will be traveling in the direction AA', and at point B is traveling in the direction BB'. The angle between the two directions of travel is θ', which is equal to the angle θ subtended by the two radii CA and CB. Because AA' and BB' are tangents to the curve, we may define curvature as follows:

$$\text{Curvature} = \frac{\theta}{\text{arc AB}}.$$

Since θ, in radians, $= \dfrac{\text{arc AB}}{r}$,

$$\text{curvature } (R) = \frac{1}{r}.$$

There are several methods of specifying curvature. The simplest method is to use the relationship between curvature (R) and radius (r) as illustrated in the above definition. Since curvature is inversely proportional to radius, it frequently is convenient to use the radius for the specification of curvature. As shown in Figure 2–2, the smaller circle, having a radius of curvature of 0.50 m, obviously has a greater curvature (a greater change in angle/unit arc length) than does the larger circle, which has a radius of curvature of 1 m. Note that, if the radius is used to specify curvature, a large degree of curvature will be represented by a small quantity and a small degree of curvature will be represented by a large quantity. To avoid this confusion, curvature should be specified in terms of the reciprocal (R) of the radius, rather than in terms of the radius itself (r).

Units of Curvature

As Bennett[1] has pointed out, there is no universally accepted name for a unit of curvature. When the radius is specified in meters, the unit *reciprocal meters* (m^{-1}) may be used.[2] Morgan[3] uses the *diopter* as a unit of curvature when the radius is expressed in meters. However, the term *diopter* has become associated with a large number of useful applications, including surface power of an ophthalmic lens (Section 2.3); the curvature of a wavefront at a specified distance from its source, that is, *vergence* (Chapter 3, Section 3.1); reduced vergence, that is, l/n and l'/n'; and focal power of a lens or of an optical system (Chapter 3, Section 3.1). The use of the diopter as a unit of curvature of an *optical surface* especially causes confusion with diopters of *surface power*. It is best, therefore, to restrict the use of the term diopter to vergence, reduced vergence, surface power, and focal power of ophthalmic lenses.

The Sagitta as a Unit of Curvature

Another method of specifying curvature is to use the *sagitta*, which in Latin means "arrow." As shown in Figure 2–3, the sagitta, s, is the distance between a point on the circle and the midpoint of a chord of the circle. The relationship between the sagitta, the chord, and the radius of a circle can

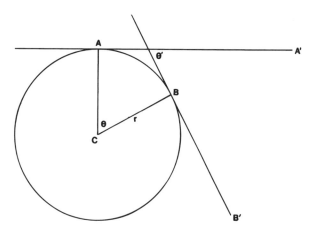

FIGURE 2–1.   **Curvature (see text for explanation).**

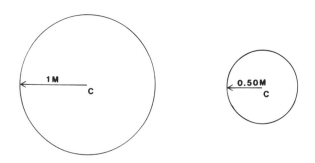

FIGURE 2–2.   **The smaller circle has the greater curvature (C = center).**

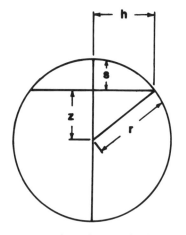

FIGURE 2–3.   **The sagitta as unit of curvature.**

be derived from this figure. With use of the relationship between the sides of a right triangle,

$$r^2 = h^2 + z^2$$
$$z^2 = r^2 - h^2$$
$$z = \pm\sqrt{r^2 - h^2}.$$

Since $s = r - z$,

$$s = r \pm \sqrt{r^2 - h^2}. \tag{2.1}$$

In practice, the *minus* root of this expression is used, because the plus root results in the diameter minus the sagitta. The expression is the *exact* formula for the value of the sagitta, s.

It is also possible to derive an *approximate* formula:

$$r^2 = h^2 + (r - s)^2$$
$$r^2 = h^2 + r^2 - 2rs + s^2.$$

When the quantity s is small in relation to r, as in the case of an ophthalmic lens, the quantity s^2 may be dropped from the formula. By transposition, we have

$$2rs = h^2$$

or

$$s = \frac{h^2}{2r}. \tag{2.2}$$

EXAMPLE
Calculate the sagitta of a glass surface having a refracting power of 15.00 D, 42 mm in diameter, and having an index of refraction of 1.523, first by using the exact formula and then by using the approximate formula.

1. By using the exact formula, $s = r - \sqrt{r^2 - h^2}$.
   Since

$$F = \frac{n' - n}{r} = \frac{1.523 - 1}{r} = \frac{0.523}{r},$$

$$r = \frac{0.523}{F} = \frac{0.523}{15} = 0.0349 \text{ m}.$$

$$h = 0.021 \text{ m},$$

   that is, one-half the chord, and

$$s = 0.0349 - \sqrt{(0.0349)^2 - (0.021)^2}$$
$$= 0.0349 - \sqrt{0.00122 - 0.00044}$$
$$= 0.0349 - \sqrt{0.00078}$$
$$= 0.0349 - 0.0279$$
$$= 0.0070 \text{ m} = 7.0 \text{ mm}.$$

2. By using the approximate formula, $s = h^2/2r$,

$$s = \frac{(0.021)^2}{2(0.0349)} = \frac{0.00044}{0.0698}$$
$$= 0.0063 \text{ m} = 6.3 \text{ mm}.$$

When working with highly curved surfaces, such as those found in contact lenses, the *exact* expression for calculating s must be used, since s is not small in relation to r (that is, the sagittae of the surfaces are not small in relation to their radii).

When considering the curvature of one of the surfaces of an ophthalmic lens, the chord length (equal to $2h$) is considered as the *aperture*, or width, of the lens. As shown in Figure 2–4, if two lens surfaces have the same aperture, the surface having the steeper curvature will have the longer sagitta.

2.2. Surfaces of Revolution

Most surfaces placed on ophthalmic lenses are surfaces of revolution, which are formed by rotating a plane curve about an axis within its plane. A *spherical surface* is generated by rotating a circle or an arc about one of its diameters, as shown in Figure 2–5. The intersection of any plane passing through

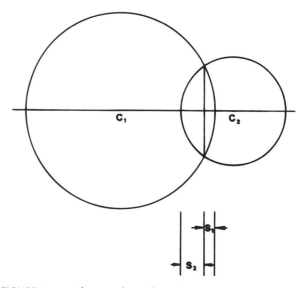

FIGURE 2–4. **When two lenses have the same aperture, the circle having the steeper curvature has the longer sagitta (C = center).**

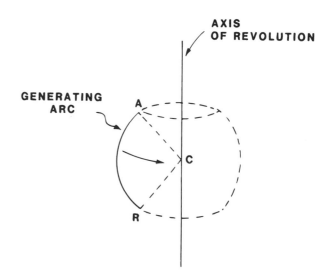

FIGURE 2–5. **A spherical surface can be generated by the rotation of an arc, AR, about an axis of revolution that passes through the center of curvature.**

a spherical surface is always a circle. A *great circle* is formed on a spherical surface when it is intersected by a plane passing through the center of the sphere, and the curvature along any great circle is equal to the curvature of the generating circle. The shortest distance between two points on a spherical surface is the flattest arc connecting them. This distance lies along a great circle through the two points. (This concept is useful for navigational purposes, to plot the course between two points on the surface of the earth.)

A *plane surface* has zero curvature and may be considered as a special case of a spherical surface, having an infinite radius.

A *cylindrical surface* is generated by rotating a straight line about another straight line that is parallel to it. As illustrated in Figure 2–6, this is the simplest surface of revolution. The curvature of a cylinder is zero along any line parallel to the axis of revolution and a maximum along the line of intersection of the surface by a plane that is perpendicular to the axis of revolution. The axis meridian (the meridian of zero curvature) and the meridian of maximum curvature are always at right angles to each other and are known as the *principal meridians*.

A *toric surface* is generated by rotating a circle or an arc about an axis that lies in the same plane but does not pass through the center of curvature of the arc. This is illustrated in Figure 2–7. The curvature of a toric surface varies from a minimum in one *principal meridian* to a maximum in the other; the two principal meridians are 90° apart. If the axis about which the toric surface is generated is beyond the center of curvature of the arc, as shown in Figure 2–7A, a sur-

face having the shape of a *doughnut*, or *tire*, is generated. For this surface, the shorter radius is in the vertical meridian and the longer radius goes around it. If the axis is closer than the center of curvature of the circle or arc, as shown in Figure 2–7B, a surface having the shape of a *barrel* is generated, having the shorter radius of curvature in the horizontal meridian. If the arc or circle is oriented concave toward the axis, a *capstan* surface is generated, as shown in Figure 2–7C. A sphere is a special case of a toric surface, in which the axis passes through the center of curvature of the arc or circle.

Referring again to the diagrams in Figure 2–7 depicting the three types of toric surfaces, the *outer* surface of each of

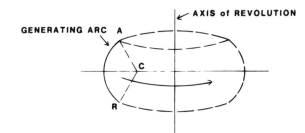

A   DOUGHNUT OR TIRE TORIC SURFACE FORMATION

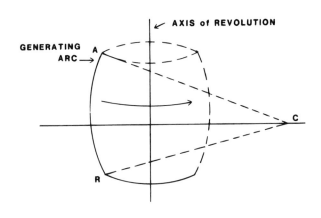

B   BARREL TORIC SURFACE FORMATION

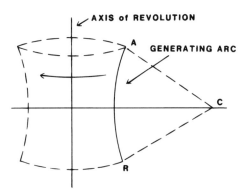

C   CAPSTAN TORIC SURFACE FORMATION

FIGURE 2–7.   **Toric surface formation. A, a doughnut, or tire, surface; B, a barrel surface; C, a capstan surface.**

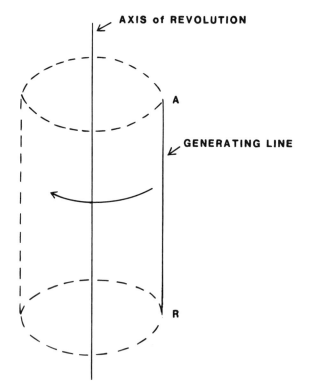

FIGURE 2–6.   **A cylindrical surface is generated by the rotation of a line about an axis of revolution that passes through the center of curvature.**

these diagrams demonstrates the *positive* form of the toric surface, and the *inner* surface of each diagram portrays the *negative* form of the toric surface. The tire formation (Figure 2–7A) is the one that is the most commonly used in ophthalmic lens construction: For it and the barrel form (Figure 2–7B), the radii of curvature in the two principal meridians are *both positive* (for the outer surface) or *both negative* (for the inner surface). However, in the case of the capstan form (Figure 2–7C), for either the outer or inner surface, the radii of curvature in the two principal meridans have *opposite* signs. This form is rarely used in ophthalmic lens construction.

2.3. Relationship between Curvature and Refracting Power of a Surface

Although the form of a surface is defined by specifying its curvature, the refracting power of a surface depends on both the curvature and the index of refraction of the material forming the surface. In geometrical optics the relationship between surface power, curvature, and index of refraction is given by the equation

$$F = \frac{n' - n}{r}, \tag{2.3}$$

where F is the refracting power in diopters, r is the radius of curvature of the surface in meters, n is the index of refraction of the medium through which light passes before reaching the surface, and n' is the index of refraction of the medium on the emergent side of the surface. Clinical optics deals almost entirely with air/glass or air/plastic surfaces, and because the index of refraction of air is unity, it is customary to define F by the relationship

$$F = \frac{n - 1}{r}, \tag{2.4}$$

where n is the index of refraction of the glass or plastic and the light is moving from the air to the surface of the lens.

2.4. The Lens Measure

The refracting power of a surface may be determined by an instrument called the *lens measure*, lens clock, or lens gauge. As shown in Figure 2–8, the lens measure has two fixed pins and a central, spring-loaded, movable pin. The position of the movable pin in relation to the fixed pins is indicated by a pointer that is activated by a system of gears. If the instrument is placed on a flat surface, the protrusion of the central pin is equal to that of the fixed pins with the result that the scale reading is zero. If placed on a convex surface, the protrusion of the central pin is less than that of the fixed pins, but if placed on a concave surface the protrusion of the central pin is greater. As shown in Figure 2–9, since the chord length (the distance between the two outer pins) has a constant value for the instrument, the position of the central pin indicates the sagitta, s, of the surface.

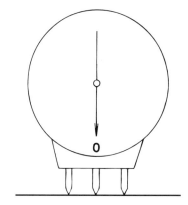

FIGURE 2–8.   **The lens measure on a flat surface.**

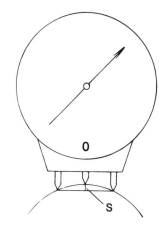

FIGURE 2–9.   **The lens measure on a convex surface. The position of the central pin measures the sagitta of the surface.**

For the lens measure to provide a direct reading of diopters of refracting power of a surface, it is necessary to state the relationship between refracting power, index of refraction, sagitta, and chord length (h being equal to one-half the chord length). This can be done by rewriting Equations 2.2 and 2.4 in terms of the value of r and by solving for the value of F.

Rearranging the terms in Equation 2.2 we have

$$r = \frac{h^2}{2s},$$

and rearranging the terms in Equation 2.4 we have

$$r = \frac{n - 1}{F}.$$

Substituting for r in both equations, we get

$$\frac{h^2}{2s} = \frac{n - 1}{F},$$

which we solve for F:

$$F = \frac{2(n - 1)s}{h^2}. \tag{2.5}$$

If for a given lens measure the distance, h (one-half the chord length), is equal to 1 cm and the instrument is calibrated for an index of refraction of 1.523, the movement of the central pin for each diopter of refracting power of the surface can be determined by solving Equation 2.5 for s and substituting the values of h and n:

$$
\begin{aligned}
s &= \frac{h^2 F}{2(n-1)} \\
&= \frac{(0.01)^2}{2(1.523-1)} \\
&= \frac{0.0001}{1.046} \\
&= 0.0000956 \text{ m, or } 0.0956 \text{ mm.}
\end{aligned}
$$

Some lens measures are calibrated for an index of refraction of 1.53 rather than 1.523; as a result, the reading is in error, slightly high.

Another instrument used in ophthalmic laboratories to measure curvature is the *curve gauge*. A curve gauge is a brass template having curved edges with curvatures corresponding to dioptric values marked on the gauge (Figure 2–10). These gauges are used for checking the curvature of surfacing tools, and the dioptric value marked on the gauge represents the refracting power for glass of index 1.53 with a curvature equal to that of the gauge.

When either a lens measure or a curve gauge is calibrated for an index of refraction other than that of the material being used, the correct power of the surface can be determined by the use of a conversion factor that is derived as follows:

$$
F_C = \frac{n_c - 1}{r},
$$

where F_C = the surface power for which the curve gauge is calibrated, and n_c = the index of refraction for which the curve gauge is calibrated.

$$
F_T = \frac{n_t - 1}{r},
$$

where F_T = the true surface power, and n_t = the index of refraction of the material being used. Setting both of the above equations equal to r, and then equal to each other, we have

$$
\frac{n_t - 1}{F_T} = \frac{n_c - 1}{F_C}
$$

and

$$
F_T = F_C \frac{n_t - 1}{n_c - 1}. \tag{2.6}
$$

For example, when a lens measure or curve gauge calibrated for an index of refraction of 1.53 is used for a material having an index of refraction of 1.523, the conversion factor is

$$
\frac{1.523 - 1}{1.53 - 1} = 0.986,
$$

with the result that a reading of +5.00 D would indicate that the true power of the surface is

$$
+5.00\,(0.986) = +4.93 \text{ D.}
$$

If CR-39 plastic, having an index of refraction of 1.498, is the material, the conversion factor is

$$
\frac{1.498 - 1}{1.53 - 1} = 0.940.
$$

2.5. Lens Form: Spherical Lenses

The term *form*, when applied to an ophthalmic lens, refers to the relationship between the front and back surface curvatures of a lens. For a lens of a given power, an infinite number of forms are possible. Some of these are shown in Figure 2–11. The simplest form for a lens is *plano-convex* or *plano-concave* (Figure 2–11A), in which one surface is flat and the other is either convex or concave. Another simple lens form is the *bi-convex* or *bi-concave* (Figure 2–11B), having half the power on the front surface and half on the back surface.

With few exceptions, modern ophthalmic lenses have convex front surfaces and concave back surfaces (Figures 2–11C and D). Such lenses are sometimes referred to as *bent* lenses. The earliest bent lens, introduced early in this century, was the *periscopic* lens. This lens had a back surface power of –1.25 D (for plus lenses) or a front surface power of +1.25 D (for minus lenses). A later development was the *meniscus* lens, having a –6.00 D back surface power (for plus lenses) or a front surface power of +6.00 D (for minus lenses).

2.6. Lens Form: Cylindrical and Toric Lenses

Cylindrical and toric lenses, used for the correction of astigmatism (or, more often, for the correction of astigmatism combined with myopia or hyperopia), may also exist in an

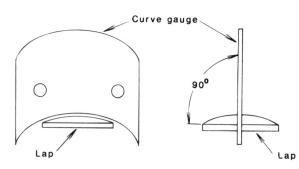

FIGURE 2–10. **The curve gauge, used to check the curvature of a surfacing lap.**

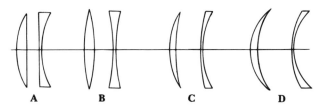

FIGURE 2–11.   **Spherical lens forms. A, plano-convex and plano-concave; B, bi-convex and bi-concave; C, periscopic; D, meniscus.**

infinite number of forms. Some of these forms are shown in Figure 2–12. For a patient who has astigmatism but no myopia or hyperopia, the simplest form of lens is the *plano-cylinder*, having one flat surface (either front or back) and one cylindrical surface. The cylindrical surface has plano power in one principal meridian and plus or minus power in the opposite principal meridian (plus if the cylinder is on the front surface, and minus if it is on the back surface). Diagrams of plus and minus cylindrical lenses are shown in Figure 2–13.

For a patient who has either myopia or hyperopia in addition to astigmatism (the usual situation) a spherical surface is ground on one side of the lens and a toric surface on the other. Traditionally, the toric surface has been ground on the front surface of the lens. However, because a toric back surface decreases the amount of meridional magnification (a difference in the induced size of the retinal image in the two principal meridians) compared with

that obtained by a toric front surface, the standard procedure in recent years has been to grind the toric surface on the back and the spherical surface on the front. Diagrams of toric surfaces are shown in Figure 2–14.

2.7. Lens Blanks and Base Curves

A lens manufacturer makes (or obtains) optical glass in the form of *rough blanks*. A rough blank is a relatively thick, molded piece of optical glass that must be ground and polished on both sides. Once one of the surfaces has been ground and polished, it is called a *semifinished blank*. When both the front and back surfaces have been ground and polished, it is ready to be cut, edged, and mounted in a frame, and is called an *uncut lens*.

In discussing the physical form of a lens, the term *base curve* is widely used. The word *curve* is commonly used, perhaps erroneously, in the sense of surface power. The term *base curve* has several nuances of meaning, but refers to the standardized curvature ground onto the lens by the manufacturer for a grouping of lens powers. It is a common manufacturing practice to group lenses into ranges of powers and to make all lenses within a particular group with the same curvature on one surface.

The selection of base curve is made when the lens is in the semifinished stage, in which case the base curve is always on the *finished* side of the lens. For example, for a spherical meniscus lens in plus power, the back surface of the lens is surfaced with a –6.00 D spherical curve, but the front surface remains unfinished. When toric surfaces were routinely ground on the front surface of the lens, the flatter of the two curvatures was considered to be the base curve. However, for the recently introduced negative toric lenses, the manufacturer continued to finish the front side of the lens, in this case using a spherical surface for the base curve.

The monochromatic lens aberrations (particularly oblique astigmatism and curvature of image) can be minimized by the careful selection of base curves. A lens designed to minimize these aberrations is called a *corrected curve*, or *best-form* lens. The first corrected-curve lenses introduced in the U.S. were the *Orthogon* lens (Bausch & Lomb) and the *Tillyer* lens (American Optical). Lens design and corrected-curve lenses are discussed in Chapter 6.

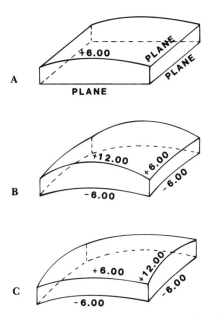

FIGURE 2–12. **Cylindrical and toric lens forms. A, plus plano-cylinder front surface and flat back surface; B, plus toric front surface and concave spherical back surface with net power in the vertical meridian of zero; C, plus toric surface and spherical back surface with net power in the horizontal meridian of zero.**

FIGURE 2–13. **Perspective drawings of minus and plus cylinders.**

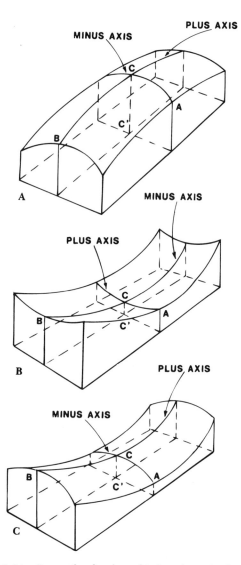

FIGURE 2–14.   **Perspective drawings of toric surfaces. A, plus power in both principal meridians; B, minus power in both principal meridians; C, plus power in one principal meridian and minus power in the other.**

2.8. Specification of Cylinder Axes

The axis of a cylindrical or toric lens is specified in such a way that when you face the patient (or the front surfaces of a pair of ophthalmic lenses) the axis increases in a *counter-clockwise* direction, from 1° to 180°, as shown in Figure 2–15. Astigmatism is said to be *with the rule* if the minus axis of the correcting cylinder is at 180° or within 30 degrees of 180°, and is said to be *against the rule* if the minus axis of the correcting cylinder is at 90° or within 30 degrees of 90°. Astigmatism is said to be *oblique* if the minus axis of the correcting cylinder is between 30° and 60° or between 120° and 150°. With-the-rule, against-the-rule, and oblique astigmatism are illustrated in Figure 2–16.

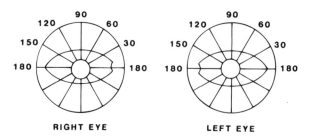

FIGURE 2–15.   **Specification of cylinder axes (facing the patient).**

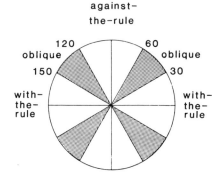

FIGURE 2–16.   **With-the-rule, against-the-rule, and oblique astigmatism for minus-cylinder notation.**

2.9. Prescription Writing and Transposition

When writing the prescription for an ophthalmic lens, the spherical power of the lens is given first, then the cylindrical power and the cylinder axis. For example, the prescription

$$-2.00\,\text{DS} \; -0.50\,\text{DC axis } 180$$

indicates that the spherical component of the prescription is −2.00 D, the cylindrical component is −0.50 D, and the cylinder axis is 180°. In practice, *DS* and *DC* are omitted, and the letter "x" is used to specify *axis*:

$$-2.00 \; -0.50 \times 180.$$

Because a toric surface may be ground either on the front or on the back of the lens, the prescription for a lens may be written in either the *plus-cylinder* form or the *minus-cylinder* form. The above prescription is written in the minus-cylinder form. However, if the cylinder is to be ground on the front of the lens, the prescription is written as follows:

$$-2.50 \; +0.50 \times 90.$$

The relationship between the spherical and cylindrical components of an ophthalmic lens can be visualized by the use of *optical crosses*, also known as *power diagrams*. For a given lens, three crosses are drawn, the two limbs of each cross representing the principal meridians of the lens. For the cross used to represent the spherical component, the power is the same in both principal meridians. For the cross used to represent the cylindrical component, the maximum power of the cylinder is specified in the meridian 90° from the axis meridian, and the power in the axis meridian is specified as zero (since there is *no* power in the axis meridian of a cylindrical lens). The optical crosses shown in Figure 2–17 represent the lens prescription in minus-cylinder form (–2.00 –0.50 x 180) (A); and the prescription for the same lens in plus-cylinder form (–2.50 +0.50 x 90) (B). Note that, for both sets of optical crosses, the *total* power in the horizontal meridian (combining spherical and cylindrical components) is –2.00 D, and the *total* power in the vertical meridian is –2.50 D. Note also that, for the minus-cylinder form, the total power in the *most plus* meridian is selected as the spherical power, but for the plus-cylinder form the total power in the *least plus* meridian is selected as the spherical power.

Considering another example, the lens prescription for a patient having hyperopia and astigmatism is

$$+1.00 -0.75 \text{ x } 30.$$

This prescription is written in the minus-cylinder form. However, if the lens is to be manufactured in the plus-cylinder form, the laboratory technician will have to transpose the prescription to the plus-cylinder form. The optical crosses shown in Figure 2–18 represent the prescription as written in the minus-cylinder form (A); note that the total power in the 30° meridian is +1.00 D, and the total power in the 120° meridian is +0.25 D. To write a prescription for this lens in the plus-cylinder form, the power in the meridian of least plus power is selected as the spherical power, and the difference between that power and the power in the most plus meridian is selected as the cylindrical power. Thus, the prescription in plus-cylinder form (B) is

$$+0.25 +0.75 \text{ x } 120.$$

There are many instances in which it is necessary to *transpose* a lens prescription from minus-cylinder form to plus-cylinder form, or vice versa. For example, optometrists routinely use minus-cylinder refractors or phoroptors and therefore write lens prescriptions in the minus-cylinder form. When a lens is to be made in the form of a front surface cylinder, it is necessary for the laboratory to transpose the prescription into plus-cylinder form (as indicated in the above example). Conversely, ophthalmologists routinely use plus-cylinder refractors or phoroptors and therefore write prescriptions in plus-cylinder form; when a lens is to be made in the form of a back surface cylinder, it is necessary for the laboratory to transpose the prescription into minus-cylinder form.

Three-Step Rule for Transposition

To transpose a sphero-cylindrical prescription from minus-cylinder form to plus-cylinder form or vice versa, the following three-step rule may be used:

1. Add the sphere power and the cylinder power algebraically, to obtain the new spherical power.
2. Change the sign of the cylinder (from minus to plus, or from plus to minus).
3. Rotate the cylinder axis 90°.

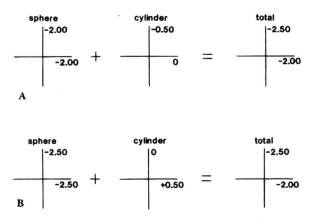

FIGURE 2–17.   Optical crosses (power diagrams). A, for the prescription –2.00 –0.50 x 180; B, for the prescription –2.50 +0.50 x 90.

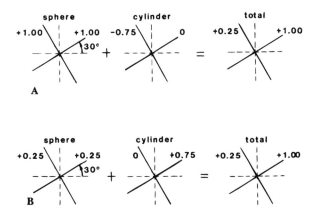

FIGURE 2–18.   Optical crosses (power diagrams). A, for the prescription +1.00 –0.75 x 30; B, for the prescription +0.25 +0.75 x 120.

Inspection of the examples given in the optical crosses shown in Figures 2–17 and 2–18 shows that, by using the three-step rule, the prescription –2.00 –0.50 x 180 may be transposed to –2.50 +0.50 x 90, and the prescription +1.00 –0.75 x 30 may be transposed to +0.25 +0.75 x 120. When using the three-step rule, the novice should check the work by means of optical cross diagrams.

The Crossed-Cylinder Form

A *crossed-cylinder* lens is one having a plus cylinder ground on the front surface and a minus cylinder ground on the back surface, with the axes of the two cylinders 90° apart. An example of a crossed-cylinder lens is

$$+0.50 \text{ DC x } 90 \text{ combined with } -0.50 \text{ DC x } 180.$$

Optical crosses representing the prescription for this lens are shown in Figure 2–19. Note that the total power of this lens in the horizontal meridian is +0.50 D, and the total power in the vertical meridian is –0.50 D. In optometric practice, crossed cylinders are used in refining the axis and

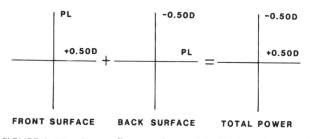

FIGURE 2–19. **Power diagrams for a +0.50 D/–0.50 D crossed cylinder.**

power of the patient's cylindrical correction, and are also used for near-point testing (for example, to determine the power of a tentative bifocal addition).

The following rule may be used to transpose a sphero-cylindrical prescription to a crossed-cylinder prescription:

1. Find both the plus-cylinder and minus-cylinder forms of the prescription.
2. Connect the extremes.

For example, if a lens prescription, written first in the minus-cylinder form and then in the plus-cylinder form, is

$$+0.50\,DS\ -1.00\,DC \times 180$$

$$-0.50\,DS\ +1.00\,DC \times 90,$$

connecting the extremes results in the prescription

$$+0.50\,DC \times 90 \text{ combined with } -0.50\,DC \times 180.$$

Note that this is the prescription given above, as an example of a crossed-cylinder lens.

When a prescription has been written in the crossed-cylinder form, the following rule may be used to transpose it into the sphero-cylindrical form:

1. Use the cylindrical power you encounter first as the spherical power.
2. For the cylindrical power, change the sign of the new spherical power and add it algebraically to the second cylinder power.
3. For the cylinder axis, use the axis of the second cylinder.

Continuing with the above example, for the lens whose crossed-cylinder prescription is

$$+0.50\,DC \times 90 \text{ combined with } -0.50\,DC \times 180,$$

when we apply this rule we obtain the sphero-cylindrical prescription

$$+0.50\,DS\ -1.00\,DC \times 180,$$

and, using the original three-step rule, this can be transposed into the plus-cylinder prescription

$$-0.50\,DS\ +1.00\,DC \times 90.$$

Each of these sphero-cylindrical prescriptions is similar to the corresponding sphero-cylindrical prescription (for the same lens) given above, which corroborates the correctness of the result. The result may also be checked by means of the optical cross diagrams shown in Figure 2–19.

Since transposition between minus-cylinder and plus-cylinder forms may be encountered routinely in optometric practice, the student is advised to memorize the three-step rule for sphero-cylindrical transposition. However, the transposition into (and out of) the crossed-cylinder form is not encountered routinely; if rules for these transpositions are forgotten, one can easily use optical crosses to make the transposition.

OPTICAL CHARACTERISTICS

2.10. Basic Terminology

Optic Axis

The optic axis of a lens is an imaginary line connecting the centers of curvature of the two surfaces of the lens, which is also normal to both of the surfaces, as shown in Figure 2–20. Although the great majority of ophthalmic lenses possess only one line that is normal to both surfaces, and therefore have a true optic axis, there are a number of possible lens forms that have more than one line normal to both surfaces and for this reason do not possess a true optic axis. In all these special cases, the two surfaces are plane parallel or spherical concentric in one or both of the principal meridians. As shown in Figure 2–21, lens forms not possessing a true optic axis include a lens having plane parallel surfaces (A) and a lens having concentric spherical surfaces (B). Figure 2–22 illustrates other lens forms that have no natural

optic axis, but are characterized by a single plane that contains all lines normal to both lens surfaces. These lenses have a cylindrical surface on the front side and a plano surface on the rear side and their axis of revolution is parallel to the plano lens surface. All the lines normal to both lens surfaces are contained in a single plane that is normal to the plano lens surface and passes through the axis of revolution (A); a lens that has a cylindrical surface on the front side and a spherical surface on the rear side and whose center of curvature falls on the axis of revolution of the cylindrical surface. The single plane normal to the axis of revolution that contains the center of curvature of the spherical surfaces also contains all lines that are normal to both lens surfaces (B); a lens with a spherical surface on the front side and a toric surface on the rear side and whose center of curvature of the spherical surface falls on the axis of revolution of the toric surface. If the plane normal to the axis of revolution at this point contains the center of curvature of the generating arc

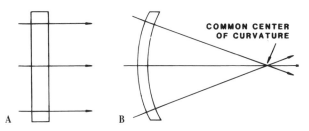

of the toric surface, this single plane contains an infinite number of lines that are perpendicular to both lens surfaces (C); a lens that has a toric surface on the front side and a spherical surface on the rear side and whose center of curvature of the generating arc of the toric surface traces a path that passes through the center of curvature of the spherical surface. The lines that are normal to both surfaces fall in a single plane that passes through the center of curvature of the spherical surface and the axis of revolution (D).

FIGURE 2–20. The optic axis (the line normal to both lens surfaces, passing through the centers of curvature of the surfaces).

FIGURE 2–21. Lenses that have no natural optic axis. A line normal to one surface at any point is also normal to the other surface. A, lens with plane parallel surfaces; B, lens with concentric spherical surfaces.

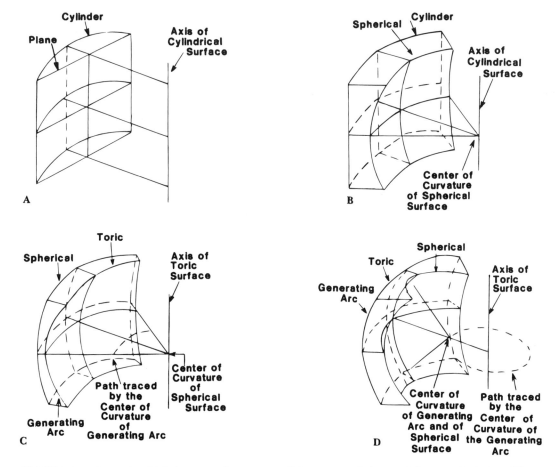

FIGURE 2–22. Lenses in which the two surfaces are parallel or concentric in one of the two principal meridians. Any line in the meridian section that is normal to one surface is normal to the other.

Optical Center

The term *optical center* is used in geometrical optics in connection with spherical lenses to designate the point on the optic axis intersected by the path of a ray of light between the two surfaces that, after refraction by the second surface, is parallel to its path before incidence at the first surface (Figure 2–23). Although for the bi-convex and bi-concave lenses shown in Figure 2–23 the optical center is located within the lens, for any *bent* ophthalmic lens the optical center falls outside the lens.

The optical center of a lens can be found by using the following method of construction (Figure 2–24).

1. Draw a line from the center of curvature of one surface to the surface, and let the point of intersection of this line with the surface be called A.
2. Draw another line parallel to the first line, passing through the other center of curvature and intersecting the other surface at a point designated as B.
3. Draw a line connecting points A and B. The point at which this line or its extension crosses the optic axis is the optical center of the lens. Any ray directed toward this point will, after passing through the lens, continue in the same direction as it had before entering the lens.

It is also possible to find the position of the optical center mathematically by using the formula

$$A_1O = \frac{r_1(d)}{r_1 - r_2} = \frac{F_2(d)}{F_1 + F_2}, \qquad (2.7)$$

where A_1 = the front vertex of the lens, O = the optical center, d = the lens thickness, r_1 and r_2 = radii of front and back surfaces, and F_1 and F_2 = refracting power of front and back surfaces.

EXAMPLE 1
If we have a lens in which $F_1 = F_2 = +4.00$ D, having a thickness of 4 mm, then

$$A_1O = \frac{4(0.004)}{4 + 4} = \frac{0.016}{8} = 0.002 \text{ m.}$$

$$A_1O = 2 \text{ mm.}$$

Therefore, the optical center O lies midway between the front and back surfaces of the lens.

EXAMPLE 2
If the front surface power is +4.00 D, and the back surface power is plano, with a thickness of 4 mm, then

$$A_1O = \frac{0(0.004)}{4 + 0} = 0.$$

This indicates that the optical center is at the front vertex, or apex, of the lens.

EXAMPLE 3
If the front surface power is +9.00 D and the back surface power is –5.00 D, with a thickness of 4 mm, then

$$A_1O = \frac{-5(0.004)}{9 - 5} = \frac{-0.02}{4} = -0.005 \text{ m.}$$

$$= -5.0 \text{ mm.}$$

The minus sign indicates that the optical center is 5.0 mm anterior to the front surface of the lens.

Vertices or Poles

The points on the front and back surface of a lens that are penetrated by the optic axis are called the front and back *vertices*, or *poles*, of the lens. When ophthalmic lenses were made only in flat, "unbent" forms (plano-convex, plano-concave, bi-convex, and bi-concave), the optical center was either on one surface of the lens (coinciding with the front or back pole or vertex) or within the lens. Although the optical center of a modern ophthalmic lens is usually not located on or within the lens (as already discussed) it is a common, although incorrect, practice to use the term op-

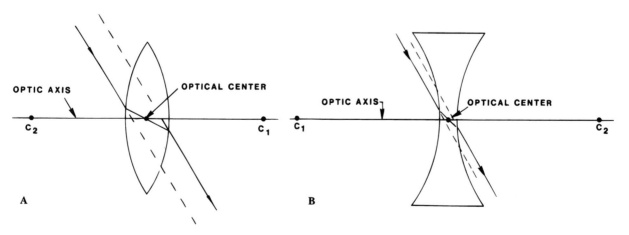

FIGURE 2–23.   **The optical center. A, of a plus lens; B, of a minus lens.**

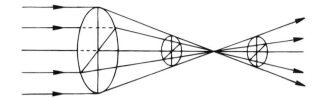

FIGURE 2–25.   Image formation by a spherical lens. A point image is formed at the secondary focal plane of the lens, but at any other plane a blur circle is formed.

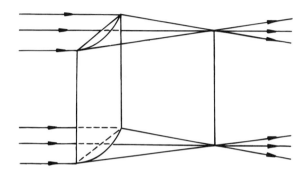

FIGURE 2–26.   Image formation by plano plus cylinder. The point image is replaced by a focal line located in the vertical meridian, formed by the refraction of rays in the horizontal meridian.

FIGURE 2–24.   Graphical method of locating the optical center of a lens.

tical center, rather than the term pole or vertex, when referring to the point on the lens penetrated by the optic axis.

2.11. Image Formation by a Spherical Lens

From geometrical optics we know that, when parallel rays of light from a distant object point are incident upon a convex spherical lens, a point image is formed on a screen placed in the secondary focal plane of the lens. As shown in Figure 2–25, if the screen is placed some distance in front of or behind the secondary focal plane of the lens, a *blur circle* is formed on the screen. As shown, the size of the blur circle increases with the distance between the screen and the secondary focal plane of the lens. The size of the blur circle also depends on the diameter of the aperture of the lens; the blur circle increases as the size of the aperture increases. A blur circle is formed only when the aperture is *circular* in form—for an elliptical or square aperture, the blur circle is elliptical or square in shape.

2.12. Image Formation by Cylindrical and Toric Lenses

If the convex spherical lens shown in Figure 2–25 is replaced by a convex plano-cylindrical lens, the point image for a point object will be replaced by a *focal line*, as shown in Figure 2–26. The axis of the cylindrical lens shown in this diagram is located in the vertical meridian, with the result that the focal line (located in the vertical meridian) is formed by refraction of rays in the horizontal meridian. Since no refraction occurs in the vertical meridian, the length of the

focal line (for rays coming from a distant axial point) is equal to the diameter of the aperture. If the screen is placed in front of or behind the position of the focal line, a *blur ellipse*, rather than a blur circle, is formed. For any position of the screen, the extent of the ellipse in the axis meridian is equal to the length of the focal line (and also equal to the diameter of the aperture), but the extent of the ellipse in the power meridian of the lens increases with increasing distance from the plane of the focal line.

If the convex plano-cylindrical lens is replaced by a convex *toric* lens, not one, but two focal lines are formed (Figure 2–27). In this diagram, the horizontal meridian is the meridian of greatest refraction, with the result that the vertical focal line, V (formed by refraction of rays in the horizontal meridian), is formed closer to the lens than the horizontal focal line, H (formed by refraction of rays in the vertical meridian). If the screen is placed at a short distance in front of or behind either of the two focal lines, a blur ellipse is formed, and its major axis is parallel to the focal line in question. If the screen is placed at the point along the optic axis of the lens where the vergence of the refracted rays is midway between that of the two focal lines, the *circle of least confusion*, C, is formed.

2.13. Terminology and Basic Concepts of Image Formation by a Lens

The following terminology is important to understand image formation by spherical, cylindrical, and toric lenses.

FIGURE 2–27.   **Image formation by a sphero-cylindrical lens having its greatest refraction in the horizontal meridian. Note that the refraction in the vertical meridian forms the horizontal focal line, and the refraction in the horizontal meridian forms the vertical focal line. The circle of least confusion is located at such a point that its dioptric power is midway between that of the two focal lines.**

Homocentric

A homocentric bundle of rays is one in which all rays meet, after refraction by the lens, at a common point. This occurs when a bundle of rays from a single object point is refracted by a spherical lens, if aberrations are neglected (Figure 2–25). Synonyms for homocentric are *monocentric* and *stigmatic* (the root *stigmatic* means "point").

Astigmatic

An astigmatic bundle of rays is one in which all rays from a single object point fail to meet, after refraction by the lens, at a common point, but form two line images perpendicular to one another (Figure 2–27). This occurs when a bundle of rays is refracted by a cylindrical or toric lens. Synonyms for astigmatic are *nonhomocentric* and *nonmonocentric*.

Conoid of Sturm

The conoid of Sturm is the entire three-dimensional figure formed by the bundle of rays refracted by a toric lens (shown in Figure 2–28). This includes, for various positions of the screen, the vertical (V) and horizontal (H) focal lines, blur ellipses, and the circle of least confusion (C). The lens shown in Figure 2–28 has a power of +2.00 DS –1.00 DC x 180, and

the vertical focal line (V) is located 50 cm from the lens, the horizontal focal line (H) is located 100 cm from the lens, and the circle of least confusion (C) is located 67 cm from the lens.

Interval of Sturm

The interval of Sturm is the dioptric or physical distance between the two focal lines. The focal line nearest the lens is called the *primary* focal line; that farthest from the lens is called the *secondary* focal line.

2.14. Dimensional Aspects of the Conoid of Sturm

The positions or locations of each of the focal lines may be found by applying the familiar thin lens formula

$$F = L' - L, \qquad (2.8)$$

to each principal meridian. In this formula, F refers to the refracting power in the meridian under consideration, L' refers to the image vergence, and L refers to the object vergence. If the physical distance of each focal line from the lens is desired, it may be found by solving the thin lens formula for image vergence and then taking the reciprocal of the image vergence.

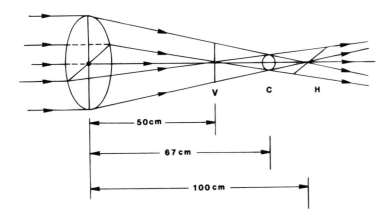

FIGURE 2–28. **The conoid of Sturm. For a lens having the prescription +2.00 –1.00 x 180, the vertical focal line is located 50 cm from the lens, the horizontal focal line is located 100 cm from the lens, and the circle of least confusion is located 67 cm from the lens.**

Expressions for lengths of the primary and secondary focal lines and for the diameter of the circle of least confusion can be derived with the aid of Figures 2–29 and 2–30. These diagrams represent the refraction of an astigmatic lens with its principal meridians located in the horizontal and vertical meridians. Plus power exists in both meridians, with the greatest amount of plus power in the horizontal meridian. For an object point on the optic axis, a vertical focal line (V′V″) is located at a distance l_1' from the lens and a horizontal focal line (H′H″) is located at a distance l_2' from the lens. The circle of least confusion (C′C″) is located at a distance l_c' from the lens. Figure 2–30 shows the top and side views of the astigmatic imagery shown in Figure 2–29.

From Figures 2–29 and 2–30, we may derive formulas for the lengths of the focal lines, by use of similar triangles. In Figure 2–30B, triangles MNH and V′V″H are similar. Therefore,

$$\frac{V'V''}{MN} = \frac{VH}{QH} = \frac{l_2' - l_1'}{l_2'}$$

$$V'V'' = \frac{l_2' - l_1'}{l_2'}(MN)$$

$$V'V'' = \frac{\dfrac{1}{L_2'} - \dfrac{1}{L_1'}}{\dfrac{1}{L_2'}}(MN)$$

$$V'V'' = \frac{L_1' - L_2'}{L_1'}(MN).$$

Since the distance MN is equal to the aperture size, the length of the primary focal line is given by the expression

$$\frac{L_1' - L_2'}{L_1'} \text{ (aperture size).} \qquad (2.9)$$

In Figure 2–30A, triangles POV and H′H″V are similar. Therefore,

$$\frac{H'H''}{OP} = \frac{VH}{QH} = \frac{l_2' - l_1'}{l_1'}$$

$$H'H'' = \frac{l_2' - l_1'}{l_1'}(OP)$$

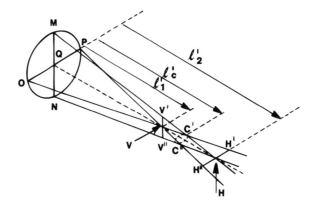

FIGURE 2–29. **Diagram used for determining the positions and lengths of the focal lines and the position and size of the circle of least confusion.**

$$H'H'' = \frac{\dfrac{1}{L_2'} - \dfrac{1}{L_1'}}{\dfrac{1}{L_1'}}(OP)$$

$$H'H'' = \frac{L_1' - L_2'}{L_2'}(OP).$$

Since OP represents the aperture size, the length of the secondary focal line is given by the expression

$$\frac{L_1' - L_2'}{L_2'} \text{ (aperture size).} \qquad (2.10)$$

Note that, for a circular aperture, OP = MN, but, for a noncircular aperture, OP ≠ MN. Note also that the circle of least confusion (discussed below) is a circle *only* for a circular aperture.

The position (l_c') and length (C′C″) of the circle of least confusion can also be found by similar triangles. In Figure 2–30A, triangles POV and C′C″V are similar, and in Figure 2–30B triangles MNH and C′C″H are similar. Therefore,

$$\frac{C'C''}{PO} = \frac{C'C''}{MN} = \frac{l_c' - l_1'}{l_1'} = \frac{l_2' - l_c'}{l_2'}$$

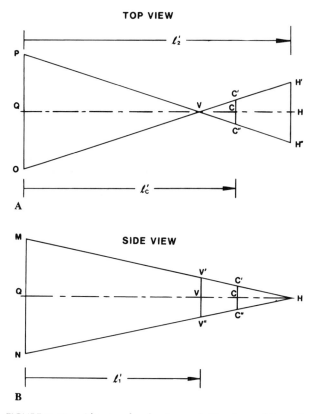

TOP VIEW

A

SIDE VIEW

B

FIGURE 2–30. **Diagram showing top and side views of the astigmatic imagery shown in Figure 2–29.**

or

$$(l_c')(l_2') - (l_1')(l_2') = (l_1')(l_2') - (l_c')(l_1')$$

$$(l_c')(l_1') + (l_c)(l_2') = (l_1')(l_2') + (l_1')(l_2')$$

$$l_c'(l_1' + l_2') = 2l_1'l_2'$$

$$l_c' = \frac{2(l_1')(l_2')}{l_1' + l_2'} \tag{2.11}$$

$$l_c' = \frac{2 \dfrac{1}{L_1' + L_2'}}{\dfrac{1}{L_1'} + \dfrac{1}{L_2'}}$$

$$l_c' = \frac{2}{L_1' + L_2'}, \tag{2.12}$$

which provides the location of the circle of least confusion.

The dioptric value of the circle of least confusion is therefore

$$L_c' = \frac{L_1' + L_2'}{2}. \tag{2.13}$$

Since

$$\frac{C'C''}{MN} = \frac{l_c' - l_1'}{l_1'},$$

then

$$C'C'' = \frac{l_c' - l_1'}{l_1'} (MN).$$

Substituting the value of l_c' in Equation 2.12,

$$C'C'' = \frac{\dfrac{2}{L_1' + L_2'} - l_1'}{l_1'} (MN)$$

$$C'C'' = \frac{\dfrac{2}{L_1' + L_2'} - \dfrac{1}{L_1'}}{\dfrac{1}{L_1'}} (MN)$$

$$C'C'' = \frac{2L_1' - L_1' + L_2'}{L_1'(L_1' + L_2')} \left(\frac{L_1'}{1}\right) (MN)$$

$$C'C'' = \frac{L_1' - L_2'}{L_1' + L_2'} (MN).$$

Therefore, the diameter of the circle of least confusion may be found by the expression

$$\frac{L_1' - L_2'}{L_1' + L_2'} \text{ (aperture size)}. \tag{2.14}$$

EXAMPLE
Given a lens, +3.50 –0.75 x 140, with a diameter of 50 mm and a point object at a distance of 1 m in front of the lens, find the following:

1. The location of the line foci.
2. The lengths of the focal lines.
3. The location of the circle of least confusion.
4. The diameter of the circle of least confusion.

1a. Location of the primary focal line (formed by the meridian with +3.50-D power):

$$L_1' = L + F_1$$
$$= -1.00 + 3.50 = +2.50 \text{ D}.$$

$$l_1' = \frac{1}{L_1'} = \frac{1}{+2.50} = 0.4 \text{ m}$$
$$= 40 \text{ cm behind the lens}.$$

1b. Location of the second focal line (formed by the meridian with +2.75-D power):

$$L_2' = L + F_2$$
$$= -1.00 + 2.75 = +1.75 \text{ D}.$$

$$l_1' = \frac{1}{L_2'} = \frac{1}{+1.75} = 0.555 \text{ m}$$
$$= 55.5 \text{ cm behind the lens}.$$

2a. Length of the first focal line:

$$\frac{L_1' - L_2'}{L_1'} \text{ (aperture size)} = \frac{(+2.50 - 1.75)50}{+2.50}$$
$$= \frac{(0.75)50}{+2.50} = 15 \text{ mm}.$$

2b. Length of the second focal line:

$$\frac{L_1' - L_2'}{L_2'} \text{ (aperture size)} = \frac{(2.50 - 1.75)50}{+1.75}$$

$$= \frac{(0.75)50}{+1.75}$$

$$= 21.4 \text{ mm.}$$

3. Location of the circle of least confusion:

$$L_c' = \frac{L_1' + L_2'}{2} = \frac{2.50 + 1.75}{2}$$

$$= \frac{+4.25}{2} = +2.125 \text{ D.}$$

$$l_c' = \frac{1}{L_c'} = \frac{1}{+2.125} = 0.471 \text{ m}$$

$$= 47.1 \text{ cm behind the lens.}$$

4. Diameter of the circle of least confusion:

$$\frac{L_1' - L_2'}{L_1' + L_2'} \text{ (aperture)} = \frac{(2.50 - 1.75)50}{(2.50 + 1.75)}$$

$$= \frac{.75 \times 50}{+4.25} = 8.8 \text{ mm.}$$

In any plane perpendicular to the optic axis of a lens, other than the circle of least confusion, the rays of light are spread over a relatively large area (as shown in Figure 2–27), whereas they are most highly concentrated at the circle of least confusion. For this reason, when presented with a distant object, a patient who has uncorrected hyperopic astigmatism can maximize his visual acuity by accommodating in such a way that the circle of least confusion (for each point on the object) is located on the retina. This is analogous to the situation that occurs when light is refracted by a spherical lens, in which the greatest concentration of light (and the best visual acuity) occurs when the image for each point on the object is placed on the retina. For a single line object, depending on its orientation, the patient may be able to maximize visual acuity by placing one of the line foci of the interval of Sturm on the retina. For a more complex configuration, the patient can accommodate in such a way as to manipulate the interval of Sturm on the retina in order to maximize visual acuity. The manipulation of accommodation may be a source of asthenopia (eyestrain) for a person with uncorrected astigmatism.

2.15. Misconceptions about Astigmatic Image Formation

The student can easily be misled into believing that the entire conoid of Sturm is formed simultaneously, and that some of the light makes up each focal line, some makes up the circle of least confusion, and some makes up the blur ellipses. However, the conoid of Sturm should be thought of in terms of the *progression of the bundle of rays* with time, after refraction by the lens. As the bundle of rays progresses with time (very rapidly indeed), the first focal line, blur ellipses, the circle of least confusion, additional blur ellipses,

and the second focal line are all formed in succession (assuming a screen oriented perpendicular to the optic axis of the lens is placed at each of these points). This is analogous to what happens when light is refracted by a spherical lens. As the bundle of rays progresses with time, blur circles of decreasing size, then the point image, then blur circles of increasing size are sequentially formed (again, assuming a screen has been placed at each position where an image is desired).

Another misconception is that, somehow, the image of the *whole object* consists of the two focal lines and the circle of least confusion. The conoid of Sturm is formed for a *point object*, just as the point image for a spherical lens is formed for a point object. Because, for a spherical lens, each point on the surface of an object forms a point image or a blur circle, it follows that, for an astigmatic lens, each point forms a conoid of Sturm with two line foci, blur ellipses, or the circle of least confusion. The resultant image of a whole object is made up of the totality of the images formed for all object points (for a specified image plane). The *clock dial* (or *sunburst dial*), used in the clinical testing of astigmatism, serves as a good example of the concept that an object can be considered as being made up of an infinite number of points, each of which may form a point image or a blur circle (in the case of a spherical optical system) or a focal line or any other configuration in the conoid of Sturm (in the case of a cylindrical optical system).

The clock dial test for astigmatism consists of a chart with radiating lines representing the numbers on the face of a clock. Before beginning the test, the patient's eye is *fogged*, that is, sufficient plus lens power is placed before the eye to make sure that the entire interval of Sturm (if astigmatism exists) is located in front of the retina. If the patient has *no astigmatism*, each object point will form a point image in front of the retina, with the result that all the lines on the clock dial appear equally clear. If the patient *does* have astigmatism, the line (on the clock dial) that appears the most distinct is the one parallel to the principal meridian of the eye that has the greatest refractive power. The minus-cylinder lens correcting the eye's astigmatism has its axis position perpendicular to the direction of the clearest line on the retina. Minus-cylinder power should be increased until the patient reports that all the radial lines are equally distinct. This technique provides the cylindrical correction, that is, the correction for the astigmatic portion of the refractive error.

Figure 2–31 shows (A) a simplified clock dial with the lines represented as a series of point objects. For an astigmatic optical system, each point object forms a conoid of Sturm. If the principal meridians are horizontal and vertical, the astigmatic imagery at the vertical line focus (B) and the astigmatic imagery at the horizontal line focus (C) are represented. It is obvious that, if the power in the vertical meridian is greater than the power in the horizontal meridian (with-the-rule astigmatism), the clearest line on the clock dial is the *vertical* line; if the power in the horizontal meridian is greater than that in the vertical meridian (against-the-rule astigmatism), the clearest line on the clock dial is the *horizontal* line.

A. OBJECT (SIMPLIFIED CLOCK DIAL)

B. IMAGE AT VERTICAL LINE FOCUS

C. IMAGE AT HORIZONTAL LINE FOCUS

FIGURE 2–31.   **A simplified clock dial, illustrating image formation by a sphero-cylindrical lens.**

2.16. The Spherical Equivalent

Spherical equivalent power is defined as the average (or *nominal*) spherical power of a cylindrical or sphero-cylindrical lens. It is determined, for a sphero-cylindrical lens, by algebraically combining one-half the cylindrical power with the spherical power.

There are a number of situations in optometric practice in which it is helpful to convert a lens formula or prescription into the spherical equivalent form. For example, how can the following lens formulas be compared to determine which has the most overall plus power?

(A) +2.00 DS −1.00 DC x 180,

(B) +3.00 DS −2.00 DC x 180.

By algebraically combining one-half of the cylindrical power with the spherical power, for each of the two formulas, we have

(A) +2.00 DS + (−0.50 DS) = +1.50 DS,

(B) +3.00 DS + (−1.00 DS) = +2.00 DS.

The second formula (B) has 0.50-D more plus spherical equivalent power than the first formula. As shown in Figure 2–28, the spherical equivalent power of the lens is represented by the *dioptric value of the circle of least confusion.*

One situation in which the spherical equivalent concept is used is when, for one reason or another, a practitioner decides to ignore or to reduce the cylindrical component of the patient's refraction and prescribes the spherical equivalent as a way to position the circle of least confusion on the retina. For example, if a patient's refractive finding is −2.00 DS −0.50 DC x 180, and if the practitioner decides not to prescribe the cylinder power, the spherical equivalent, −2.25 DS, is likely to be prescribed. Even though the patient has 0.50 D of uncorrected astigmatism, the circle of least confusion would then fall on the retina (with accommodation relaxed).

Occasionally a practitioner finds that a patient has a large amount of previously uncorrected astigmatism and decides to *reduce* (but not completely ignore) the cylindrical correction. This may be done particularly if the cylinder has an oblique axis. For example, if the refractive finding is +2.00 DS −3.00 DC x 45, the practitioner may decide to prescribe only −2.00 D of cylinder power. In this case, the lens to prescribe, as a way to place the circle of least confusion on the retina, is found by algebraically adding one-half the *cylinder reduction* to the original sphere power to obtain the new sphere power. The prescribed lens power is, thus, +1.50 DS −2.00 DC x 45. The original lens formula, +2.00 DS −3.00 DC x 45, and the modified prescription both have a spherical equivalence of +0.50 D.

The Jackson crossed-cylinder lens, which is frequently used in refraction for determining the axis and power of the cylindrical component, is an example of a lens that has zero spherical equivalent power. A +0.50 D/−0.50 D Jackson crossed-cylinder lens (+0.50-D cylinder on the front surface and −0.50-D cylinder on the back surface, with the axes 90° apart), when transposed to the sphero-cylindrical form, can be expressed as either

−0.50 DS +1.00 DC

or

+0.50 DS −1.00 DC.

In either case, use of the rule for determining spherical equivalent power shows that the crossed-cylinder lens has a spherical equivalent power of *zero.* The placement of a Jackson crossed-cylinder lens before the eye, therefore, allows us to change the power in each of the principal meridians without changing the average, or spherical equivalent, power.

The concept of spherical equivalent power is also useful when we wish to compare refractive findings obtained by different forms of instrumentation or by more than one examiner. For example, when a newly developed automatic refraction system is being evaluated, it is customary to compare the results obtained in routine clinical refraction in terms of the spherical component (i.e., the spherical portion of the lens formula), the spherical equivalent power, the cylinder power, and the cylinder axis.

2.17. Power in an Oblique Meridian of a Cylindrical Lens

Since a cylindrical lens has its maximum refracting power in one meridian (the power meridian) and has zero power in the meridian at right angles (the axis meridian), it is reasonable to assume that in any oblique meridian the refracting power lies somewhere between zero and that of the power meridian. However, a cylindrical lens forms a clear image only for each of the two focal lines; each line is perpendicular to the principal meridian that forms the line. There are only two focal lines because two incident rays from a given object point reunite after refraction *only* if they lie in a principal meridian. Any two rays, from a single object point, that lie in an *oblique* meridian will fail to reunite after refraction. Such rays are said to exhibit "skew" convergence or divergence.

Is it possible to talk of refracting power in a given oblique meridian when there is no clear image formed by the lens in that meridian? If the diopter is the reciprocal of focal length, does it follow that diopters of power exist only when a clear image is present? Using the theorems developed by the Swiss mathematician Leonard Euler (1707–1783) concerning the curvatures of two normal sections intersecting each other at right angles at a point of the curved surface, Southall[4] derived an equation for the curvature along a meridian of a cylindrical surface other than a principal meridian, such that

$$R_\alpha = R_c \sin^2 \alpha, \qquad (2.15)$$

where R_c is the maximum curvature and α is the angle from the axis meridian to the unknown oblique meridian. It should be understood that this equation results in only an approximation, since the curvature R_α is not constant along the entire oblique meridian. For a normal section along an oblique meridian of a cylindrical surface, the resulting curve is *elliptical.* If only a small, central portion of the curve in an oblique meridian is considered, we may assume that the curvature of this small portion is *circular.* This assumption is valid for ophthalmic lenses because the area of the cylindrical surface used is only a small portion of the complete cylinder from which it is taken.

Since curvature is related to surface power, we can derive a relationship for F_α as follows:

$$F = (n' - n)R$$

or

$$R = \frac{F}{n' - n}$$

$$R_\alpha = \frac{F_\alpha}{n' - n} = R_C \sin^2 \alpha$$

$$\frac{F_\alpha}{n' - n} = \frac{F_c \sin^2 \alpha}{n' - n}$$

or

$$F_\alpha = F_C \sin^2 \alpha, \qquad (2.16)$$

where F_C is the cylinder power and α is the angle from the axis to the meridian in question. For any two meridians on a cylindrical surface of power F_C that are 90° apart, that is, meridians that are α and $\alpha + 90$ from the cylinder axis,

$$F_\alpha = F_C \sin^2 \alpha$$

$$F_{\alpha + 90} = F_C \sin^2(\alpha + 90) = F_C \cos^2 \alpha.$$

Therefore, the algebraic sum of the powers in the two perpendicular meridians is

$$F_\alpha + (F_{\alpha + 90}) = F_C \sin^2 \alpha + F_C \cos^2 \alpha.$$

$$= F_C(\sin^2 \alpha + \cos^2 \alpha)$$

$$= F_C(1)$$

$$F_\alpha + (F_{\alpha + 90}) = F_C.$$

Thus, the algebraic sum of the powers in any two meridians perpendicular to each other on a cylindrical surface is constant and equal to the total power of the cylinder.

Although, in the strictest sense, power, as traditionally defined, does not exist in an oblique meridian of a cylindrical surface, the sine square law has many useful applications. Bennett and Rabbetts[5] have used the term *notational power* to denote the power in the oblique meridian of a cylindrical surface, calculated by the sine square equation. This equation is sufficiently accurate for determining sagittal depths and thicknesses of oblique meridians for ophthalmic lenses of average dimension. Keating and Carroll[6] showed that the sine square law is related to *minimizing the blur* or *maximizing the modulation transfer function* for meridional refraction of a line object.

Long and Haine[7] showed that the sine square law is applicable to laser refraction. It is possible to refract oblique meridians and reconstruct the refraction in conventional notation (sphere, cylinder, and axis) using the sine square law. Although meridional refraction does not provide a clear image, it does provide the position of "best focus" in each of several preselected meridians.

Keating[8] stated that dioptric power exists in an off-axis meridian and has a *curvature* component and a *torsional* component. The torsional component can be demonstrated when one works with oblique meridians in a number of routine optometric procedures such as the "skewed reflex" seen in retinoscopy, misalignment of the mire images in keratometry, and the scissors motion occurring in lensometry.

The references cited above indicate that the approximations arrived at by the sine square law provide accurate numerical results under the conditions for which it is applied. One should, however, recognize the unique nature of oblique power, as well as its limitations. Specifically, the prismatic effect at any point along an oblique meridian of a sphero-cylindrical lens cannot be calculated by use of the power determined by the sine square formula (see Chapter 4).

Southall's derivation ($R_\alpha = R_c \sin^2 \alpha$) was used to derive the formula for the power in the oblique meridian of a cylindrical lens. This formula can also be derived from first principles on the basis of the diagram shown in Figure 2–32. Referring to this diagram, the line segment CB represents the axis meridian (the meridian of zero power) of a cylindrical surface. CA represents the power meridian, and CP represents an oblique meridian at an angle α from the axis

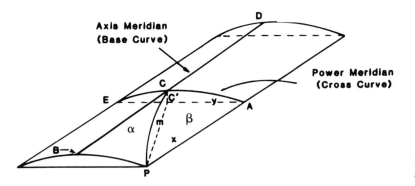

FIGURE 2–32.   Diagram for derivation of the power in an oblique meridian of a plano-cylinder.

meridian. If F_P is defined as the refractive power in the oblique meridian, CP, and if F_C is the power in the power meridian, CA, it follows from Equation 2.5 that

$$F_P = 2(n-1)\frac{CC'}{m^2}$$

and

$$F_C = 2(n-1)\frac{CC'}{y^2}.$$

By solving the latter equation for CC' and substituting the result in the former,

$$F_P = F_C \frac{y^2}{m^2},$$

but $y^2 = m^2 \sin^2\alpha$; therefore,

$$F_P = \frac{F_C\, m^2 \sin^2\alpha}{m^2}$$

$$F_p = F_C \sin^2\alpha. \qquad (2.17)$$

In calculating the power in an oblique meridian of a cylindrical surface, it is convenient to use a table of values of $\sin^2\alpha$, such as may be found in any book of mathematical tables, or to use a pocket calculator. However, if one simply remembers representative values of $\sin^2\alpha$, a graph can be sketched showing the sine square values in all meridians of a cylindrical surface, as shown in Figure 2–33.

Approximate values of $\sin^2\alpha$ can be obtained by using $\alpha/90$ instead of $\sin^2\alpha$ (Table 2–1).

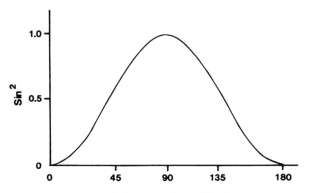

FIGURE 2–33.   Graph showing values of $\sin^2$ from 0° to 180°.

TABLE 2–1
Values of $\sin^2\alpha$ for Various Angles, with Use of the Approximation $\sin^2\alpha = \alpha/90$

Angle (°)	Sin²	α/90
0	0.00	0.00
30	0.25	0.33
45	0.50	0.50
60	0.75	0.67
90	1.00	1.00

2.18. Power in an Oblique Meridian of a Toric Lens

As with a cylindrical lens, the concept of the power in an oblique meridian of a toric lens has a limited meaning, but the concept of surface power in an oblique meridian of a toric surface is useful in calculating the difference between center thickness and edge thickness. In Figure 2–34, CA and CB represent the principal meridians of a toric surface. CC" represents a line perpendicular to the surface and is the vertex depth for the arc CP. C'C" is the vertex depth of the arc AP, and CC' is the vertex depth of the arc CA. The plane PAA' is parallel to the plane CC"B containing arc CB, and the curvature of the arc AP is assumed to be the same as that of arc CB. With use of Equation 2.4 again,

$$F_A = 2(n-1)\frac{CC'}{y^2},$$

$$F_B = 2(n-1)\frac{C'C''}{x^2},$$

and

$$F_P = 2(n-1)\frac{CC''}{m^2}.$$

Since CC" = CC' + C'C", one can solve the first two equations for CC' and C'C", and substitute in the third equation. Thus,

$$F_P = \frac{y^2 F_A + x^2 F_B}{m^2}.$$

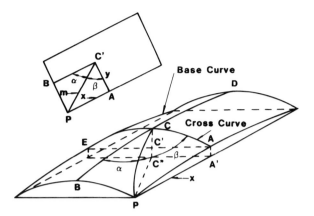

FIGURE 2–34. **Diagram for derivation of the power in an oblique meridian of a sphero-cylindrical lens.**

But

$$y^2 = m^2 \sin^2 \alpha$$

and

$$x^2 = m^2 \sin^2 \beta;$$

therefore,

$$F_P = F_A \sin^2 \alpha + F_B \sin^2 \beta. \qquad (2.18)$$

Since

$$\sin^2 \beta = 1 - \cos^2 \beta = 1 - \sin^2 \alpha,$$

then

$$F_P = F_B + (F_A - F_B) \sin^2 \alpha. \qquad (2.19)$$

Equation 2.19 may be arrived at empirically by solving Equation 2.17 a number of times. F_B is sometimes referred to as the spherical component, and $(F_A - F_B)$ as the cylindrical component of the toric surface. By thus analyzing the toric surface into spherical and cylindrical components one may restate Equation 2.19:

$$F_P = F_S + F_C \sin^2 \alpha, \qquad (2.20)$$

where F_S and F_C are the powers of the spherical and cylindrical components, respectively. Applications of Equations 2.17 and 2.20 in calculating lens thickness are discussed in Chapter 3.

2.19. Obliquely Crossed Cylinders

If two or more cylindrical lenses are placed in apposition, they may be resolved into a single sphero-cylindrical lens whose principal meridians are 90° apart. The easiest way to visualize what takes place is to plot sine square curves for each of the cylindrical lenses on a graph and then summate the two curves. This is shown in Figure 2–35, for the special case of two plano-cylinders of the same power with their plus axes 90° apart (+3.00 DC x 180 and +3.00 DC x 90). When the sine square curves for these two cylinders are summated, the result is a *straight line*, representing a spherical value of +3.00 D. However, when we plot sine square curves for two cylinders of equal power that do not have their plus axes 90° apart (+3.00 DC x 180 and +3.00 DC x 120), summation of the two curves results in a third sine square curve representing a sphero-cylindrical power, as nearly as can be determined by inspection, of +1.00 DS +3.00 DC x 150 (Figure 2–36). The minimum and maximum positions of the resultant sine square curve lie at approximately 150° and 60°. These positions represent the principal meridians for the resultant sphero-cylindrical lens.

Vector Analysis Method

A more precise method of resolving obliquely crossed cylinders involves the use of *vector analysis*. However, the method described in this chapter differs from ordinary vector analysis in that all angles are *doubled*. Suppose that we have two cylindrical lenses, having powers F_1 and F_2, whose axes are separated by the angle gamma (γ), with gamma defined as the *acute* angle between the two axes, measured in a counterclockwise direction from F_1 to F_2. In plotting the angle 2γ (twice the angle between the two cylinder axes) for vector analysis, the angle is always laid out in a counterclockwise direction from the axis of cylinder F_1 to the axis of cylinder F_2.

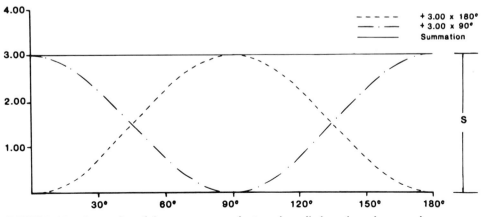

FIGURE 2–35. **Summation of sine square curves for two plus cylinders of equal power whose axes are 90° apart.**

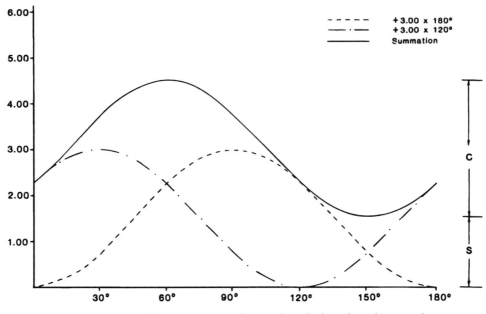

FIGURE 2–36.   **Summation of sine square curves for two plus cylinders of equal power whose axes are not 90° apart.**

As shown in Figure 2–37, the axes of cylinders F_1 and F_2 are chosen in such a way that the angle γ between the axes of the two cylinders is the *acute* angle (rather than the obtuse angle) between the two axes. The power of cylinder F_1 is then plotted along the *x*-axis to the right of the origin, and the power of cylinder F_2 is plotted at an angle 2γ. Construction lines are then drawn parallel to F_1 and F_2 and a diagonal line is drawn from the origin. The length of the diagonal line is equal to the power of the resultant cylinder, and the angle between the diagonal line and the line representing the axis of cylinder F_1 (which we call 2θ) is equal to *twice* the angle between the axis of the resultant cylinder and the axis of the cylinder F_1. (When using this system, both cylinders must have the *same sign*, so that the resultant cylinder axis falls between the axes of the cylinders F_1 and F_2. If the cylinders both have the same power, the resultant cylinder axis is halfway between the two original axes; if one cylinder is stronger than the other, the resultant axis falls closer to the axis of the stronger cylinder.)

Using the vector analysis method, we may determine the power and axis of the resultant cylinder, but the spherical component must be determined mathematically.

Mathematical Method

Vector analysis can be used to derive mathematical formulas for the cylinder axis, cylinder power, and spherical power. By dropping a perpendicular from the end of the vector representing the resultant cylinder to the *x*-axis (Figure 2–38), one can derive an expression to find angle 2θ. In Figure 2–38, where $a = OP$ and $b = NO$, then, in triangle MOP,

$$\tan 2\theta = \frac{a}{F_1 + b},$$

in triangle NOP,

$$\sin 2\gamma = \frac{a}{F_2},$$

and

$$a = F_2 \sin 2\gamma.$$

In triangle NOP,

$$\cos 2\gamma = \frac{b}{F_2},$$

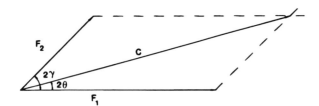

FIGURE 2–37.   **Diagram for using the vector method of obtaining the angle 2θ and the cylinder power.**

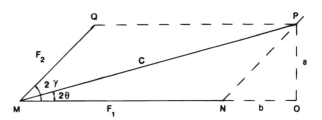

FIGURE 2–38.   **Diagram for derivation of formulas for cylinder axis and power.**

and

$$b = F_2 \cos 2\gamma,$$

with the result that

$$\tan 2\theta = \frac{F_2 \sin 2\gamma}{F_1 + F_2 \cos 2\gamma}. \qquad (2.21)$$

The angle θ is the resultant cylinder axis, measured in a counterclockwise direction from the axis of cylinder F_1.

A formula for determining the power of the resultant cylinder, C, may be derived as follows:

In triangle MOP,

$$\sin 2\theta = \frac{a}{C},$$

and

$$C = \frac{a}{\sin 2\theta},$$

Since $a = F_2 \sin 2\gamma$, substituting,

$$C = \frac{F_2 \sin 2\gamma}{\sin 2\theta}. \qquad (2.22)$$

Now that we have expressions for determining the power and axis of the resultant cylinder, it is necessary only to determine the *spherical* component of the lens formula. The final spherical component includes the spherical components of the two original sphero-cylindrical lenses and the spherical power of the resultant sphero-cylindrical lens. An expression for the resultant spherical power can be derived from Figure 2–39. In this diagram, the dashed lines (which can be labeled S_1 or S_2 and S_3 or S_4) are perpendicular to one another and represent the principal meridians of the resultant sphero-cylindrical lens. As explained in Section 2.17, for a cylinder of any power, the power in any two oblique meridians lying at right angles to each other adds up to the total power of the cylinder. If we forget about F_2 for the moment and consider only the powers F_1, S_1, and S_3,

$$S_1 + S_3 = F_1,$$

and if we forget about F_1 and consider only the powers F_2, S_3, and S_4,

$$S_2 + S_4 = F_2,$$

it then follows that

$$S_1 + S_3 + S_2 + S_4 = F_1 + F_2.$$

Since S_1 and S_2 combine to make up the resultant sphere power, S, and since S_3 and S_4 combine to make up the power of the resultant sphere plus the power of the cylinder, $S + C$, therefore

$$S_1 + S_2 = S$$

and

$$S_3 + S_4 = S + C.$$

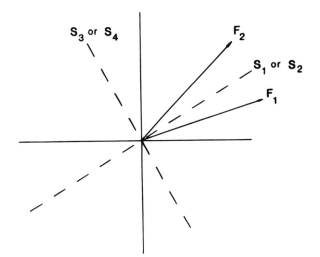

FIGURE 2–39.   **Diagram for the derivation of a mathematical expression for the resultant spherical power.**

Substituting,

$$S + (S + C) = F_1 + F_2$$
$$2S + C = F_1 + F_2$$
$$S = \frac{F_1 + F_2 - C}{2}. \qquad (2.23)$$

To the resultant sphere power, we must add the spherical components of the original lens formulas.

The procedure for combining obliquely crossed cylinders is illustrated by an example, showing first the vector analysis method and then the mathematical method.

EXAMPLE

Given the obliquely crossed cylinders, plano +2.50 DC x 30 and plano −2.00 DC x 140, find the resultant spherocylindrical lens.

The first procedure is to put both cylinders in the same form, either plus or minus. The most common procedure is to put them both into plus-cylinder form:

plano +2.50 DC x 30

and

−2.00 DS +2.00 DC x 50.

The two cylinders are plotted in the form of a vector diagram (Figure 2–40) as follows:

1. $F_1 = +2.50$ D, $F_2 = +2.00$ D, $\gamma = 50° − 30° = 20°$, and $2\gamma = 40°$.
2. Measuring counterclockwise, F_1 is plotted (2.5 units long) along the x-axis, to the right of the origin, and F_2 is plotted (2.0 units long) at an angle of 40°.
3. The angle θ may be found by *direct measurement* from the vector diagram, with use of a protractor. Using the method of direct measurement, the angle 2θ is found to be approximately 18°, with the result that θ is approximately 9°.
4. Since the angle θ is defined as the acute angle between the axis of cylinder F_1 and the axis of the resultant

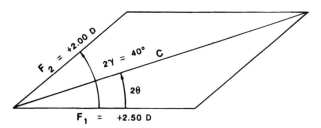

FIGURE 2–40.   **Two cylinders in plus cylinder form, +2.50 DC x 30 and +2.00 DC x 50, plotted in the form of a vector diagram.**

cylinder, the axis of the resultant cylinder is equal to 30° + 9°, or 39°.

5. The power, C, of the resultant cylinder may be found by direct measurement from the vector diagram. By direct measurement, it is found to be approximately +4.23 D.
6. The sphere resulting from the two obliquely crossed cylinders is found by Equation 2.23.

$$S = \frac{F_1 + F_2 - C}{2}$$
$$= \frac{+2.50 + 2.00 - 4.23}{2}$$
$$= +0.135 \text{ D.}$$

7. Adding the –2.00 DS from one of the original lens formulas (the other had plano sphere power), the formula for the resultant lens is approximately

(–2.00 DS + 0.135 DS) +4.25 DC x 39

or

–1.865 DS +4.25 DC x 39.

Rounding off, we get

–1.87 DS +4.25 DC x 39.

The sphero-cylindrical result of obliquely crossed cylinders can also be determined by calculation.

1. When the angle θ is found by calculation, Equation 2.21 is used:

$$\tan 2\theta = \frac{F_2 \sin 2\gamma}{F_1 + F_2 \cos 2\gamma}$$
$$= \frac{2 \sin 40}{2.5 + 2 \cos 40}$$
$$= \frac{1.286}{4.032} = 0.319$$
$$2\theta = 17.69°$$
$$\theta = 8.85°$$

Hence, the resultant plus-cylinder axis is 30° + 8.85° = 38.85°.

2. To find the power of the resultant cylinder by calculation, Equation 2.22 is used:

$$C = \frac{F_2 \sin 2\gamma}{\sin 2\theta}$$

$$= \frac{1.286}{0.304} = +4.23 \text{ D.}$$

3. The sphere resulting from the two obliquely crossed cylinders is found by the use of Equation 2.23:

$$S = \frac{F_1 + F_2 - C}{2}$$
$$= \frac{2.50 + 2.00 - 4.23}{2}$$
$$= +0.135 \text{ D.}$$

4. When the +0.135 DS is added to the –2.00 DS from the original lens formula, the total sphere power is –1.865 D.
5. The total resultant sphero-cylinder has a power of –1.865 DS +4.23 DC x 38.85, or approximately –1.87 DS +4.25 DC x 39.

When both cylinders have the same sign, the resulting axis is between the two original axes, and if the two cylinders are of equal power, the resultant axis is halfway between the two; if they are of unequal powers, the resultant axis is shifted toward the axis of the stronger of the two cylinders. In our examples, the axis of the resultant cylinder was closer to F_1 than to F_2, as expected, since the cylinder F_1 was slightly stronger than F_2 (Figure 2–41).

Polar Coordinate Method

In 1950, American Optical Company[9] described a vector analysis system for resolving obliquely crossed cylinders by using a polar coordinate plot in which the labeled meridians were only half as large as the corresponding real angles. For an angle of 30° (labeled on the polar plot), the actual angle is 60°. With use of this system, it is not necessary to multiply angle γ by 2 or to divide angle 2θ by 2, as is done with the vector analysis method illustrated by Figure 2–37.

Humphrey Instruments[10] reintroduced this type of coordinate system in 1976 to explain how the astigmatic properties of an eye can be measured by means of the Humphrey Vision Analyzer without requiring an azimuthal rotation of any optical elements (*azimuthal rotation* is a rotation like that of the hands of a clock). The Humphrey Vision Analyzer is a computer-assisted instrument for subjective refraction, in

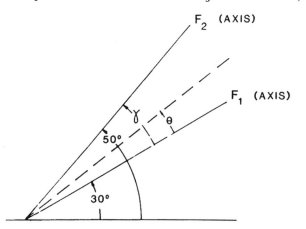

FIGURE 2–41.   **Diagram showing the position of the resultant axis for the two cylinders plotted in Figure 2–40.**

which any cylindrical correction can be created by a combination of two crossed cylinders, one having axes oriented at 45° and 135°, and the other having axes oriented at 90° and 180°. During the testing procedure, the axes of the two crossed cylinders remain in these positions (even though their powers may be altered).

A vector, when confined to a given plane, can be represented by two numbers: (1) the length or magnitude of the vector, and its angle with respect to some axis in the given plane, or (2) the components of the vector along two directions in the plane, usually the horizontal (x) and the vertical (y) axes. At first glance, cylindrical lenses appear to be vectors since they can be described in terms of both a magnitude and a direction. But closer examination shows that they are not vectors—they do not obey the vector addition law. For example, the combination of the two cylinders +1.00 DC axis 180 and +1.00 DC axis 90, having their axes 90° apart, results in *no cylindrical power* rather than the expected result (by vector analysis) of 1.41 D.

Humphrey's method permits cylindrical measurements to behave like simple vectors so that they can be added in

the ordinary manner. The only difference between the Humphrey diagram (Figure 2–42) and a conventional polar coordinate plot is that the angular scale indicates angles that are only *one-half* the size of the angles one would measure with a protractor: An angle measuring 90° with a protractor would be labeled 45° on the Humphrey diagram. For example, suppose we wish to combine the following two lenses:

(A) +5.00 DS –3.00 DC x 30,
(B) –3.00 DS + 2.00 DC x 80.

Cylinders may be stated in either plus or minus cylinder form, but both cylinders must have the *same sign*. Therefore, transposing the formula for lens A, we have

(A) +2.00 DS +3.00 DC x 120,
(B) –3.00 DS +2.00 DC x 80.

Steps to resolve obliquely crossed cylinders with use of the Humphrey diagram are shown in Figure 2–43.

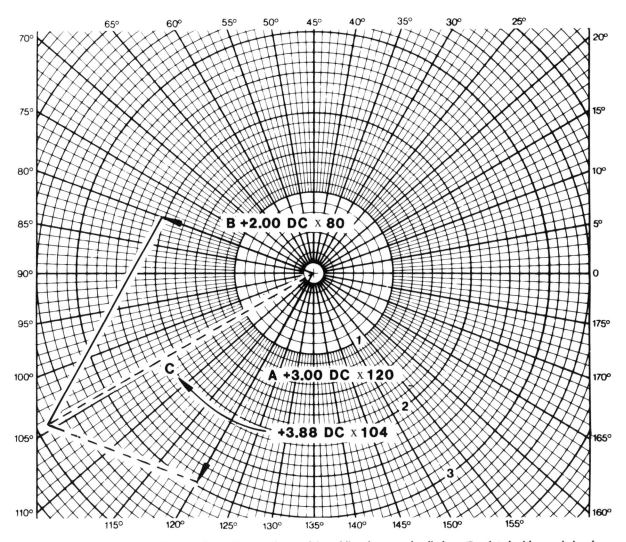

FIGURE 2–42.   Humphrey's polar coordinate diagram for resolving obliquely crossed cylinders. (Reprinted with permission from Humphrey Instruments, San Leandro, CA.)

FIGURE 2–43. **Steps required for resolving obliquely crossed cylinders using the Humphrey diagram. (Reprinted with permission from Humphrey Instruments, San Leandro, CA.)**

Step 1. Construct a box format (A).

Step 2. Write the two lens powers in the box (B).

Step 3. Compute the equivalent sphere for each lens and enter it in the appropriate box (C). For this example, the equivalent sphere for lens A is

$$+2.00 +3.00/2 = +3.50 \, \text{D},$$

and the equivalent sphere for lens B is

$$-3.00 +2.00/2 = -2.00 \, \text{D}.$$

Step 4. Add the equivalent spheres for lenses A and B in the appropriate box (D).

Step 5. Plot the value of the two cylinders on the Humphrey diagram (Figure 2–42), plotting each cylinder at an axis that is actually *twice* the real angle.

Step 6. Complete the vector parallelogram. The length and direction of the diagonal, *C*, represent the resultant cylinder power and axis. Enter the values of the resultant cylinder power and axis in the appropriate boxes (E). In this example, the vector sum is

$$+3.88 \, \text{DC} \times 104$$

Step 7. Compute the resultant sphere value, using the following formula:

$$S_R + C_R/2 = SE_{SC},$$

where S_R = the resultant sphere power, C_R = the resultant cylinder power, and SE_{SC} = the spherical equivalent of the resultant sphero-cylinder power. Transposing, we have

$$S_R = SE_{SC} - C_R/2$$

In this example,

$$S_R = +1.50 - 3.88/2$$
$$= +1.50 - 1.94$$
$$= -0.44 \, \text{D}.$$

This value is placed in the appropriate box (F). The formula of the resultant sphero-cylinder is therefore

$$-0.44 \, \text{DS} +3.88 \, \text{DC} \times 104.$$

2.20. Astigmatism from Lens Tilt

Figure 2–44 shows that when a homocentric pencil of light is incident normally along the optical axis of a spherical lens, the refracted pencil of light is stigmatic (A), but if the lens is pantoscopically tilted so that the pencil of light is obliquely incident upon the optical axis of the lens at its front pole (B), the refracted pencil will be astigmatic. The astigmatism occurs simply as a result of the obliquity of the incident light. Not only is a cylindrical component introduced, but the spherical power also changes.

The spherical refraction produced by the lens increases in power, and the cylinder that is generated has the same sign as that of the original sphere. The axis of the resulting cylinder is parallel to the axis of rotation of the lens. For example, if a plus lens is *pantoscopically* tilted (tilted inward toward the cheekbone) so that the wearer looks through the pole of the lens obliquely, plus cylinder is induced, and since the axis of rotation is horizontal, the axis of the induced plus cylinder is

A

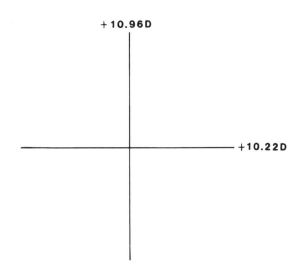

ANGLE of VERTICAL LENS TILT

B

FIGURE 2–44.   **Astigmatism caused by lens tilt.** A, a homocentric pencil of light incident normally along the optic axis of a spherical lens; B, the lens is rotated around a horizontal meridian with the result that the lens is tilted in the vertical meridian with respect to the homocentric bundle of incident light. The obliquity of incidence in the vertical meridian increases the power of the vertical meridian as compared with that of the horizontal meridian, with the result that the refracted pencil is astigmatic. The refracted rays in the vertical meridian form a horizontal focal line, H; the refracted rays in the horizontal focal line form a vertical focal line, V.

horizontal. Likewise, if a minus lens is pantoscopically tilted, a minus cylinder is induced, with its axis horizontal.

For small values of angle α, the power of the new sphere is given by the expression

$$S' = S_o\left(1 + \frac{\sin^2 \alpha}{2n}\right), \qquad (2.24)$$

where S' = the power of the new sphere, S_o = the power of the original sphere, and α = the angle of obliquity. If the index of refraction of the glass or plastic is assumed to be 1.50, Equation 2.24 then becomes

$$S' = S_o\left(1 + \frac{\sin^2 \alpha}{3}\right). \qquad (2.25)$$

The induced cylinder is given by the expression

$$C = S'\tan^2 \alpha. \qquad (2.26)$$

EXAMPLE
For a +10.00-D spherical lens, whose index of refraction is 1.50, tilted 15° around the horizontal axis, the power of the new sphere is

$$S' = 10\left(1 + \frac{\sin^2 15}{3}\right)$$

$$= 10\left(1 + \frac{0.2588^2}{3}\right)$$

$$= 10(1 + 0.067/3) = 10(1 + 0.022)$$

$$= +10.22 \text{ D},$$

and the power of the cylinder is

$$C = S'\tan^2 \alpha$$

$$= 10.22 \tan^2 15$$

$$= 10.22(0.2679)^2$$

$$= 10.22(0.072)$$

$$= +0.74 \text{ D}.$$

This lens behaves (as shown in the power diagram in Figure 2–45) as if it had the formula +10.22 DS +0.74 DC x 180.

Pantoscopic tilt results in a change in power (spherical and cylindrical) *only* when the optic axis of the lens fails to go through the center of rotation of the eye (which is considered to be 14 mm behind the corneal apex). By making certain approximations, a very simple relationship can be demonstrated between the pantoscopic tilt of a lens and the level at which the center must be placed to cause the optic axis to pass through the center of rotation of the eye. Referring to Figure 2–46, the point E lies directly in front of the pupil when the eyes are in the primary position, and the line CE lies in the primary horizontal plane of the head. When the angle α is expressed in degrees,

$$\sin \alpha = \sin \gamma = \frac{EF}{EC}$$

$$EF = EC(\sin \gamma).$$

Since $\sin 1° = 0.0175$,

$$EF = EC(0.0175),$$

and if EC is assumed to have a value of 27 mm,

$$EF = 27 (0.0175)$$

$$= 0.4725$$

$$= \text{approximately } 0.5. \qquad (2.27)$$

+**10.96D**

+**10.22D**

FIGURE 2–45.   **Power diagram indicating the sphero-cylindrical power that results when a +10.00 D spherical lens is tilted 15° around the horizontal meridian.**

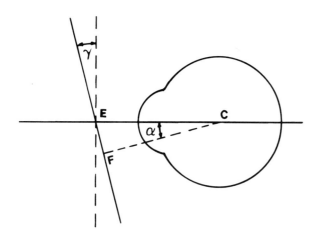

FIGURE 2–46. **Diagram used to establish the relationship between the amount of pantoscopic tilt and the level of the optical center so that the optic axis of the lens can pass through the center of rotation of the eye.**

Therefore, to make the optic axis of the lens pass through the center of rotation of the eye, the amount, in millimeters, the optical center must be lowered from the pupillary level is approximately equal to *one-half the pantoscopic tilt, in degrees*. The distance EC varies somewhat from one patient to another, but from a practical point of view, there is little to be gained by treating this distance as a variable.

2.21. The Maddox Rod

The Maddox rod is actually a series of glass or plastic rods (Figure 2–47) designed for use in phoria measurement. The patient views a small, intense source of light (*muscle light*) with the Maddox rod placed in front of one eye and sees a streak, or line oriented in the direction perpendicular to the orientation of the rods (Figure 2–48). (The same effect can be produced by the use of a single rod, which makes multiple rods unnecessary.) However, use of a single rod requires very precise positioning of the patient's eye; with multiple rods, the patient's eye may be located behind any of the rods. The rods are usually *red* to encourage dissociation of the two eyes and to make the streak of light more noticeable.

FIGURE 2–47. **The Maddox rod.**

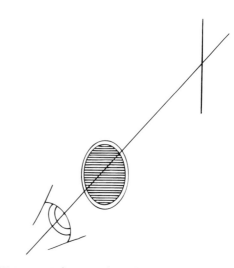

FIGURE 2–48. **When a patient views an intense source of light through a Maddox rod, he or she sees a streak of light, oriented in the direction perpendicular to the direction of the rods.**

Each of the individual rods acts as a plano-cylindrical lens. As shown in Figure 2–49, if a single Maddox rod has its axis oriented vertically, rays of light *are not* refracted in the direction parallel to the axis of the rod (the axis meridian of the cylinder), but are refracted in the meridian perpendicular to the axis of the rod (the power meridian of the cylinder), which forms a focal line in the vertical meridian (parallel to the axis of the rod). Thus, one might expect the streak produced by the Maddox rod to be located parallel to the axis of the rod. However, this does not happen. As already noted, the streak is oriented in the meridian *perpendicular* to the direction of the orientation of the rods. Why?

Although we tend to think of a plano-cylindrical lens as forming only one focal line, it actually forms *two* focal lines.

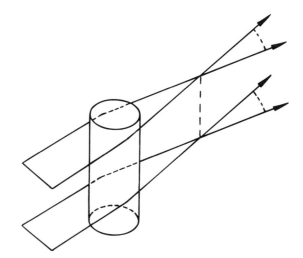

FIGURE 2–49. **A single Maddox rod, acting as a plano-cylindrical lens. Light is not refracted in the direction parallel to the axis of the rod (the cylinder axis meridian) but is refracted in the direction perpendicular to the axis of the rod (the power meridian) and forms a focal line parallel to the axis of the rod. A second focal line is formed at *infinity*.**

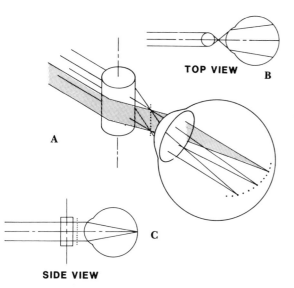

FIGURE 2–50. **When a single Maddox rod is placed in front of the eye, the first focal line is too close to the eye to be focused by the eye's optical system, and is therefore "wasted"; however, parallel rays of light in the meridian parallel to the axis of the rod *are* focused and form a focal line perpendicular to the axis of the rod.**

However, the focal line parallel to the power meridian of the lens is formed at infinity, just as the image formed by a plano-spherical lens, for parallel incident rays, is formed at infinity. The focal line formed at infinity can be seen only if it is focused on a screen by a converging optical system. The *patient's eye* acts as the converging system that focuses the focal line on the retina (the screen).

This explanation accounts for the appearance of the streak, seen perpendicular to the direction of orientation of the Maddox rod or rods, but what about the *other* focal line? Why does the patient not see it? The image formed by the power meridian of the rod is so close to the eye that the resultant vergence brought about by the rod (having a radius of curvature of only 2 or 3 mm) is so great that the eye is completely incapable of focusing it on the retina. This focal line is therefore "wasted," and the patient sees only the line that is formed at infinity.

As a schematic illustration of how the Maddox rod functions, consider a single Maddox rod having a power of +40.00 DC axis 90, placed 3 cm in front of the patient's cornea (Figure 2–50). A bundle of rays from a distant object point, incident upon the Maddox rod, forms a vertical line focus 5 mm in front of the cornea. With the patient's cornea located so close to the vertical focal line, what effect does the optical system of the eye have on the vergence in the horizontal meridian? The eye's optical system has little or no effect. There is nearly *infinite* vergence of rays in the horizontal meridian in the corneal plane, since it is so close to the vertical focal plane of the cylindrical lens. Compared with the nearly infinite vergence for incident rays, the 60-D change in vergence brought about by the optical system of the eye is insignificant. However, in the vertical meridian, the situation is entirely different. In this meridian, the eye's optical system refracts the parallel rays and forms a horizontal focal line on the retina.

References

1. Bennett, A. G. *Ophthalmic Lenses.* The Hatton Press, London, p. 12, 1968.
2. Fincham, W. A. H., and Freeman, M. H. *Optics,* 9th edition. Butterworths, London, p. 62, 1980.
3. Morgan, M. W. *The Optics of Ophthalmic Lenses.* Professional Press, Chicago, p. 14, 1978.
4. Southall, J. P. C. *Mirrors, Prisms and Lenses,* 3rd edition. Macmillan, New York, pp. 300–306, 1933.
5. Bennett, A. G., and Rabbetts, P. B. Refraction in Oblique Meridians of the Astigmatic Eye. *Br. J. Physiol. Opt.,* Vol. 32, pp. 59–77, 1976.
6. Keating, M. P., and Carroll, J. P. Blurred Imagery and the Sine Squared Law. *Am. J. Optom. Physiol. Opt.,* Vol. 53, pp. 66–69, 1976.
7. Long, W. F., and Haine, C. L. The Endpoint of the Laser Speckle Pattern in Meridional Refraction. *Am. J. Optom. Physiol. Opt.,* Vol. 52, pp. 582–586, 1975.
8. Keating, M. P. Dioptric Power in an Off-Axis Meridian: The Torsional Component. *Am. J. Optom. Physiol. Opt.,* Vol. 63, pp. 830–838, 1986.
9. *Transposition of Obliquely Crossed Cylinders.* Bureau of Visual Science. American Optical Co., Southbridge, MA, 1950.
10. *Adding an Over-Refraction to a Prescription Using the Humphrey Diagram.* Operator's Manual Application Note 017.0, Humphrey Instruments, San Leandro, CA, 1976.

Questions

1. What is the sagittal depth of a surface of –5.00 D that has a 50-mm diameter? Index of refraction is 1.523.

2. The radius of curvature of a surface is 5.25 cm. If the refracting power is 13.30 D, what is the index of refraction?

3. What is the reading of a lens measure calibrated for 1.530 when "clocking" a surface whose refracting power is +5.00 D, if the index of refraction of the glass is 1.523?

4. A fused bifocal has a front surface power of +13.00 D as measured by a lens measure calibrated for a refractive index of 1.53. The index of refraction of the major portion is 1.523 and the index of refraction of the segment is 1.69. What is the actual front surface power of the major portion and of the segment?

5. A lens measure graduated for spectacle crown glass with an index of refraction of 1.53 is placed on the surface of a steel sphere 40 cm in diameter. What reading does it give?

6. A lens gauge is used on a surface of –4.00 D having an index of 1.50. The lens gauge reading on the surface is –5.00 D. For what index of refraction is the lens gauge calibrated?

7. A lens gauge is calibrated for a glass with an index of refraction of 1.50. An infinitely thin bi-convex lens of +7.00 measures only +2.50 on each surface when measured with the lens gauge. Find the index of refraction of the glass.

8. The curved surface of a convex plano-cylindrical lens mates exactly with the curved surface of a –3.00 D

plano-cylindrical lens made with glass of index 1.45. When placed together with their axes parallel, the combination has +1.00 D along the power meridian. What is the index of refraction of the glass of the convex plano-cylindrical lens?

9. If the index of the material from which a contact lens is made is 1.42, and the radius of curvature of the front surface is 6 mm, what is the refracting power of this surface?

10. The back surface of a lens is –3.00 D. The front surface measures +6.50 D in the vertical and +9.00 D in the horizontal. Write the prescription for the lens.

11. (a) Calculate the power in the meridian 30 degrees from the axis of a –6.00-D cylinder. (b) What is the power 30 degrees from the power meridian?

12. What is the power in the 0, 30, 45, 60, 90, 120, 150, and 180 meridians of the following lenses?
    (a) –2.00 DS +4.00 DC x 120
    (b) +4.00 DC x 180/–2.00 DC x 60

13. A lens gauge calibrated for a refractive index of 1.523 is placed on a cylindrical surface with a radius of curvature of 10 cm, such that the line connecting the three legs makes an angle of 30° with the cylinder axis. What would be the reading of the lens gauge?

14. Locate the focal lines and circle of least confusion for the following lenses:
    (a) +10.00 DS –5.00 DC x 90
    (b) +5.00 DS –10.00 DC x 90
    (c) +5.00 DS –5.00 DC x 90
    (d) –5.00 DS –5.00 DC x 90
    (e) +3.00 DS –6.00 DC x 90

15. For a point object at infinity, an unknown lens has a vertical line focus at 33 1/3 cm and a horizontal line focus at 50 cm behind the lens. What is the prescription?

16. The meridian of least refractive power of a patient's astigmatic eye is 30°. When the patient's eye is fogged, what line appears clearest on a clock dial?

17. A parallel pencil of light falls axially on a lens having a power of +3.00 DS –2.00 DC axis 90. What is the power of the lens that, placed at the circle of least confusion, would restore the emergent light to parallelism in both meridians (Assume both lenses to be infinitely thin.)?

18. Find the sphero-cylindrical resultant equivalent of the following combination of obliquely crossed cylinders:
    (a) +4.00 DC x 20/–2.75 DC x 65
    (b) +2.00 DC x 20/+3.00 DC x 70
    (c) –1.75 DC x 120/+1.25 DC x 135
    (d) +4.00 DC x 80/–2.00 DC x 135
    (e) +2.25 DC x 40/–4.00 DC x 115

19. With +3.00 D in the vertical meridian and +1.00 D in the horizontal meridian, what is the prescription written in the crossed-cylinder form?

20. A lens with a power of +7.00 DS +2.50 DC x 50 has a –3.00-D surface on the back side. What is the lowest surface power on the front surface?

21. The fixed legs of a lens measure calibrated for spectacle crown glass, $n = 1.523$, are separated by 22 mm when the instrument is new, but, after wear, become separated by 24 mm. What must be the index of refraction of a glass for the instrument to give the correct surface power?

22. A –10.00-D spherical lens with an index of 1.50 has pantoscopic tilt of 10°. The pole of the lens lies directly in front of the pupil when the head is in the primary position. Through the polar area, what is the effective power of the lens?

23. What is the spherical equivalence of a lens that has a power of +5.00 DS –3.00 DC x 90?

24. The axes of two cylinders, one +2.00 D and the other +3.50 D, are crossed with the axis of a +3.25 D cylinder encountered first, as measured counterclockwise from the horizontal meridian. The resultant sphero-cylinder produced has a cylinder power of +4.00 D. What is the resultant spherical component of the sphero-cylinder?

25. A prescription of +1.00 DS –3.50 DC x 120 is indicated by a patient's subjective refractive finding. Since the patient has not previously worn a cylinder lens, a decision is made to prescribe only 2.00 D of the cylinder. What is the prescription ordered from the laboratory?

26. A lens gauge placed on a cylindrical surface reads +1.00 D. When the gauge is rotated 30 degrees, it reads +3.00 D. If neither position of the lens gauge is along a principal meridian, what is the power of the cylindrical surface?

27. Light from infinity is focused by a sphero-cylindrical lens into two line images located at distances of 10 cm and 20 cm from the lens. If a –1.00 DS is placed in contact with the sphero-cylinder, what is the length of the interval of Sturm?

CHAPTER THREE

Power Specification and Measurement

A number of methods can be used to specify the refracting power of an ophthalmic lens. The methods are (1) approximate power (also called nominal power), according to which the power of a lens is specified in terms of its front and back surface powers without regard to thickness; (2) back vertex power and front vertex power, according to which the power of a lens is specified in terms of the refracting power for emergent rays at its back surface or front surface; (3) equivalent power, according to which the power of a "thick" lens or optical system is specified in terms of the power of a single thin lens; and (4) effective power, according to which the power of a lens depends on its distance from the wearer's eye. Of all the methods of power specification, only *back vertex power* is used routinely by optical laboratories and practitioners.

Although the practitioner can determine approximate power by the use of the lens gauge and can determine front vertex power by means of hand neutralization with trial lenses, all methods routinely employed in modern optometric practice involve the measurement of back vertex power. Instrumentation for the measurement of back vertex power includes the lensometer or vertometer, the projection lensometer, and the automatic (computerized) lensometer.

POWER SPECIFICATION

3.1. Refractive Power

Although designers of lenses used in cameras and other optical instruments have always described these lenses in terms of *focal length*, ophthalmic lenses are described in terms of *refracting power*. Refracting power is defined as the change in vergence that occurs when light passes through a lens.

Light consists of waves that, in a medium such as air or glass, advance perpendicularly to their own wavefronts. If a wavefront is flat (plane), the paths of the waves are parallel. However, if the wavefront has a convex curvature, as when light emanates radially from a point source, the wave paths are divergent; if the wavefront has a concave surface, the wave paths converge to a focus. All that any lens can do is to produce a change in vergence on the surface of an incident wave. The power of a lens describes the extent of this change.

The unit used for specifying the power of a spectacle lens is the *diopter*, abbreviated by the letter D. As noted by Levene,[1] a French ophthalmologist, F. Monoyer, suggested the term in 1872 at an ophthalmologic congress in Heidelberg. Originally the term diopter described the refracting power of a lens in air with a focal length of 1 m. As mentioned in Chapter 2, Section 2.1, the term diopter has also been used to describe the curvature of a surface—the diopter of curvature is equal to the reciprocal of the radius of the surface in meters. Thus, if the radius of a spherical refracting surface is 0.5 m, its curvature is 2 D.

The term diopter is also used to describe the curvature of a wavefront at a specified distance from its focus or its source. The reciprocal of this distance expressed in meters is commonly called *vergence*, and the unit of vergence is the diopter. The term *reduced distance*, either in object space or in image space, is the actual distance divided by the index of refraction of the medium, such as

$$\frac{l}{n} \quad \text{or} \quad \frac{l'}{n'}.$$

Reduced vergence is the reciprocal of reduced distance. That is,

$$\frac{1}{l/n} \quad \text{or} \quad \frac{1}{l'/n'},$$

which can be written as

$$\frac{n}{l} \quad \text{or} \quad \frac{n'}{l'}.$$

If we let

$$L = \frac{n}{l}, \text{ and } L' = \frac{n'}{l'},$$

then L and L' are examples of reduced vergence, expressed in terms of the diopter. The fundamental expression for the refractive power, F, of an optical system is that it is equal to the reduced image vergence, L', minus the reduced object vergence, L, or

$$F = L' - L. \tag{3.1}$$

Hence, refractive power is the ability to produce a *change in reduced vergence.*

Equation 3.1 is useful in dealing with thin-lens, object-image relationships. When applied to single spherical refracting surfaces, the expression for power becomes

$$F = \frac{n'}{l'} - \frac{n}{l} = \frac{n' - n}{r}, \tag{3.2}$$

and since, for an object at infinity,

$$l' = f'$$

and

$$F = \frac{n'}{f'} = \frac{n' - n}{r},$$

and since, for an image at infinity,

$$l = f$$

and

$$F = \frac{-n}{f} = \frac{n' - n}{r},$$

therefore,

$$F = \frac{n'}{f'} = \frac{-n}{f}. \tag{3.3}$$

Many methods of specifying power of ophthalmic lenses have been used. The following are the most common methods.

3.2. Approximate Power

The approximate power of an ophthalmic lens is given by the simple formula

$$F_A = F_1 + F_2, \tag{3.4}$$

where F_1 and F_2 are the front and back surface powers, as measured by the lens measure (lens clock) as shown in Figure 3–1. The lens measure indicates the correct surface power *only* if the lens is made of the same material for which the lens measure has been calibrated (see Chapter 2, Section 2.4). Significant errors occur if a lens measure calibrated for an index of refraction of 1.53 or 1.523 is used without a correcting factor for measuring the surface power of a CR-39 plastic lens ($n = 1.498$) or a High-Lite glass lens ($n = 1.70$). *Thickness* does not enter into the approximate power formula because this formula results in the correct power only for a lens of zero thickness. Since most ophthalmic lenses cannot be considered to be infinitely thin, a more accurate expression for lens power, such as back vertex power, front vertex power, and equivalent power, is required.

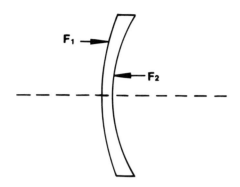

FIGURE 3–1.   **Front and back surface powers, as measured by the lens clock.**

3.3. Back Vertex Power

When an ophthalmic lens is ordered from a laboratory, the power of the lens is specified as *back vertex power*. The back vertex power of a lens is defined as the reciprocal of the reduced distance from the back pole of the lens to the secondary focal point (the reduced distance is the actual distance divided by the index of refraction). An expression for the back vertex power of a lens in air is shown in Figure 3–2. Back vertex power is shown as the reciprocal of the distance A_2F'. By using the general equation for refraction at a single spherical surface,

$$\frac{n'}{l'} = \frac{n}{l} + \frac{n' - n}{r},$$

for the second surface of the lens (where n is the index of refraction of the lens and 1 is the index of refraction of the surrounding air), we obtain the equation

$$\frac{1}{f_v} = \frac{n}{O' - t} + \frac{1 - n}{r_2} = F_V$$

$$\frac{1}{f_v} = \frac{n}{O' - t} + F_2. \qquad (3.5)$$

When applied to the first surface, we obtain the equation

$$\frac{n}{O'} = \frac{1}{\infty} + \frac{n - 1}{r_1}$$

$$\frac{n}{O'} = F_1. \qquad (3.6)$$

Solving Equation 3.6 for O' (note that $O' = n/F_1$), and substituting in Equation 3.5,

$$F_V = \frac{1}{f_v}$$

$$= \frac{n}{\dfrac{n}{F_1} - t} + F_2 = \frac{\dfrac{F_1}{n}(n)}{F_1\left(\dfrac{n}{F_1} - t\right)}$$

$$F_V = \frac{F_1}{1 - \dfrac{t}{n}F_1} + F_2. \qquad (3.7)$$

However,

$$\frac{F_1}{1 - F_1\left(\dfrac{t}{n}\right)} = F_1 + F_1^2\left(\frac{t}{n}\right) + F_1^3\left(\frac{t}{n}\right)^2 + ...$$

This is an infinite series in which each term gets smaller and smaller, and in ophthalmic optics only the first two terms of the series are used. The back vertex power of a lens, then, can be stated either in terms of the exact formula (Equation 3.7) or in terms of the approximate formula,

$$F_V = F_1 + F_2 + F_1^2\frac{t}{n}. \qquad (3.8)$$

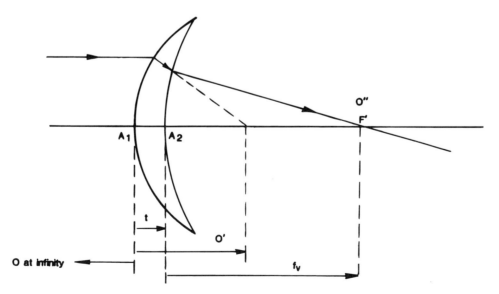

FIGURE 3–2.   **Diagram for derivation of the expression for the back vertex power of a lens.**

Either the exact formula or the approximate formula may be used if F_1 and F_2 are given and one wants to find F_v. However, the exact formula is easier to use if F_v and F_2 are known and one wants to find F_1, since the use of the approximate formula in this situation requires solving a quadratic equation.

Although the power of a lens may be stated in terms of either back vertex power, front vertex power, or equivalent power, there are two important reasons for using *back vertex power* for specifying the power of an ophthalmic lens:

1. Since the back vertex power is measured from the back pole of the lens (an easy-to-locate reference point) to the secondary focal point, we can to place the lens in any position we wish, as long as we choose a suitable power to place the secondary focal point of the lens at the far point of the eye (the concept of the far point of the eye is discussed in Chapter 5). Whether the lens is placed in the "spectacle plane" or is placed on the cornea (a contact lens), we can specify its back vertex power to make it have the desired effect.
2. Use of back vertex power allows unlimited freedom in terms of lens form—the *bend* (cross-section shape) of the lens. Back vertex power allows us to use any form of lens both in examining and in fitting the patient; and all we have to do is make the secondary focal point of the lens coincide with the far point of the eye. An instrument known as the *lensometer*, or *vertometer*, is used to measure back vertex power. Use of this instrument is discussed later in this chapter.

3.4. Front Vertex Power (Neutralizing Power)

One method of measuring the power of an ophthalmic lens is by "neutralizing" it with a lens from a trial case. Two lenses are said to neutralize each other if, when placed in contact, their total refracting power is zero. Strictly speaking, when one lens is neutralized by another the implication is not only that their focal lengths are equal in magnitude, but that the secondary focal point of the known lens is coincident with the primary focal point of the unknown lens. These conditions are realized in the case of a plano-convex and a plano-concave lens placed with their surfaces in contact (Figure 3–3).

The commonly used procedure of placing a trial case lens (calibrated in terms of back vertex power) with its back pole in contact with the front pole of a spectacle lens to neutralize the lens measures the *front vertex power* of the spectacle lens. Front vertex power (also called *neutralizing power*) is defined as the negative reciprocal of the reduced distance from the front pole of the lens to its primary focal point.

An expression for neutralizing power can be derived in a manner similar to that for back vertex power. Neutralizing power is the negative reciprocal of the distance A_1F in Figure 3–4. By using the general equation for refraction at a spherical surface, the refraction at the first surface is given by

$$\frac{n}{O'} = \frac{1}{f_N} + \frac{n-1}{r_1}$$

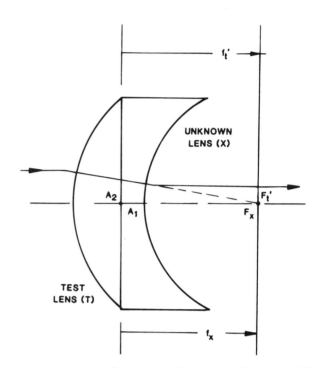

FIGURE 3–3.   **Neutralizing power. The secondary focal point of the known lens is coincident with the primary focal point of the unknown lens.**

$$\frac{1}{-f_N} = F_1 - \frac{n}{O'} = F_N \tag{3.9}$$

and the refraction at the second surface is given by

$$\frac{1}{\infty} = \frac{n}{O'-t} + \frac{1-n}{r_2}$$

$$\frac{1}{\infty} = \frac{n}{O'-t} + F_2. \tag{3.10}$$

Solving Equation 3.10 for O' (note that $O' = t - n/F_2$), and substituting in Equation 3.9,

$$F_N = \frac{1}{-f_N} = F_1 - \frac{n}{O'}$$

$$= F_1 - \frac{n}{t - \dfrac{n}{F_2}} = F_1 - \frac{n\left(\dfrac{F_2}{n}\right)}{\left(t - \dfrac{n}{F_2}\right)\dfrac{F_2}{n}}$$

$$= F_1 - \frac{F_2}{\left(t - \dfrac{n}{F_2}\right)\left(\dfrac{F_2}{n}\right)}$$

$$F_N = F_1 + \frac{F_2}{1 - \dfrac{t}{n}F_2}. \tag{3.11}$$

However,

$$\frac{F_2}{1 - \dfrac{t}{n}F_2} = F_2 + F_2^2\frac{t}{n} + F_2^3\left(\frac{t}{n}\right)^2 + \dots.$$

FIGURE 3–4.   **Diagram for derivation of the expression for the front vertex power (neutralizing power) of a lens.**

Dropping all but the first two terms of the series, we can state the neutralizing power of a lens in terms of the approximate formula,

$$F_N = F_1 + F_2 + F_2^2 \frac{t}{n}. \qquad (3.12)$$

Comparison of Approximate Power, Back Vertex Power, and Neutralizing Power

The following examples illustrate the differences between approximate power, back vertex power, and neutralizing power.

EXAMPLE 1

Given a lens for which $F_1 = +6.00$ D, $F_2 = -7.00$ D, $t = 2.0$ mm, and $n = 1.523$, find F_A, F_V, and F_N.

For approximate power,

$$F_A = +6.00 - 7.00 = -1.00 \text{ D}.$$

For back vertex power,

$$F_V = +6.00 - 7.00 + 36\frac{0.002}{1.523}$$
$$= +6.00 - 7.00 + 0.047$$
$$= -0.95 \text{ D}.$$

For neutralizing power,

$$F_N = +6.00 - 7.00 + 49\frac{0.002}{1.523}$$
$$= +6.00 - 7.00 + 0.06$$
$$= -0.94 \text{ D}.$$

EXAMPLE 2

Given a lens for which $F_1 = +16.00$ D, $F_2 = -4.00$ D, $t = 7.5$ mm, and $n = 1.523$, find F_A, F_V, and F_N.

For approximate power,

$$F_A = +16.00 - 4.00 = +12.00 \text{ D}.$$

For back vertex power,

$$F_V = +16.00 - 4.00 + 256\frac{0.0075}{1.523}$$
$$= +16.00 - 4.00 + 1.26$$
$$= +13.26 \text{ D}.$$

For neutralizing power,

$$F_N = +16.00 - 4.00 + 16\frac{0.0075}{1.523}$$
$$= +16.00 - 4.00 + 0.08$$
$$= +12.08 \text{ D}.$$

As shown by these examples, for low-powered, fairly thin lenses, the differences between approximate power, back vertex power, and neutralizing power are relatively small; but for thick, high-powered lenses, the differences can be large. The error involved in using hand neutralization for the lens in Example 2, rather than using the lensometer or vertometer, is 1.18 D. For meniscus ophthalmic lenses, the front vertex power is less than the back vertex power.

3.5. Equivalent Power

Many optical devices are constructed with a series of lenses separated by air or arranged with a series of curved surfaces separated by media having different refractive indices. Most of these complex systems are *symmetrical*; that is, the centers of curvature of the surfaces all fall on a common optical axis.

On occasion it is conceptually and mathematically convenient to express the result of a complex optical system in terms of an imaginary single, thin lens that would produce an image of a distant object of the same size and at the same position as produced by the system. Replacing an optical system with an imaginary single thin lens allows the application of simple object-image relationships to the equivalent lens.

The focal length of the thin lens that will produce an image size and an image position similar to those produced by the system is called *equivalent focal length*. The reciprocal of the equivalent focal length in meters is defined as the *equivalent power*.

To determine the position of the thin equivalent lens with respect to the system, the location of the principal planes of the system must be known. In a symmetrical optical system there is only a single pair of planes which have the property that, in these planes, the magnification is positive unity (+1); that is, the object and the image of the object are the same size, and the image is erect. These planes are called the *principal planes*, and the points of intersection of the optical axis with these planes form the *principal points* of an optical system.

The plane associated with the object space is called the *primary principal plane*, and the plane associated with the image space is called the *secondary principal plane*. The distance from the primary principal point (P) of the system to the primary focal point (F) is known as the *primary equivalent focal length*, and the distance from the secondary principal point (P′) to the secondary focal point (F′) is called the *secondary equivalent focal length*. The reciprocal of the secondary equivalent focal length is known as the *equivalent power* of the system.

Thus, if a single, thin lens with a secondary focal length of P′F′ is situated at P′, it achieves the effect of the lens system (Figure 3–5). The secondary focal length, as measured from this single, thin lens, is equal to the secondary equivalent focal length of the system as measured from the secondary focal point. Equivalent power is frequently referred to as *principal plane refraction*.

The following is a useful method of conceptualizing the principal planes of an optical system. When any ray in either object space or image space goes through the focal point associated with that respective space, in the opposite space there is a ray parallel to the optical axis of the system. The rectilinear portions of the ray in these two spaces intersect in a point on the principal plane with which the respective focal point is associated. Therefore, as shown in Figure 3–6, the ray going through F intersects the parallel ray in the image space on the primary principal plane (H), and the ray going through F′ intersects the parallel ray in the object space of the secondary principal plane (H′).

The formula for calculating the equivalent power of any two optical elements may be derived from the thick lens diagram shown in Figure 3–7. The lens shown in this diagram is assumed to be in air. In the similar triangles JA_1F_1' and KA_2F_1':

$$\frac{h_1}{h_2} = \frac{f_1'}{f_1' - t}.$$ (a)

In the similar triangles $OP'F_s'$ and KA_2F_s':

$$\frac{h_1}{h_2} = \frac{f_E'}{l_2'}.$$ (b)

Therefore,

$$\frac{f_E'}{l_2'} = \frac{f_1'}{f_1' - t}.$$ (c)

EQUIVALENT THIN LENS

FIGURE 3–5.   **The equivalent power of a lens system is equal to the power of a single, thin lens placed at the secondary principal plane of the system.**

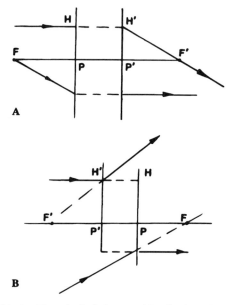

FIGURE 3–6.   **The principal planes and focal points of an optical system. A, a converging system; B, a diverging system.**

Refraction at the second surface may be expressed as

$$\frac{1}{l_2'} - \frac{n}{f_1' - t} = \frac{1}{f_2'}$$

or

$$\frac{1}{l_2'} = \frac{1}{f_2'} + \frac{n}{f_1' - t}.$$ (d)

If Equation (d) is divided by Equation (c), we obtain

$$\frac{1}{f_E'} = \frac{1}{f_2'} + \frac{n}{f_1'} - \frac{1(t)}{f_1'(f_2')}.$$

Multiplying the last term in the above expression by n/n, we have

$$\frac{1}{f_E'} = \frac{1}{f_2'} + \frac{n}{f_1'} - \left(\frac{1(t)(n)}{f_1'(f_2')(n)}\right).$$

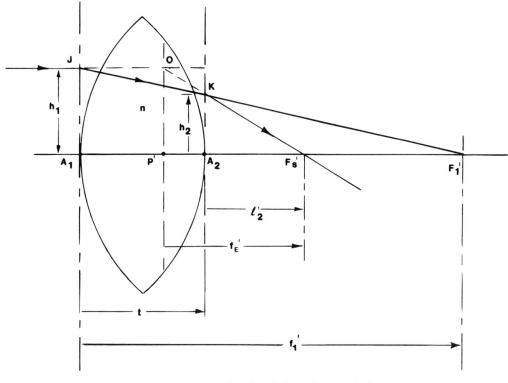

FIGURE 3–7.   **Diagram for deriving the formula for equivalent power.**

Rearranging the last term,

$$\frac{1}{f_E'} = \frac{1}{f_2'} + \frac{n}{f_1'} - \left(\frac{1}{f_2'}\right)\left(\frac{n}{f_1'}\right)\left(\frac{t}{n}\right).$$

The above equation may be restated as

$$F_E = F_1 + F_2 - cF_1F_2 \qquad (3.13)$$

and

$$F_E = \frac{-n}{f_E} = \frac{n'}{f_E'}, \qquad (3.14)$$

where F_1 = the power of the first element; F_2 = the power of the second element; c = the reduced distance from the secondary principal point of the first element to the primary principal point of the second element, that is,

$$c = \frac{P_1'(P_2)}{n_2}, \qquad (3.15)$$

where n_2 is the index of refraction of the intervening medium; f_E = the primary equivalent focal length, that is, PF; and f_E' = the secondary equivalent focal length, or $P'F'$. When Equation 3.13 is used for two thin lenses in air, F_1 and F_2 represent the powers of each lens, respectively, and c represents the distance between the lenses; but when Equation 3.13 is used for a thick lens, F_1 and F_2 represent the surface powers of the lens and c represents the reduced thickness, t/n, of the lens.

When the equivalent power formula is used to express the power of an ophthalmic lens, the resulting infinitely thin lens, with the power F_E, is located at the secondary principal plane (H') of the lens (Figure 3–8). Unfortunately, there is no easy way to determine the location of the secondary principal plane of a lens. An additional problem is that the principal planes move backward or forward as the *form* of the lens is changed. For these reasons, the concept of equivalent power is seldom used for ophthalmic lenses, but it *is* used in the case of most complex optical systems, such as those used in low-vision aids. The various methods of specifying focal lengths are shown in Figure 3–9.

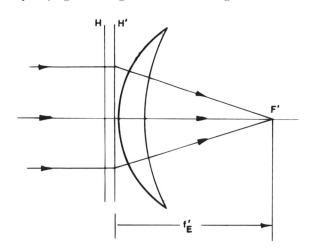

FIGURE 3–8.   **Equivalent power. A thin lens located at H', having a focal length of f_e', would have the same effect as the thick lens.**

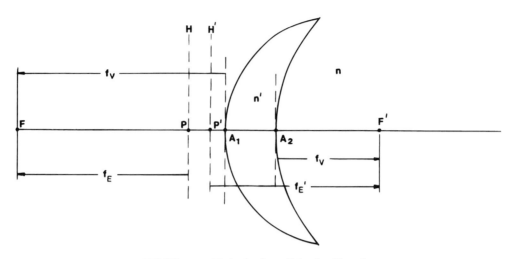

FIGURE 3–9. **Methods of specifying focal lengths.**

The relationships between equivalent power, back vertex power, and front vertex power are illustrated in the following example.

EXAMPLE
Given a +5.00 D lens and a +8.00 D lens, separated (in air) by a distance of 12.5 mm, find (1) equivalent power; (2) back vertex power; (3) front vertex power; (4) the positions of the principal planes.

1. To find the equivalent power of the system,

$$F_E = F_1 + F_2 - cF_1F_2$$

$$= +5.00 + 8.00 - \frac{0.0125}{1}(5.00)\,(8.00)$$

$$= +13.00 - 0.50 = +12.50 \text{ D}.$$

2. To find the back vertex power of the system,

$$F_V = \frac{F_1}{1 - \dfrac{t}{n}F_1} + F_2$$

$$= \frac{5}{1 - \dfrac{0.0125}{1}(5.00)} + 8.00$$

$$= \frac{5.00}{0.9375} + 8.00$$

$$= 5.33 + 8.00 = +13.33 \text{ D}.$$

3. To find the front vertex power of the system,

$$F_N = \frac{F_2}{1 - \dfrac{t}{n}F_2} + F_1$$

$$= -\frac{8.00}{1 - \dfrac{0.0125}{1}(8.00)} + 5.00$$

$$= \frac{8.00}{0.9} + 5.00$$

$$= 8.89 + 5.00$$

$$= +13.89 \text{ D}.$$

4. To find the positions of the principal planes of the system,

$$F_E = \frac{1}{f_E{}'},$$

$$f_E{}' = \frac{1}{F_E} = \frac{1}{12.5} = 0.08 \text{ m} = 8 \text{ cm}$$

$$f_E = -\frac{1}{F_E} = -\frac{1}{12.5} = -0.08 \text{ m} = -8 \text{ cm}$$

$$F_V = \frac{1}{f_V}$$

$$f_V = \frac{1}{F_V} = \frac{1}{+13.33}$$

$$= 0.075 \text{ m} = 7.5 \text{ cm}$$

$$F_N = -\frac{1}{f_N}$$

$$f_N = -\frac{1}{+13.89}$$

$$= -0.072 \text{ m} = -7.2 \text{ cm}.$$

If e = distance from the first lens to P, and if e' = distance from the second lens to P', then

$$e = f_N - f_E$$

$$= -7.2 - (-8) = 0.8 \text{ cm},$$

and

$$e' = f_V - f_E{}'$$

$$= 7.5 - 8$$

$$= -0.5 \text{ cm}.$$

These results indicate that the primary principal point lies 0.8 cm to the right of the +5.00-D lens, and the secondary principal point lies 0.5 cm to the left of the +8.00-D lens.

3.6. Effective Power

The effective power of a lens may be defined as the ability of the lens to focus parallel rays of light at a given plane. Although the term has several slightly different uses, its major use is to indicate the change in lens power required if a lens is moved from one position to another in front of the patient's eye. Plus lenses are more effective (i.e., bring about more change in vergence than needed) and minus lenses are less effective (bringing about less change in vergence than needed) as they are moved farther from the eyes. Suppose, for example, that a test lens located at a distance of 15 mm in front of the patient's cornea produces the desired optical effect and has a back vertex power of +10.00 D. Parallel rays of light are focused 10 cm behind the lens, as illustrated by lens A in Figure 3–10. If, however, the patient selects a frame that causes the spectacle lens to be located at B (say, 10 mm in front of the patient's cornea), parallel rays no longer are focused at plane F by test lens A. A lens whose back vertex power is equal to that of lens B must now be used to focus parallel rays at F. The back focal length f_B of lens B is equal to the back focal length f_A minus the distance d. In this case, $f_A = 0.10$ m and $d = 0.005$ m, so

$$f_B = f_A - d$$
$$= 0.10 - 0.005 = 0.095 \text{ m}$$

and

$$F_B = \frac{1}{0.095} = +10.53 \text{ D}$$

In other words, the *effective power* (its ability to focus parallel rays of light in plane F) of a lens with reference to position B is +10.53 D.

With the aid of the relationships shown in Figure 3–10, we may derive a formula for use in determining the required power of a lens, when the lens is moved from its original position, A, to a second position, B.

$$f_B = f_A - d$$
$$F_B = \frac{1}{f_A - d}$$
$$= \frac{1}{\dfrac{1}{F_A} - d}$$
$$F_B = \frac{F_A}{1 - dF_A}. \qquad (3.16)$$

In this equation, d is given a plus sign if the lens is moved toward the eye (as in the above example), and is given a minus sign if the lens is moved away.

Using Equation 3.16 to solve the example, we have

$$F_B = \frac{+10}{1 - 0.005(+10)} = +10.53 \text{ D}.$$

Back vertex power as defined above is simply the ability of a lens to focus *parallel rays* with reference to its back pole. Thus the term effective power is frequently used synonymously with back vertex power. It is convenient to use back vertex power because ophthalmic lenses are placed in the spectacle plane, at a fixed distance from the cornea, and back vertex power gives the effective power of the lens in the spectacle plane.

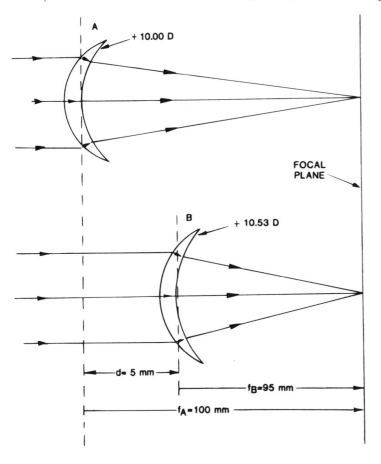

FIGURE 3–10. **Diagram illustrating the required change in lens power to cause parallel rays to focus in the same plane when the lens is moved in both fore and aft directions along the optic axis.**

POWER MEASUREMENT

3.7. Reference Points

The *Major Reference Point* (MRP) has been defined by Fry[2] as "the point on the lens that has the prismatic effect that is called for in the prescription." However, this term is not applicable to all state-of-the-art lenses, such as progressive addition lenses, with the result that the ANSI Z80.1-1995 recommendations[3] introduce the following terms that are consistent with international practice and *replace* the term Major Reference Point:

> The *Distance Reference Point* is the point on the lens, as specified by the manufacturer, at which the distance sphere power, cylinder power, and axis position must be measured.
>
> The *Near Reference Point* is the point on a lens, as specified by the manufacturer, at which the power of the add is measured.
>
> The *Fitting Point* is the point on a lens, as specified by the manufacturer, which is used as a reference point for positioning the lens in front of the wearer's eye.
>
> The *Prism Reference Point* is the point on a lens, as specified by the manufacturer, at which the prism value of the finished lens is to be measured. In nonaspherical single-vision and standard multifocal lenses, the prism reference point and the fitting point are assumed to coincide.

3.8. Hand Neutralization

As stated in Section 3.4, two lenses are said to neutralize each other if, when placed in contact, their combined power is zero. Before the invention of the lensometer, optometrists routinely used hand neutralization to verify the powers of prescription lenses received from the laboratory. For some years after the lensometer became available it was used mainly by laboratories; many practitioners preferred to use hand neutralization.

With practice, hand neutralization gives fairly accurate findings on minus lenses and low-powered plus lenses, but it becomes less accurate with moderate and high plus lenses. Despite its limitations, hand neutralization is a highly useful procedure to estimate the power of a lens quickly when a lensometer is not readily available.

Since ophthalmic lenses are calibrated in *back vertex power*, the object of neutralization is to find this power. To do this the *back* pole of the trial lens must be in contact with the *back* pole of the unknown lens. However, since ophthalmic lenses typically have *concave* back surfaces, it may be impossible to place the back pole of the trial lens in contact with the back pole of the unknown lens, and any measurement thus obtained would be in error. To avoid an air space between the two lenses, the neutralizing lenses are usually held so that contact occurs between the back pole of the neutralizing lens and the front pole of the unknown lens (Figure 3–11). This measurement gives the *front vertex power*. An examination of the formulas for back

and front vertex powers indicates that these powers differ from one another as the form and thickness are changed. For lenses of low power and for negative lenses, the front and back vertex powers are nearly the same. With strong positive lenses, however, the front vertex power is invariably weaker than the back vertex power, and thus the power found by neutralization is somewhat less than the back vertex power.

Hand Neutralization of Spherical Lenses

With experience, it is possible to estimate very closely the required power of the neutralizing lens. To neutralize an unknown spherical lens, the following procedure is used:

1. The lens is held at arm's length with the back surface of the lens facing the observer, who views through the lens a target that is approximately 6 m from the lens. The target must have both vertical and horizontal contours: A large cross, a large square, or a 20/400 letter E are adequate targets. To minimize the effects of aberra-

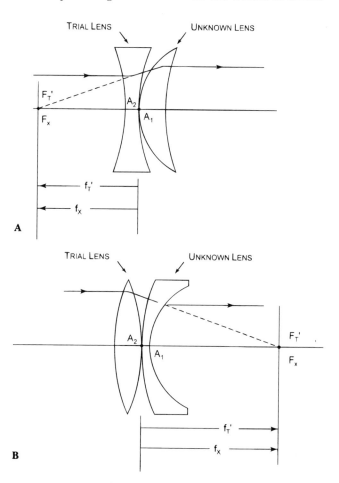

FIGURE 3–11.   **Hand neutralization by a trial lens. A, neutralization of an unknown plus lens; B, neutralization of an unknown minus lens.**

tions the observer should direct attention principally to the *transverse* motion of the image seen through the central zone of the lens and take care that the contact does not scratch the lenses, especially when plastic lenses are neutralized.

2. The observer slowly moves the lens, both vertically and horizontally, noting whether the transverse movement of the target appears to be in the same direction as that of the movement of the lens, or in the opposite direction. Movement in the *same* direction (*with* motion) indicates that the lens is a *minus* lens (Figure 3–12); movement in the *opposite* direction (*against* motion) indicates that the lens is a *plus* lens (Figure 3–13) as long as the distance from the lens to the observer's eye is less than the focal length of the lens. If the distance from the lens to the observer's eye is *longer* than the focal length of the lens, the observer sees *with* motion, and the image is inverted.

3. The observer then selects a lens of the opposite power and places it with its back surface in contact with the front surface of the unknown lens. Both lenses are slowly moved vertically and horizontally, and the judgment of *with* or *against* motion is again made. Figure 3–3 shows a minus lens being neutralized. If the neutralizing lens is of insufficient power, *with* motion will be seen; if the neutralizing lens is too great in power, *against* motion will be seen; and if the neutralizing lens is of the correct power, *no* motion will be seen—the lens is neutralized. For example, if no motion is seen when a +4.00-DS lens is used as the neutralizing lens, the power of the unknown lens is –4.00 DS.

The stronger the lens to be neutralized, the slower the speed of the motion; the closer the power of the neutralizing lens to that of the unknown lens, the faster the speed of the motion. Since the lens to be neutralized was a *spherical* lens, the same speed (and direction) of motion would be expected in both the vertical and horizontal meridians.

Hand Neutralization of Cylindrical and Sphero-Cylindrical Lenses

If the unknown lens is a cylindrical or sphero-cylindrical lens, the speed (and possibly also the direction) of motion will differ in different meridians. To neutralize a cylindrical or a sphero-cylindrical lens, the following procedure is used:

1. As with the spherical lens, the lens is held at arm's length with the back surface of the lens facing the observer, who views through the lens, at a distance of approximately 6 m, a target having vertical and horizontal contours.

2. The observer then rotates the lens, and *scissors motion* is seen. As shown in Figure 3–14, the vertical and horizontal lines of a cross target are seen within the lens as being displaced from their positions as viewed outside the lens (A); when the lens is oriented so that the two limbs of the cross are parallel to the principal meridians of the lens, the limbs of the cross seen within the lens appear to be parallel to (and continuous with) the limbs seen outside the lens (B).

3. Once the orientation shown in Figure 3–14B has been found, in which both limbs of the cross are continuous in-

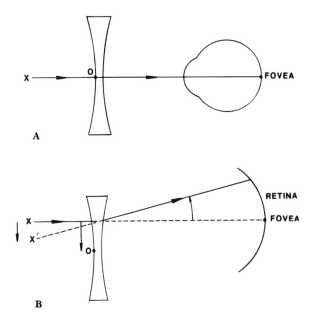

FIGURE 3–12.   **Hand neutralization. *With* motion, for a minus lens.**

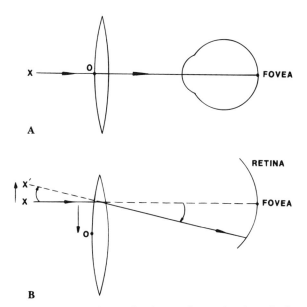

FIGURE 3–13.   **Hand neutralization. *Against* motion, for a plus lens.**

side and outside the lens, further rotation of the lens shows that the scissors motion itself possesses either *with* or *against* motion. If the line seen inside the lens rotates *with* the direction of the rotation, the line target is parallel to the minus-cylinder axis (Figure 3–15), whereas if the line inside the lens rotates *against* the direction of rotation, the line target is parallel to the plus cylinder axis (Figure 3–16). Since ophthalmic lens prescriptions are routinely specified in terms of minus cylinders, the observer is interested in finding the position of the *minus*-cylinder axis.

4. Once the two principal meridians have been located, the power in each meridian is neutralized separately with use of spherical lenses. Once the power of the lens in each principal meridian has been found (the power is the *opposite* of that of the

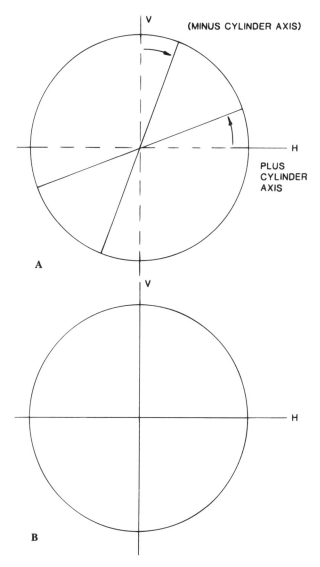

A

B

FIGURE 3–14.   **Hand neutralization of a lens containing cylindrical power. A, off-axis, showing scissors motion; B, on-axis.**

neutralizing lens), the prescription of the lens is written in minus-cylinder form. For example, if the lens is neutralized in the horizontal meridian with a −3.00 DS and in the vertical meridian with a −2.00 DS (indicating that the power of the unknown lens is +3.00 D in the horizontal meridian and +2.00 D in the vertical meridian), the prescription of the unknown lens is

$$+3.00 \, \text{DS} - 1.00 \, \text{DC} \times 180$$

A recommended procedure is always to neutralize the *minus axis* meridian first. Thus, this meridian will always have the most plus (or least minus) power, and the difference in power between the two principal meridians will become the cylindrical power of the lens. The power diagrams shown in Figure 3–17, based on this example, should aid in understanding this procedure.

5.   The major difficulty involved in hand neutralization is the determination of *cylinder axis*. This may be done by drawing a line with a grease pencil or a felt pen on the back surface of the lens while firmly holding the lens in

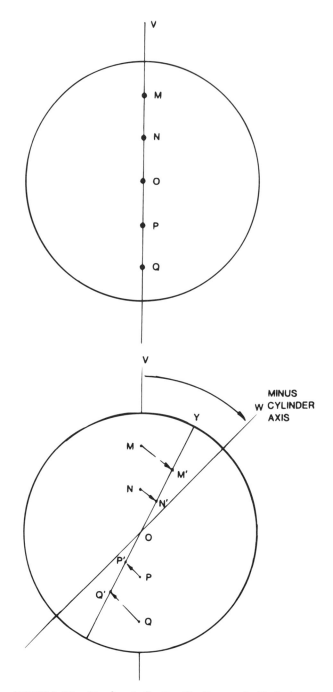

FIGURE 3–15.   **Hand neutralization. The line seen inside the lens rotates *with* the direction of rotation of the lens, and the line target is parallel to the minus cylinder axis.**

the position in which the line of the cross representing the axis is continuous within and outside the lens. Then measure the axis by means of a lens protractor. This procedure involves an inherent error of approximately ±5 degrees.

6.   An additional difficulty involved in hand neutralization is that of marking the optical center, or pole, of the lens. This is done by placing a small dot on the lens at the point where the two lines of the cross meet inside the lens (when the lens is held at such an orientation that the two lines are continuous within and outside the lens). Again, this requires

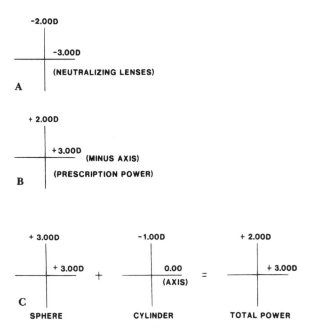

FIGURE 3–17.   Power diagrams illustrating the process of hand neutralization. A, power of neutralizing lenses; B, power of lens being neutralized; C, power diagrams for sphere power, cylinder power, and total power of lens being neutralized. With this procedure, the lens formula can easily be written in minus cylinder form.

FIGURE 3–16.   **Hand neutralization. The line seen inside the lens rotates *against* the direction of rotation of the lens, and the line target is parallel to the plus cylinder axis.**

a steady hand and involves a certain amount of error. However, "spotting" or "centering" machines are available for marking the cylinder axis and the pole of the lens. (These instruments were the precursors of the modern lensometer.)

If a lens (spherical, cylindrical, or sphero-cylindrical) contains *prism*, the lines of the cross seen through the lens (when the principal meridians of the lens have been found) are displaced in one direction or the other, perhaps even outside the lens. When one looks through a prism, the image of a

given object is displaced *toward the apex* of the prism. With this information the direction of the base of the prism in the unknown lens can be determined. For example, as shown in Figure 3–18, if the observer is neutralizing the right lens of a pair of glasses and the vertical line seen is displaced toward the right (as one looks through the ocular side of the lens), the prism in the unknown lens is a *base-in* prism (A). To measure the amount of base-in prism, *base-out* neutralizing prisms are used to find the amount of base-out prism power necessary to cause the vertical line of the cross to be undeviated by the lens (Figure 3–18B).

3.9. The Lensometer

The *lensometer*, or *vertometer*, shown in Figure 3–19, is an optical instrument designed for the purpose of measuring the vertex power of a spectacle lens. As shown in Figure 3–20, the basic elements of the lensometer include a *focusing sys-*

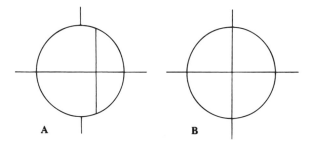

FIGURE 3–18.   **Hand neutralization of a lens containing prism. A, vertical line is displaced to the right (looking through the ocular side of the right lens), indicating base-in prism; B, the base-in power is neutralized by means of a trial case prism having base-out prism power.**

FIGURE 3–19.   **The lensometer.**

tem and an *observation system.* The focusing system consists of a light source, a movable target, a *standard lens* (collimating lens), and a lens stop with a small central aperture. Depending on the particular instrument, the target may be in the form of a cross (usually having a single line oriented in one direction and triple lines oriented in a direction 90° away), as shown in Figure 3–21, or the target may have a series of small dots or points arranged in a circular pattern, as shown in Figure 3–22.

When one uses the lensometer with the target consisting of two perpendicular lines, the target must be rotated until the perpendicular lines are parallel to the two principal meridians of the lens being neutralized. When the target is in focus for one principal meridian, the image of the line (or

lines) seen clearly are oriented *perpendicularly* to that principal meridian. The cylinder axis can then be read directly from the cylinder axis scale. The *cylinder power* is the dioptric difference between the power readings found for the two line images. For example, in Figure 3–23 the lens has a power of +1.00 DS –2.00 DC x 120. The appearance of the lensometer target for the "most plus" meridian is shown in part A (the scale reading shows +1.00 D and the single line in the 30° meridian is in focus). Figure 3–23B shows the appearance of the target in the "least plus" meridian (the scale reading at –1.00 D and the triple lines in the 120° meridian in focus).

When one uses the lensometer with a target formed of dots arranged in a circle, the target itself is not rotated. When cylindrical power is present, each dot source forms its own conoid of Sturm with two line foci—each focal line is oriented perpendicularly to the principal meridian for which the target is in focus. The power wheel of the lensometer can be adjusted, sequentially, until each line image is clearly focused. The cylinder axis is then determined by projecting the orientation of the line images on a cylinder axis scale. As with the lensometer, which has perpendicular line targets, the *cylinder power* is the dioptric difference between the power readings found for the two perpendicular line foci. For the lens with a power of +1.00 DS –2.00 DC x 120 (described above), Figure 3–24 shows the appearance of the lensometer target for the "most plus" meridian (A) (the scale reading shows +1.00 D and each dot elongated to form a line in the 30° meridian). Figure 3–24B shows the appearance of the target in the "least plus" meridian (a scale reading of –1.00 D and each dot forming a line parallel to the 120° meridian).

In the lensometer, the power of the standard lens must be greater than that of any lens to be measured; usually the power of the lens is +20.00 D to +25.00 D. The lens stop (lens rest) is designed to hold the unknown lens with its back surface against the stop to make possible the measurement of *back vertex power.* The lens stop is located at the secondary focal plane of the standard lens. Placing the lens stop in this position linearly relates the movement of the target from its zero position to the *back vertex power* of the lens being neutralized.

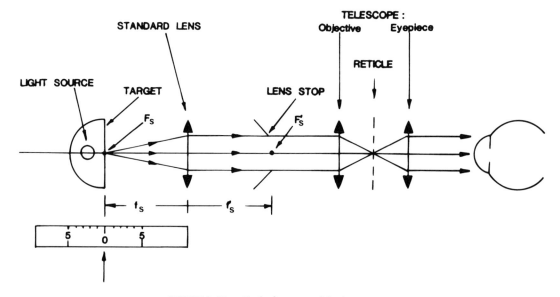

FIGURE 3–20.   **Optical system of the lensometer.**

When the lens stop is located at the secondary focal plane of the standard lens, the apparent size of the image of the target remains constant. This phenomenon occurs because the equivalent power of the combination of the standard lens and the spectacle lens, acting together as a thick lens, remains equal to the equivalent power of the standard lens with no lens before the lens stop. The observation system consists of a low-powered Keplerian telescope with an objective lens, a reticle located in the secondary focal plane of the objective lens, and

an adjustable eyepiece. The reticle (Figure 3–25) usually contains a set of crosshairs for focusing, a prism scale, and a cylinder axis scale (the latter only when a dot target is used).

With no lens before the lens stop, the zero position of the target is the anterior focal plane of the standard lens. In this position, light emerging from the standard lens is parallel, and it enters the objective lens of the telescope parallel, which results in a clear image of the target on the reticle. If the eyepiece is properly adjusted, the observer sees a clear image.

As mentioned earlier, the movement of the target from its zero position is directly proportional to the back vertex power of the lens being tested. This can be demonstrated by the application of the Newtonian equation involving the extra-focal distances x and x', in which $xx' = ff'$. In the lensometer, the displacement of the target from the anterior focal point (F_S) of the standard lens is equal to the distance x_S. The displacement of the image from the secondary focal point (F_S') of the standard lens is equal to the distance x_S'. When a lens is neutralized in a lensometer, the secondary focal length of the lens under test is equal to the distance x_S'.

Under all conditions, to have a clearly focused image on the reticle, the rays forming the image must be parallel when they impinge on the objective lens. For the rays to emerge parallel from a test lens, the rays must leave the secondary focal point of the test lens (for plus lenses) or be headed for the secondary focal point of the test lens (for minus lenses).

When a concave lens is placed in the instrument (Figure 3–26), light rays from the target diverge. For the target to be seen clearly, it must be moved farther away from the standard lens by means of a drum provided for this purpose.

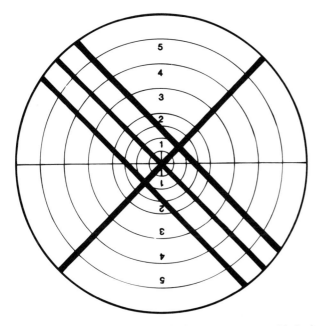

FIGURE 3–21. **Lensometer target having a cross pattern with single and triple lines.**

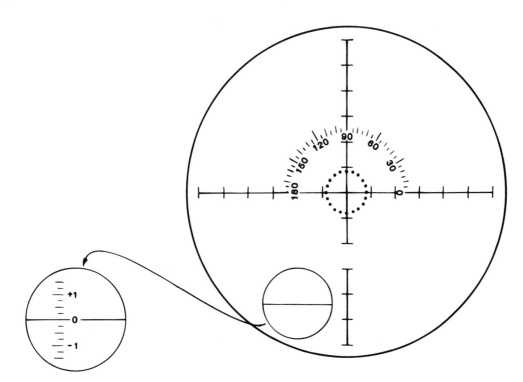

FIGURE 3–22. **Lensometer target having a circular dot pattern.**

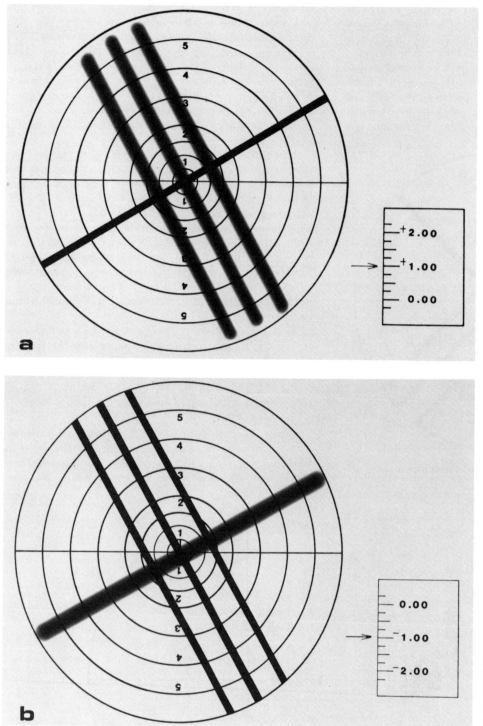

FIGURE 3–23. **Appearance of lensometer target having a cross pattern, for a lens having the power +1.00 DS –2.00 DC x 120. A, for the "most plus" meridian; B, for the "least plus" meridian.**

The distance through which the lens is moved, x_S, is such that the distance x_S' (from the lens stop to the image position) is equal to the secondary focal length of the lens (f_T') being tested (i.e., as the lens will be worn before the eye).

On the other hand, when a convex lens is placed in the instrument (Figure 3–27), rays from the target converge, with the result that the target must be moved closer to the standard lens. The distance through which the target must be moved is such that the distance, x_S', from the lens stop

to the new position of the image of the target, is now equal to the secondary focal length, f_T', of the lens being tested (i.e., as the lens will be worn before the eye).

For both the concave test lens and the convex test lens, the distance shown as x_S' may appear to be equal to the *primary* focal length, f_T. However, it is actually equal to the *secondary* focal length, f_T', when the lens is worn before the eye because, when one measures a lens in the lensometer, the light travels from the back of the lens to the front.

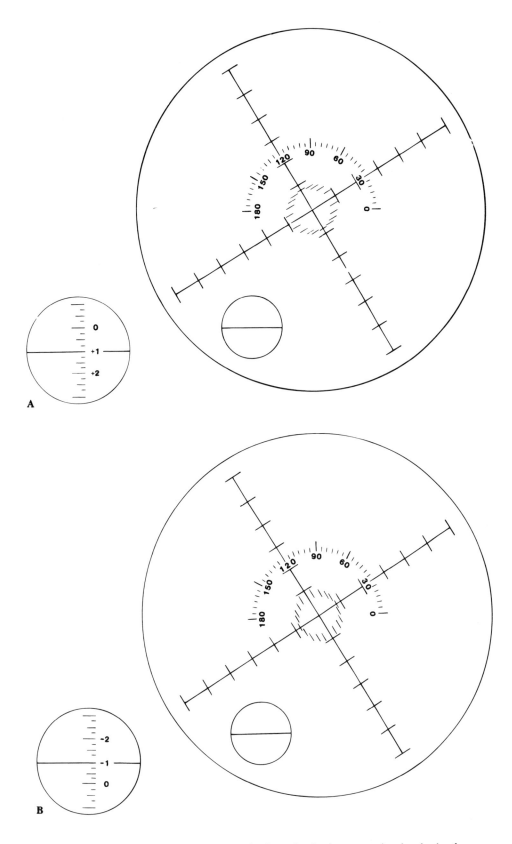

FIGURE 3–24.   Appearance of lensometer target having a circular dot pattern, for a lens having the power +1.00 DS –2.00 DC x 120. A, for the "most plus" meridian; B, for the "least plus" meridian.

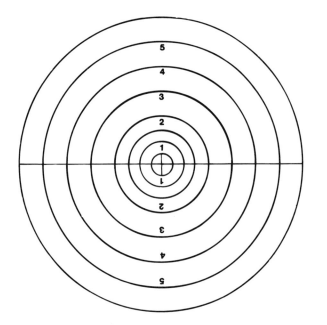

FIGURE 3–25. **Appearance of the reticle target in the telescope eyepiece.**

Calibration of the Lensometer

The calibration of the lensometer is based on the Newtonian formula

$$xx' = ff',$$

where x is the distance from the primary focal plane of the lens to the object, and x' is the distance from the secondary focal plane of the lens to the image. When this formula is applied to the standard lens, we have

$$x_S x_S' = f_S f_S'$$

Since, for the lensometer, $f_S' = -f_S$,

$$x_S x_S' = -f_S^2$$

and

$$x_S = -\frac{f_S^2}{x_S'}.$$

As the lens is worn before the eye,

$$x_S' = -f_T'.$$

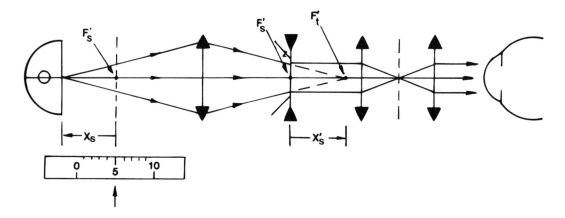

FIGURE 3–26. **When a concave lens is placed in the lensometer, the target must be moved farther from the standard lens.**

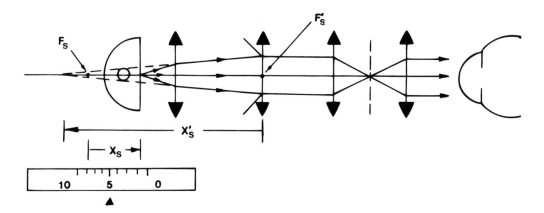

FIGURE 3–27. **When a convex lens is placed in the lensometer, the target must be moved closer to the standard lens.**

We now substitute,

$$x_S = \frac{f_S^2}{f_T'}.$$

Since $1/f_T'$ = back vertex power, we have

$$x_S = f_S^2 F_V. \qquad (3.17)$$

Note, in the above formula, that since f_S^2 is a constant, F_V changes with x_S in a *linear* manner, as already discussed. A given amount of rotation of the measuring drum brings about an equal change, in diopters, over the whole range of the instrument, with the result that the numbers on the measuring drum are *equally spaced*.

If the unknown lens is placed with its *front* surface against the lens stop, *front* vertex power can be measured. When this is done, although the power readings can be taken directly from the power scale, the cylinder axis readings must be modified by subtracting the axis reading from 180° (unless the principal meridians are 180° and 90°). For example, if a lens having a back vertex power of +2.00 DS –1.00 DC x 120 is placed on a lensometer with its front surface against the lens stop, the lens reading is +2.00 DS –1.00 DC x 60. Subtracting 60° from 180°, we get 120°, which was the original axis.

A displacement of the image of the target from the center of the reticle indicates the power and direction of the prismatic effect of the lens at its position in front of the lens stop. The telescope through which the target image is viewed is a Keplerian telescope, which inverts the image of the target, with the result that, although base-up prism normally displaces the image downward, toward the apex of the prism, the inversion of the image of the target by the telescope causes the image to be displaced in the *upward* direction. In other words, the displacement of the image is in the *same* direction as that of the base of the prism.

Extent of Target Movement

The extent of the target movement required to measure a lens of a given power depends on the power of the standard lens, as illustrated by the following examples:

EXAMPLE 1
For a lensometer fitted with a standard lens having a power of +20.00 D, what is the extent of the target movement in measuring a lens having a power of +1.00 D?

$$\begin{aligned} x_S &= f_S^2(F_V) \\ &= (0.05^2)(1) \\ &= (0.0025)(1) \\ &= 0.0025 \text{ m} = 2.5 \text{ mm.} \end{aligned}$$

Since the amount of target movement is the same for a diopter on *any* part of the power scale, the example shows that the amount of target movement for a lensometer with a +20.00-D standard lens is 2.5 mm per diopter of power of the unknown lens.

EXAMPLE 2
If the above lensometer is moved from a +20.00-D reading to a –20.00 D reading, how far does the target move?

$$\begin{aligned} x_S &= (0.05^2)(40) \\ &= (0.0025)(40) \\ &= 0.1 \text{ m} = 10 \text{ cm.} \end{aligned}$$

The total extent of target movement, therefore, for a lensometer having a +20.00-D standard lens is 10 cm (100 mm).

EXAMPLE 3
Given a lens having the prescription

$$+3.00 \text{ DS} - 6.00 \text{ DC x } 180,$$

how far does the target move in measuring the power in the two principal meridians with a lensometer that is fitted with a standard lens of +25.00 D? (Note that this lens has a refracting power of +3.00 D in the horizontal meridian and –3.00 D in the vertical meridian and the difference in power between the two principal meridians is 6.00 D.) The amount of movement will be

$$\begin{aligned} x_S &= f_S^2 F_V \\ &= (0.04)^2(6) \\ &= 0.0016(6) \\ &= 0.0096 \text{ m} = 9.6 \text{ mm.} \end{aligned}$$

Operation of the Lensometer

Operation of the lensometer to verify the prescription of a pair of glasses involves the following steps:

1. The first procedure, before placing the glasses in the instrument, is to focus the eyepiece. Beginning with the eyepiece completely out (turned all the way to the left), one turns the eyepiece slowly inward and views the crosshairs until they are in sharp focus. One may then verify the focus by turning the power drum (usually located on the right-hand side of the instrument) until the image of the cross target or the dot target is in sharp focus. When this occurs, the power drum reading should be 0.00 D, and both the image of the target and the crosshairs should be sharply focused.

2. Then place the glasses in the instrument with the right lens in the lens stop, with the *back* surface of the lens against the stop. After activating the spring-loaded clamp that holds the lens in place, center the lens (approximately) in the lens stop by moving the glasses from side to side and moving the stage (on which the glasses rest) up or down, as required.

3. If the instrument is equipped with a target having a single line in one direction and triple lines in the direction 90° away, turn the power drum until the target is in sharp focus. (Whether to turn the drum in the minus or plus direction is determined by noting the direction of motion of a distant object seen through the lens, as in hand neutralization.) When both sets of lines are in sharp focus for the same setting of the power drum, as shown in Figure 3–28 (or when the two sets of lines are equally blurred, as shown in Figure 3–29), the lens is a *spherical* lens.

4. If either the single line or the triple line target comes into focus separately, turn the power drum to the setting where the line or lines in the *most plus* meridian are in focus. At this point rotate the axis scale, if necessary, until the *single line* is in sharp focus (Figure 3–23A). The power drum reading at this point indicates the spherical power of the lens. Then turn the power

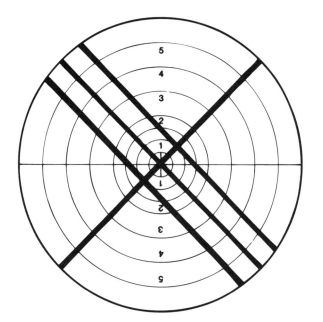

FIGURE 3–28. **Lensometer target with the two sets of lines in sharp focus.**

FIGURE 3–29. **Lensometer target with the two sets of lines equally blurred.**

drum in the minus direction until the triple lines are in focus (Figure 3–23B). The difference between this reading and the first reading of the power drum indicates the power of the cylinder, and the axis scale provides the cylinder axis. The lens prescription is then recorded in the minus-cylinder form.

5. During the process of adjusting the power drum for each of the two principal meridians, the operator should *center* the lens, so that the target is centered with respect to the reticle scale. Once the lens has been centered, the lens is "spotted," by using the spring-loaded, inked, spotting device. Spotting enables the operator to measure the distance between the centers of the two lenses, once the prescription for both lenses has been determined.

6. If the instrument is equipped with a target in the form of a circular array of dots, all the dots come into sharp focus simultaneously if the lens is a spherical lens. However, if the lens contains cylindrical power, there will be a power drum setting at which each dot is elongated in one meridian, and another setting at which each dot is elongated in the opposite meridian. With the lensometer, the procedure is to first find the *most plus* position of the power drum in which the dots are in focus (although elongated), as shown in Figure 3–24A. The power drum reading at this point is the spherical power. Then move the drum in the minus direction until the dots are in focus but elongated in the opposite direction, as shown in Figure 3–24B. Rotate the axis scale until the axis indicator is parallel to the direction of elongation of the dots. The difference between the two readings is the cylinder power, and the axis scale reading provides the minus-cylinder axis.

7. Now loosen the lens clamp and move the glasses along the stage until the left lens is in front of the lens stop (*without changing the height of the stage*), and repeat procedures 2 through 5. Since the height of the stage has not been changed, one can determine the presence of a vertical prismatic effect. If, when the target is in focus and centered in the horizontal direction, the center of the target is above or below the center of the reticle scale, vertical prism is present. By using the prism scale in the reticle, one can determine the amount and direction of the base of the prism. If the center of the target is displaced upward with regard to the center of the prism scale, base-up prism is present; if the target is displaced downward, base-down prism is present. The amount of prism is indicated on the prism scale— each unit on the scale usually represents 1 prism diopter.

If *prism* has been ground into the lens being tested, it may be impossible to center the lens in the lensometer (i.e., so that the perpendicular line target or the dot target is centered with respect to the reticle scale in the lensometer eyepiece). In such a case, the center of the perpendicular line target or dot target will be displaced to one side or the other (for horizontal prism), upward or downward (for vertical prism), or obliquely (for oblique prism). If this occurs, rotate the eyepiece of the instrument so that the reticle scale intersects the center of the perpendicular line or dot target (as shown in Figure 3–30). The reticle scale should then coincide with the base–apex line of the prism. The concentric circles in the reticle scale indicate the *amount* of prism, and the *direction* of the prism base is given by the direction of the center of the lensometer target with respect to the center of the reticle scale. For example, if, for the *right* eye, the lensometer target is displaced temporally, resulting in a scale reading of 2 prism diopters (as shown in Figure 3–31), the result is 2 prism diopters *base out.*

3.10. Lensometer Calibration, Alignment, and Measurement Errors

In the daily use of a lensometer, the operator should be aware of the following points, which are important to ensure that the instrument is functioning properly:

1. *Adjustments and Calibration.* The *eyepiece* of the instrument must be adjusted to the eye of the individual operator

FIGURE 3–30. **Measuring a lens containing oblique prism. The eyepiece of the lensometer is rotated so that the reticle scale is coincident with the base–apex line of the prism, and the amount of the prism and the direction of the base are then read and recorded.**

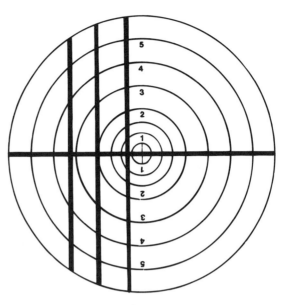

FIGURE 3–31. **Measuring a lens containing horizontal prism. The eyepiece is rotated so that the reticle scale is coincident with the base–apex line of the prism, and the amount of the prism and the direction of the base are then read and recorded.**

by using the procedure described in the previous section. This is particularly important when more than one person is routinely using the instrument. The *zero setting* of the lensometer is also important. When the eyepiece is correctly adjusted and the target is clearly focused, the dioptric scale reading should be zero with no test lens in the instrument. If the dioptric scale reading is *not* zero, the scale setting is incorrect. For many lensometers the scale can be reset to the correct reading.

A properly calibrated lensometer should not only read zero with no lens in place, but should also read correctly for high-powered (i.e., higher than 10.00-D) plus and minus lenses. Precision test lenses are available from some of the major lens manufacturers to check the accuracy of the lensometer. An error that is always in the same direction, that is, either too much plus or too much minus (for strong plus lenses and minus lenses), indicates that the *lens stop* is in an incorrect position. If both strong plus lenses and strong minus lenses read too high or too low, the power of the standard lens is likely to be incorrect. Cylinder axis errors and misalignment of the marker device or the lens platform can be checked by the use of cylindrical test lenses.

The *centration of the reticle* may be checked by rotating the reticle. If the reticle is properly centered, the center of the reticle should remain stationary during rotation. To check for *centration of the target*, the center of the target image, as the target is rotated, should coincide with the center of the reticle. If the target is not centered, errors in prism measurement occur.

2. *Measurement Problems.* Measurement of the power of a *contact lens* may be a problem. If the lens stop is large and the back surface of the contact lens is steeply curved, the back pole of the contact lens does lie in the plane of the lens stop, but *in front* of the stop. An error is thus induced in the measurement of back vertex power.

If the front surface of the contact lens is placed against the lens stop, *front vertex power* is measured. With the front surface of the contact lens against the lens stop, the front

pole of the contact lens lies *behind* the plane of the lens stop. In most cases, the distance from the plane of the lens stop is smaller when the front surface is placed against the stop than the distance when the back surface is placed against the stop. Therefore, the error is greater for *back* vertex power than for *front* vertex power (Figure 3–32). Although the measurement error is smaller for front vertex power than that for back vertex power, since contact lens powers are specified in back vertex power, they must also be *measured* in terms of back vertex power. Several aperture devices have been manufactured to assist in placing the back pole of the contact lens in the plane of the lens stop. Some lensometers are equipped with special lens holders that assist measuring of back vertex power.

The measurement of *bifocal* or *trifocal additions* also presents a problem because the lensometer is designed to measure lenses that are intended for distance vision. A bifocal addition is intended for near vision (see Chapter 8, Multifocal Lenses).

3.11. Projection Lensometers

With the projection lensometer (Figure 3–33) the operator views the target on a screen, rather than through a telescope. Focusing is not necessary, and this arrangement has the advantage that two or more people may look at the target at the same time. The glasses to be verified are placed in a horizontal (rather than a vertical) position. In all other respects, the operation of the instrument is similar to the operation of a standard lensometer.

The projection lensometer is particularly convenient for verifying *contact lens* power, since the contact lens is simply placed (back surface downward) on the lens stop. On the other hand, with a standard lensometer, a contact lens must

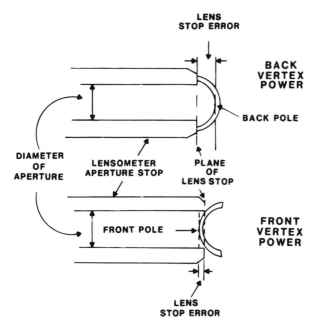

FIGURE 3–32.   **Measuring the power of a contact lens.** Because of the small radius of curvature, the back pole of the contact lens cannot be placed in the plane of the lens stop.

be placed in a vertical position against the lens stop, a procedure not only inconvenient, but one that may result in pressure being put on the contact lens, which tends to cause flexure of the lens while the reading is taken.

3.12. Automatic Lensometers

A number of completely automatic lensometers have recently been introduced (Figure 3–34). An automatic lensometer contains a microcomputer that processes the data, displays the result, and provides a printout of the measurement, including sphere, cylinder, axis, and prism power. The latest model of the Humphrey Automatic lensometer includes a spectrometer that displays and prints out the spectral transmittance curve of the tested lens for midrange ultraviolet light (UV-B), long wavelength ultraviolet light (UV-A), and the visible spectrum.

Each of these instruments employs a different principle in determining the measurements. They are designed to rapidly measure the back vertex power in all meridians and to select the meridians of maximum and minimum power (the principal meridians).

The process of checking and analyzing ophthalmic lenses occurs automatically and rapidly, which saves substantial time and effort. The automatic lensometer also eliminates the human errors involved in reading the scale and the arithmetic errors that could occur in subtracting the two readings to obtain the cylinder power. In addition, any controversy over the variability of measurements obtained by different operators can be resolved.

Automatic instruments are expensive. Since an optometrist uses a lensometer only intermittently during the working day, a decision whether or not to purchase an automatic instrument involves weighing the cost against the sav-

FIGURE 3–33.   **A projection lensometer.**

FIGURE 3–34.   **An automatic lensometer.**

ing in time and the possibility of greater accuracy. However, a high-volume optical laboratory routinely makes use of one or more lensometers continuously throughout the day; since the verification of spectacles is a demanding task, requiring a high level of concentration, the use of automatic instruments in a laboratory can be justified on the basis of improvement in the efficiency of the verification process.

RELATIONSHIPS BETWEEN LENS POWER AND LENS THICKNESS

Lens thickness is often an important consideration in the selection of the materials used in designing a patient's eyewear. Since a minus lens is thicker in the periphery than at the center, the dispenser will often want to exert some control over the *edge thickness* of the lens; and since a plus lens is thicker at the center than in the periphery, the dispenser may want to exert some control over the *center thickness* of a plus lens. Thickness usually becomes an important factor for lens prescriptions of about ±4.00 D or more. However, different problems are presented by minus and plus lenses. For a minus lens, an edge thickness that is greater than necessary detracts from the cosmetic effect of the lenses, but does not usually create a problem of excess weight unless the lens is very large. For a plus lens, a center thickness greater than necessary detracts from the cosmetic effect of the glasses and often causes the glasses to be unduly heavy. The problem of lens weight can, of course, be controlled to a great extent by using plastic lenses which, as pointed out in Chapter 1, have a specific gravity of a little more than half that of glass lenses.

3.13. The Approximate Sagitta Formula

Chapter 2, Section 2.1 (with reference to Figure 2–3) explained that the sagitta, s, of a lens surface having a radius of curvature r and a half chord length h is given by the formula

$$s = \frac{h^2}{2r}.$$

By making use of the relationship between the radius of curvature and the refracting power of a surface,

$$F = \frac{n-1}{r},$$

we have

$$s = \frac{Fh^2}{2(n-1)}$$

and

$$F = \frac{2(n-1)s}{h^2}. \tag{3.18}$$

In this formula, the distance s is measured from the arc to the chord, and is positive if measured toward the right and negative if measured toward the left.

Given the sagitta of each of the surfaces of a lens, together with the chord length and the index of refraction of the material, we can determine the refracting power of each lens surface and, by algebraically adding the two surface powers, determine the approximate power of the lens.

EXAMPLE
Given a round lens (Figure 3–35) having the sagittae $s_1 = 4.8$ mm and $s_2 = 2.8$ mm, a diameter (chord length)

of 40 mm, and an index of refraction of 1.50, find the approximate power of the lens.

For the front surface of the lens,

$$F_1 = \frac{2(n-1)s_1}{h^2}$$
$$= \frac{2(1.50-1)(0.0048)}{(0.02)^2}$$
$$= +12.00 \text{ D},$$

and for the back surface,

$$F_2 = \frac{2(1-1.50)(0.0028)}{(0.02)^2}$$
$$= -7.00 \text{ D}.$$

We find the approximate power by adding the two surface powers,

$$F_A = +12.00 - 7.00 = +5.00 \text{ D}$$

The *lens measure*, used to determine the refracting power of a lens surface, is constructed so that it has a constant chord length, $2h$, and is calibrated for a specific index of refraction. The above example, therefore, could also be solved by using the lens measure.

3.14. Formula Relating Power to Center Thickness and Edge Thickness

An approximate formula relating the power of an ophthalmic lens to the difference between center thickness and edge thickness may be derived with the help of Figure 3–36. As shown in this figure, the center thickness (also called polar thickness), t_C, and the edge thickness, t_P, can be related to the sagittae, s_1 and s_2, by the formula

$$t_C = s_1 + t_P - s_2,$$

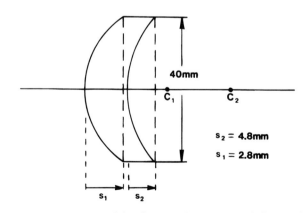

FIGURE 3–35. **Determining the approximate power of a lens on the basis of the sagittae and chord length.**

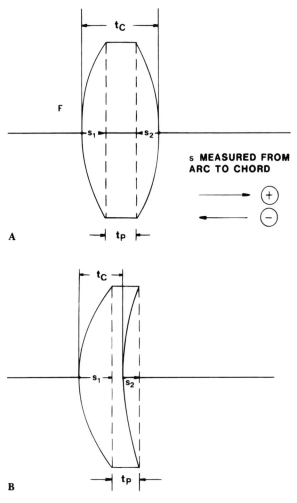

s MEASURED FROM
ARC TO CHORD

$\longrightarrow$ $(+)$

$\longleftarrow$ $(-)$

FIGURE 3–36.   **Diagram for derivation of a formula relating the power of an opthalmic lens to the difference between the center thickness and the edge thickness.**

or

$$t_C - t_P = s_1 - s_2, \qquad (3.19)$$

remembering that s is negative when measured (from arc to chord) toward the left. Solving Equation 3.18 for s, we have

$$s = \frac{Fh^2}{2(n-1)},$$

and substituting this value for s_1 and s_2, we have

$$
\begin{aligned}
t_C - t_P &= \frac{F_1 h^2}{2(n-1)} - \frac{F_2 h^2}{2(1-n)} \\
&= \frac{F_1 h^2}{2(n-1)} + \frac{F_2 h^2}{2(n-1)} \\
&= \frac{(F_1 + F_2)h^2}{2(n-1)}.
\end{aligned}
$$

Since $F_1 + F_2$ is equal to approximate power, F_A, we have

$$t_C - t_P = \frac{F_A h^2}{2(n-1)}. \qquad (3.20)$$

The use of this formula is demonstrated by the following example.

EXAMPLE

Given a round lens, 50 mm in diameter, having a power of +1.00 D and an index of refraction of 1.523, what is the difference between the center thickness and edge thickness ($t_C - t_P$) of this lens?

$$
\begin{aligned}
t_C - t_P &= \frac{+1(0.025)^2}{2(0.523)} \\
&= 0.0005975 \text{ m} \\
&= \text{approx. } 0.6 \text{ mm.}
\end{aligned}
$$

On the basis of this result, we can state the following *general rule*: For every diopter of refracting power, with a 50-mm lens blank, there will be a change in thickness of 0.6 mm between the center and the edge. Although this rule does not always give a precise result, it provides an approximate result, for both plus and minus lenses, to predict an increase or a decrease in thickness.

The Exact Sagitta Formula

When s is not small in relation to r, that is, when we are dealing with a *highly curved surface*, use of the approximate sagitta formula,

$$s = \frac{Fh^2}{2(n-1)},$$

gives a result that is considerably less than the true value. In such a case, the sagittal values of s_1 and s_2 in the formula

$$t_C - t_P = s_1 - s_2$$

must be calculated by the exact formula,

$$s = r - \sqrt{r^2 - h^2}.$$

An example illustrates the difference in results when the approximate formula is used instead of the exact formula to calculate sagittae and lens thickness.

EXAMPLE

A lens has the following parameters: F_1 = +12.00 D, F_2 = –6.00 D, n = 1.523, edge thickness (t_P) = 1.0 mm, and lens diameter = 60 mm. What will be the center thickness, t_C, (1) using the approximate sagitta formula and (2) using the exact sagitta formula?

1. Using the approximate sagitta formula,

$$
\begin{aligned}
s_1 &= \frac{Fh^2}{2(n-1)} \\
&= \frac{+12(0.03)^2}{2(1.523-1)} \\
&= \frac{+12(0.0009)}{1.046} \\
&= 0.0103 \text{ m} \\
&= 10.3 \text{ mm.}
\end{aligned}
$$

$$s_2 = \frac{Fh^2}{2(1-n)}$$

$$= \frac{-6\,(0.03)^2}{2(1-1.523)}$$

$$= \frac{-6\,(0.0009)}{1.046}$$

$$= 0.00516 \text{ m} = 5.16 \text{ mm.}$$

$$t_C - t_P = s_1 - s_2$$

$$t_C = s_1 - s_2 + t_P$$

$$= 10.3 - 5.16 + 1.0$$

$$= 6.14 \text{ mm.}$$

2. Using the exact sagitta formula,

$$s_1 = r - \sqrt{r^2 - h^2}.$$

$$= \frac{1.523 - 1}{F} - \sqrt{\left(\frac{1.523-1}{F}\right)^2 - h^2}$$

$$= \frac{0.523}{12} - \sqrt{\left(\frac{0.523}{12}\right)^2 - (0.03)^2}$$

$$= 0.0436 - \sqrt{0.001899 - 0.0009}$$

$$= 0.0436 - \sqrt{0.001}$$

$$= 0.0436 - 0.03162$$

$$= 0.01198 \text{ m} = 11.98 \text{ mm.}$$

$$s_2 = r - \sqrt{r^2 - h^2}.$$

$$= \frac{1.523 - 1}{F} - \sqrt{\left(\frac{1.523-1}{F}\right)^2 - h^2}$$

$$= \frac{-0.523}{-6} - \sqrt{\left(\frac{-0.523}{-6}\right)^2 - (0.03)^2}$$

$$= 0.0872 - \sqrt{0.007598 - 0.0009}$$

$$= 0.0872 - \sqrt{0.0067}$$

$$= 0.0872 - 0.08185$$

$$= 0.00535 \text{ m} = 5.35 \text{ mm.}$$

$$t_C - t_P = s_1 - s_2$$

$$t_C = s_1 - s_2 + t_P$$

$$= 11.98 - 5.35 + 1.0$$

$$= 7.63 \text{ mm.}$$

By comparing the approximate value (6.14 mm) and the exact value (7.63 mm), we can determine the percentage error resulting from the use of the approximate formula:

$$\text{Percent error} = \frac{(7.63 - 6.14)100}{7.63}$$

$$= 19.51\%.$$

This demonstrates that, for highly curved surfaces, when lens thickness is determined by the use of the approximate sagitta formula, a large error results.

3.15. Thickness Calculations for Cylindrical and Sphero-Cylindrical Lenses

For a plano-cylindrical lens, Figure 3–37 shows that along the *axis* meridian, thickness has a constant value; along the *power* meridian, thickness changes in the same manner that it does for a spherical lens. The thickness at any point, P, lying in an oblique meridian, OP, may be determined by either of two methods. For each of these methods, either the center thickness or the thickness of a specific peripheral point on the lens must be known. For example, if the edge thickness is known, the center thickness may be found by applying Equation 3.20 to the power meridian of the lens.

1. The first method uses the perpendicular distance from the peripheral point, P, to the cylinder axis. If the peripheral point is described in relation to a specified point, O, on the cylinder axis along an oblique meridian at an angle, α, to the cylinder axis, as shown in Figure 3–38, the perpendicular distance from point P to point C on the cylinder axis is found by the use of the equation

$$CP = OP \sin \alpha$$

The value of CP is then substituted for h, and the full power of the cylinder is used for F in Equation 3.20:

$$t_C - t_P = \frac{F_C (CP)^2}{2(n-1)}$$

2. Using the second method, the power of the cylinder in the oblique meridian is calculated from the equation

$$F_\alpha = F_C \sin^2 \alpha,$$

and the distance OP is substituted for h, while the value of F_α is substituted for F in Equation 3.20:

$$t_C - t_P = \frac{F_\alpha (OP)^2}{2(n-1)}$$

Section 2.14 explained that the concept of refracting power in an oblique meridian of a cylindrical lens is controversial because a cylindrical lens has refracting power only in the *power meridian* (having zero power in the axis merid-

FIGURE 3–37.   **For a plano-cylindrical lens, thickness has a constant value along the axis meridian, but changes in the same manner as for a spherical lens in the power meridian.**

AXIS

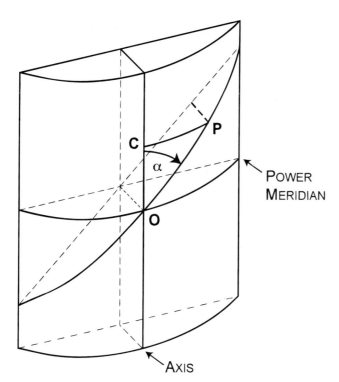

FIGURE 3–38.   **Determining the perpendicular distance from a peripheral point, P, to a point, C, on the cylinder axis.**

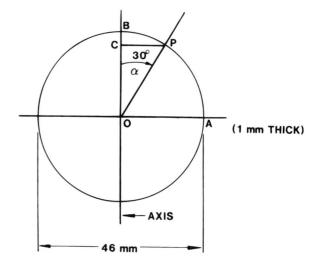

FIGURE 3–39.   **Determination of the thickness at point P along an oblique meridian, OP, of a cylinder.**

ian). However, the concept of refracting power in an oblique meridian is useful—and completely valid—to calculate the *thickness* at a point in an oblique meridian of a lens.

Both these methods for determining the thickness in an oblique meridian of a cylindrical lens are illustrated by the following example.

EXAMPLE

Given a 46-mm round lens, centered in the eyewire, having a power of +5.00 DC axis 90, an index of refraction of 1.523, and an edge thickness of 1.0 mm at the *thinnest point* along the edge, find the thickness at a point, P, located at the edge of the lens and such that a line drawn from this point to the center of the lens subtends an angle (α) of 30° from the cylinder axis (Figure 3–39).

For either method of solving the problem, we must first find the center thickness, t_C. Note that for a plus cylinder the thinnest point along the edge of the lens will be the point where the cylinder power meridian meets the edge of the lens, specified as point A. Therefore, for the power meridian (the 180° meridian),

$$t_C - t_P = \frac{h^2 F}{2(n-1)}$$

$$t_C = \frac{h^2 F}{2(n-1)} + t_P$$

$$= \frac{(0.023)^2(+5)}{2(1.523-1)} + 0.001$$

$$= \frac{0.002645}{1.046} + 0.001$$

$$= 0.00253 + 0.001$$

$$= 0.00353 \text{ m} = 3.53 \text{ mm}.$$

Using the first method, the distance CP, or h, is found as follows:

$$CP = OP \sin \alpha$$

$$= OP \sin 30$$

$$= 23(0.5) = 11.5 \text{ mm}.$$

Since all points along the axis have the same thickness, that is,

$$t_O = t_C = t_B,$$

we can find the thickness at point t_P as follows:

$$t_C - t_P = \frac{h^2 F}{2(n-1)}$$

$$t_P = t_C - \frac{h^2 F}{2(n-1)}$$

$$= 0.00353 - \frac{(0.0115)^2(+5)}{1.046}$$

$$= 0.00353 - 0.00063$$

$$= 0.0029 \text{ m} = 2.9 \text{ mm}.$$

Using the second method, the power along OP is found as follows:

$$F_\alpha = F_C \sin^2 \alpha = (+5)\sin^2 30°$$

$$= (+5)(0.25) = +1.25 \text{ D}.$$

Since the distance OP is 23 mm, we can find the thickness at P by

$$t_P = t_C - \frac{h^2 F_\alpha}{2(n-1)}$$

$$= 0.00353 - \frac{(0.023)^2(+1.25)}{1.046}$$

$$= 0.00353 - 0.00063$$

$$= 0.0029 \text{ m} = 2.9 \text{ mm},$$

which gives the same result as the first method.

Either of these two methods may be used to calculate thickness changes in cylindrical lenses. If the perpendicular distance from the peripheral point is found, the full power of the cylinder must be used in Equation 3.20. However, if the oblique distance from a perpendicular point is used, the power along the oblique meridian must be used in Equation 3.20.

To determine the thickness at a point in the periphery of a *sphero-cylindrical* lens, it is necessary to consider both the spherical and cylindrical components. Using F_S to designate the spherical power and F_C to designate the cylinder power, we can determine the thickness resulting from both the spherical and cylindrical components at a peripheral point P, located at a distance h from the center of the lens along a meridian oriented at α degrees from the cylinder axis, by use of the formula

$$t_C - t_P = \frac{h^2(F_S + F_C \sin^2 \alpha)}{2(n-1)} \qquad (3.21)$$

References

1. Levene, J. R. *Clinical Refraction and Visual Science.* Butterworths, London, p. 45, 1977.
2. Fry, G. A. The Major Reference Point in Single Vision Lenses. *Amer. J. Optom. Arch. Am. Acad. Optom.*, Vol. 24, pp. 1–7, 1947.
3. *American National Standards for Ophthalmics: Prescription Ophthalmic Lenses—Recommendations.* ANSI Z80.1-1995. American National Standards Institute, New York, 1995.

Questions

1. A ray incident upon a refracting surface of index 1.50 is headed toward a point on the optic axis 20 cm behind the surface. After refraction by the surface, it emerges parallel to the optic axis. What is the refracting power of the surface?

2. A 7-mm-thick lens has a +16.00 D front surface and a −6.00 D back surface. If it is made of glass of index of refraction 1.523, what is its back vertex power?

3. A lens has back vertex power of +4.00 D and an ocular surface of −6.00 D. If the lens is 3.00 mm thick and the index of refraction is 1.50, what is the front surface power?

4. If the power of the front surface of a lens with an index of refraction of 1.523 is +12.00 D and its center thickness is 10 mm, determine the power of the back surface to make the lens have
   (a) zero approximate power
   (b) zero vertex power
   (c) zero neutralizing power
   (d) +10.00 D vertex power

5. A −10.00-D lens gives the desired optical effects when in a given position in front of the eye. What new lens, 8 mm nearer the eye, will give the same result?

6. A lens with the power +13.00 DS −3.00 DC x 180, gives the desired correction when in a given position in front of the eye. If the lens is to be worn 5 mm closer to the eye, what lens power is necessary to give the same result?

7. The equivalent power of a thick lens is +12.50 D. The back vertex power is +15.00 D. What is the distance of the second principal plane from the back vertex of the lens?

8. By hand neutralization, a single-vision lens is neutralized along the 15° meridian by a +2.25-D trial lens and along the 105° meridian by a +0.50-D trial lens. What is the prescription of the lens being neutralized?

9. A certain lensometer manufactured to have a standard lens of +20.00 D was accidentally fitted with a +25.00-D standard lens. With the target in focus, the wheel was adjusted to read zero power when no lens was before the lens stop. If a +12.50-D lens is placed before the lens stop, what will be the reading on the wheel with the target again in focus?

10. A lensometer with a standard lens of +20.00 D is incorrectly constructed in that the lens rest is 1 cm too close to the standard lens. With no lens before the lens stop, the wheel is adjusted to read zero. If a +20.00-D lens is placed before the lens rest, what will be the reading when the target is again brought into focus?

11. In using a lensometer-type instrument, the target moves 8 mm when one focuses between the two principal meridians of a lens with the power +3.00 DS +5.00 DC x 90. What is the power of the "standard lens" in the instrument?

12. The standard lens of a lensometer is +20.00 D. The single line (sphere) of the target is in focus 10 mm behind the plano position. The triple or cylinder line is in focus 5 mm in front of the plano position. If the axis indicator is 90°, what is the lens prescription?

13. A lens of unknown power is placed in a vertometer and the target is moved until the image of the target is seen clearly on the reticle. The distance from the standard lens to the target is 60 mm. The power of the standard lens is +20.00 D. What is the power of the unknown lens?

14. A front surface bifocal lens is placed with the ocular surface against the lens stop of a lensometer. Through the distance portion of the lens the readings are as follows: single-line reading, +2.00 D; triple-line reading, +3.25 D; axis-dial reading, 15; single-line reading through the segment portion, +4.25 D. With the lens reversed (the front surface against the lens stop) the readings are as follows: single-line reading through the distance portion, +2.25 D; single-line reading through the segment portion, +4.25 D. What is the prescription of this lens?

15. A lens with a center thickness of 3 mm is measured with calipers. The minimum edge thickness is 2 mm in the 30° meridian and the maximum edge thickness is 5 mm in the 120° meridian. The lens is 40 mm in diameter and has an index of 1.50. Write the prescription for this lens.

16. What is the edge thickness of a 42-mm, −3.75-D lens with a 0.7-mm center thickness? The index of refraction is 1.523.

17. What is the center thickness of a 50-mm, +4.00-D lens with a 2-mm edge thickness? The index of refraction is 1.523.

18. What is the highest minus power possible for a 40 mm-diameter flat blank that is 5 mm thick? The center thickness of the finished lens is to be 1 mm thick. The index of refraction is 1.523.

19. If the vertex power of a lens is required to be +4.00 D and, on request, the center thickness was increased from 5 mm to 8 mm without consideration for this change, what will be the resultant change in power? The back surface power is –10.00 D and the index of refraction is 1.523.

20. A meniscus lens has surface powers of +10.00 D and –6.00 D. The lens is circular, its diameter is 40 mm, and its edge thickness is 0.5 mm. The index of refraction is 1.5. Find the thickness of the thinnest flat plate of glass from which the lens can be ground.

21. The secondary principal plane of a thick lens is inside the lens, 2 cm from the second surface, and the equivalent power of the lens is +10 D. What is the back vertex power?

22. If the front surface of a lens has a true power of +12.00 D, the center thickness is 6 mm, and the index is 1.50, for the lens to have zero vertex power, what is the true power of the back surface?

CHAPTER FOUR

Ophthalmic Prisms and Decentration

In geometrical optics we learn that a prism has the property of changing the direction of a beam of incident light without changing the vergence of the light. Although the primary function of an ophthalmic lens is to compensate for a refractive anomaly by changing the vergence of incident light, it is sometimes necessary to incorporate a prismatic component in the lens to compensate for an anomaly of binocular vision. The prismatic component may be placed with its base-apex meridian in any desired direction: in the horizontal meridian (as base-in or base-out prism), in the vertical meridian (as base-up or base-down prism), or in any oblique meridian.

An obvious method of incorporating prismatic power into an ophthalmic lens is to grind the prism into the lens during the surfacing process. However, even a spherical or cylindrical lens induces prismatic power whenever the visual axis passes through any point in the lens other than its optical center. Thus, a second method of providing prismatic power in an ophthalmic lens is to *decenter* the lens.

In this chapter, the terminology and optical properties of prisms are presented first, followed by discussions of units of measurement, the effects of prisms on the eyes, prismatic effects of spherical and cylindrical lenses, the resolving of oblique prisms, prescribing prism by decentration, the effects of prism power on the thickness of a lens, and the use of Fresnel Press-on prisms (Optical Sciences Group).

4.1. Terminology

A *prism* is defined as a portion of a transparent isotropic substance included between two polished, nonparallel surfaces, called *refracting surfaces*. Although we usually think of a prism as having flat surfaces, ophthalmic prisms usually have curved rather than flat surfaces, and may be used in conjunction with spherical, cylindrical, or sphero-cylindrical power.

The intersection of the refracting surfaces (extended if necessary) forms a line known as the *edge*, or *apex*, of the prism. Any section through the prism in a plane perpendicular to the edge is called a *principal section*. The included angle between the two refracting surfaces lying in a principal section is known as the *aptical*, or *refracting* angle, denoted by the Greek letter β (beta). The thick side of the prism, which subtends the aptical angle, is called the *base* of the prism. If any point on the refracting edge of a prism is taken as the apex, a principal section through that point intersects either refracting surface, which forms a line known as the *base-apex* line. The importance of the base-apex line is that it fixes the direction of the plane in which the deviation produced by the prism takes place. In ophthalmic practice, the convention is to use the base of the prism to specify its setting in relation to the eye. This is known as the *base setting*, with the apex lying 180 degrees from the base.

In Figure 4–1, the plane of the paper is a principal section, and the edge of the prism is a line extending perpendicularly in front of (or behind) the paper, at the apex. Figure 4–2 is a perspective view of a plano-prism with plane surfaces, indicating the refracting angle, β, the edge, and the base-apex direction. Ophthalmic optics is concerned only with rays of light traveling in principal sections. Other rays, called *skewed* rays, and are of no interest.

4.2. Refracting Power of a Prism

The angle of deviation of light brought about by a prism is denoted by the Greek letter ε (epsilon). As shown in Figure 4–3, rays of light are always deviated toward the *base* of the prism. However, for an observer viewing an object through the prism, the object appears to be displaced toward the *apex* of the prism.

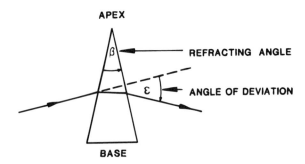

FIGURE 4–1.   A principal section of a prism. The edge of the prism is perpendicular to the plane of the paper, at the apex.

With the aid of Figure 4–4, it is possible to derive the formula for the refracting power of a thin prism. When rays of light strike the first face, AB, of the prism, there is a change in the speed of light, but since the rays of light strike the prism at an angle of 90°, there is no deviation of the light. However, when light strikes the second face, BC, of the prism, there is deviation of the light, since it does not strike the face at a 90° angle. Constructing a perpendicular to the surface BC, we can indicate the refracted ray, which makes an angle, ε, from the incident ray. By inspection of the diagram, we

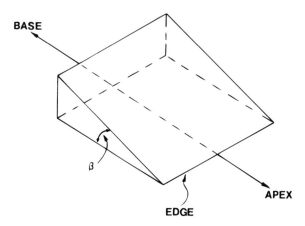

FIGURE 4–2.   A perspective view of a plano-prism.

FIGURE 4–3.   The action of an opthalmic prism.

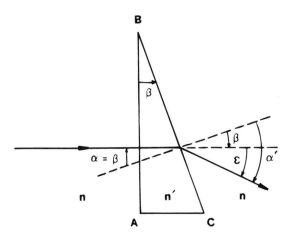

FIGURE 4–4.   Diagram for deriving the formula for refraction by a thin prism.

note that we can find two additional angles that are equal to the refracting angle, β. We also note that the angle of refraction at the surface BC is equal to angle β plus angle ε. Applying Snell's law,

$$n \sin \alpha = n' \sin \alpha'.$$

Since, in this diagram, α is equal to β and α' is equal to $\beta + \varepsilon$, we have

$$n' \sin \beta = n \sin(\beta + \varepsilon).$$

If we now limit our consideration to thin prisms, having refracting angles of about 10° or less, we can make the approximation that an angle (in radians) is equal to its sine, with the result that

$$n'\beta = n\beta + n\varepsilon.$$

For a thin prism in air, $n = 1$, and the index of refraction of the material from which the prism is made can be represented by n (rather than n'). The above equation then becomes

$$n\beta = \beta + \varepsilon$$

and

$$\varepsilon = \beta(n - 1) \tag{4.1}$$

In this formula, the angles ε and β may be expressed in either radians or degrees. For a medium having an index of refraction of 1.50, in air, this formula reduces to

$$\varepsilon = \beta(1.5 - 1) = \frac{\beta}{2},$$

indicating that the angle of deviation of an ophthalmic prism is equal to half the refracting angle of the prism.

4.3. Specification of the Power of an Ophthalmic Prism

Although the refracting angle, β, of a prism is always specified in *degrees*, the angle of deviation, ε, or *refracting power* of an ophthalmic prism, is usually specified in *prism diopters*. A prism diopter is defined as a deviation of 1 unit at a distance of 100 units. Although any unit can be used, it is convenient to think of the deviation in *centimeters*, in which case the prism diopter can be defined as a deviation of 1 cm at a distance of 1 m.

To derive an expression for the deviation brought about by a prism, in prism diopters, we begin with Equation 4.1, which states that the deviation in degrees is equal to the refracting angle of the prism times the index difference,

$$\varepsilon° = \beta°(n - 1).$$

Referring now to Figure 4–5, we have an angle of deviation, $\varepsilon°$, such that the displacement is x units for a distance of 100 units (A). Inspection of the diagram shows that

$$\tan \varepsilon° = \frac{x}{100}$$

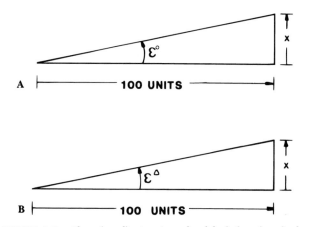

FIGURE 4–5.   The prism diopter. A, angle of deviation given in degrees; B, angle of deviation given in prism diopters.

or

$$x = 100 \tan \varepsilon°.$$

If we now state the angle of deviation in terms of prism diopters (B), we can substitute ε for x (since we have defined a prism diopter as a deviation of 1 unit at a distance of 100 units), with the result that

$$\varepsilon^\Delta = 100 \tan \varepsilon°, \tag{4.2}$$

$$\varepsilon^\Delta = 100 \tan \beta°(n - 1), \tag{4.3}$$

and

$$\tan \beta° = \frac{\varepsilon^\Delta}{100(n - 1)}. \tag{4.4}$$

Equation 4.4 is not an exact expression but, as will be shown later, involves very little error for small angles. Although the angle ε can be stated in either degrees or prism diopters, the refracting angle of the prism, β, is always stated in degrees. The prism diopter differs from the degree or the radian because the prism diopter is a unit of *tangent measurement*, whereas the degree and the radian are units of *arc measurement*. As illustrated in Figure 4–6, a radian is the angle subtended by an arc that is equal to the radius of a circle. In this diagram, the length of the arc BC is equal

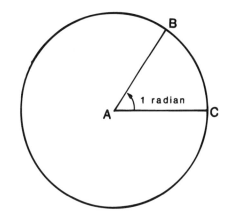

FIGURE 4–6.   An angle of 1 radian. The length of the arc BC is equal to the length of the radius, AB or AC.

to either of the radii of the circle, AB or AC. Since there are 2π radians in a circle, we can say that

$$1 \text{ radian} = \frac{180}{\pi} = 57.5°$$

and that

$$1° = \frac{\pi}{180} = 0.0175 \text{ radian}.$$

Another unit of arc measurement is the *centrad*, which is defined as the angle subtended by an arc equal to 1/100th of the radius of a circle (or, simply, equal to 1/100th of a radian). The relationship between the centrad and the prism diopter is illustrated in Figure 4–7. It can be seen that, for small angles, the centrad and the prism diopter are essentially equal.

Relationship between Degrees and Prism Diopters

For small angles, an angle specified in degrees may be converted to prism diopters, or vice versa, with very little error. In the case of the conversion of degrees to prism diopters,

$$1° = 0.0175 \text{ radian}$$
$$= 1.75 \text{ centrads}$$

and

$$1° = 1.75 \text{ prism diopters.} \tag{4.5}$$

In the case of conversion from prism diopters to degrees,

$$1 \text{ prism diopter} = 1 \text{ centrad}$$
$$= \frac{1}{1.75°}$$

and

$$1 \text{ prism diopter} = 0.57°. \tag{4.6}$$

As shown in Figure 4–8, as an angle increases in size, the tangent of the angle (which is analogous to prism diopters) increases more rapidly than the angle itself (the arc angle, expressed in degrees, centrads, or radians). We may now ask: How large must an angle be before it is no longer accurate to assume that prism diopters and centrads are equal?

Reference to Table 4–1 indicates that the error involved in assuming that prism diopters and centrads are equal increases from –0.1% for an angle of 10° to –8.3% for an angle of 30° and to –55.8% for an angle of 57.3° (which is equal

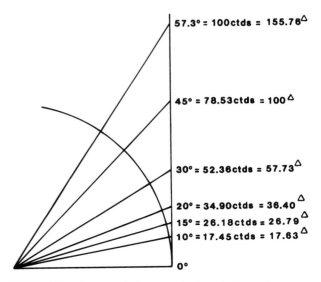

FIGURE 4–8.   **As an angle increases in size, the tangent measurement (prism diopters) increases more rapidly than the arc measurement (degrees, radians, or centrads).**

to 100 centrads, or 1 radian). Since ophthalmic prisms are almost never prescribed in powers greater than 5 prism diopters (2.9°) for each eye or a total of 10 prism diopters (5.7°) for both eyes, the error involved in making the conversion is not significant.

The measurement of phorias and fusional vergences, however, involves the use of prisms in powers as high as 25 to 40 prism diopters (14.04°–21.8°), with the result that an error on the order of 1% to 1.5% is involved in these measurements if one makes the assumption that prism diopters are equal to centrads. The matter is further complicated by the fact that rotary prisms used in phoroptors or refractors are located at a great enough distance from the eyes to bring about a decrease in the *effectivity* of such prisms when used for testing near-vision distances (discussed in Section 4.17).

4.4. Relationship between Refracting Angle and Angle of Deviation

As stated in Equation 4.1, the angle of deviation of a prism is related to the refracting angle by the expression

$$\varepsilon° = \beta°(n - 1)$$

FIGURE 4–7.   **The relationship between A, the centrad (arc measurement), and B, the prism diopter (tangent measurement) (Not to scale).**

TABLE 4-1
Comparison of Degrees, Centrads, and Prism Diopters[a]

Degrees	Centrads	Prism Diopters	Percentage Error[b]
10	17.45	17.63	−0.1
15	26.18	26.79	−0.8
20	34.90	36.40	−1.4
30	52.36	57.73	−8.3
45	78.53	100.00	−27.3
57.3	100.00	155.76	−55.8

[a]Where centrads = degrees/0.573, and prism diopters = 100 tan $\varepsilon°$.
[b]If it is assumed that prism diopters are equal to centrads.

with the result that for a medium having an index of refraction of 1.5, in air,

$$\varepsilon° = \frac{\beta°}{2},$$

and for ophthalmic crown glass, having an index of refraction of 1.523,

$$\varepsilon° = \beta°(0.523).$$

If $\beta = 1°$,

$$\varepsilon° = 1(0.523)$$
$$= 0.523$$

since

$$\varepsilon^\Delta = 100 \tan\beta(n - 1)$$

when $\beta = 1°$,

$$\tan\beta = 0.0175,$$

and

$$\varepsilon^\Delta = 100(0.0175)(0.523)$$
$$\varepsilon^\Delta = 0.915.$$

As a rule, for crown glass having an index of refraction of 1.523, a prism having a refracting angle of 1 degree produces *approximately 1 prism diopter* of deviation.

4.5. Effects of Prisms on Movements of the Eyes

The effects of prisms on movements of the eyes may be considered in terms of either *monocular* or *binocular* effects, and binocular effects may be considered in terms of resultant *horizontal* prismatic effects or in terms of resultant *vertical* prismatic effects.

Monocular Prismatic Effects

If one looks at a distant object with one eye occluded while a prism is introduced before the eye, the image of the object is displaced toward the apex of the prism. To look at the image of the object, a person's eye must move through an angle equal to the angle of deviation of the prism (Figure 4–9). Base-in prism causes the eye to move outward (abduction), and base-out prism causes the eye to move inward (adduction).

Binocular Prismatic Effects

If, with both eyes open, one looks at a distant object while a base-in prism is placed before the right eye and a base-out prism of equal amount is placed before the left eye, to look at the object, both eyes move to the *right* by an equal amount, and the lines of sight of the two eyes remain parallel. The movements of the eyes in which both eyes move in the same direction and of an equal amount are called *conjugate* movements, or *version* movements.

However, if a small amount of base-out prism is placed before each eye, to see a single image, both eyes move *inward* by the same amount. Similarly, base-in prism placed before each eye causes the eyes to move *outward*. Eye movements in which the eyes move toward one another (convergence) or away from one another (divergence) are called *disjunctive* movements, or *vergence* movements.

If prisms bring about only conjugate movements, the *resultant prismatic effect* is considered to be equal to zero. However, if prisms cause a disjunctive or vergence movement, the *resultant prismatic effect* is the extent of the disjunctive movement.

Resultant Horizontal Prismatic Effects

When prisms are placed before each eye with their bases in the same direction for each eye (that is, both base-in or both base-out), the resultant prismatic effect can be found by adding the powers of the prisms (base-in added to base-in, or base-out added to base-out). If the bases are in opposite directions but of different powers, the power of the weaker prism is subtracted from that of the stronger prism, and the remainder is the resultant prismatic effect. These principles are illustrated below by examples.

EXAMPLE 1
Given the prisms placed before the eyes,

OD 3 prism diopters, base-out
OS 3 prism diopters, base-out.

The resultant prismatic effect is found by adding the powers of the two prisms, and is therefore 6 prism diopters, base-out.

EXAMPLE 2
Given the prisms placed before the eyes,

OD 4 prism diopters, base-in
OS 2 prism diopters, base-out.

The resultant prismatic effect is found by subtracting the power of the weaker prism from that of the smaller prism, and is therefore 2 prism diopters, base-in, OD.

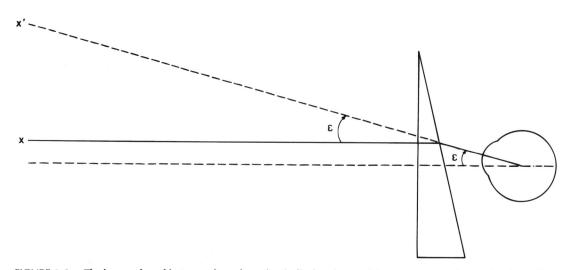

FIGURE 4–9.   **The image of an object seen through a prism is displaced toward the apex at an angle equal to the angle of deviation of the prism.**

Resultant Vertical Prismatic Effects

When vertical prisms are placed before each eye with their bases in the *same direction* for each eye but are of different powers, the resultant vertical prismatic effect is found by subtracting the power of the weaker prism from that of the stronger prism. The base of the resultant vertical prismatic effect is expressed as applying to the eye with the stronger prism. If the bases are in *opposite directions*, the resultant vertical prismatic effect is found by numerically adding the powers of the two prisms. Since a base-up effect for one eye is the same as a base-down effect for the other eye, the total prismatic effect may be expressed with respect to either eye (base-up for one eye or base-down for the other eye). These principles are illustrated by examples.

EXAMPLE 1
Given the prisms placed before the eyes,

OD 3 prism diopters, base-up
OS 1 prism diopter, base-up.

The resultant prismatic effect is found by subtracting the power of the weaker prism from that of the stronger prism, and is therefore 2 prism diopters, base-up, OD.

EXAMPLE 2
Given the prisms placed before the eyes,

OD 2 prism diopters, base-down
OS 2 prism diopters, base-up.

The resultant prismatic effect is found by adding the powers of the two prisms and can therefore be expressed as 4 prism diopters, base-down, OD, or as 4 prism diopters, base-up, OS.

4.6. Prentice's Rule

A spherical lens can be considered as being made up of an infinite number of prisms stacked base-to-base (for a plus lens) or apex-to-apex (for a minus lens), as shown in

Figure 4–10. For both plus and minus lenses, the power of a prism increases from the pole of the lens toward the periphery. For a given lens, the prismatic effect is a function of both the distance of the point from the pole of the lens and the power of the lens. This relationship, based on the definition of the prism diopter and illustrated in Figure 4–11, is called *Prentice's rule*. As shown in this illustration, an incident ray from a distant object passing through a lens at a distance, d, from the lens pole, C, crosses the optic axis at the secondary focal point of the lens. For small angles,

$$\tan \varepsilon = \varepsilon_{\text{rads}} = \frac{d_{\text{m}}}{f_{\text{v}'}} = d_{\text{m}}F_{\text{v}}$$

and

$$\varepsilon_{\text{rads}} = d_{\text{m}}F_{\text{v}}$$
$$\varepsilon_{\text{centrads}} = 100d_{\text{m}}F_{\text{v}}$$
$$= d_{\text{cm}}F_{\text{v}}$$

or, since for thin prisms, prism diopters are equal to centrads,

$$\varepsilon_{\text{prism diopters}} = d_{\text{cm}}F_{\text{v}}. \qquad (4.7)$$

Prentice's rule simply states that the prismatic effect at any point on a spherical lens is equal to the distance of the point from the pole of the lens, in centimeters, multiplied by the power of the lens, or

$$P = dF, \qquad (4.8)$$

where P = the prismatic power, in prism diopters; d = the distance from the lens pole, in centimeters; and F = the refracting power of the lens.

EXAMPLE
A pair of spectacles having the prescription +3.00 DS, each eye, fits on the wearer's face in such a way that when used for distance vision the foveal line of sight for each eye passes through a point 5 mm nasal to the optical center, or pole, of the lens. What is the prismatic effect encountered by each eye?

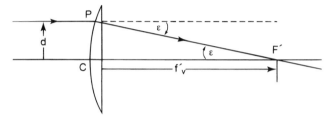

FIGURE 4–10. **A spherical lens considered as an infinite number of prisms stacked base-to-base (plus lens) or apex-to-apex (minus lens).**

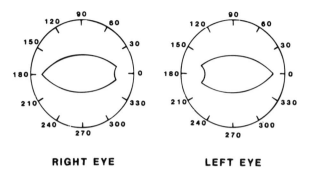

RIGHT EYE   **LEFT EYE**

FIGURE 4–12. **The base of a prism can assume any position on a circle, varying in notation from 0° to 360°.**

FIGURE 4–11. **Diagram used to derive Prentice's rule.**

$$P = dF$$
$$= 0.5\,(+3.00)$$
$$= 1.5 \text{ prism diopters}$$

In addition to being able to calculate the amount of prismatic power induced by an ophthalmic lens, it is important to know the direction of the *base* of the prism. Specification of the direction of the base of a prism differs from specification of the axis of a cylinder, in the following manner. The position of the axis of a cylinder can be properly specified by using only the *upper half* of a circle (from 0° to 180°), with the zero position to the examiner's right, looking toward the patient, and with degree values increasing in a counterclockwise direction. Since the cylinder axis extends across the entire lens, the meridians 90° and 270° represent the same cylinder axis position. However, the base of a prism can assume *any position* on a circle and, hence, can vary in notation from 0° to 360°, as shown in Figure 4–12.

Although for a cylinder 0° and 180° identify the same axis position, by convention 180° is preferred to 0°. By contrast, a prism base has *opposite* effects if specified at 0° (base-in for the right eye or base-out for the left eye) as opposed to 180° (base-out for the right eye and base-in for the left eye).

Oblique directions of prisms are most often described clinically in terms of horizontal and vertical components, using the cardinal directions, up, down, in, and out. *Base-in* means the base of the prism is toward the nose (nasally); *base-out* means the base is away from the nose (temporally). For convenience, a circle for specifying the base of a prism is often divided into four quadrants, as shown in Figure 4–13. For the *right eye*, in the 0° to 90° quadrant, the base is *up and in*; for the 90° to 180° quadrant, it is *up and out*; for the 180° to 270° quadrant, it is *down and out*; and for the 270° to 360° quadrant, it is *down and in*. For the *left eye* the

quadrants are reversed, 0° to 90°, *up and out*; 90° to 180°, *up and in*; 180° to 270°, *down and in*; and 270° to 360°, *down and out*.

Another system, often used in England, is illustrated in Figure 4–14. In this system, two 180° scales are used, one corresponding to the upper hemicircle and the other to the lower hemicircle. The zero position for the upper hemicircle starts on the right-hand side, and the zero position for the lower hemicircle starts on the left-hand side. Using the system illustrated in Figure 4–12, a prism for the right eye, with a base located at 210°, is expressed in the English system as "30° down and out." However, throughout this book, the system of notation using the *entire 360°* is used.

At any point other than the optical center, or pole, of a spherical lens, prism is induced according to Prentice's rule. The prismatic effect is found, as shown in the above example, simply by multiplying the distance (in centimeters) separating the point in question from the optical center by the power of the lens. The direction of the base-apex line of the prism lies along the line connecting the point in question to the optical center. The direction of the base is found by examining the *change in thickness* immediately surrounding the point along the line connecting the point to the optical center. The prism base direction is always the direction of *increasing thickness*. It is important to examine only the thickness changes on the line segment immediately surrounding the point in question. The direction of the base is then *projected on a circle*; the remainder of the thickness changes of the lens are ignored.

One situation in which induced prismatic power is of importance occurs when a spectacle wearer *converges* to read while wearing lenses that are "centered" for the interpupillary distance (PD). As shown in Figure 4–15, a wearer of plus lenses experiences a *base-out* (temporalward) prismatic effect when converging to read (A), and a wearer of minus lenses experiences a *base-in* (nasalward) prismatic effect when converging to read (B), assuming in both cases that the lenses are centered for the distance PD. The amount and direction of this effect is shown in the following examples using Prentice's rule.

EXAMPLE 1

Given a patient whose prescription is

OD +3.00 DS
OS +3.50 DS

FIGURE 4-13.   A circle for specifying the base of a prism may be divided into four quadrants.

FIGURE 4-14.   The English system of prism base notation, using two hemicircles.

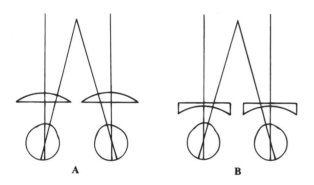

FIGURE 4-15.   Prismatic effects caused by convergence of the eyes (when the lenses are centered for distance vision). A, base-out prismatic effect from plus lenses; B, base-in prismatic effect from minus lenses.

and a distance PD of 64 mm and a near PD of 60 mm. If the lenses are centered for the distance PD, what is the prismatic effect experienced for reading, for each eye separately and for both eyes?

OD $P = 0.2(3) = 0.6$ prism diopter, base-out.
OS $P = 0.2(3.5) = 0.7$ prism diopter, base-out.

Both eyes: $P = 0.6 + 0.7 = 1.3$ prism diopters, base-out.

EXAMPLE 2
Given a patient whose prescription is

OD −5.00 DS
OS −6.00 DS

and a distance PD of 70 mm and a near PD of 65 mm. If the lenses are centered for the distance PD, what is the total prismatic effect for near work?

OD $P = 0.25(5) = 1.25$ prism diopter, base-in.
OS $P = 0.25(6) = 1.50$ prism diopter, base-in.

Both eyes: $P = 1.25 + 1.50 = 2.75$ prism diopters, base-in.

When a patient looks upward or downward (through a point in each lens above or below the lens pole), a vertical prismatic effect is induced, as shown in the next example.

EXAMPLE 3
Given a patient whose prescription for reading is

OD +2.00 DS
OS +2.00 DS.

Since the lenses are worn only for reading, they are centered for the near PD. However, when the patient reads, each line of sight passes through a point in the lens 5 mm below the pole of the lens. What is the vertical prismatic effect for each eye and for both eyes (Figure 4-16)?

OD $P = 0.5(2) = 1$ prism diopter, base-up.
OS $P = 0.5(2) = 1$ prism diopter, base-up.

In considering the vertical prismatic effect for both eyes, we are not concerned with the total prismatic effect (as in the case when adding base-in or base-out effects for the two eyes) but with the *resultant* prismatic effect. We ask the question: Is there a greater vertical prismatic effect for one eye than for the other eye? In this example, the vertical prismatic effect is the same for each eye, so the resultant vertical prismatic effect is zero.

If, on the other hand, the patient's reading prescription is +2.00 DS for the right eye and +3.00 DS for the left eye, the vertical prismatic effect experienced by the left eye is

$P = 0.5(3) = 1.5$ prism diopters, base-up,

and the resultant prismatic effect is

1.5 base-up − 1.0 base-up,

or

0.5 prism diopter, base-up, left eye.

4.7. Oblique Prismatic Effects

The discussion of prismatic effects, so far, has been limited to effects in which the base-apex line is located in either the horizontal or the vertical meridian. However, oblique prismatic effects occur whenever the line of sight passes through a portion of the lens not horizontally or vertically in line with the pole of the lens. Such an effect is illustrated in the two diagrams in Figure 4-17, in which the line of sight passes, respectively, through points A, B, C, and D, each equidistant from the center, O, for a plus lens, P (A), and for a minus lens, M (B). Considering the plus lens first, the prismatic effect for each point is equal to the distance (AO, BO, CO, or DO) multiplied by the power of the lens. Since the lens is a plus lens, the thickness decreases from point O outward. As we examine the thickness changes

FIGURE 4–16.   **A base-up prismatic effect is induced when a wearer of plus lenses reads through a point below the pole of the lens.**

immediately surrounding points A, B, C, and D, the region central to each point is thicker than the region peripheral to each point. Hence, the base direction is projected toward the center, O, and *through* point O on a circle surrounding the lens. For a plus lens, the projection must be made through the center, toward the perimeter of the circle.

For the minus lens, the prismatic effect for each point is equal to the distance (AO, BO, CO, or DO) multiplied by the power of the lens. Since the lens is a minus lens, the thickness increases from the point O outward. As we examine the thickness immediately surrounding points A, B, C, and D, the region immediately peripheral to each point is thicker than the region immediately central to each point. Hence, the base direction is projected on a circle surrounding the lens. The following example illustrates the procedures used in locating the base direction of a prismatic effect for plus and minus lenses.

EXAMPLE

Given a patient wearing a plus lens before the right eye and a minus lens before the left eye (Figure 4–18). Assume the patient moves his eyes to the point P on each lens, by looking 2 cm to the left and 1 cm upward from the pole, C. In each diagram, the direction of the base of the prism is indicated by an arrow. Inspection of the diagram for the right lens (Figure 4–18A) indicates that the tangent of angle θ is 0.5, with the result that angle θ = 180° plus 26.6°, or 206.6°; hence, the base of the prism is located at 206.6°. For the left lens (Figure 4–18B), angle θ is equal to 26.6°, with the result that the base of the prismatic effect is located at 26.6°.

Horizontal and Vertical Components of Oblique Prisms

Another method of specifying the power of an oblique prism is to resolve the prism into horizontal and vertical components. Referring to Figure 4–19, ε represents an oblique prism with its base at θ, and ε_h and ε_v are its horizontal and vertical components. Expressions for these components are

$$\text{horizontal component, } \varepsilon_h = \varepsilon \cos \theta \qquad (4.9)$$

$$\text{vertical component, } \varepsilon_v = \varepsilon \sin \theta. \qquad (4.10)$$

In a similar fashion, two prismatic effects or components, one horizontal and one vertical, can be reduced to a single prismatic effect by the use of vector analysis. Since

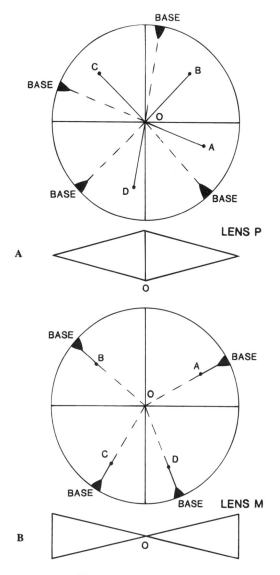

FIGURE 4–17.   **Oblique prismatic effects. A, for a plus lens; B, for a minus lens.**

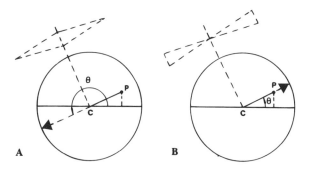

FIGURE 4–18.   **Oblique prismatic effects for a patient wearing a plus lens before the right eye, A, and a minus lens before the left eye, B.**

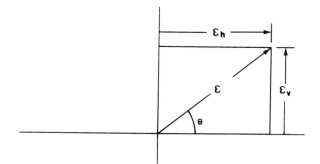

FIGURE 4-19.   **Prismatic effects considered in terms of horizontal and vertical components.**

$$\varepsilon_h = \varepsilon \cos \theta,$$

$$\varepsilon = \frac{\varepsilon_h}{\cos \theta}, \qquad (4.11)$$

and since

$$\varepsilon_v = \varepsilon \sin \theta,$$

$$\varepsilon = \frac{\varepsilon_v}{\sin \theta}. \qquad (4.12)$$

If both ε_h and ε_v are known, the prismatic effect, ε, can be found with use of the Pythagorean theorem,

$$\varepsilon = \sqrt{\varepsilon_h^{\,2} + \varepsilon_v^{\,2}}. \qquad (4.13)$$

EXAMPLE 1

What are the horizontal and vertical prismatic components of a prism having a power of 3 prism diopters base at 120°, placed before the right eye?

Since the base falls in the second quadrant, the bases of the horizontal and vertical components will be out and up, respectively. Since the angle of the prism base is 60 degrees less than the horizontal meridian (that is, $120° = 180° - 60°$), the value of θ will be 60°.

$$\sin \theta = \frac{\varepsilon_v}{\varepsilon} \text{ and } \cos \theta = \frac{\varepsilon_h}{\varepsilon}.$$

$$\sin 60 = \frac{\varepsilon_v}{3}$$

$$0.866 = \frac{\varepsilon_v}{3}$$

$$\varepsilon_v = 2.6 \text{ prism diopters, base-up,}$$

and

$$\cos 60 = \frac{\varepsilon_h}{3}$$

$$0.5 = \frac{\varepsilon_h}{3}$$

$$\varepsilon_h = 1.5 \text{ prism diopters, base-out.}$$

EXAMPLE 2

What single prism can replace the combination of a prism having a power of 4 prism diopters base-in and a prism having a power of 2 prism diopters base-down, for the right eye?

The base of the single prism will fall in the fourth quadrant:

$$\varepsilon = \sqrt{\varepsilon_h^{\,2} + \varepsilon_v^{\,2}}$$

$$= \sqrt{16 + 4}$$

$$= \sqrt{20}$$

$$= 4.47 \text{ prism diopters}$$

Let angle θ be the angle from the prism base to the 360° meridian. Consequently,

$$\sin \theta = \frac{\varepsilon_v}{\varepsilon}$$

$$= \frac{2}{4.47}$$

$$= 0.447$$

and

$$\theta = 26.58°,$$

with the result that the direction of the prism base is

$$360° - 26.58° = 333.42°.$$

Hence, the single prism can be specified as:

4.47 prism diopters, base at 333.42°.

4.8. Obliquely Crossed Prisms

If a lens contains two prisms crossed at oblique angles, each prism is treated separately, being resolved into horizontal and vertical components, and these are then added (or subtracted as the case may be).

EXAMPLE

Given a right lens having obliquely crossed prisms (Figure 4-20), one having a power of 2 prism diopters, base at 30°, and the other having a power of 3 prism diopters, base at 240°. Resolve the total prismatic effect into horizontal and vertical components.

For the 2-prism diopter prism having its base at 30°,

$$\varepsilon_h = \varepsilon \cos \theta = \varepsilon \cos 30$$

$$= 2(0.866)$$

$$= 1.732 \text{ prism diopters, base-in,}$$

and

$$\varepsilon_v = \varepsilon \sin \theta = \varepsilon \sin 30$$

$$= 2(0.5) = 1 \text{ prism diopter, base-up.}$$

For the 3-prism diopter prism having its base at 240°,

$$\varepsilon_h = \varepsilon \cos \theta = \varepsilon \cos 60$$

$$= 3(0.5) = 1.5 \text{ prism diopters, base-out.}$$

and

$$\varepsilon_v = \varepsilon \sin \theta = \varepsilon \sin 60$$

$$= 3(0.866)$$

$$= 2.598 \text{ prism diopters, base-down.}$$

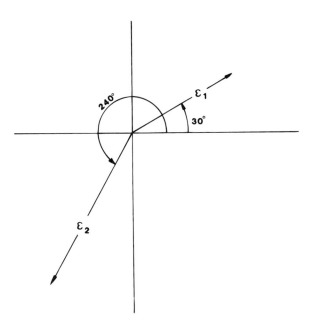

FIGURE 4–20. **Obliquely crossed prisms (right lens).**

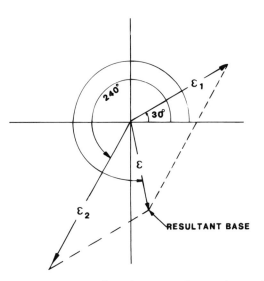

FIGURE 4–21. **Construction of a vector diagram for resolving obliquely crossed prisms.**

The total prismatic effect is therefore

1.732 base-in – 1.5 base-out =
0.232 prism diopter, base-in,

combined with

2.598 base-down – 1 base-up =
1.598 prism diopters, base-down.

An alternative method of resolving obliquely crossed prisms involves the construction of a vector diagram. Figure 4–21 shows such a diagram, and uses the above example. First, a vector is constructed for the first prism, 2 units long and at an angle of 30°. A vector is then constructed for the second prism, 3 units long and at an angle of 240°. A parallelogram is then constructed, and the diagonal of the parallelogram represents the power and the base direction of the resultant prism.

4.9. Effective Power of a Prism in an Oblique Meridian

The amount of deviation of light caused by a prism (or the displacement of an object seen through the prism), refers to the deviation or displacement in the base-apex meridian. However, there are occasions to need the effect (effective power) of a prism in a meridian other than the base-apex meridian, in particular the horizontal and vertical meridians.

Referring to Figure 4–22, if one looks through a base-down prism at a cross target, the horizontal line of the cross appears to be displaced upward. If the observer stands at a distance of 1 m from the target, the amount of displacement in centimeters is equal to the power of the prism.

Rotating the prism so that the base is in the position shown in Figure 4–23 displaces the horizontal and vertical lines of the cross. Referring to the diagram,

$$\cos\alpha_1 = \frac{\varepsilon_v}{\varepsilon}$$

and

$$\cos\alpha_2 = \frac{\varepsilon_h}{\varepsilon},$$

and by solving for ε_v, and ε_h, we can find the amount of vertical and horizontal displacement caused by the prism:

$$\varepsilon_v = \varepsilon \cos\alpha_1$$

and

$$\varepsilon_h = \varepsilon \cos\alpha_2.$$

As a general expression, therefore, the effective power of a prism in a meridian other than the base-apex meridian (Figure 4–24) is equal to the power of the prism times the cosine of the angle between the specified meridian and the base-apex meridian,

$$\varepsilon_\alpha = \varepsilon \cos\alpha. \qquad (4.14)$$

The use of Equation 4.14 is illustrated by the following examples:

EXAMPLE 1
What is the prismatic effect along a direction that is 30 degrees from the base-apex direction of a prism whose power is 3 prism diopters?

$$\varepsilon_\alpha = \varepsilon \cos\alpha$$
$$= 3\cos 30$$
$$= 3(0.866)$$
$$= 2.598 \text{ prism diopters.}$$

TARGET

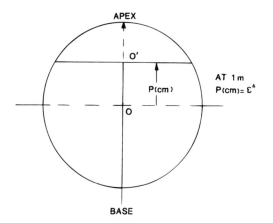

FIGURE 4–22. **Displacement caused by a prism in a principal section.**

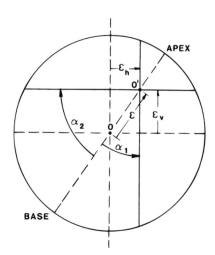

FIGURE 4–23. **Displacement caused by a prism in an oblique meridian.**

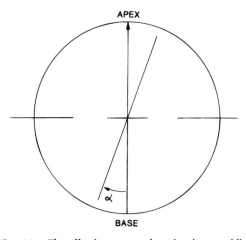

FIGURE 4–24. **The effective power of a prism in a meridian other than the base-apex meridian.**

EXAMPLE 2
For a prism of any power, what is the prismatic effect along a line perpendicular to the base-apex direction?

$$\varepsilon_\alpha = \varepsilon \cos \alpha$$
$$= \varepsilon \cos 90$$
$$= \varepsilon(0)$$
$$= 0.$$

EXAMPLE 3
For a prism of any power, what is the prismatic effect along a line 180 degrees from the base-apex direction?

$$\varepsilon_\alpha = \varepsilon \cos \alpha$$
$$= \varepsilon \cos 180$$
$$= \varepsilon(-1)$$
$$= -\varepsilon.$$

4.10. Specification of Prismatic Effects: The Prism Reference Point

When a prescription is written without any specification for prism, no resultant prismatic effects are expected when the patient's eyes are in the *primary position*, that is, with the eyes looking straight ahead with the head erect. To accomplish this, the optical centers (poles) of the lenses should be located directly in front of the centers of the pupils. Prisms are often incorporated into spectacle prescriptions to manage ocular motility problems. The amount of prism desired can often be obtained by mounting the spectacle lenses in such a way that the visual axes no longer pass through the poles of the lenses.

The American National Standards Institute (ANSI) Z80.1-1995 *Prescription Ophthalmic Lenses—Recommendations*[1] has defined the *prism reference point* as the point on the lens, as specified by the manufacturer, at which the prism value of the finished lens is to be measured. When no prism is prescribed, this is the optical center of the lens; but if prism is prescribed, the prism reference point is the point on the lens manifesting the amount and direction of prism called for in the prescription. In either case, the prism reference point should fall directly in front of the center of the patient's pupil. Implicit in the definition of prism reference point is that the point has not only the prism called for in the prescription, but also the *correct refracting power*. The location of the prism reference point is usually specified in relation to the *geometric center* of the lens.

4.11. Specification of Lens and Frame Sizes

Since January 1962, all frames made by members of the Optical Manufacturers' Association have been measured and designated by the *boxing system*. According to this system, the size of the frame (and the size of the lens within the frame) is specified by giving the horizontal and vertical dimensions of a rectangle that circumscribes the lens, as shown in Figure 4–25. The A measurement is the horizontal distance between the two vertical tangents at the lens bevel, and the B measurement is the vertical distance between the two horizontal tangents at the lens bevel. The horizontal A measurement is usually greater than the B measurement, and the difference between them is termed the *difference*. The horizontal A measurement is usually given as the *eye size* of the frame. The horizontal distance between the tangents at the lens bevels of the nasal side of each lens is called the *distance between lenses* (DBL). This measurement is the shortest distance between the two lenses.

The *geometric center* of the frame aperture (or of the lens that fills it) is defined as the geometric center of the circumscribing rectangle, and is easily found by constructing the diagonals of the "box": The intersection of the diagonals is the geometric center. The intersection of the perpendicular bisectors of the horizontal and vertical (A and B) dimensions also determines the geometric center.

Distance between Centers

The distance between centers (DBC) is the distance between the geometric centers of the two apertures of the frame. This distance is often called the *frame PD*. The A measurement added to the DBL always gives the frame PD.

Effective Diameter

An additional specification provided by the frame manufacturer is the effective diameter, *ED* (Figure 4–26). The effective diameter of a lens is twice the distance from the geometric center to the peak of the lens bevel that is farthest from the geometric center. This measurement is useful in determining the *minimum blank size*, which is the smallest possible finished uncut lens size from which a finished lens having a particular prescription can be cut. The minimum blank size is determined by doubling the amount of decentration and adding the product to the effective diameter: The minimum blank size is therefore given by the expression

minimum blank size = ED + 2 (decentration).

If the minimum blank size exceeds the finished uncut lens size currently available for a particular prescription, oversize blanks must be ordered or the decentration must be provided by grinding prism onto the lenses.

EXAMPLE
Given the prescription OD +2.00 DS, OS +2.00 DS, PD = 66 mm, finished lens size = 54 by 45 mm, ED = 60 mm, and DBL = 20 mm. What is the minimum blank size?

Since the frame PD is 74 mm (54 + 20) and the patient's PD is 66 mm, the decentration per lens is 4 mm inward,

minimum blank size = 60 + 2(4) = 68 mm.

Realistically, it is best to make an allowance beyond the minimum blank size because the peripheral portions of the blank may not be suitable because of defects at the edge of the blank. As lens and frame sizes have increased from year to year, the sizes of single-vision blanks have not kept up with the increase in the sizes of frames being used. Frequently, additional charges are made for providing oversize blanks or for grinding in the decentration.

Every optometrist should keep a current list of the readily available finished lenses including their prescrip-

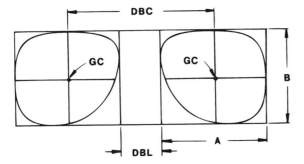

FIGURE 4–25. **The boxing system. The eye size is specified by giving the horizontal and vertical dimensions of a rectangle that circumscribes the lens. GC = geometric center.**

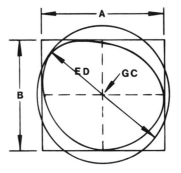

FIGURE 4–26. **The effective diameter (ED) of a lens is twice the distance from the geometric center (GC) to the peak of the lens bevel that is farthest from the geometric center.**

tion ranges and sizes. If a prescription can be filled from finished lenses kept in stock by the laboratory, extensive delays in obtaining the finished lenses as well as unexpected additional charges can be avoided.

Lens Shape

The shape of a lens is the contour made by the perimeter of the lens when the front surface of the lens is observed perpendicularly. The trade name of a frame implies a specific, unique shape. Currently, no standardization exists for defining lens shape. The manufacturer of a given frame must make available *formers* (also called *patterns*) for use by laboratories in edging lenses to fit the frame. Under the boxing system, the center chuckhole of the former falls at the geometric center of the rectangle enclosing the former. Thus, the geometric center of the former and that of the lens coincide. A line running through the centers of the three chuckholes on the former gives the orientation of the 0° to 180° line (Figure 4–27). Manufacturers usually identify formers by trade name or by a number.

4.12. Prismatic Power and Thickness

An expression for the change in thickness of a plano-prism between two points on the prism, P and Q, can be derived with the aid of Figure 4–28. In this diagram, a line parallel to the base has been constructed, extending from Q, as well as an additional line parallel to the flat face of the prism. Using Equation 4.4, relating the refracting angle of the prism to its deviation in prism diopters,

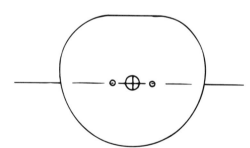

FIGURE 4–27.   **The 0° to 180° line of a former.**

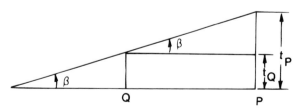

FIGURE 4–28.   **Diagram for derivation of the relationship between prism power and change in thickness across the prism.**

$$\tan \beta° = \frac{\varepsilon}{100(n' - n)}.$$

Referring to the upper triangle in Figure 4–28,

$$\tan \beta° = \frac{t_P - t_Q}{\overline{QP}},$$

and setting the two right-hand terms equal to each other,

$$\frac{t_P - t_Q}{\overline{QP}} = \frac{\varepsilon}{100(n' - n)},$$

and

$$t_P - t_Q = \frac{\overline{QP}(\varepsilon)}{100(n' - n)}. \tag{4.15}$$

For a plano-prism, the thickness difference between two points, P and Q (P is thicker than Q), is equal to the distance between the two points times the power of the prism in prism diopters, divided by 100 times the index difference.

EXAMPLE
If a 1 prism diopter prism is ground on a 50-mm lens blank having an index of refraction of 1.523, what is the thickness difference from one edge to the other?

$$t_P - t_Q = \frac{50(1)}{100(1.523 - 1)}$$

$$= 0.956 \text{ mm}.$$

As a rule, for a prism ground on a 50-mm blank, with $n = 1.523$, the thickness change across the prism is approximately *1 mm per prism diopter of power.*

4.13. Thickness of a Lens/Prism

If a spherical ophthalmic lens contains prism power, calculations concerning thickness must include the thickness difference (between two points) resulting from the spherical lens power in addition to that caused by the prismatic power. One method of creating prism power is to *decenter* the lens. As shown in Figure 4–29, decentering is done by mounting an ophthalmic lens in a frame such that the pole, C, of the lens does not coincide with the geometric center (i.e., the lens is decentered) (A). A decentered lens can be considered as a composite lens made up of a centered lens and an attached prism "on its back." By drawing a dashed line through the lens (B) we are able to distinguish between thickness changes caused by the *lens* and those caused by the *prism*.

The point C', shown in Figure 4–29B, is used as a reference point, and is equivalent to the optical center (or pole) of the lens itself, without the prism behind it. The stated amount of prismatic effect (i.e., the amount found by verifying the lens with a lensometer) is the prismatic effect at the point C', which is solely a result of the *prism* component. At any other point on the lens, the prismatic effect will be different than that at point C', because the *lens* component produces an additional prismatic effect at all points other than the point C'.

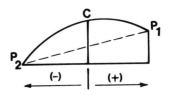

FIGURE 4–30.   **Sign convention for changes in thickness of a decentered lens (a lens/prism).**

FIGURE 4–31.   **Calculation of the thickness at the geometric center of +5.00-DS decentered lens to obtain 2 prism diopters of base-out prism.**

FIGURE 4–29.   **When a lens is decentered, it becomes a lens/prism. The diagonal line makes it possible to differentiate the thickness difference caused by the lens from that caused by the prism.**

The following expression indicates the thickness difference caused by the lens only, between the point C at the geometric center and a peripheral point P, by using Equation 3.20,

$$t_C - t_P = \frac{F_A h^2}{2(n - 1)}.$$

The thickness difference between points C and P caused by the prism only, applied to Equation 4.15, is

$$t_C - t_P = \frac{\overline{CP}\varepsilon}{100(n - 1)},$$

with the result that the equation for the thickness difference for the combination of the lens and the prism becomes

$$-t_P = \frac{\overline{CP}^2 F_A}{2(n - 1)} - \frac{\overline{CP}\varepsilon}{100(n - 1)}. \qquad (4.16)$$

As shown in Figure 4–30, we can establish a *sign convention* for use with this formula. If the point in question (P) is *thicker* than the prism at point C, the distance CP has a *plus* sign, but if the point is on a part of the prism that is *thinner* than the prism at point C, the distance CP has a *minus* sign. In other words, if the peripheral point, P, is located toward the *base* of the prism, CP has a plus sign, but if P is located toward the *apex* of the prism, CP has a minus sign.

EXAMPLE 1
Given a left lens with the prescription +5.00 DS, decentered to obtain 2 prism diopters, base-out, at the geometric center of the lens. If the lens has a horizontal diameter of 40 mm, a nasal edge thickness of 1 mm, and an index of refraction of 1.50, what is the thickness at the geometric center of the lens?

As shown in Figure 4–31, the lens (for the left eye) is decentered *out* to obtain base-out prism at the geometric center.

$$t_C - t_P = \frac{(-0.02)^2(+5)}{2(1.5 - 1)} - \frac{(-0.02)(2)}{100(1.5 - 1)}$$

$$t_C - 0.001 = 0.002 - (-0.008)$$

$$t_C = 0.0038 = 3.8 \text{ mm}.$$

The process may be less confusing if Equation 3.20 and Equation 4.15 are solved separately, and then the thickness differences are combined (keeping in mind, for each equation, whether C or P is thicker).

An Important Point. For any decentered lens, the difference in edge thickness along the base-apex direction can be attributed solely to the prism. Because a decentered lens is a centered lens with a prism on its back side, use of Equation 4.15 when the edge thicknesses along the base-apex meridian are known allows calculation of the prismatic effect at the geometric center of the lens.

EXAMPLE 2
A –5.00-D lens, 50 mm in diameter, has a nasal edge thickness of 4 mm and a temporal edge thickness of 1 mm. If the index of refraction is 1.50, what is the prismatic effect at the geometric center?

If we consider this lens/prism as a centered –5.00 D lens with a prism on its back, all the prismatic effect at the geometric center of the lens is caused solely by the prism component, and

$$t_P - t_Q = \frac{\overline{QP}(\varepsilon)}{100(n' - n)}$$

$$0.004 - 0.001 = \frac{0.05\varepsilon}{100(0.5)}$$

$$0.05\varepsilon = 0.15$$

$$\varepsilon = 3 \text{ prism diopters}$$

Therefore, the –5.00 D lens has 3 prism diopters of base-in prism at its geometric center.

4.14. Prismatic Effects of Cylindrical Lenses

Prentice's rule can be applied to a cylindrical lens whose axis is either horizontal or vertical. As shown in Figure 4–32, to find the prismatic effect at a point, P, on a cylindrical lens, a line is drawn from P, perpendicular to the

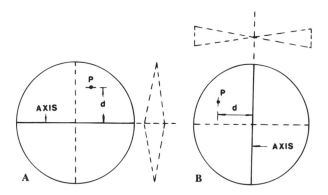

FIGURE 4–32.   **Determining the prismatic effect at a point, P, on a cylindrical lens whose axes are horizontal and vertical.**

cylinder axis, and the prismatic effect is found by multiplying the distance, d (in centimeters), by the power of the cylinder. For a plus cylinder, the base is toward the cylinder axis; for a minus cylinder, the base is away from the cylinder axis.

The same principle applies for a cylindrical lens whose axis is *not* horizontal or vertical (Figure 4–33). A line is drawn from the point, perpendicular to the cylinder axis. (Note that the sine square rule for calculating the power in an oblique meridian of a cylindrical lens *cannot* be used for calculating prismatic effects because the deviation occurs only in the plane of a *principal section*.) The perpendicular distance, d, from the point in question to the cylinder axis may be determined by construction or by calculation.

Using the construction method, we draw a diagram to scale (Figure 4–33), indicating the horizontal and vertical meridians of the lens, the cylinder axis, and the point, P. We can then construct a triangle with x' and y' as the horizontal and vertical legs, and d as the hypotenuse. The prismatic effect is then equal to the distance, d, multiplied by the power, F_C, of the cylinder. Since the prismatic effect along the hypotenuse of the triangle is equal to dF_C, the horizontal and vertical components of the prismatic effect may be found by use of the expressions

$$\text{horizontal component} = x'(F_C),$$

$$\text{vertical component} = y'(F_C).$$

The diagram shown in Figure 4–34 may be used to derive a formula for calculating the prismatic effect at a point, P, on a cylindrical lens. The sign convention requires that the angle θ always be measured from the *nasal* (toward the temporal) side of the lens. This means that for a *right* lens, the angle θ is the same as the cylinder axis, but for a *left* lens the angle θ is equal to $180°$ minus the cylinder axis. The derivation is done on the basis of the similar triangles PNL and OKL. In triangle PNL,

$$d = (y + w)\cos\theta,$$

and in triangle OKL,

$$w = x\tan\theta.$$

Substituting for w,

$$d = (y + x\tan\theta)\cos\theta,$$

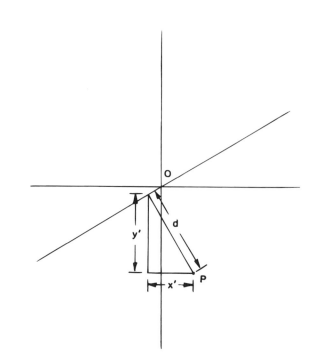

FIGURE 4–33.   **Construction method for determining the prismatic effect at a point, P, on a cylindrical lens.**

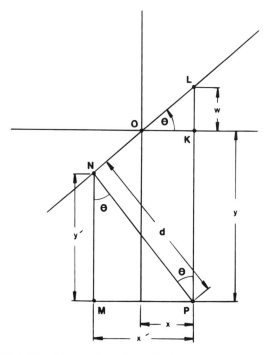

FIGURE 4–34.   **Diagram for deriving the formula for calculating the prismatic effect at a point, P, on a cylindrical lens.**

or

$$d = y\cos\theta + x\tan\theta\cos\theta$$

and, since

$$\tan\theta\cos\theta = \sin\theta,$$

$$d = y\cos\theta + x\sin\theta. \tag{4.17}$$

In this formula, the following sign convention must be used: If P is located nasally from the origin, O, x has a *plus* sign; if P is located temporally from O, x has a *minus* sign; if P is located below O, y has a *plus* sign; and if P is located above O, y has a *minus* sign. For the angle θ, when θ is acute, both sine and cosine are plus, but when θ is obtuse, sine is plus and cosine is minus.

We may also derive formulas for the horizontal and vertical components of the prismatic effect. For the horizontal component,

$$\varepsilon_h = F_c(x'),$$

but in triangle MNP,

$$\sin\theta = x'/d, \text{ and } \therefore x' = d\sin\theta.$$

Therefore,

$$\varepsilon_h = F_c(d\sin\theta). \qquad (4.18)$$

For the vertical component,

$$\varepsilon_v = F_c(y'),$$

but in triangle NMP,

$$\cos\theta = y'/d, \text{ and } \therefore y' = d\cos\theta.$$

Therefore,

$$\varepsilon_v = F_c(d\cos\theta). \qquad (4.19)$$

The following sign convention applies to the horizontal and vertical components: ε_h is positive for base-out and negative for base-in; ε_v is positive for base-up and negative for base-down.

For a single *sphero-cylindrical* lens, it is necessary to find the horizontal and vertical components for the sphere, as well as for the cylinder, and to add (or subtract) them to find the total prismatic effect in each meridian. Thus,

$$\text{total horizontal prism } = \varepsilon_{hc} + \varepsilon_{hs} \qquad (4.20)$$

and

$$\text{total vertical prism } = \varepsilon_{vc} + \varepsilon_{vs}. \qquad (4.21)$$

The two components are combined algebraically, adding base-in to base-in, base-out to base-out, base-up to base-up, and base-down to base-down. Base-in is subtracted from base-out (and vice versa), and base-up is subtracted from base-down (and vice versa). The procedure is then repeated for the second lens.

Resultant Prismatic Effect (Prismatic Imbalance) between Right and Left Eyes

As noted in Section 4.5, when we consider prismatic effects for the two eyes we are concerned with *resultant* prismatic effects or with prismatic *imbalance* between the two eyes. For horizontal prismatic effects, when the base of the prism is either *in* or *out* for *both* eyes, the resultant horizontal prismatic effect is found by adding the two amounts of the prism. However, for an equal amount of base-in for one eye and base-out for the other eye, the eyes simply

make a *conjugate* (sideways) shift, to one side or the other, with no change in convergence. For vertical prismatic effects, an equal amount of base-up or base-down prism for each eye simply requires the eyes to make a conjugate movement (downward for base-up or upward for base-down), with the result that the prismatic effects cancel each other. However, when the bases of vertical prism have opposite directions, such as base-up on the right eye and base-down on the left eye, the resultant vertical prismatic imbalance is found by adding the amounts of the prism. Base-up prism in front of the right eye causes the right eye to turn downward, and base-down prism in front of the left eye causes the left eye to turn upward. The result is *vertical divergence*. These effects are illustrated by the following examples:

OD 2 base-out, OS 2 base-out,
total effect = 4 base-out.

OD 3 base-out, OS 2 base-in,
total effect = 1 base-out.

OD 1 base-down, OS 1 base-down,
total effect = zero.

OD 1 base-down, OS 2 base-up,
total effect = 3 base-down OD
or 3 base-up OS.

The calculation of prismatic effects experienced by a wearer of sphero-cylindrical lenses is illustrated by the example below.

EXAMPLE

Assume the prescription

OD +6.00 DS –3.00 DC x 140
OS +2.00 DS –3.00 DC x 120.

When reading, the wearer looks through a point in each lens 11 mm down and 2.5 mm in (Figure 4–35). What are the prismatic effects for each eye, in the horizontal and vertical meridians, and what are the combined effects for both eyes?

For the *right eye* (Figure 4–35A), with use of the sign convention, x and y both have *positive* signs. For the *sphere*,

A   **RIGHT LENS**   **B**   **LEFT LENS**

FIGURE 4–35. **Prismatic effect occurring when wearer looks downward 11 mm and inward 2.5 mm (each eye) to read.**

$$\varepsilon_h = F_s(x)$$
$$= +6(0.25) = +1.50$$
$$= 1.50 \text{ prism diopters, base-out.}$$

$$\varepsilon_v = F_s(y)$$
$$= +6(1.1) = +6.60$$
$$= 6.60 \text{ prism diopters, base-up.}$$

For the *cylinder*,

$$d = y\cos\theta + x\sin\theta$$
$$= 1.1\cos 140 + 0.25\sin 140$$
$$= -0.8426 + 0.1607 = -0.6819.$$

$$\varepsilon_h = F_c(d\sin\theta)$$
$$= -3(-0.6819)(0.428)$$
$$= 1.315$$
$$= 1.315 \text{ base-out.}$$

$$\varepsilon_v = F_c(d\cos\theta)$$
$$= -3(-0.6819)(-0.766)$$
$$= -1.567$$
$$= 1.567 \text{ base-down.}$$

The total horizontal prismatic effect is given by

$$\varepsilon_{hs} + \varepsilon_{hc} = 1.5 \text{ base-out} + 1.315 \text{ base-out}$$
$$= 2.815 \text{ base-out.}$$

The total vertical prismatic effect is given by

$$\varepsilon_{vs} + \varepsilon_{vc} = 6.60 \text{ base-up} + 1.567 \text{ base-down}$$
$$= 5.033 \text{ base-up.}$$

For the left eye (Figure 4–35B), with use of the sign convention, both x and y are again positive. For the *sphere*,

$$\varepsilon_h = F_s(x)$$
$$= 2(0.25) = +0.50$$
$$= 0.50 \text{ prism diopter, base-out.}$$

$$\varepsilon_v = F_s(y)$$
$$= 2(1.1) = 2.2$$
$$= 2.2 \text{ prism diopter, base-out.}$$

For the *cylinder*,

$$d = y\cos\theta + x\sin\theta$$
$$= 1.1\cos 60 + 0.25\sin 60$$
$$= 1.1(0.5) + 0.25(0.866)$$
$$= +0.7665 \text{ cm.}$$

$$\varepsilon_h = F_c(d\sin\theta)$$
$$= -3(0.7665)(0.866) = -1.99$$
$$= 1.99 \text{ prism diopters, base-in.}$$

$$\varepsilon_v = F_c(d\cos\theta)$$
$$= -3(0.7665)(0.5) = -1.15$$
$$= 1.15 \text{ prism diopters, base-down.}$$

The total horizontal prismatic effect is

$$\varepsilon_{hs} + \varepsilon_{hc} = 0.5 \text{ base-out} + 1.99 \text{ base-in}$$
$$= 1.49 \text{ prism diopters, base-in.}$$

The total vertical prismatic effect is

$$\varepsilon_{vs} + \varepsilon_{vc} = 2.2 \text{ base-up} + 1.15 \text{ base-down}$$
$$= 1.05 \text{ base-up.}$$

To find the resultant prismatic effect for both eyes:

resultant horizontal effect

$$= 2.815 \text{ base-out} + 1.49 \text{ base-in}$$
$$= 1.325 \text{ prism diopters, base-out, right eye.}$$

resultant vertical effect

$$= 5.033 \text{ base-up} + 1.05 \text{ base-up}$$
$$= 3.983 \text{ prism diopters, base-up, right eye.}$$

4.15. Decentration

As described in Section 4.11, when the boxing system is used, the geometric center of the lens coincides with the geometric center of the rectangle enclosing the lens. To control prismatic effects, the pole of the lens is usually displaced from the geometric center. The displacement of the pole of the lens from the geometric center is called *decentration*. A *centered* lens is one in which the pole falls at the geometric center; a *decentered* lens is one in which the pole is not located at the geometric center.

Lenses are decentered to control prismatic effects. Decentration is used both to *create* prismatic effects and to *avoid* prismatic effects. When prismatic power is required in a prescription, it often can be obtained by decentration. When decentration *cannot* provide the desired prismatic effect, prism power may be *ground* on the lens by surfacing procedures. By grinding one surface at an appropriate angle to the other surface, differences in thickness occur across the opposing edges of a lens and create the prismatic effect. When the prism is ground into a lens, the surface powers and thickness must also provide the correct back vertex power. Whether a finished lens has been decentered to provide prism or prism has been provided by grinding, if properly done the prismatic effect is the same. Even if grinding is used to produce a prismatic effect, the finished lens will behave as if it were a decentered lens. However, the optical center of the lens may not even be located on the lens.

Decentering a finished, uncut lens is usually more economical than grinding prism onto a lens. Decentration is done when the prismatic effect required is not large, or when the power of the lens is sufficiently great so that only a small amount of decentration is needed. If a large amount of prism is required, the prism must be produced by grinding. When prismatic power is produced by grinding, the surface powers may be chosen to optimize selected performance parameters of the lens/prism combination.

The following examples illustrate the use of decentration in relation to the prism reference point.

Decentration of Spherical Lenses

EXAMPLE 1

Given the following prescription,

OD –4.00 DS
OS –4.00 DS

PD = 64 mm, eye size = 48 mm, DBL = 20 mm, find (1) the locations of the prism reference points of the lenses as related to the geometric centers; (2) the amount and direction of the decentration.

(1) Since the frame PD is 68 mm (48 + 20) and the patient's PD is 64 mm, the centers of the pupils each fall 2 mm in from the geometric center. Hence, the prism reference point for each lens should be located 2 mm inward from the geometric center of the lens.

(2) The prism reference point is placed before the center of the pupil by decentration. Since no prism is prescribed, the only point having zero prismatic effect on the lens is the pole of the lens. Consequently, the pole must be placed, for each lens, in front of the center of the pupil. In the finished lenses, the poles are located 2 mm inward, for each lens, from the geometric center. Hence, decentration is 2 mm in for each lens.

EXAMPLE 2

Given the prescription

OD –4.00 DS with 1 prism diopter, base-in
OS –4.00 DS with 1 prism diopter, base-in

PD = 64 mm, eye size = 50 mm, DBL = 20 mm, find (1) the location of the prism reference points of the lenses as related to the geometrical centers; (2) the amount and direction of the decentration.

(1) Since the frame PD is 70 mm (50 + 20) and the patient's PD is 64 mm, the center of each pupil is located 3 mm inward from the geometric center of the lens. Therefore, the prism reference points should fall 3 mm in from the geometric center for each lens.

(2) For this problem it is easier to calculate the decentration in two distinct steps. The first step is to move the pole of the lens to the center of the pupil, which initially gives a *zero* amount of prism. In this problem, the pole of each lens is first moved 3 mm inward. For the second step, the pole of each lens is moved to provide the appropriate amount of prism before the center of the pupil. One prism diopter, base-in, is required for each eye; by use of Prentice's rule, the pole of a –4.00 D lens must be displaced 2.5 mm to provide 1 prism diopter of prism. The direction of the displacement must be *out* to achieve a base-in effect for each eye wearing a minus lens.

In the first step, the pole is moved *3 mm in* from the geometric center; in the second step, the pole is moved *2.5 mm out* from the center of each pupil. The net position of these two movements leaves the pole of each lens resting 0.5 mm in from the geometric center. Hence, the decentration is *0.5 mm in* for each lens.

EXAMPLE 3

Given the prescription

OD –4.00 DS with 1 prism diopter, base-out
OS +2.00 DS with 1 prism diopter, base-out

PD = 64 mm, eye size = 48 mm, DBL = 20 mm, find (1) the location of the prism reference point for each lens relative to the geometric center, (2) the amount and direction of decentration for each lens.

(1) Since the frame PD is 68 mm (48 + 20) and the patient's PD is 64 mm, the center of each pupil is located 2 mm inward from the geometric center of the lens. Therefore, the prism reference points are positioned *2 mm in* from the geometric center for each lens.

(2) Using the two-step method described in Example 2, the first step is to position the pole of each lens before the center of the pupil, which provides zero prismatic effect initially. In the first step, the pole is moved *2mm in* from the geometric center for each lens. In the second step, the pole is then moved from the position in front of the center of the pupil, for each eye, to provide the appropriate amount of prism. For the right eye, since 1 prism diopter, base-out, is required, the pole of the –4.00 D lens must be displaced 2.5 mm, and the direction of the displacement must be *in* to achieve a base-out effect. In the first step, the pole was moved *2 mm in* from the geometric center and, in the second step, the pole was moved an additional *2.5 mm in*. The final position for these two movements is therefore *4.5 mm in* from the geometric center of the lens. Hence, the *decentration* for the right lens is *4.5 mm in*.

Since 1 prism diopter, base-out, is also needed for the left eye, in the second step, the pole of the +2.00 D lens must be moved 5 mm from the center of the pupil. The direction of the displacement must be *out* to provide a base-out effect before the left eye. For the left lens, in the first step, the pole was moved *2 mm in* from the geometric center, and, in the second step, the pole was moved *5 mm out* from the center of the pupil. The net position of the pole for these two movements is *3 mm out* from the geometric center. Therefore, for the left lens, the decentration is *3 mm out*.

EXAMPLE 4

A +6.00 D lens, intended for the right eye, is to have a prismatic effect of 3 prism diopters base-down and 2 prism diopters base-in. What is required decentration to bring about this prismatic effect?

The direction of the decentration can be found by visualizing where the prism reference point must be placed in relation to the optical center of the lens. *Change in thickness* about the prism reference point is the sole concern. In this example, the base-*down* and base-*in* prism are required for the right lens. Inspection of Figure 4–36 shows that for these prismatic effects to occur, the prism reference point must fall in the *upper left* quadrant of the lens, and hence the optical center will have to be moved *downward* and *inward* from the prism reference point.

The following rule is helpful in determining the direction of decentration to induce a given prismatic effect. If a lens (or a meridian of a lens) has *plus* power, the required decentration is in the *same* direction as that of the base of the prism; if a lens (or meridian of a lens) has *minus* power, the required decentration is in the direction *opposite* to the base of the prism.

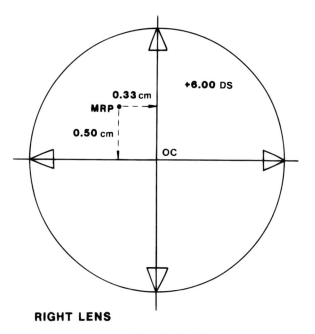

RIGHT LENS

FIGURE 4–36.   **A +6.00 D sphere, for the right eye, is to have a prismatic effect of 3 prism diopters, base-down, and 2 prism diopters, base-in. For these prismatic effects to occur, the prism reference point must fall in the upper left quadrant of the lens.**

In the above example, the *amount* of decentration can be determined by the use of Prentice's rule,

$$\varepsilon = dF,$$

or

$$d = \frac{\varepsilon}{F}.$$

Therefore,

$$d_v = \frac{3}{6} = 0.50 \text{ cm downward}$$

and

$$d_h = \frac{2}{6} = 0.33 \text{ cm inward.}$$

Hence, the required decentration is 0.50 cm down and 0.33 cm in.

Decentration of Plano-Cylindrical Lenses

EXAMPLE 1

Given a right lens with the formula +3.00 DC axis 180. In what direction, and how much, must the lens be decentered to produce, at the prism reference point, (1) 1 prism diopter, base-down, or (2) 2 prism diopters, base-up?

Since the prismatic effect of a cylindrical lens is always perpendicular to the cylinder axis (see Section 4.14), a cylindrical lens may be decentered to create a prismatic effect *only* when the prescribed base direction coincides with the direction of the power meridian. Therefore, a cylinder whose axis is horizontal, as the one in this example, can be decentered to produce only a *vertical* prismatic effect (base-up or base-down), whereas

a cylinder whose axis is vertical (90°) can be decentered to produce only a *horizontal* prismatic effect (base-in or base-out). The solutions to this example, therefore, are as follows:

(1) To induce 1 prism diopter, base-down, the lens must be decentered (with use of Prentice's rule)

$$d = \frac{\varepsilon}{F} = \frac{1}{3} = 0.33 \text{ cm downward.}$$

(2) To induce 2 prism diopters, base-up, the lens must be decentered

$$d = \frac{\varepsilon}{F} = \frac{2}{3} = 0.67 \text{ cm upward.}$$

EXAMPLE 2

Given a right lens with the formula –2.00 DC axis 30. In what direction, and how much, must the lens be decentered to produce, at the prism reference point, (1) 1 prism diopter, base at 120°, or (2) 2 prism diopters, base at 300°?

Since the prismatic effect of a cylindrical lens is perpendicular to the cylinder axis, a cylinder whose axis is 30° can be decentered to produce a prismatic effect whose base is *only* 120° or 300° (Figure 4–37).

(1) To induce 1 prism diopter, base at 120°, the lens must be decentered

$$d = \frac{\varepsilon}{F} = \frac{1}{-2} = 0.5 \text{ cm in the 300° direction.}$$

(2) To induce 2 prism diopters, base at 300°, the lens must be decentered

$$d = \frac{\varepsilon}{F} = \frac{2}{-2} = 1.0 \text{ cm in the 120° direction.}$$

It is rare that the power meridian of a plano-cylindrical lens coincides exactly with the base-apex meridian of the prescribed prism. Therefore, if prismatic power is required in a plano-cylinder, it must usually be obtained by

FIGURE 4–37.   **The lens, –2.00 DC axis 30, can be decentered to produce a prismatic effect whose base is either at 120° or at 300°.**

a *surfacing* operation; that is, by grinding the refractive surfaces of the lens at the inclination to one another that is required to produce the desired prismatic effect.

Decentration of Sphero-Cylindrical Lenses Whose Principal Meridians Are Horizontal and Vertical

EXAMPLE

Given a right lens with the formula +2.50 DS –4.50 DC axis 90. In what direction, and how much, must the lens be decentered to produce, at the prism reference point, 1 prism diopter base-up and 1 prism diopter base-in?

The first step is to determine the power in each of the two principal meridians, so that we may apply Prentice's rule to each meridian, and use the rule-of-thumb for the direction of decentration. As shown in Figure 4–38, the power in the vertical meridian is +2.50 D and that in the horizontal meridian is –2.00 D.

$$d_v = \frac{\varepsilon}{F_v} = \frac{1}{2.5} = 0.4 \text{ cm upward}$$

and

$$d_h = \frac{\varepsilon}{F_h} = \frac{1}{-2} = 0.5 \text{ cm outward.}$$

The decentration is therefore 0.4 cm upward and 0.5 cm outward.

Decentration of Sphero-Cylindrical Lenses Whose Principal Meridians Are Oblique

When the principal meridians are oblique, a *graphic* method provides a much simpler method of arriving at a solution than a purely mathematic approach. Using the graphic method, the lens is considered in the crossed-cylinder form. The desired prism is first resolved into components lying along the two principal meridians. The decentration is calculated separately for each principal meridian, and is then expressed in terms of vertical and horizontal components. To demonstrate both methods, the following example is solved first by the graphic method and then by the mathematic method.

EXAMPLE

Given a left lens with the formula +3.00 DS –1.00 DC axis 30. In what direction, and how much, must the lens be decentered to produce, at the prism reference point, 1 prism diopter base-up and 3 prism diopters base-in?

GRAPHIC METHOD. With the aid of Figures 4–39 and 4–40, the graphic method is used in the following manner:

1. Construct vertical and horizontal lines that intersect the two principal meridians (30° and 120°) at point R, as shown in Figure 4–39.
2. Using a convenient scale, mark off line segments RV to correspond to the direction and amount of the speci-

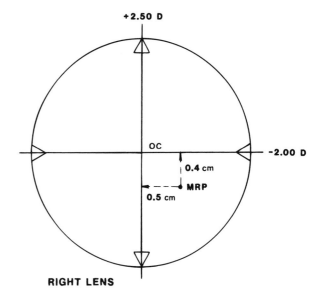

RIGHT LENS

FIGURE 4–38.   **Decentration of the lens, +2.50 DS –4.50 DC axis 90, to produce a prismatic effect of 1 prism diopter, base-up, and 1 prism diopter, base-in.**

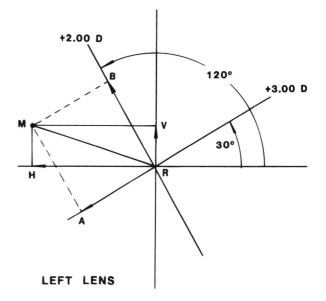

LEFT LENS

FIGURE 4–39.   **Resolving the prismatic effect, 1 prism diopter, base-up, and 3 prism diopters, base-in, for the lens +3.00 DS –1.00 DC axis 30, into components parallel and perpendicular to the cylinder axis. RV = 1.00 prism diopter; RH = 3.00 prism diopters; RA = 2.12 prism diopters; RB = 2.35 prism diopters.**

fied vertical prismatic effect and RH to correspond to the direction and amount of the specified horizontal prismatic effect:

RV = 1 prism diopter base-up.
RH = 3 prism diopters base-in.

3. Complete the rectangle RVMH.
4. Draw the diagonal RM. This represents the single resultant prismatic effect.
5. From point M, drop perpendiculars to the two principal meridians, and thus form line segments MA and MB.

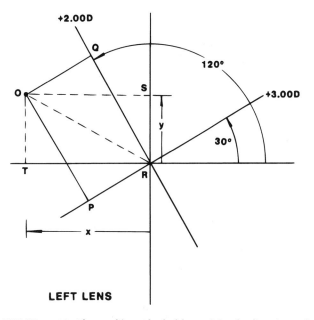

+2.00D

Q

120°

O

S

+3.00D

30°

y

T

R

P

x

LEFT LENS

FIGURE 4-40.   **The graphic method of determining the direction and amount of decentration to produce a prismatic effect of 1 prism diopter base-up and 3 prism diopters base-in, for the lens +3.00 DS –1.00 DC axis 30. RQ = 1.18 cm; RP = 0.706 cm; RS = 0.72 cm up; RT = 1.22 cm in.**

6. The single original prism can now be resolved into prism components RA, with its base at 210° and RB, with its base at 120°. The lengths of line segments RA and RB represent the amount of prism along the two principal meridians. These are:

$$\varepsilon_{210} = 2.12 \text{ prism diopters,}$$

and

$$\varepsilon_{120} = 2.35 \text{ prism diopters.}$$

7. The decentration required to produce the prismatic effect can now be determined by the use of Prentice's rule. Along the 210° meridian,

$$d = \frac{\varepsilon}{F} = \frac{2.12}{3} = 0.7067 \text{ cm,}$$

and along the 120° meridian,

$$d = \frac{\varepsilon}{F} = \frac{2.35}{2} = 1.18 \text{ cm.}$$

8. Draw a second diagram (Figure 4–40), and again construct vertical and horizontal lines that intersect the two principal meridians (30° and 120°) at point R.

9. Using a convenient scale, lay off the decentration along each principal meridian such that

RP = 0.7067 cm along 210° meridian,

and

RQ = 1.18 cm along the 210° meridian.

10. Complete the rectangle QRPO, the corner O representing the position of the required optical center.

11. Drop perpendiculars from point O to the horizontal meridian (point T) and to the vertical meridian (point S).

12. The lengths of line segments RT and RS represent the amounts of horizontal and vertical decentration, respectively:

$$RS = y = 0.72 \text{ cm upward,}$$

and

$$RT = x = 1.22 \text{ cm inward.}$$

MATHEMATIC METHOD. In Section 4.14, the total horizontal prismatic effect at a point in the periphery of a sphero-cylindrical lens was given by the expression

$$\text{total horizontal prism} = \varepsilon_{hs} + \varepsilon_{hc}$$

or

$$\varepsilon_h = xF_s + F_c(y\cos\theta + x\sin\theta)\sin\theta \qquad (4.22)$$

and the total vertical prismatic effect at a point in the periphery was given by the expression

$$\text{total vertical prism} = \varepsilon_{vs} + \varepsilon_{vc}$$

or

$$\varepsilon_v = yF_s + F_c(y\cos\theta + x\sin\theta)\cos\theta. \qquad (4.23)$$

The letters y and x are the vertical and horizontal decentrations of the optical center from the geometric center required to produce the specific prism at the prism reference point, R. Equations 4.22 and 4.23 can be expanded as follows:

$$\varepsilon_h = yF_c\sin\theta\cos\theta + x(F_s + F_c\sin^2\theta) \qquad (4.24)$$

and

$$\varepsilon_v = y(F_s + F_c\cos^2\theta) + xF_c\sin\theta\cos\theta, \qquad (4.25)$$

These expressions form a pair of simultaneous equations. Solving these equations simultaneously or by transformation, we find that

$$x = \frac{\varepsilon_h F_s + \varepsilon_h F_c\cos^2\theta - \varepsilon_v F_c\sin\theta\cos\theta}{F_s(F_s + F_c)} \qquad (4.26)$$

and

$$y = \frac{\varepsilon_v F_s + \varepsilon_v F_c\sin^2\theta - \varepsilon_h F_c\sin\theta\cos\theta}{F_s(F_s + F_c)}. \qquad (4.27)$$

Note that the sign convention developed in Section 4.14 is used in Equations 4.26 and 4.27. The angle θ is measured from the nasal side of the lens temporally to the axis; ε_h is positive for base-out and negative for base-in; and ε_v is positive for base-up and negative for base-down. When y is positive, the decentration is up; when y is negative, the decentration is down. When y is positive, the decentration is out; when x is negative, the decentration is in.

The mathematic method is now used as an alternate method of solving the above example: Given a left lens with the formula +3.00 DS –1.00 DC axis 30. In what direction, and how much, must the lens be decentered to produce, at the prism reference point, 1 prism diopter base-up and 3 prism diopters base-in?

$$y = \frac{\varepsilon_v F_s + \varepsilon_v F_c \sin^2\theta - \varepsilon_h F_c \sin\theta \cos\theta}{F_s(F_s + F_c)}$$

$$= \frac{(1)(3) + (1)(-1)\sin^2 150 - (-3)(-1)\sin 150 \cos 150}{+3(3-1)}$$

$$= \frac{3 + (-0.25) + 1.299}{6} = \frac{4.049}{6} = 0.675 \text{ cm (upward).}$$

$$x = \frac{\varepsilon_h F_s + \varepsilon_h F_c \cos^2\theta - \varepsilon_v F_c \sin\theta \cos\theta}{F_s(F_s + F_c)}$$

$$= \frac{(-3)(3) + (-3)(-1)\cos^2 150 - (1)(-1)\sin 150 \cos 150}{+3(3-1)}$$

$$= \frac{-9 + 2.25 - 0.433}{6} = \frac{-7.183}{6} = -1.197 \text{ cm (inward).}$$

4.16. Effects of Prisms on the Eyes

The effects that prisms have on the eyes, already referred to in Section 4.5, may be understood by performing a number of experiments with prisms. Either trial case prisms or square plastic prisms may be used.

EXPERIMENT 1

Occlude one eye. While you look at a distant object (such as a letter on a Snellen chart), place a 10 prism diopter prism, base-down, in front of your open eye. This brings about the situation shown in Figure 4–41. Light rays from the object are deviated toward the base of the prism, with the result that the object appears to be displaced toward the *apex* of the prism. If you choose to keep looking at the object, your eye *must* move upward. Indeed, it is difficult *not* to allow the eye to move upward. If someone else looks behind the occluder, he or she will see that your occluded eye *also* moves upward. This is a *conjugate* movement, that is, a movement in which both eyes move in the same direction.

EXPERIMENT 2

Repeat Experiment 1, but with both eyes open. Diplopia (double vision) will occur. You will be able to look at either the upper or the lower image of the object, but you will be unable to fuse them into one.

EXPERIMENT 3

Repeat this experiment, again with both eyes open, but with only a 2 prism diopter prism, base-down. Although you may briefly see double, the images will quickly coalesce into one because a *vertical fusional vergence* movement has been made. The eye seeing through the prism turns upward to keep the images on the foveas of each eye. Since the visual system's ability to make vertical fusional vergence movements is not very great, any prism stronger than 3 or 4 prism diopters (base-down or base-up) usually results in diplopia, as in Experiment 2. A vergence movement, in which one eye turns in one direction and the other eye makes no movement or moves in the opposite direction, is called a *disjunctive* movement.

EXPERIMENT 4

With both eyes open, while watching a distant object, place a 5 prism diopter prism, base-out, in front of each eye (Figure 4–42). Although the distant object may blur slightly, it will remain single because the eyes make a *positive fusional vergence* movement (A). This, again, is a disjunctive movement, since the eyes move in opposite directions (one to the right, the other to the left). The object may appear to blur because the accommodative mechanism has been stimulated to maintain single binocular vision.

EXPERIMENT 5

Repeat Experiment 4 but with the prism oriented in the base-in direction (Figure 4–42B). Since 10 prism diopters is about the maximum amount of *negative fusional vergence* (fusional divergence) of which the eyes are capable, you will probably see double in this experiment. If you continue to see single, repeat the experiment with stronger prisms (e.g., 7 or 8 prism diopters for each eye). Diplopia will most likely occur.

EXPERIMENT 6

Again while looking at a distant object, place a 5 prism diopter prism in front of each eye with the bases in the same direction—first with both bases to the right, then with both bases to the left, and then with both bases up and again with both bases down. In each case, single vision remains because the eyes make a *conjugate* movement (to the left with base-to-the-right prism, and to the right with base-to-the-left prism, downward with base-up, or upward with base-down).

Summarizing, there are two kinds of eye movements that can occur when prisms are used: (1) conjugate

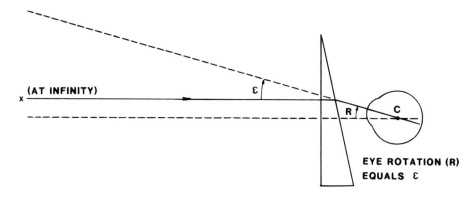

FIGURE 4–41. **A 10 prism diopter prism, base-down, causes light rays to be deviated toward the base of the prism, with the result that the object appears to be displaced toward the apex.**

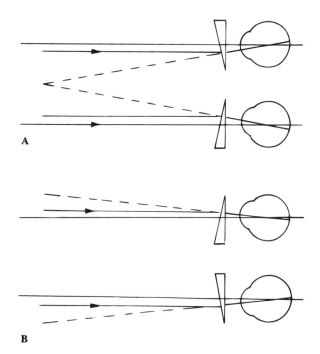

B

FIGURE 4–42. **A, a 5 prism diopter, base-out prism in front of each eye causes the eyes to make a positive fusional vergence movement; B, a 5 prism diopter, base-in prism in front of each eye causes the eyes to make a negative fusional vergence movement.**

movements (also called *version movements*), in which both eyes move in the same direction, and (2) disjunctive movements (also called *vergence movements*), in which the two eyes move in opposite directions.

4.17. Effectivity of a Prism

We can speak of the effectivity (or *effective power*) of a prism, just as we can talk about the effective power of a lens. As a lens is moved away from the eye its effective power increases (for a plus lens) or decreases (for a minus lens) (discussed in Chapter 3). When we speak of the effectivity of a prism, we are concerned with the *angular rotation* of the eye (inward, outward, upward, or downward) in relation to the power of the prism.

The effectivity of a prism for a distant object is illustrated in Figure 4–43. As shown in this diagram (A), the rotation of the eye (R) is equal to the angle of deviation of the prism (ε), with the result that, for distance fixation, there is no loss in effectivity.

The situation existing for near vision is shown in Figure 4–43B. As shown in this diagram, angle R is smaller than angle ε, so the prism has lost effectivity. Note that, in this diagram, h represents the distance between the prism and the center of rotation for the eye, and p represents the distance from the prism to the object of regard. A formula for determining the effectivity of a prism, when used for near vision, may be derived as follows:

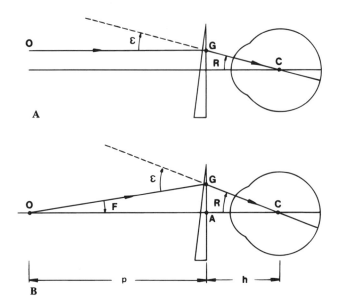

A

B

FIGURE 4–43. **Diagram for use in deriving the formula for the effectivity of a prism. Note that for a distant object, A, there is no loss of effectivity; for a near object, B, a loss of effectivity occurs.**

$$\text{angle } \varepsilon = \text{angle } R + \text{angle } F$$
$$\text{angle } F = \text{angle } \varepsilon - \text{angle } R$$
$$\tan R = \frac{\overline{AG}}{h}, \text{ and } \tan F = \frac{\overline{AG}}{p}$$
$$\overline{AG} = h \tan R = p \tan F$$
$$hR = pF \text{ (for small angles only)}$$
$$F = \frac{hR}{p}.$$

Substituting $\varepsilon - R$ for F,

$$\varepsilon = R + \frac{hR}{p}.$$
$$\varepsilon = R(1 + h/p)$$
$$= R(p + h)$$
$$R = \frac{\varepsilon p}{(p + h)}. \tag{4.28}$$

EXAMPLE
What is the effectivity of a prism of 15 prism diopters located 25 mm in front of the center of rotation of the eye, when the wearer reads at a distance of 40 cm from the prism?

$$R = \frac{15(0.40)}{0.40 + 0.025}$$
$$= \frac{6}{0.425}$$
$$= 14.12 \text{ prism diopters.}$$

The prism, therefore, has lost approximately 1 prism diopter of effectivity. Since prisms are usually prescribed in powers of no more than a few prism diopters, this loss of effectivity, for near vision, usually presents no problem. It does, however, assume some importance for rotating prisms used in refractors or phoroptors, since these prisms are used in powers exceeding 15 prism diopters. Also, the value of h is greater for refractors and phoroptors than for a spectacle lens, since Risley prisms are located several millimeters in front of the lens apertures. If the object is located at infinity, R is equal to ε. If h approaches zero in value, the value of R approaches that of ε.

4.18. Risley Prisms

Risley prisms, also called *rotary prisms*, are prisms used in refractors or phoroptors to measure phorias and fusional vergences. Each Risley prism is made up of two prisms, one behind the other, which are geared so that they rotate together when a knurled knob is turned. The carrier in which the two prisms are mounted may be positioned with the knurled knob oriented either vertically or horizontally. When the knob is oriented vertically (as shown in Figure 4–44), *base-in* or *base-out* prism power is introduced; when the knob is oriented horizontally, *base-up* or *base-down* prism is introduced.

When the knob is oriented vertically and is turned so that the scale reading is zero (as in Figure 4–45), one of the prisms is oriented in the base-in position and the other is oriented in the base-out position, so that no horizontal prismatic

effect is present (A). When the knob is turned in the *base-in* direction, the prisms rotate in opposite directions (one clockwise, the other counterclockwise), but both bases rotate in a *nasalward* direction and cause the desired base-in effect. Similarly, when the knob is turned in the *base-out* direction, the prisms again rotate in opposite directions, but in such a way that both bases move *temporally* and cause a base-out effect. As shown in (B) and (C), in the two extreme positions, after a rotation of 90 degrees for each prism, a maximum amount of base-in or base-out prismatic effect is obtained; if each prism has a power of 15 prism diopters, the maximum achievable effect is 30 prism diopters. The same applies, of course, for the introduction of base-up or base-down prism.

In Figure 4–46, P_1 and P_2 represent the positions of the base-apex lines of the two prisms as base-in or base-out prism power is introduced. If the length of the line P_1 (or P_2) is equal to the power of 1 prism unit, the length of the line ε_h indicates the power of a prism unit for that position of the base-apex line. For example, when P_1 is oriented vertically, $\varepsilon_h = 0$, but when P_1 is oriented horizontally, $\varepsilon_h = P_1$. For any position of P_1 and P_2 *for each prism,*

$$\varepsilon_h = P \sin\theta, \qquad (4.29)$$

and the deviation for *both* prisms can be represented by

$$2\varepsilon_h = P_1 \sin\theta + P_2 \sin\theta$$
$$= (P_1 + P_2)(\sin\theta),$$

FIGURE 4–44. **Risley prisms oriented vertically so that base-in or base-out prism power can be introduced.**

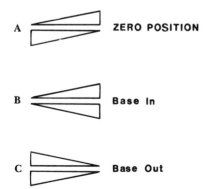

FIGURE 4–45 **Introduction of horizontal prism. A, no prismatic effect; B, maximum base-in effect; C, maximum base-out effect.**

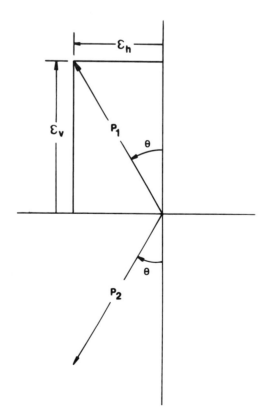

FIGURE 4–46. **Diagram for derivation of the formula for the deviation caused by a pair of Risley prisms.**

since

$$P_1 = P_2,$$

$$2\varepsilon_h = 2P\sin\theta. \qquad (4.30)$$

As for the vertical prismatic effect, ε_v, for any position of the prisms, the values of ε_v are equal for the two prisms, but opposite in direction. These values, therefore, cancel each other, so the only resulting prismatic effect is base-in or base-out.

The same principle applies, of course, to the use of Risley prisms in producing vertical prismatic effects. With the knob oriented horizontally, the amount of base-up or base-down prismatic effect that is introduced is given by the equation

$$2\varepsilon_v = 2P\sin\theta, \qquad (4.31)$$

with the lateral components canceling each other.

4.19. Fresnel Press-on Prisms

In 1970, the Optical Sciences Group of San Rafael, California, developed a series of *Fresnel Press-on prisms*—thin, plastic, membrane prisms ranging in powers from 0.5 to 30 prism diopters. These prisms are an adaptation of the hand-ground lenses designed by the French engineer and physicist Augustine Fresnel in 1821. Fresnel's lenses were originally used for lighthouse beacons. Since refraction occurs only at the surface of an optical element and depends primarily on the angle between the two surfaces, the intervening (nonrefracting) portion of a conventional optical element can be removed without appreciably affecting the refracting power. The angle between the two surfaces remains constant across the prism.

The Fresnel Press-on prism consists of a series of identical small plastic prisms lying parallel and adjacent to each other on a thin plastic base membrane (Figure 4–47). Each small prism (B) has the same deviation power as the conventional prism shown in (A). However, the Fresnel Press-on prism is only 1 mm thick, or about one-tenth the thickness of a solid conventional prism of the same power.

Fresnel Press-on prisms are made of a specially formulated plasticized polyvinyl chloride (PVC) material with a refractive index of 1.525, very close to that of ophthalmic crown glass. The prisms are manufactured by a process of injection or compression molding, using molds cut usually from brass. Only one surface of the membrane is impressed with the prismatic grooves; the other surface is flat. The resulting flat surface of the thin flexible membrane can be applied without adhesive material to the back surface of a conventional glass lens.

The prisms are designed for in-office application. First, the membrane is cut to conform to the size and shape of the lens. Then it is applied to the back surface of the lens while the lens and membrane are immersed in water. After drying, the membrane is highly adherent to the glass surface and can be removed only by immersing the lens in water and peeling off the membrane.

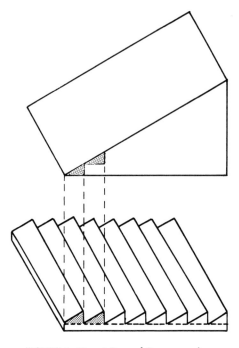

FIGURE 4–47.   **A Fresnel Press-on prism.**

Press-on prisms can be used clinically as a permanent correction—for example, as a substitute for conventional prisms when the required prism power is not available or is subject to a long delay. However, these prisms are applied most commonly for temporary use, such as in diagnosing a binocular vision problem or as an aid in orthoptic training. They are also useful when an oculomotor condition varies with time—in a situation in which the amount of prism required may undergo frequent changes.

The greatest advantages of Press-on prisms are their thinness, their lightness of weight, and their in-office application. Their disadvantages include a slight loss of visual acuity and contrast (for the wearer) and the striated appearance (to observers) of the grooves.

There are a number of reasons for loss in visual acuity. As with conventional prisms, Fresnel prisms suffer from *distortion* and *chromatic aberration*. A comparison of distortion for conventional prisms and for Fresnel prisms has been made by Adams et al.[2] They broke the complex aberration of distortion into five simple distortions:

1. Horizontal magnification
2. Vertical magnification
3. Curvature of vertical lines
4. Asymmetric horizontal magnification
5. Change in vertical magnification with horizontal angle

They found that the Fresnel membrane prisms produced substantially less horizontal and vertical magnification and slightly less curvature of vertical lines than the conventional prisms. Conventional prisms demonstrated slightly less asymmetric horizontal magnification and change of vertical magnification with horizontal angle than the Fresnel prisms.

A second source of visual acuity loss is *scattering of light*, caused by the grooves. The scattering of light causes both a loss of contrast and the presence of bothersome reflections. The most important factor determining resolution is the width of the grooves. Resolution improves with decreasing groove width, but if the grooves are *too* narrow, diffraction becomes a problem. The striated appearance can be improved to some extent by use of a lightly tinted or photochromic lens.

When a prismatic component is to be included in a patient's prescription, the advantages and disadvantages of Press-on prisms should be carefully weighed to determine the suitability of using Press-on prisms.

References

1. *American National Standard for Ophthalmics: Prescription Ophthalmic Lenses—Recommendations.* ANSI Z80.1-1995. American National Standards Institute, New York, 1995.
2. Adams, A. J., Kapash, R. J., and Barkan, E. Visual Performance and Optical Properties of Fresnel Membrane Prisms. *Am. J. Optom. Arch. Am. Acad. Optom.*, Vol. 48, pp. 289–297, 1971.

Questions

1. What is the refracting angle of a prism of 1 prism diopter having the following indices of refraction?
   (a) 1.42
   (b) 1.53
2. Compute the prismatic power in the 60th meridian of a prism of 3 prism diopters, base at 90°.
3. A patient wears +2.00 DC x 180, with the cylinder axis passing through the geometric center. During reading, the patient's lines of sight pass through the lens 10 mm down and 2 mm in from the geometric center of the lens. What is the prismatic effect?
4. Compute the equivalent prism for the following combinations of prisms:
   (a) OD 2 prism diopters, base-out/4 prism diopters, base-down
   (b) OS 2 prism diopters, base-up/1 prism diopters, base-in.
5. Compute the horizontal and vertical components of the following prisms:
   (a) OD 3 prism diopters, base at 30°
   (b) OS 2 prism diopters, base at 240°.
6. A Risley prism consisting of two prisms of 12 prism diopters is mounted before a patient's eye. Each prism is rotated 30° from the zero position. What is the prismatic effect obtained in front of the eye?
7. The refracting angle of a prism is 8° and the index of refraction is 1.55. What deviation does it produce, in degrees, for a pencil of light from infinity?
8. The refracting angle of a prism is 10° and the index of refraction is 1.65. What is the deviation in prism diopters produced for a pencil of light from infinity?

9. Compute the horizontal and vertical prismatic effects for a point located 12 mm below and 2 mm in from the geometric center of each of the following lenses:
   (a) OD +3.00 DS
   (b) OS –2.00 DC x 90
   (c) OD +2.00 DC x 180
10. Calculate the vertical and horizontal prismatic effects for the given points on the following lenses:
    (a) 10 down and 2 in: OD +5.00 DS/–2.00 DC x 45
    (b) 10 down and 5 out: lens same as in (a)
    (c) 5 up and 5 in: OS –5.00 DS/+2.00 DC x 120.
11. A prescription is as follows:
    OD –2.50 DS
    OS +2.00 DS/–5.00 DC x 30.
    If the reading points are 10 mm below and 3 mm in each from the distance optical centers, what are the vertical and horizontal prismatic imbalances for each eye at the reading level?
12. The pole of a finished lens is located 5 mm directly below point A and 10 mm nasalward of point B. Point A has a prismatic power of 2 prism diopters base-up and point B has a prismatic power of 3 prism diopters base-in. What is the refracting power (R_x) of this lens?
13. When a patient looks through a point 6 mm above the optical center of one of his spectacle lenses at an object 6 m away, he discovers that the image of the object is displaced 12 cm upward. On looking through a point 8 mm to his left of the optical center at the same object, the image is displaced 24 cm to his right. What is the refracting power (R_x) of the above lens?
14. If a 15-prism diopter lens is placed 25 mm in front of the center of rotation of the patient's eye, what is the actual rotation made by the eye when the person views an object 20 cm from the prism?
15. Given:
    OD +2.00 DS with 1 prism diopter, base-in
    OS +4.00 DS with 1 prism diopter, base-in
    frame size = 48 mm
    DBL = 20 mm
    PD = 62 mm.
    After the lens is cut, the decentration is found to be 8 mm in on the right lens. Where is the prism reference point on the right lens located?
16. If a +6.00 D lens (index = 1.50) has been decentered in 4 mm and the horizontal box size of the finished lens is 56 mm, what is the difference in edge thickness along the horizontal meridian?
17. A prescription of +4.00 D is made up into a lens with an effective diameter of 50 mm. If the unfinished blank is 60 mm, what is the maximum prismatic effect obtainable by decentration at the geometric center of the finished lens?
18. Given the following:
    a right lens = +6.00 D
    index of refraction = 1.5
    size of lens = 50.0 mm round
    nasal thickness = 1.0 mm
    temporal thickness = 2.8 mm

edge thickness at the 90° meridian = edge thickness at the 270° meridian.

In relation to the geometric center, where is the horizontal location of the pole?

19. A frame has the following boxed dimensions:
    horizontal (A) = 54 mm
    vertical (B) = 48 mm
    effective diameter (ED) = 59 mm
    DBL = 16 mm
    If the patient's PD is 64 mm, what is the minimum blank size required if no allowance is made for cutting and edging operations?

20. The R_x:
    OD –2.50 DS/1 prism diopter, base-out
    OS +5.00 DS/1 prism diopter, base-out
    The prism is obtained by decentration:
    PD = 60/56 mm
    DBL = 20 mm
    horizontal box size = 42 mm
    What is the decentration (amount and direction) of the right and left lenses, respectively?

21. A single-vision, uncut +3.00-D sphere, 60 mm round, with knife edges, is decentered to produce 3 prism diopters, base-out before the left eye. The index of refraction is 1.50. What is the approximate thickness at the prism reference point?

22. Two finished lenses ($n = 1.50$) have a power of +5.00 D, a round shape with a diameter of 60 mm, and a 1-mm minimum edge thickness. During surfacing and finishing, lens A was not decentered, but lens B was decentered 4 mm in. Assuming spherical surfaces, what is the thickness at the geometric center of lens A in comparison to that of lens B?

23. A tangent scale is constructed to measure prism diopters at 100 cm. If this scale is moved to 80 cm to obtain the correct dioptral value of the prism, the reading must be multiplied by what factor?

24. A patient wears a lens on the left eye of +2.00 DS – 4.00 DC x 135. What is the prismatic effect induced when the patient looks 1 cm straight up from the optical center?

25. Two thin prisms are crossed with their bases at an angle of 60 degrees to each other. The first produces a deviation of 3 prism diopters and the second a deviation of 5 prism diopters. What is the deviation in prism diopters produced by the combination?

CHAPTER FIVE

The Correction of Ametropia

The first four chapters of this text considered ophthalmic lenses with little or no reference to particular eyes for which the lenses were intended. Although a detailed presentation of the optical system of the human eye is more suitable for a textbook on physiological optics, this chapter discusses the concepts and principles involved in the use of lenses for the correction of ametropia ("correction" is misleading; neither ophthalmic lenses nor contact lenses "correct" ametropia—the term compensate is more appropriate).

The power of a lens for the compensation of ametropia depends not only on the optical properties of the eye (specifically, the location of the "far point" of the eye), but also on the distance between the correcting lens and the eye. The required lens power, therefore, may change significantly when an ametrope is compensated for with contact lenses rather than glasses. A discussion of the use of lenses for the compensation of ametropia requires a discussion of *accommodation*. The phrase "with accommodation at rest" is an integral part of any definition of emmetropia or ametropia. Thus, emmetropia, myopia, and hyperopia are defined in terms of the positions of the *far point of accommodation* and the *near point of accommodation*. The accommodative state of the eye varies with the mode of correction (glasses vs. contact lenses), varies from one eye to the other with anisometropia, and varies in the two principal meridians of the eye with astigmatism.

An additional concept in a discussion of the correction of ametropia with lenses is the change in retinal image size brought about by the correcting lens. The change in retinal image size is of little consequence when spherical ametropia is about the same amount for both eyes, but it can often become a significant problem when astigmatism or anisometropia is present.

5.1. The Schematic Eye

The refractive state of a given eye is determined by the values of the individual refractive components of the eye and their relationships with one another. Refractive components are corneal refracting power, anterior chamber depth, lens refracting power, and the axial length of the eye. The values of refractive components are determined by their radii of curvature (in the case of the cornea and the lens) and by their indices of refraction. For the healthy eye, the indices are thought to show little variation from one eye to another, but the radii of curvature of the cornea and the lens, as well as the anterior chamber depth and the axial length of the eye, are known to vary widely from one eye to another.

The refractive components of the eye and its focal points, principal points, and nodal points are generally characterized in terms of a *schematic eye*. Such "paper and pencil" eyes are useful in performing a number of calculations relative to the optics of the eye and are particularly useful for calculations involving *magnification*.

Although a large number of schematic eyes have been designed, the best known, and most detailed, is the "exact" schematic eye (Figure 5–1) designed by Gullstrand.[1] This schematic eye differs from others by stipulating indices of refraction and radii of curvature for both the nucleus and the cortex of the lens, and by representing the cornea as having both front and back surfaces. Gullstrand supplied values for all constants of this eye, in both the unaccommodated and the accommodated state. Representative values, in the unaccommodated state, are given in Table 5–1. As shown in Figure 5–1, the principal planes of this eye are located just behind the cornea, and the nodal planes straddle the posterior surface of the lens. The total refracting power of the eye is 58.64 D, and the refractive state is 1.00 D of hyperopia.

Gullstrand's "simplified" schematic eye, shown in Figure 5–2, represents the lens as having just one pair of refracting surfaces and a single index of refraction. In addition, it represents the cornea as having a single refracting surface and the radius of the anterior surface increased slightly to compensate for the small amount of refraction that would occur at its posterior surface. The constants of this eye are shown in Table 5–2; the index of refraction of the aqueous and vitreous are the same as those given for the exact schematic eye (1.336), but the index of refraction of the lens (1.413) is greater than that for either the nucleus or the cortex of the lens for the "exact" schematic eye. One advantage of the simplified eye is that the values of many of its components are easy to remember—the radii of curvature of the cornea and the two lens surfaces are, respectively, 7.8, 10.0, and 8.0 mm, and the anterior chamber depth and the lens thickness are both 3.6 mm. Convenient numbers for the anterior focal length of the eye (measured from the cornea) and the axial length of the eye are, re-

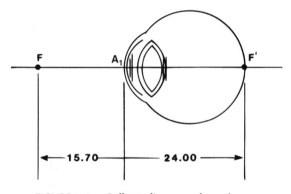

FIGURE 5–1.   **Gullstrand's exact schematic eye.**

TABLE 5–1
Schematic Eye Data (Unaccommodated)

		Gullstrand's Exact Schematic Eye	Gullstrand's Simplified Schematic Eye
Indices	Cornea	1.376	—
	Aqueous	1.336	1.336
	Lens cortex	1.386	—
	Lens nucleus	1.406	1.413
	Vitreous	1.336	1.336
Positions	Cornea, anterior	0	0
	Cornea, posterior	0.5 mm	—
	Lens, anterior	3.6 mm	3.6 mm
	Lens, posterior	7.2 mm	7.2 mm
Radii	Cornea, anterior	7.7 mm	7.8 mm
	Cornea, posterior	6.8 mm	—
	Lens, anterior	10.0 mm	10.0 mm
	Lens, posterior	–6.0 mm	–6.0 mm
Powers	Cornea	43.05 D	42.74 D
	Lens	19.11 D	21.76 D
	Complete eye	58.64 D	60.48 D
Focal points	Anterior (A_1F)	–15.70 mm	–14.99 mm
	Posterior (A_1F')	24.38 mm	23.90 mm
Axial length		24.00 mm	23.90 mm

SOURCE: Adapted from H. H. Emsley, *Visual Optics*, Vol. 1, Hatton Press, London, 1963, pp. 343–348.

TABLE 5–2
Principal Point and Nodal Point Data for Gullstrand's Simplified Schematic Eye*

		Unaccommodated Eye (mm)	*Accommodated Eye (mm)*
Principal points	A_1P	1.6	1.8
	A_1P'	1.9	2.1
	F_1P	16.6	14.4
Nodal points	A_1N	7.1	6.6
	A_1N'	7.4	7.0

* Data rounded to first decimal place.
SOURCE: Adapted from H. H. Emsley, *Visual Optics*, Vol. 1, Hatton Press, London, 1963, p. 436.

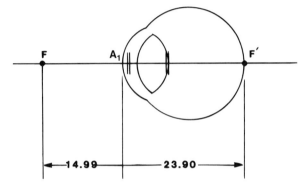

FIGURE 5–2. **Gullstrand's simplified schematic eye.**

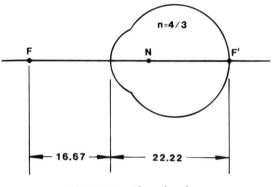

FIGURE 5–3. **The reduced eye.**

spectively, 15 and 24 mm, and the total refracting power of the eye can be considered as 60 D (even though the value given for the exact schematic eye is somewhat less than this amount and that given for the simplified schematic eye is somewhat more).

The "reduced eye," shown in Figure 5–3, is further simplified. The total refraction of the reduced eye is considered to take place at the front surface of the cornea, located about 2 mm behind the "real" cornea (actually the location of a single principal point), and the eye is considered to have a single nodal point located about 7 mm behind the "real" cornea.

5.2. Emmetropia and Ametropia

In a discussion of ametropia, consideration is given to a single eye and accommodation is assumed to be at rest, with the result that the refractive power (or vergence) of the eye is at its minimum value.

An *emmetropic* eye is one in which, with accommodation at rest, infinity and the retina are conjugate points, that is, one in which parallel incident rays of light come to a focus on the retina. A standard emmetropic eye (such as Gullstrand's schematic eye) has a standard refractive power and a standard axial length. As shown in Figure 5–4, emmetropia may result when an eye has (1) a standard refractive power and a standard axial length, (2) an excessive refractive power and a shorter than normal axial length, or (3) a deficient refractive power and an excessive axial length.

An *ametropic* eye is defined as an eye in which, with accommodation at rest, infinity and the retina are *not* conjugate, or as one in which parallel rays of light fail to come to a focus on the retina. If parallel rays of light focus in front of the retina, the eye is *myopic;* if they focus behind the retina, the eye is *hyperopic.*

An eye with *axial ametropia* (Figure 5–5) is one that has the standard refractive power but an axial length that is either too long, having axial myopia (A), or too short, having axial hyperopia (B). An eye having *refractive ametropia* (Figure 5–6) is one that has the "standard" axial length but one of the refractive components (the cornea or the crystalline lens) provides either excessive refractive power, which results in refractive myopia (A), or too little refractive power, which results in refractive hyperopia (B). The distinction between axial and refractive ametropia may best be understood by considering the eye as having two lengths: the *axial* length (the physical length of the eyeball) and the *focal length* of the eye's optical system, that is, the distance from the secondary principal plane to the secondary focal plane of the eye. The two lengths are shown in Figure 5–7.

If both the axial length of the eye and the secondary focal length of the eye's optical system correspond to those of the schematic eye, the eye is emmetropic (although Gullstrand's "exact" schematic eye has 1.00 D of hyperopia, we are considering the schematic eye emmetropic). If the axial length of the eye is shorter or longer than that of the schematic eye and the secondary focal length corresponds to that of the schematic eye, the eye has *axial* hyperopia or myopia, respectively. If the axial length of the eye in question corresponds to that of the schematic eye, but the focal length of the optical system is ei-

FIGURE 5–4.   **Emmetropic eyes.**

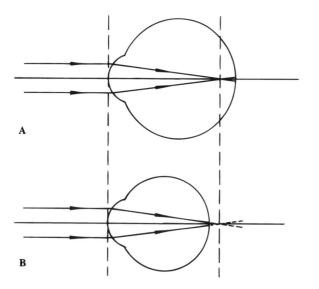

FIGURE 5–5.   **A, axial myopia; B, axial hyperopia.**

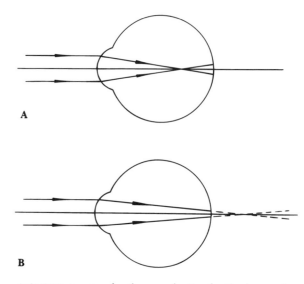

FIGURE 5–6.   **A, refractive myopia; B, refractive hyperopia.**

ther longer or shorter than that of the schematic eye, the eye has *refractive* hyperopia or myopia, respectively.

The terms axial and refractive ametropia are, to a great extent, only abstractions. Sorsby et al. found[2] that emmetropic eyes have a wide range of axial lengths, corneal retracting powers, and lens refracting powers. They also found that although eyes having ametropia up to about ±4.00 D have axial lengths within the same range as those of emmetropic eyes, eyes having ametropia in excess of ±4.00 D almost always have axial lengths outside the emmetropic range. Therefore, eyes that have low refractive errors can be considered as having a *combination* of axial and refractive ametropia, and eyes with high refractive errors (particularly those well above ±4.00 D) can be considered as having relatively pure *axial* ametropia.

A point of confusion sometimes arises in designating the refractive error of a given eye. Because a myopic eye has an excessive amount of refractive power in relation to its axial length, a myopic eye is sometimes considered to be a *plus* eye (requiring a minus lens). A hyperopic eye is deficient in refractive power in relation to its axial length and is considered a *minus* eye (requiring a plus lens). Most writers make clear whether they are referring to a myopic eye or a hyperopic eye, but stating that an eye "has a refractive error of +3.00 D" is ambiguous because that could mean either that the eye has an excess of refractive power of 3.00 D (and is therefore myopic) or that the eye requires for its correction a +3.00-D lens (and is therefore hyperopic). Such ambiguity can be avoided by stating that an eye has "3.00 D of myopia" or "3.00 D of hyperopia." In any event, the context in which the terminology is used usually makes clear the meaning.

5.3. The Far and Near Points of Accommodation

Accommodation may be defined as the adjustment of the optical system of the eye for vision at various distances, which results in the retina being conjugate to the object of

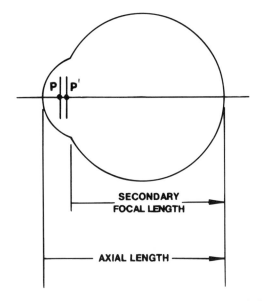

FIGURE 5–7.   **The axial length (physical length) of the eyeball compared with the secondary focal length of the eye's optical system.**

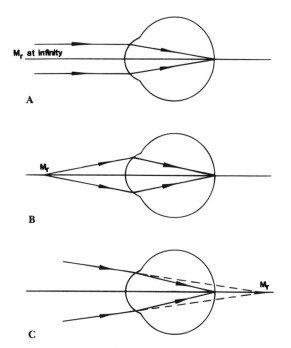

FIGURE 5–8.   **Far point of accommodation. A, for an emmetropic eye; B, for an uncorrected myopic eye; C, for an uncorrected hyperopic eye.**

regard. The *far point of accommodation* (punctum remotum, or M_r) is defined as the object point that is conjugate with the retina when accommodation is fully relaxed, in which case an object placed at the far point will be imaged on the retina. As shown in Figure 5–8, the far point of accommodation for an emmetropic eye is at infinity (A), the far point of accommodation for an uncorrected myopic eye is a *real* object point in front of the eye (B), and the far point of accommodation for an uncorrected hyperopic eye is a *virtual* object point located behind the eye (C).

The *near point of accommodation* (punctum proximum, or M_p) is defined as the object point that is conjugate to the retina with accommodation fully in play. As shown in Figure 5–9, for both an emmetropic eye (A) and an uncorrected my-

opic eye (B), the near point of accommodation is a real object point located in front of the eye; for an uncorrected hyperopic eye (C), the near point of accommodation may be either a real object point located in front of the eye or a virtual object point located behind the eye (depending on the amount of hyperopia and the amplitude of accommodation).

The amount of hyperopia that falls within the range of the patient's accommodation is known as *facultative* hyperopia; the amount of hyperopia that cannot be overcome by accommodation is called *absolute* hyperopia.

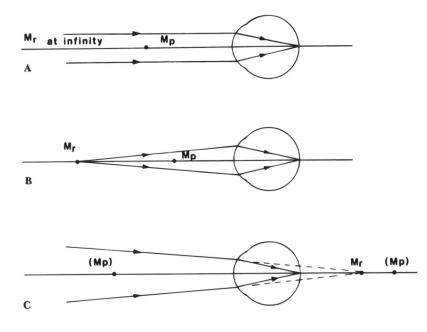

FIGURE 5–9.   **Near point of accommodation. A, for an emmetropic eye; B, for an uncorrected myopic eye; C, for an uncorrected hyperopic eye.**

5.4. The Correction of Spherical Ametropia

The function of a correcting lens, whether for myopia or hyperopia, is to artificially place the far point of the eye at infinity, with the result that infinity (rather than a real object point in front of the eye or a virtual object point behind the eye) is conjugate to the retina. For this to occur, the secondary focal point of the correcting lens must coincide with the far point of the eye. As shown in Figure 5–10, for a myopic eye (A) both the far point of the eye and the secondary focal point of the correcting lens are located *in front of* the eye. For a hyperopic eye (B) both the far point of the eye and the secondary focal point of the correcting lens are located *behind* the eye. (As mentioned earlier, the term "compensate" is more appropriate.) As also shown in Figure 5–10, the correcting spectacle lens is placed in a plane known as the *spectacle plane*, considered to be located at or near the primary focal plane of the eye (which, for Gullstrand's exact schematic eye, is 15 mm in front of the corneal apex). However, the correcting lens is more often placed *closer* to the eye than the primary focal plane, in which case the focal length for a minus lens must be longer (a lens of weaker power), and the focal length for a plus lens must be shorter (a lens of stronger power). Thus, the *effective power* of the lens is changed. As discussed in Chapter 3, Section 3.5, the change in effective power of a lens, as it is moved closer to the eye, can be determined by comparing the focal lengths without the use of a formula or by the use of the effective power formula given in Equation 3.7.

Correction of myopia and hyperopia by the use of spherical lenses is illustrated by the following examples and Figure 5–11:

EXAMPLE 1
An uncorrected myope has a far point of accommodation located 26.5 cm in front of the corneal plane. What is the required power of the correcting lens if the lens is to be located (1) 15 mm in front of the corneal apex; (2) 10 mm in front of the corneal apex? (Figure 5–11A.)

(1) The power of the correcting lens placed 15 mm from the corneal apex is the reciprocal of the secondary focal length of the lens.

$$f' = 0.265 \text{ m} - 0.015 \text{ m} = -0.25 \text{ m}.$$

$$F = \frac{1}{-0.25} = -4.00 \text{ D}.$$

(2) The focal length of the lens, if located 10 mm in front of the corneal apex, is

$$f' = -0.265 \text{ m} - 0.010 \text{ m} = -0.255 \text{ m}$$

and

$$F = \frac{1}{-0.255} = -3.92 \text{ D}.$$

Alternatively, Example 1 may be solved as an effectivity problem, with use of Equation 3.16, and a change in d of 5 mm.

$$F_B = \frac{F_A}{1 - dF_B} = \frac{-4.00}{1 - 0.005(-4.00)} = -3.92 \text{ D}.$$

EXAMPLE 2
An uncorrected hyperopic eye has a far point of accommodation located 18.5 cm behind the corneal apex. What is the required power of a correcting lens located (1) 15 mm in front of the corneal apex; (2) 20 mm in front of the corneal apex? (Figure 5-11B.)

(1) The power of the correcting lens, placed 15 mm from the corneal apex, is the reciprocal of the secondary focal length of the lens.

$$f' = 0.185 \text{ m} + 0.015 \text{ m} = +0.20 \text{ m}.$$

$$F = \frac{1}{+0.20} = +5.00 \text{ D}.$$

(2) The focal length of the correcting lens, for a 20-mm fitting distance, is

$$f' = 0.185 \text{ m} + 0.020 \text{ m} = +0.205 \text{ m}$$

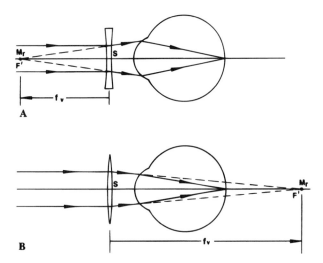

FIGURE 5–10.   Correction of ametropia. A, myopia; B, hyperopia.

FIGURE 5–11.   The effective power of a lens. A, the correction of a myopic eye and B, of a hyperopic eye with lenses located at two different distances from the corneal apex.

and

$$F = \frac{1}{+0.205} = +4.88 \text{ D.}$$

As an effectivity problem, by assigning to d a value of -5mm,

$$F_B = \frac{+5.00}{1 - (-0.005)(+5.00)} = +4.88 \text{ D.}$$

5.5. Range and Amplitude of Accommodation

Accommodation, like refraction, is normally specified as if it occurred in the *spectacle plane.* Accommodation may be specified in terms of range or amplitude. *Range of accommodation* is defined as the linear distance traversed by the point of conjugacy in moving from the far point to the near point of accommodation. It is the distance over which accommodation is available; hence, an object can be seen clearly only if located at the far point or near point of accommodation or at any point between the far and near points.

Referring to Figure 5–12, the range of accommodation (in either the uncorrected or the corrected state) is equal to the distance from the far point of accommodation to the near point of accommodation. An *emmetropic* eye that has a finite (real) near point of accommodation (Figure 5–12A) has an infinite range of accommodation (extending from infinity to the near point of accommodation). For a *myopic* eye, the far point and the near point are always *real* object points located at finite distances in front of the eye (Figure 5–12B), with the result that the range of accommodation is always less than infinity. If a *hyperopic* eye (having the far point of accommodation behind the eye) has the near point of accommodation located at a finite distance in front of the eye (Figure 5–12C), the range of accommodation is infinite, as it is for the emmetropic eye. The point of conjugacy moves (to the right) from the far point to infinity, as a *virtual* object point, and from infinity to the near point of accommodation (still moving to the right) as a *real* object point. (Because a real object can be placed only in "real" space, an object cannot be placed at the far point of accommodation of a hyperopic eye or at the near point of accommodation of a hyperopic eye if the near point is located behind the eye.)

Amplitude of accommodation is defined as the dioptric difference between the far and near points of accommodation. For an eye in either the uncorrected or the corrected state, the amplitude of accommodation is given by the expression

$$\text{amplitude of accommodation} = \frac{1}{M_r S} - \frac{1}{M_p S}, \quad (5.1)$$

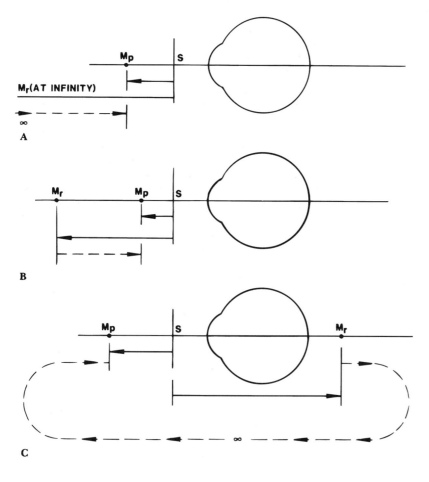

FIGURE 5–12. **The range of accommodation. A, emmetropic eye; B, myopic eye; C, hyperopic eye.**

where M_rS is the linear distance from the far point of accommodation to the spectacle plane, and M_pS is the linear distance from the near point of accommodation to the spectacle plane.

Typical values of the range and amplitude of accommodation are illustrated by the following examples and Figure 5–13:

EXAMPLE 1

Given an emmetropic eye (having its far point at infinity) with a near point of accommodation located at a distance of 10 cm in front of the spectacle plane. What are (1) the range and (2) the amplitude of accommodation?

(1) The range of accommodation extends from infinity to a distance of 10 cm from the spectacle plane; therefore, it is equal to infinity.
(2) The amplitude of accommodation

$$= \frac{1}{M_rS} - \frac{1}{M_pS}$$
$$= \frac{1}{\text{infinity}} - \frac{1}{-0.10}$$
$$= 0 + 10.00 = +10.00 \text{ D.}$$

This example shows that for an emmetropic eye with its far point of accommodation located at infinity, the *range* of accommodation is equal to infinity minus a finite number, which is, of course, still infinity. The amplitude of accommodation, on the other hand, is equal to the reciprocal of the near point of accommodation.

EXAMPLE 2

Given an uncorrected myopic eye (Figure 5–13B) with a far point of accommodation located 50 cm in front of the spectacle plane and a near point of accommodation 10 cm in front of the spectacle plane. What are (1) the range and (2) the amplitude of accommodation?

(1) The range of accommodation extends from 50 to 10 cm from the spectacle plane, and is therefore equal to 40 cm.
(2) The amplitude of accommodation

$$= \frac{1}{-0.50} - \frac{1}{-0.10}$$
$$= -2.00 + 10.00 = 8.00 \text{ D.}$$

EXAMPLE 3

Given an uncorrected hyperopic eye (Figure 5–13C) with a far point of accommodation located 50 cm behind the spectacle plane and a near point of accommodation located 10 cm in front of the spectacle plane. What are (1) the range and (2) the amplitude of accommodation?

(1) The range of accommodation extends from 50 cm behind the spectacle plane to 10 cm in front of the spectacle plane, and is therefore equal to infinity.
(2) The amplitude of accommodation

$$= \frac{1}{0.50} - \frac{1}{-0.10}$$
$$= 2 + 10 = 12.00 \text{ D.}$$

This example shows that if an uncorrected hyperopic eye has a finite, or *real*, near point of accommodation, the range of accommodation (like that of the emmetropic eye) is infinite.

EXAMPLE 4

Given an uncorrected hyperopic eye (Figure 5–13D) with a far point of accommodation located 10 cm behind the spectacle plane and a near point of accommodation located 25 cm behind the spectacle plane. What are (1) the range and (2) the amplitude of accommodation?

(1) The range of accommodation extends from 10 cm behind the spectacle plane to 25 cm behind the spectacle plane, and is therefore equal to 15 cm.
(2) The amplitude of accommodation

$$= \frac{1}{0.10} - \frac{1}{0.25}$$
$$= 10.00 - 4.00 = 6.00 \text{ D.}$$

Because both the far and near points of the eye in this example are located behind the spectacle plane, it is impossible to place a real object at either of these points.

5.6. Spectacle Refraction versus Ocular Refraction

As discussed in Section 5.4, a lens that corrects an ametropic eye (with accommodation relaxed) places the image of an infinitely distant object at the far point of the eye. The image formed by the correcting lens becomes an object for the optical system of the eye; by definition, if an object lies at the far point of the eye, the image of that object formed by the eye is focused on the retina. The amount of ametropia is indicated by the dioptric value of the distance from the far point of accommodation to the spectacle plane. As already discussed, the focal length of a correcting lens depends on the position of the lens in front of the eye. In practice, spectacle lenses are located as close to the eyes as possible—limiting factors are anatomical features such as eyelashes, eyebrows, nose, cheeks, and the mechanical fitting aspects of the frame. The typical vertex distance is approximately 13 mm, with the spectacle plane lying closer to the eye than the eye's anterior focal plane.

The power of the correcting lens, specified at the spectacle plane, is termed *spectacle refraction*. On occasion it may be useful to calculate ametropia in relation to the first principal plane of the eye, in which case the power of the lens is referred to as *ocular refraction* or as *principal plane refraction*. The objective of a clinical refraction is to determine the power of the correcting lens in the spectacle plane. Spectacle refraction is therefore of greater interest to clinicians than is ocular refraction; when reference is made by clinicians to the refractive state of the eye (without any qualification), spectacle refraction is assumed.

When a contact lens is placed on the cornea, the difference between ocular refraction and the refraction brought

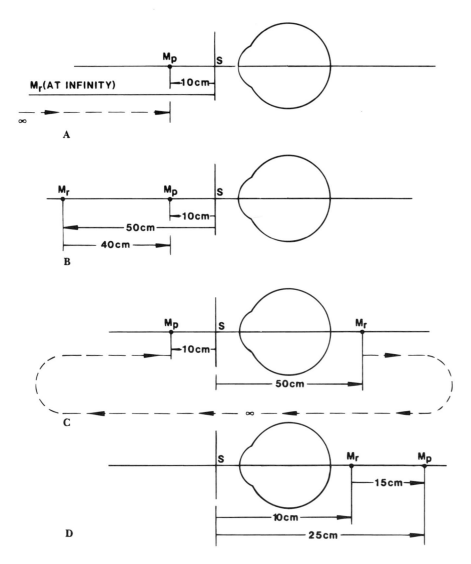

FIGURE 5–13.   **Determination of range and amplitude of accommodation. A, an emmetropic eye; B, an uncorrected myopic eye; C and D, uncorrected hyperopic eyes.**

about by the contact lens is very small because the distance between the corneal apex and the first principal plane of the eye is only slightly more than 1 mm (1.35 mm, for Gullstrand's "exact" schematic eye). A logical (but not often used) term for the power of a contact lens, specified as the power required for a lens placed in contact with the corneal apex, is *contact lens refraction*.[3]

Although the difference involved in measuring the refractive state at the spectacle plane rather than at the first principal plane of the eye is negligible for small amounts of ametropia, the difference in measurement assumes large proportions for large amounts of ametropia. This can be demonstrated by calculating the ocular refraction for eyes with spectacle refractions of +10.00 D and −10.00 D, and assuming in each case that the refractive examination was performed at a distance of 15 mm from the primary principal plane of the eye.

In Figure 5–14, for an eye whose spectacle refraction is +10.00 D, the secondary focal length of a correcting lens located at the primary principal plane of the eye is

$$10 \text{ cm} - 1.5 \text{ cm} = +8.5 \text{ cm},$$

and the refracting power of the correcting lens, or the ocular refraction, is

$$\frac{1}{+0.085} = +11.76 \text{ D}.$$

In Figure 5–15, for an eye whose spectacle refraction is −10.00 D, the secondary focal length of a correcting lens located at the primary principal plane of the eye is

$$-10 \text{ cm} - 1.5 \text{ cm} = -11.5 \text{ cm},$$

and the ocular refraction is

$$\frac{1}{-0.115} = -8.70 \text{ D}.$$

For these two examples, ocular refraction differs from spectacle refraction by more than 1.75 D for the +10.00-D hyperope and by more than 1.25 D for the −10.00-D

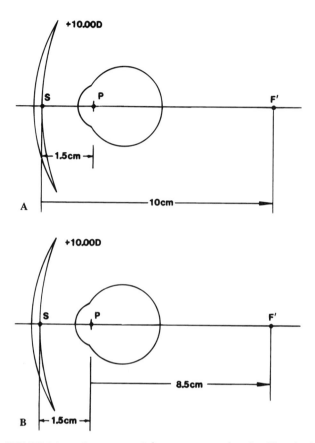

FIGURE 5–14.   **For a +10.00 D hyperope, secondary focal length of the correcting lens, A, measured from the spectacle plane, 10 cm; B, measured from the primary principal plane, 8.5 cm.**

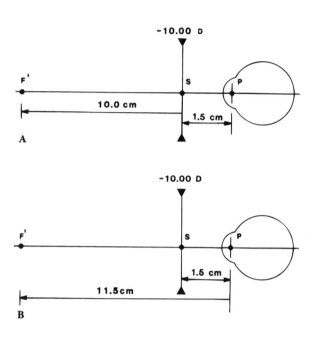

FIGURE 5–15.   **For a –10.00 D myope, secondary focal length of the correcting lens. A, measured from the spectacle plane, 10 cm; B, measured from the secondary principal plane, 11.5 cm.**

myope. For each example, if *contact lens refraction* were calculated, there would be little difference from ocular refraction.

5.7. Spectacle Accommodation versus Ocular Accommodation

For the sake of convention, accommodation is usually considered to take place at the spectacle plane. However, because it represents a *change in ocular refraction*, accommodation actually takes place at the first principal plane of the eye, and this must be considered when one determines the amount of accommodation necessary for a corrected ametrope.

The amount of ocular accommodation required of an eye (Figure 5–16) can be determined by the use of the formula

$$\text{ocular accommodation} = V_d - V_n, \qquad (5.2)$$

where V_d is the vergence of light in the principal plane for an object at a distance of 6 m (assumed to be infinity), and V_n is the vergence of light in the principal plane for an object at near distance (usually assumed to be at 40 cm). In

any near-point situation, because V_n has a less plus or greater minus value than V_d, the eye must supply the amount of accommodation equal to the difference between the two vergence values for the near-point object to be clearly focused. For example in Figure 5–17, for an emmetropic eye (A) viewing a distant object, the vergence of light at the principal plane is equal to

$$V_d = \frac{1}{\text{infinity}} = 0,$$

and the vergence for an object at a distance of 40 cm from the spectacle plane (considering a distance of 15 mm from the spectacle plane to the first principal plane of the accommodated eye), as shown in Figure 5–17B, is equal to

$$V_n = \frac{1}{-0.40 - 0.015} = -2.41 \text{ D}.$$

This is only 0.09 D less than the value of 2.50 D required for the spectacle plane.

Let us now consider the amount of ocular accommodation required for the corrected 10.00 D hyperope (Figure 5–18) and the corrected 10.00 D myope (Figure 5–19), for the 40 cm distance. For the 10.00 D hyperope (Figure 5–18A), as discussed in Section 5.6, the ocular refraction for this eye (the vergence of light at the first principal plane for an object at infinity) is

$$V_d = +11.76 \text{ D}.$$

The vergence of light at the spectacle plane for an object at 40 cm (Figure 5–18B) can be found by first adding the vergence of the light rays entering the lens (–2.50 D) to the

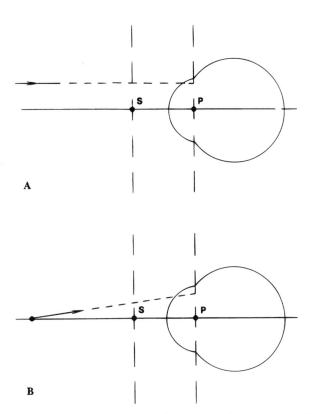

FIGURE 5–16. **A, vergence at the principal plane (P) for an object at infinity (V_d); B, vergence at the principal plane (P) for a near object (V_n).**

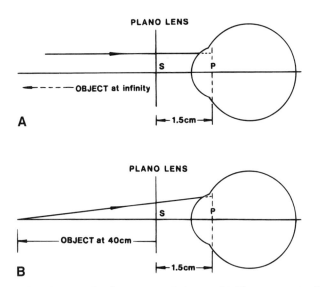

FIGURE 5–17. **Ocular accommodation required for an emmetropic eye.**

vergence impressed by the lens (+10.00 D), which results in a vergence on leaving the lens of +7.50 D. The formula applied is

$$L' = L + F$$
$$= -2.50 + 10.00$$
$$= +7.50 \text{ D}.$$

The distance from the spectacle plane to the image is found by taking the reciprocal of +7.50 D, which is +0.133 m. Subtracting from this the 15-mm fitting distance, we have

$$+0.133 - 0.015 = +0.118 \text{ m},$$

which is the distance from the principal plane to the image. Therefore,

$$V_n = \frac{1}{+0.118} = +8.47 \text{ D},$$

and ocular accommodation

$$= V_d - V_n$$
$$= +11.76 - 8.47$$
$$= +3.29 \text{ D}.$$

For the 10.00 D myope (Figure 5–19A), as discussed in Section 5.6, the ocular refraction for this eye (i.e., the vergence of light at the principal plane for a distant object) was

$$V_d = -8.70 \text{ D}.$$

The vergence of light at the spectacle plane for an object at 40 cm (Figure 5–19B) can be found by adding the vergence of the light rays entering the lens (–2.50 D) to the vergence impressed by the lens (–10.00 D), which results in a vergence on leaving the lens of –12.50 D, that is,

$$L' = L + F$$
$$= -2.50 + (-10.00)$$
$$= -12.50 \text{ D}.$$

Taking the reciprocal of –12.50 D, we have an image distance from the spectacle plane of –0.08 m. Adding to this the 15-mm fitting distance, we have

$$-0.08 - 0.015 = -0.095 \text{ m}$$

for the distance from the principal plane to the image. Therefore,

$$V_n = \frac{1}{-0.095} = -10.53 \text{ D},$$

and ocular accommodation

$$= V_d - V_n$$
$$= -8.70 - (-10.53)$$
$$= +1.83 \text{ D}.$$

Summarizing, we find that the ocular accommodation required for the 10 D hyperope is 3.29 D and that required for the 10 D myope is only 1.83 D, compared with 2.41 D of accommodation required of an emmetrope. The 10 D hyperope, therefore, must accommodate about 1.00 D *more* than the emmetrope, and the 10 D myope needs to accommodate about 0.50 D *less* than the emmetrope. We usually think of 0.25 D as the minimum change in stimulus to accommodation that would have an effect on an individual's visual functioning (a "just-noticeable-difference"

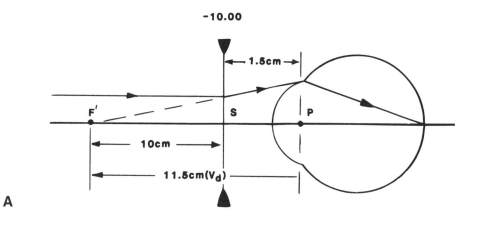

FIGURE 5–18.   Ocular accommodation required for a corrected 10.00 D hyperopic eye.

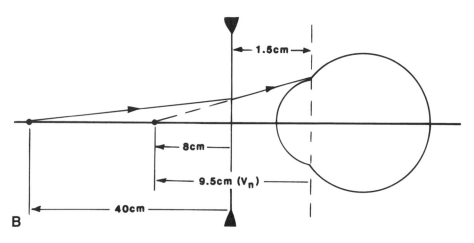

FIGURE 5–19.   Ocular accommodation required for a corrected 10.00 D myopic eye.

step); thus, as a rule, for a reading distance of 40 cm, the amount of increased accommodation for a hyperope or decreased accommodation for a myope reaches 0.25 D for about 3.00 D of hyperopia or myopia.

The increase in the amount of ocular accommodation required by the spectacle-wearing hyperope is of little consequence for the young hyperope with an adequate amplitude of accommodation. However, when the amplitude of accommodation decreases as the onset of presbyopia approaches, a 4.00 D hyperope can expect to require a bifocal addition at an *earlier age* than that of a 4.00 D myope because of the greater accommodative demand.

Because a contact lens fits on the cornea rather than about 13 mm in front of it and, therefore, is less than 2 mm in front of the first principal plane of the eye, the newly presbyopic hyperope has to accommodate *less* while wearing contact lenses than while wearing spectacles, and the newly presbyopic myope has to accommodate *more* while wearing contact lenses than while wearing spectacles. Consequently, fitting contact lenses to a myope who is an incipient presbyope may appear to hasten the onset of the presbyopia.

5.8. Accommodation and Effectivity in Anisometropia

The principle of effectivity applies also to anisometropia. We assume (according to Hering's law of equal innervation to the ocular muscles) that the two eyes accommodate equally. However, if one eye has 10 D of hyperopia and the other has 10 D of myopia, and if each eye is corrected by means of a spectacle lens for distance vision, one eye will be out of focus by more than 1.25 D (as compared to the other) when accommodating at a 40 cm distance. What actually happens in such a case is that the accommodative mechanism responds with no more than the amount of accommodation required for the myopic eye (in fact, it is well established that most people routinely exhibit a *lag of accommodation* for near work and accommodate about 0.50 or 0.75 D less than required by the stimulus).

EXAMPLE
As a more probable example, consider a patient whose distance prescription is

OD +2.00 DS
OS −4.00 DS

(1) What is the induced anisometropia at 40 cm for a young patient having a high amplitude of accommodation? (2) For a presbyopic patient, what is the power of the add, for a distance of 40 cm, that would require 1.00 D of ocular accommodation for each eye? (3) What is the induced anisometropia for an absolute presbyope who requires a +2.50 D add for a distance of 40 cm?

(1) For the young patient, we must calculate the values V_d and V_n for each eye. To calculate V_d, we first use the formula $L' = L + F$.
For the right eye, the vergence at distance is given by

$$L' = L + F$$
$$= 0 + 2.00 = +2.00 \text{ D},$$
$$l' = \frac{1}{+2.00} = +0.50 \text{ cm}$$

at the spectacle plane.

The image formed by the lens is the object for the eye; so the object distance, l (for the first principal plane of the eye), is given by

$$l = +0.50 - 0.015$$
$$= +0.485 \text{ m}.$$

Therefore,

$$V_d = \frac{1}{0.485} = +2.062 \text{ D}.$$

To find the value of V_n, we use the relationship

$$L' = L + F$$
$$= -2.50 + 2.00 = -0.50 \text{ D},$$
$$l' = \frac{1}{-0.50} = -2.00 \text{ m}$$

at the spectacle plane.

The near-object distance, l, for the principal plane of the eye is given by

$$l = -2.00 - (0.015) = -2.015 \text{ m}.$$
$$V_n = \frac{1}{-2.015} = -0.496 \text{ D}.$$

and ocular accommodation

$$= V_d - V_n$$
$$= +2.062 - (-0.496)$$
$$= 2.56 \text{ D}.$$

For the left eye, the vergence at distance is given by

$$L' = L + F$$
$$= 0 + (-4.00) = -4.00 \text{ D},$$
$$l' = \frac{1}{-4.00} = -0.25 \text{ m}$$

at the spectacle plane.

The object distance, l (for the first principal plane of the eye), is given by

$$l = -0.25 - 0.015$$
$$= -0.265 \text{ m}.$$

Therefore,

$$V_d = \frac{1}{-0.265} = -3.77 \text{ D}.$$

To find the value of V_n,

$$L' = L + F$$
$$= -2.50 + (-4.00) = -6.50 \text{ D},$$
$$l' = \frac{1}{-6.50} = -0.1538 \text{ m}$$

measured from the spectacle plane.

The near-object distance, l, measured from the principal plane of the eye, is given by

$$l = -0.1538 - (0.015) = -0.1688 \text{ m.}$$

$$V_n = \frac{1}{-0.1688} = -5.92 \text{ D.}$$

and

ocular accommodation

$$= V_d - V_n$$
$$= -3.77 - (-5.92)$$
$$= 2.15 \text{ D.}$$

The induced anisometropia at 40 cm is equal to the accommodation required by the right eye minus the accommodation required by the left eye, or,

$$2.56 - 2.15 = 0.41 \text{ D.}$$

The patient should accommodate no more than the amount required for the myopic eye, 2.15 D. If either the right eye or the left eye is clearly focused, the opposite eye will be out of focus by 0.41 D. For maximum binocular efficiency, a patient who wore this prescription and did a significant amount of near work would need for near work single-vision lenses incorporating an add of approximately +0.37 D for the hyperopic eye. The prescription for near work would be

OD +2.37 D
OS –4.00 D

(2) For the presbyopic patient who is required to use 1.00 D of ocular accommodation for each eye, at a distance of 40 cm, the relationship for

required ocular accommodation = $V_d - V_n$.

For an add of 1.00 D of ocular accommodation for each eye, $V_d - V_n$ must be equal to 1.00 D for each eye.
For the right eye in (1),

$$V_d = +2.062 \text{ and } V_d - V_n \text{ must equal } +1.00 \text{ D.}$$

Therefore,

$$V_n = V_d - 1.00 = 2.062 - 1.00$$
$$= +1.062 \text{ D,}$$

$$l_n = \frac{1}{+1.062} = +0.942 \text{ m,}$$

from the principal plane.
This distance is the reciprocal of the vergence of light, for the 40 cm distance, at the principal plane of the eye, and therefore is the distance from the principal plane to the image formed by the spectacle lens. To find the distance from the spectacle plane to the image, we must add 0.015 m to this value,

$$+0.942 + 0.015 = +0.957 \text{ m,}$$

which is the image distance from the spectacle plane; by taking the reciprocal of this distance, we can find the image vergence at the spectacle plane

$$\frac{1}{+0.957} = +1.045 \text{ D.}$$

To determine the power of the lens needed to require 1.00 D of accommodation for the right eye, we use the formula

$$L' = L + F$$
$$+1.045 = -2.50 + F$$
$$F = +3.545 \text{ D.}$$

To find the *add* needed for the right lens, we subtract the power of the distance prescription, +2.00 D

$$\text{add} = +3.545 \text{ D} - 2.00 \text{ D}$$
$$= +1.545 \text{ D.}$$

For the left eye in (1),

$$V_d = -3.77 \text{ D.}$$
$$V_d - V_n = +1.00 \text{ D.}$$
$$V_n = -3.77 - 1.00 = -4.77 \text{ D.}$$
$$l_n = \frac{1}{-4.77} = -0.2096 \text{ m.}$$

This is the distance from the principal plane of the eye to the image formed by the spectacle lens.
To find the distance from the spectacle plane to the image, we must subtract 0.015 m from this value

$$-0.2096 - (-0.015) = -0.1946 \text{ m,}$$

which is the image distance from the spectacle plane; by taking the reciprocal of this distance, we can find the image vergence at the spectacle plane

$$L_S' = \frac{1}{-0.1946} = -5.14 \text{ D.}$$

To determine the lens needed to permit 1.00 D of accommodation for the left eye, we use the formula

$$L' = L + F$$
$$-5.14 = -2.50 + F$$
$$F = -2.64 \text{ D.}$$

To find the add for the left lens, we subtract from this the power of the distance prescription, –4.00 D

$$\text{add} = -2.64 \text{ D} - (-4.00 \text{ D})$$
$$= +1.36 \text{ D.}$$

In summary, the distance prescription is

OD +2.00 DS
OS –4.00 DS

and the near prescription that would require 1.00 D of ocular accommodation for each eye is

OD +3.55 DS
OS –2.64 DS.

The difference in the powers of the lenses for the two eyes, for the distance prescription, is 6.00 D, and the difference in the powers for the near prescription requiring 1.00 D of ocular accommodation at 40 cm is 6.19 D. The induced anisometropia at 40 cm without an add is 0.41 D. This reduces to approximately 0.19 D (the difference between the powers of the adds) when each eye is permitted to accommodate 1.00 D.

(3) For the absolute presbyope wearing a +2.50 D add for 40 cm, the patient would exert no accommodation, with the result that there would be *no* induced anisometropia. The bifocal portion of the lens can be considered as a +2.50 D lens in front of the distance lens. The +2.50 D addition lens renders the rays from an object at 40 cm parallel on the distance lens (Figure 5–20). The parallel rays impinging on the distance lens are then focused at the far point and, finally, on the retina.

These three examples demonstrate that induced anisometropia is at a maximum when no add is worn, that the wearing of a bifocal add reduces the amount of induced anisometropia by reducing the amount of accommodation required, and that a maximum add (e.g., a +2.50 D add for a 40 cm reading distance) reduces the amount of induced anisometropia to zero.

5.9. Accommodation and Effectivity in Astigmatism

The concepts of accommodation and effectivity can be applied to astigmatism in the same manner in which they apply to anisometropia, if astigmatism is considered to be a special case of anisometropia, confined to one eye, with the refracting power differing in the two principal meridians. Under those conditions, the effectivity changes demonstrated for anisometropia can also be demonstrated for astigmatism.

Hofstetter[4] pointed out that the cylindrical correction necessary for distance vision may not be adequate for near work. O'Brien and Bannon[5] determined the correction for astigmatism for each of 50 eyes at both distance vision and near vision by each of three techniques and found a constant increase in the power of the cylinder, from 8% to 10%, for near vision by all three methods. The increase was always in the direction (and in the approximate amount) as expected as a result of loss of effectivity of the lens power prescribed for distance when used for an accommodating eye for near vision.

In practice, the astigmatism correction determined for distance vision is considered sufficient for correction of astigmatism at the near point. The fact is, however, that in large astigmatic errors for young persons, the astigmatic correction for distance vision represents a substantial undercorrection for near vision. If 0.25 D represents a just-noticeable-difference step, a patient who has from 3.00 to 4.00 D of astigmatism would have one meridian out of focus by about 0.25 D compared with the other meridian when accommodating for a distance of 40 cm. For example, in an extreme case (which is very unlikely to occur) in which the refraction of the eye is +5.00 D in one principal meridian and −5.00 D in the other, one meridian would be out of focus by more than 0.75 D compared with the other meridian.

In addition to changes in power of the astigmatic correction based on effectivity, changes in cylinder *axis* may occur as a result of the depression and convergence of the visual axes for near work.[6] In cases of high astigmatism, changes in the amount of the astigmatic correction, axis of the astigmatic correction, or both should be investigated. If a patient does extensive near work, a separate pair of spectacles should be prescribed, based on an examination for astigmatism (both axis and power) at the near point.

5.10. Retinal Image Size in Uncorrected Ametropia

In determining the size of the retinal image, one is concerned primarily with finding the *linear distance* between two image points that correspond to two known object points. Several methods are available for determining retinal image size. However, when dealing with an ametropic eye in the uncorrected state, the *chief ray* method has the advantage that the size of the retinal image is unaffected by *image blur* because a chief ray (Figure 5–21) passes through the center of the entrance pupil of the eye (E) with the result that it passes through the center of the retinal blur circle formed by the object point. Using the chief ray method, the retinal image size is found by determining the subtense

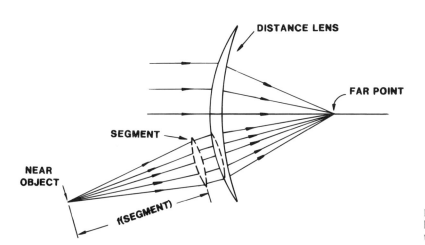

FIGURE 5–20. **With a +2.50 D addition, the rays of light from an object at 40 cm are parallel when striking the distance portion of the lens.**

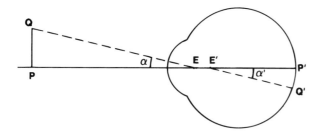

FIGURE 5–21.   **Chief ray method of determining retinal image size.**

of the retina of the angle formed at the center of the exit pupil (E′) by a pair of chief rays. The chief rays originate from a pair of object points whose separation represents the *size of the object* under consideration.

For simplicity, one of the object points (point P in Figure 5–21) is placed on the optic axis of the eye; the second object point, Q, is an off-axis point. The size of the retinal image, Q′P′, is determined by tracing the chief ray from the object point Q through the eye to the image point Q′, on the retina. The ray is directed toward the center of the entrance pupil, E, and emerges into the vitreous as if it came from the center of the exit pupil, E′.

Retinal Image Size in Uncorrected Axial Ametropia

In Figure 5–22, the angle α′ made between the optic axis and the chief ray as it emerges from the exit pupil forms a *constant ratio* with the angle α between the optic axis and the incident chief ray. The retinal image size is therefore directly proportional both to the angle that the incident chief ray makes with the optic axis, α, and to the axial length of the eye. Consequently, for a given object size, the size of the retinal image of an uncorrected axially ametropic eye varies *only* with the axial length of the eye.

As shown by the three retinal positions in Figure 5–22, the retinal image is of normal size in the emmetropic eye, smaller than normal in an axially hyperopic eye, and larger

than normal in an axially myopic eye. If the optical system of the eye (made up of the cornea, the anterior chamber, and the lens) is similar to that of the emmetropic schematic eye, the greater the amount of axial hyperopia, the smaller the retinal image, and the greater the amount of axial myopia, the larger the retinal image.

Retinal Image Size in Uncorrected Refractive Ametropia

When the ametropia is refractive rather than axial, the refractive power of the eye's optical system varies from one eye to another, but the axial length is equal to that of the standard (schematic) emmetropic eye. As shown in Figure 5–23, the power of the eye's refractive system has no effect on the angle of incidence of the chief ray as it passes through the entrance pupil, so the retinal image size is essentially the same for uncorrected refractive myopia, emmetropia, and uncorrected refractive hyperopia.

5.11. Retinal Image Size in Corrected Ametropia

Axial Ametropia

A ray passing through the primary focal point of any lens or optical system is refracted in such a way as to emerge from the optical system *parallel to the optic axis*. Therefore, as shown in Figure 5–24, if the correcting lens for an *axially ametropic eye* is placed in the primary focal plane of the eye, the size of the retinal image is determined *only* by the distance from the optic axis to the ray passing through the primary focal point of the eye. Therefore, in all cases of purely axial ametropia (whether myopia or hyperopia), the size of the retinal image formed by the combination of the eye and the correcting lens is the same as that of the emmetropic schematic eye. Consequently, if an eye has *purely axial* myopia or hyperopia,

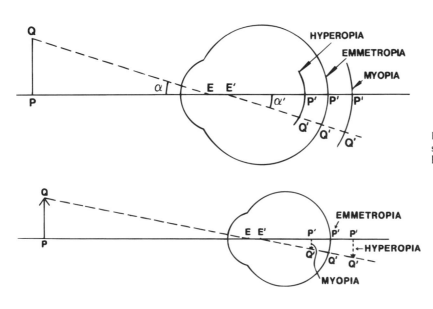

FIGURE 5–22.   **In uncorrected axial ametropia, the size of the retinal image varies only with the axial length of the eye.**

FIGURE 5–23.   **In uncorrected refractive ametropia, the size of the retinal image, in both myopia and hyperopia, is essentially the same as in the emmetropic eye. The size of the retinal image is given by the distance between the centers of the blur circles formed at points P′ and Q′ on the retina.**

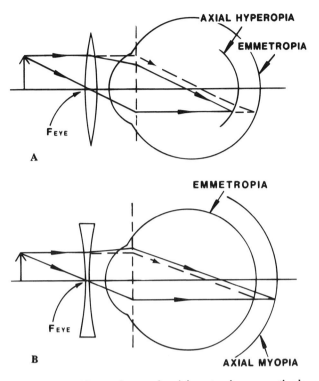

FIGURE 5–24.   **If an eye has purely axial ametropia, a correcting lens placed in the primary focal plane of the eye provides the eye with the same retinal image size as the (theoretical) emmetropic eye. A, axial hyperopia; B, axial myopia.**

a correcting lens placed at the primary focal plane of the eye provides that eye with the same retinal image size as that of the (theoretical) emmetropic eye. A comparison of Figures 5–22 and 5–24 shows, however, that for the eye in question the correcting lens *enlarges* the size of the retinal image for an axially hyperopic eye but *reduces* the size of the retinal image for an axially myopic eye.

Refractive Ametropia

When the correcting lens for an eye having refractive ametropia is placed at the primary focal point of the eye, as shown in Figure 5–25, the situation occurring for the axially ametropic eye does not prevail. Rather than the retinal image size being basically similar for myopia, emmetropia, and hyperopia, Figure 5–25A shows that the retinal image for the corrected refractively hyperopic eye is *larger* than that for the emmetropic eye; Figure 5–25B shows that the retinal image for the corrected refractively myopic eye is *smaller* than that for the emmetropic eye. However, a comparison of Figures 5–23 and 5–25 shows that for the eye in question the correcting lens *enlarges* the size of the retinal image for a refractively hyperopic eye but *reduces* the size of the retinal image for a refractively myopic eye—exactly the same situation occurring with an *axially* myopic or hyperopic eye.

Magnification by a Spectacle Lens

Although the magnification brought about by a spectacle lens is discussed in more detail in Chapter 10, two commonly used terms are defined here:

SPECTACLE MAGNIFICATION. This is the magnification brought about by a correcting lens; it compares the retinal image size with the correcting lens to that without the lens. Spectacle magnification is caused by both the power and the shape (form) of the lens. As shown in the above examples, for both axial and refractive ametropia a plus lens enlarges the retinal image size of the eye in question, but a minus lens reduces the retinal image size.

RELATIVE SPECTACLE MAGNIFICATION. This is the comparison of the size of the retinal image of the eye, with the correcting lens, to the size of the retinal image of the

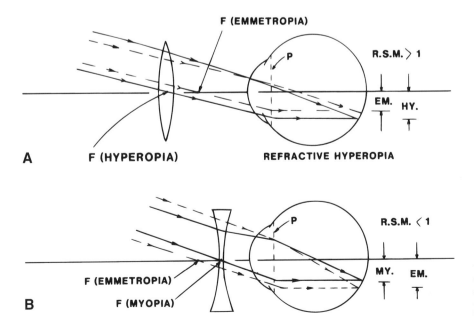

FIGURE 5–25.   **For an eye having purely refractive ametropia, the retinal image for a corrected myopic eye is smaller than that for an emmetropic eye, but the retinal image for a corrected hyperopic eye is larger than that for an emmetropic eye.**

theoretical (schematic) emmetropic eye. As discussed above and shown in Figures 5–24 and 5–25, relative spectacle magnification depends on whether the ametropia is axial or refractive. The image size is essentially the same as that for the emmetropic eye in *axial* ametropia, but is magnified in hyperopia and minified in myopia, as compared with that for the emmetropic eye, in *refractive* ametropia.

References

1. Emsley, H. H. *Visual Optics*, Vol. 1. The Hatton Press, London, pp. 323–348, 1963.
2. Sorsby, A., Benjamin, B., Davey, J. B., Sheridan, M., and Tanner, J. M. *Emmetropia and Its Aberrations: A Study of the Correlation of the Optical Components of the Eye.* Medical Research Council Special Report Series, No. 203, H. M. Stationery Office, London, 1957.
3. Grosvenor, T. *Contact Lens Theory and Practice.* Professional Press, Chicago, p. 423, 1963.
4. Hofstetter, H. W. Correction of Astigmatism for Near Work. *Am. J. Optom. Arch. Am. Acad. Optom.*, Vol. 23, pp. 121–131, 1945.
5. O'Brien, J. M., and Bannon, R. E. Accommodation and Astigmatism. *Am. J. Ophthalmol.*, Vol. 30, pp. 289–296, 1947.
6. Hughes, W. Changes in Axis of Astigmatism with Accommodation. *Arch. Ophthalmol.*, Vol. 26, pp. 742–749, 1941.

Questions

1. Given a pair of lenses:
   OD +6.00 D
   OS plano
   The lenses are 15 mm from the primary principal planes of the eyes. Assume the left eye is in focus for an object at 25 cm from the spectacle plane and that differential accommodation is impossible. What is the uncorrected ocular anisometropia?

2. Given a pair of lenses:
   OD +2.00 D
   OS −4.00 D
   Assume that the spectacle plane is 15 mm from the primary principal plane of the eyes and that differential accommodation is impossible. The target is located at 40 cm from the spectacle plane. What are the adds for the right eye and left eye, respectively, that would require 1.00 D of ocular accommodation for each eye?

3. a. The distance correction is
      OD plano
      OS −5.00 D
      The lenses are 20 mm from the primary principal planes of the eyes. The reading distance is 25 cm from the spectacle plane. The left eye is given a +2.00 D add. What must the power of the add of the right lens be so that both eyes are simultaneously in focus for the near distance? (Assume that the eyes cannot accommodate differentially.)

   b. In the above problem, what is the anisometropia for an object at 25 cm without the use of the bifocal? (Assume the eyes cannot accommodate differentially.)

4. What is the stimulus to accommodation for a person wearing a far-point correction if the lens power is +10.00 D, the distance from the lens to the primary principal plane is 15 mm, and the distance from the spectacle plane to the object is 40 cm?

5. Rework Question 4 assuming a +1.00 D bifocal add.

6. The following lens corrects an eye for infinity: +2.00 DS −7.00 DC x 90. If the horizontal meridian of the eye is in focus for an object 25 cm from the spectacle plane, what prescription is needed to bring the vertical meridian into focus? (Assume the spectacle is 20 mm from the primary principal plane of the eye and that astigmatic accommodation is impossible.)

7. The following lens corrects the eye for infinity: +3.00 DS +5.00 DC x 180. Assume the spectacle plane is 15 mm from the primary principal plane of the eye and that astigmatic accommodation is impossible. If the vertical meridian is in focus for an object 30 cm from the spectacle plane, what lens power is needed to bring the horizontal meridian into focus?

8. A 3 D hyperope has an amplitude of accommodation of 6 D. When uncorrected, where is the near point of accommodation located?

9. If the accommodative amplitude is 5 D and the far point of accommodation is 20 cm, what is the range of accommodation?

10. A patient has a punctum remotum of 100 cm when looking through a +4.00 D lens. When the patient looks through a −2.00 D lens, the punctum proximum is 20 cm. What is the amplitude of accommodation?

11. A 50-year-old patient with findings indicating an amplitude of accommodation of 3.00 D is given a bifocal prescription providing a +2.00 D add. Through the reading portion of the lenses, where is the near point of accommodation?

12. Light from a patient's retina emerges from his unaccommodated eye, passes through a +6.00 D lens, and comes to a focus 25 cm in front of his spectacle plane. What is the patient's refractive error?

13. A patient's distance subjective is +1.50 DS OU (both eyes). With trial lenses correcting the distance ametropia and an add of +2.50 D, the patient's range of clear vision at near distance is 40 to 25 cm. What is this patient's amplitude of accommodation?

14. A patient's eye, with no lens in place, has a near point of accommodation of 25 cm. The conjugate focus of the retina is located 20 cm in front of the eye when a +2.50-D lens is used and half the amplitude of accommodation is used. What is the refractive error of the eye?

15. A patient's eye, with no lens in place, has a near point of accommodation of 33 1/3 cm. The conjugate focus of the retina is located 50 cm in front of the eye when a +2.00-D lens is used and half the amplitude of accommodation is used. What is the amplitude of accommodation of the eye?

CHAPTER SIX

Aberrations and Ophthalmic Lens Design

Ophthalmic lenses are subject to a number of aberrations that degrade their performance in varying degrees. Aberrations include chromatic aberration, which occurs as a result of the heterochromatic nature of ambient light (whether sunlight or artificial light) and monochromatic aberrations, which occur whenever incident light is not confined to a narrow bundle of paraxial rays. The design of ophthalmic lenses should take these aberrations into consideration, minimizing their effects to the extent that seems to be practical.

For the most part, chromatic aberration is caused by the material from which the lens (or prism) is made and therefore can be controlled to some extent by the judicious selection of materials. Monochromatic aberrations, on the other hand, are caused less by the properties of the material than by factors such as the size of the lens aperture, the angle the incident rays make with the optic axis of the lens, and the position of the lens in relation to the eye. Monochromatic aberrations are controlled by varying the front and back surface powers and the thickness of the lens, and by varying vertex distance.

Although an understanding of the principles of lens design was evident early in the nineteenth century, the development of commercially available lenses designed to minimize monochromatic aberrations began almost a century later. During the early decades of the present century, each major lens manufacturer developed its own series of corrected curve lenses, and the responsibility of the practitioner was simply to select the trade name lens that he or she judged was the best for the patient at hand. However, in recent years, recommendations made by a committee of the American National Standards Institute and a decrease in the influence of the major lens manufacturers have combined to place a greater responsibility for ophthalmic lens design on the expertise of the individual practitioner.

6.1. Laws of Geometrical Optics

Geometrical optics concerns a number of laws that explain the way light behaves. According to the law of rectilinear propagation of light, a *ray* of light is the direction along which light travels; in a homogeneous, isotropic medium, the rays travel in a straight lines. The rays that constitute a *beam* of light behave independently—when two rays of light intersect, they continue along their course without interaction. According to the laws of reflection, the incident ray, the reflected ray, and the line normal to the reflecting surface at the point of incidence all lie in the same plane, and the angle of reflection is equal to the angle of incidence, each lying on opposite sides of normal. According to the laws of refraction, the incident ray, the refracted ray, and the line normal to the surface at the point of incidence all lie in the same plane, and the sine of the angle of incidence forms a constant ratio with the sine of the angle of refraction—a relationship known as *Snell's law.*

Geometrical optics accepts these laws as established properties of light. The laws hold true, but they involve a certain amount of oversimplification. For instance, a ray of light, although a convenient device for representing the direction of propagation of a wavefront, is an abstraction; in fact, it does not really exist. Geometrical optics and ophthalmic lens theory treat optical systems as if they were perfect imaging systems. In doing so, these studies assume (1) that all rays originating from one object point reconverge to form one conjugate image point (real or virtual) after treatment by the optical system, (2) that a plane object situated at right angles to the optical axis is imaged point for point in a similar plane in image space, and (3) that the image is an exact geometrical reproduction of the object.

The above assumptions are valid only if restricted to the following practices: (1) use of *monochromatic* light, for which the optical system has a single index of refraction and has no chromatic aberration and (2) a limit for the rays involved in image formation to only those rays whose paths throughout the system are confined to a small cylindrical region immediately surrounding the optical axis of the system (the *paraxial* region). A paraxial ray lies near the optical axis; hence, the angles and the ray heights are very small.

The sine of an angle can be expressed in terms of the angle, in radians, in the following expression:

$$\sin \alpha = \alpha - \frac{\alpha^3}{3!} + \frac{\alpha^5}{5!} - \frac{\alpha^7}{7!} \cdots$$

If the angles are small, the first term can be used without serious error. This assumption forms the basis for paraxial theory, also known as *first-order theory.* The error involved in equating the angle, expressed in radians, to its sine reaches approximately 1% for an angle of 15°. First-order theory is useful because any well-designed optical system nearly conforms to first-order calculations; hence, first-order optical imagery provides a reference against which to measure the extent of the aberrations.

In actual practice, extending the limits of effective rays beyond the paraxial region is often necessary. The failure of rays to arrive at unique positions based on object point–image point correspondence of first-order theory creates various aberrations that either impair the quality of the image or deform the image.

An approximate conception of the deviation (aberration) from perfect image formation can be obtained by using the first and second numbers of the expression for sin α, that is,

$$\sin \alpha = \alpha - \frac{\alpha^3}{3!}.$$

This approximation is called *third-order theory* and provides accuracy to four decimal places for values as high as 23°, or about 0.4 radian.

Seidel's[1] mathematically complicated calculations of third-order monochromatic theory addressed five aberrations: spherical aberration, coma, oblique astigmatism, curvature of image, and distortion. In Seidel's calculations, the aberrations, that is, the departure from the imagery produced by paraxial (Gaussian) theory, are delineated by five different sums, S_1, S_2, S_3, S_4, and S_5, which are the coefficients of the terms of the equations. When the more oblique rays perform as those in the paraxial region, the value of each of the five terms is zero. If Seidel's first condition, S_1, is satisfied (i.e., if $S_1 = 0$), no spherical aberration is present. If his second condition is satisfied ($S_2 = 0$), no coma exists; if the third condition is satisfied ($S_3 - S_4 = 0$), the oblique astigmatism is eliminated; if the fourth condition is satisfied ($S_3 = S_4 = 0$), curvature of image is eliminated; and if $S_5 = 0$, distortion is eliminated. Each succeeding term is meaningless unless the preceding terms have been satisfied, that is, reduced to zero.

Seidel's mathematical expressions provide the lens designer with approximate criteria for initial construction of the image. However, an accurate representation of the image is completed by trigonometrically tracing pertinent rays through the system. (Computers have reduced the time and effort necessary for such a process.) Basic understanding of aberrations is required to evaluate the performance of ophthalmic lenses and to provide some insight into the problems confronting the lens designer. Each aberration is discussed below as if it were the only aberration present and as if no interaction occurs among aberrations.

CHROMATIC ABERRATION AND ACHROMATIC LENSES

6.2. Chromatic Aberration

Chromatic aberration occurs solely as a result of the nature of the *material* from which a lens or prism is made and is caused by the material having differing indices of refraction for light of differing wavelengths. Chromatic aberration can be considered as *longitudinal* (axial) or as *transverse* (lateral) aberration.

Longitudinal (axial) chromatic aberration means that the secondary focal length of a lens is different for each of the monochromatic constituents of white light. If white light is incident upon a lens (Figure 6–1) and if filters are successively used to isolate various wavelengths, the shortest wavelength (violet) undergoes the greatest refraction and the longest wavelength (red) undergoes the least refraction. Because longitudinal chromatic aberration requires an optical system that *changes the vergence* of incident light, this type of aberration is not produced by a prism (unless the prism also has refracting power).

The *bichrome* test, a test used to determine the endpoint in subjective refraction, takes advantage of the longitudinal chromatic aberration of the eye. One side of the chart is projected through a red filter and the other side through a green filter, with the result that if the eye is in focus for the yellow portion of the spectrum (to which the eye is most sensitive) the red and green charts will appear to be equally distinct. However, if the red side of the chart is more sharply focused than the green side, the eye is relatively *myopic* for yellow light; if the green side of the chart is more sharply focused, the eye is relatively *hyperopic* for yellow light.

Transverse (lateral) chromatic aberration, in the case of a lens, can be expressed as (1) differences in the image size (linear magnification) of chromatically formed images or (2) angular dispersion (differences in prismatic effects). Whether expressed in linear or angular terms, transverse chromatic aberration occurs because the equivalent focal length of a lens is different for components of light having different refractive indices.

1. *Linear Magnification Differences.* Because the secondary focal length of a lens is different for each of the monochromatic constituents of white light, the axial image positions of the constituents differ; hence, for an extended object, their image sizes differ (Figure 6–2). When ex-

pressed in this manner, transverse chromatic aberration is often referred to as *chromatic difference in magnification.* If the longitudinal chromatic aberration of a lens has been corrected by the use of an achromatic doublet (see Section 6.7), transverse chromatic aberration may still be present. Even though the blue-colored image occupies the same position on the axis of the lens as the red-colored image, the principal planes for the blue and red light are not located in the same positions, with the result that the two images are not the same size.

2. *Differences in Prismatic Effects.*

a. *Lenses.* The transverse chromatic aberration of a lens can be expressed in terms of the differences in prismatic effects created, for example, by blue and red light. Referring to Figure 6–3, the prismatic effect for blue light is equal to dF_F, and the prismatic effect for red light is equal to dF_C, with d being the distance from the optic axis of the lens. Expressed in prism diopters, the lateral chromatic aberration is therefore equal to

$$dF_F - dF_C = d(F_F - F_C).$$

b. *Prisms.* Because a prism does not change the vergence of light, it does not manifest axial chromatic aberration. It does, however, manifest angular dispersion (lateral chromatic aberration), as shown in Figure 6–4. The angular dispersion is defined as the difference in prismatic effects for blue and red light, that is,

$$\varepsilon_F - \varepsilon_C.$$

Chromatic aberration is discussed further in Section 6.4 (for prisms) and in Section 6.6 (for lenses).

Because of the presence of chromatic aberration, a wearer of high-powered lenses may occasionally see *color fringes* around objects. The amount of chromatic aberration depends on the material of which the lens is made. For ex-

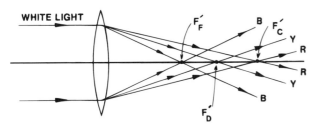

FIGURE 6–1.   **Longitudinal (axial) chromatic aberration.**

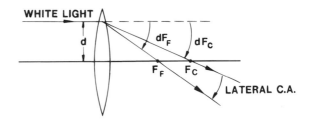

FIGURE 6–3.   **Transverse chromatic aberration (C.A.) expressed as the difference in prismatic effects created by red and blue light.**

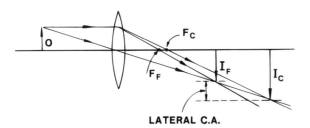

FIGURE 6–2.   **Transverse (lateral) chromatic aberration (C.A.); also referred to as the chromatic difference in magnification.**

FIGURE 6–4.   **A prism can manifest transverse chromatic aberration (C.A.) but cannot manifest longitudinal chromatic aberration.**

ample, chromatic aberration is relatively high for *flint* glass, used for the manufacture of some bifocal segments.

Because chromatic aberration requires light containing a range of wavelengths, it does not occur with *monochromatic* light. However, light falling upon an ophthalmic lens is very seldom monochromatic, with the result that all substances from which lenses and prisms are made are subject to chromatic aberration. Because chromatic aberration is caused by the material itself, it cannot be reduced or eliminated by changing the form (the amount of *bend*) of the lens. However, it can be controlled by the use of a *doublet*, which is a lens made of two kinds of glass. Chromatic aberration does not occur in reflection because the angle of reflection is the same for all wavelengths of light; nor does it occur when light is refracted by parallel plates of glass.

6.3. Chromatic Dispersion

When we specify the index of refraction of a substance, we normally specify the index for the *helium d* line. This is the Fraunhofer line that has a wavelength of 587.56 nm. For example, ophthalmic crown glass is specified as having an index of refraction of 1.523. This is the index of refraction of the helium d line. The index of refraction of the d line, n_d, is defined as follows:

$$n_d = \frac{\text{velocity of helium light in a vacuum}}{\text{velocity of helium light in the medium}}.$$

To discuss chromatic dispersion, we must consider the index of refraction of two additional spectral lines: n_C refers to the index of refraction of the Fraunhofer C line, at the red end of the spectrum and having a wavelength of 656.27 nm; n_F refers to the index of refraction of the Fraunhofer F line, at the blue end of the spectrum, having a wavelength of 486.13 nm.

Mean refractivity is given by the expression

$$n_d - 1,$$

and *mean dispersion* is given by the expression

$$n_F - n_C.$$

Usually, although not always, the higher the mean refractive index n_d, the greater the mean dispersion ($n_F - n_C$). The *dispersive power* of a medium is given by the ratio of mean dispersion to mean refractivity

$$\frac{n_F - n_C}{n_d - 1}.$$

The reciprocal of dispersive power is known as *refractive efficiency*, or *constringence*, and is indicated by the letter V (also called the *Abbe number*)

$$V = \frac{n_d - 1}{n_F - n_C}. \tag{6.1}$$

In comparing the Abbe numbers of two media, if the media have the same dispersion, the one having the higher mean refractivity has the higher Abbe number; but if the two media have the same refractivity, the medium having the

lower mean dispersion has the higher Abbe number (and the lower dispersive power).

The advantage of using the Abbe number (rather than the dispersive power) to specify chromatic dispersion of a lens is that it is expressed as a *number greater than unity*, and the most desirable lens materials are those with higher Abbe numbers. For example, the Abbe number of ophthalmic crown glass is 58.9; that of flint glass is 30.

6.4. Chromatic Aberration in Prisms

As shown in Section 6.2, the transverse chromatic aberration of a prism can be expressed as the difference in the deviating power of the prism for the Fraunhofer F and C lines, or

$$\text{transverse chromatic aberration} = \varepsilon_F - \varepsilon_C.$$

Because the refracting angle and the deviating power of a prism are related by the expression

$$\varepsilon^\circ = \beta^\circ(n - 1),$$

it follows that

$$\varepsilon_d = \beta(n_d - 1)$$
$$\varepsilon_F = \beta(n_F - 1)$$
$$\varepsilon_C = \beta(n_C - 1)$$

and

$$\varepsilon_F - \varepsilon_C = \beta(n_F - 1) - \beta(n_C - 1).$$

Since

$$\beta = \frac{\varepsilon_d}{n_d - 1}$$

$$\varepsilon_F - \varepsilon_C = \frac{\varepsilon_d(n_F - 1)}{n_d - 1} - \frac{\varepsilon_d(n_C - 1)}{n_d - 1}.$$

$$\varepsilon_F - \varepsilon_C = \frac{\varepsilon_d(n_F - n_C)}{n_d - 1}.$$

Since

$$\frac{1}{V} = \frac{n_F - n_C}{n_d - 1},$$

$$\varepsilon_F - \varepsilon_C = \frac{\varepsilon_d}{V}. \tag{6.2}$$

This equation tells us that the chromatic dispersion of a prism is equal to the deviation of the d line divided by the Abbe number of the material from which the prism is made. For example, for a prism made of crown glass having an Abbe value of 60, and having a deviating power of 5 prism diopters,

$$\frac{\varepsilon_d}{V} = \frac{5}{60} = 0.08 \text{ prism diopter.}$$

For a prism made of a given material, the chromatic dispersion increases in direct proportion to the power of the prism.

Because the transverse chromatic aberration of a prism is equal to

$$\varepsilon_F - \varepsilon_C,$$

and since Equation 6.2 shows that

$$\varepsilon_F - \varepsilon_C = \frac{\varepsilon_d}{V},$$

it follows that the transverse chromatic aberration of a prism is equal to

$$\frac{\varepsilon_d}{V}.$$

6.5. Achromatic Prisms

An achromatic prism is a prism that produces deviation without dispersion and is constructed by placing two prisms made of different materials in direct contact with the bases oriented in opposite directions. Such a prism can be made achromatic for two wavelengths, usually for the F and C lines. The rays of light for the two wavelengths for which the prism is achromatic emerge parallel, as shown in Figure 6–5. To be achromatic, the chromatic dispersion of the two prisms must be equal, or

$$\frac{\varepsilon_1}{V_1} = \frac{\varepsilon_2}{V_2}.$$

Since the prisms have their bases in opposite directions, the final deviation, ε, is given by

$$\varepsilon = \varepsilon_1 - \varepsilon_2$$

and

$$\varepsilon_1 = \frac{V_1}{V_2}(\varepsilon_2) = \frac{V_1}{V_2}(\varepsilon_1 - \varepsilon)$$

and also

$$\varepsilon_2 = \frac{V_2}{V_1}(\varepsilon_1) = \frac{V_2}{V_1}(\varepsilon_2 + \varepsilon).$$

The deviating powers of the two prisms are given by the derived expressions

$$\varepsilon_1 = \frac{V_1 \varepsilon}{V_1 - V_2} \qquad (6.3)$$

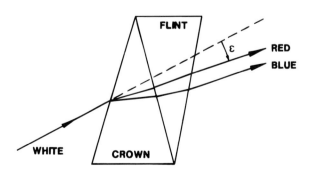

FIGURE 6–5.   **An achromatic prism.**

and

$$\varepsilon_2 = \frac{V_2 \varepsilon}{V_1 - V_2}, \qquad (6.4)$$

which can be used to design an achromatic prism.

EXAMPLE
Given two prisms, one having an index of refraction of 1.50 and an Abbe number of 60 and the other having an index of refraction of 1.60 and a nu value of 40, design an achromatic prism having a power of 2 prism diopters.

$$\varepsilon_1 = \frac{60(2)}{60 - 40} = 6 \text{ prism diopters}$$

and

$$\varepsilon_2 = \frac{40(2)}{60 - 40} = 4 \text{ prism diopters.}$$

Chromatic aberration is responsible for the color fringes sometimes seen with high-power prisms during phoria and fusional vergence testing. However, for the low-power prism components that are occasionally used in ophthalmic lenses (usually no stronger than 2 or 3 prism diopters), chromatic aberration is seldom a problem. Chromatic doublets are not seriously considered as ophthalmic appliances because both thickness and weight are unacceptable.

6.6. Chromatic Aberration in Lenses

Longitudinal Chromatic Aberration

The formula for the longitudinal chromatic aberration of a lens can be derived by using the lens maker's formula for the Fraunhofer d, F, and C lines:

$$F_d = (n_d - 1)(R_1 - R_2),$$
$$F_C = (n_C - 1)(R_1 - R_2),$$
$$F_F = (n_F - 1)(R_1 - R_2).$$

Therefore,

$$F_F - F_C = (n_F - 1)(R_1 - R_2) - (n_C - 1)(R_1 - R_2),$$
$$F_F - F_C = (n_F - n_C)(R_1 - R_2).$$

Since

$$R_1 - R_2 = \frac{F_d}{n_d - 1},$$

$$F_F - F_C = \frac{n_F - n_C}{n_d - 1}(F_d).$$

Since

$$\frac{n_F - n_C}{n_d - 1} = \frac{1}{V},$$

$$F_F - F_C = \frac{F_d}{V}. \qquad (6.5)$$

This expression shows that, as with a prism, the longitudinal chromatic aberration of a lens varies directly with power. For example, for a –6.00-D lens having an Abbe number of 60,

$$\text{longitudinal chromatic aberration} = \frac{-6}{60} = -0.10 \text{ D.}$$

Transverse Chromatic Aberration

In Section 6.2, the angular expression for transverse chromatic aberration (for a lens) was

$$d(F_F - F_C).$$

Since in Equation 6.5

$$F_F - F_C = \frac{F_d}{V},$$

the transverse chromatic aberration of a lens can therefore be expressed as:

$$\text{transverse chromatic aberration} = d\frac{F_d}{V}. \quad (6.6)$$

6.7. Achromatic Lenses

A lens is considered to be achromatic, that is, free of longitudinal chromatic aberration, if the focal lengths are the same for the F and C lines. For a lens to be achromatic, two lenses of different materials, one convex and one concave, each having different Abbe values, must be used (Figure 6–6). The power of each lens must be such that

$$F_T = F_1 + F_2$$

and

$$\frac{F_1}{V_1} = \frac{-F_2}{V_2},$$

or

$$F_1 = \frac{V_1}{V_2}(-F_2)$$

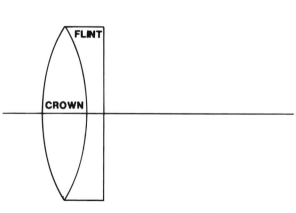

FIGURE 6–6.   **An achromatic lens.**

and

$$-F_2 = \frac{V_2}{V_1}(F_1).$$

Substituting,

$$F_1 = F_T - F_2 = F_T + \frac{V_2}{V_1}(F_1)$$

and

$$F_2 = F_T - F_1 = F_T + \frac{V_1}{V_2}(F_2).$$

The refracting powers are given by the derived expressions. For the first lens,

$$F_1\left(\frac{V_1 - V_2}{V_1}\right) = F_T$$

and

$$F_1 = \left(\frac{V_1}{V_1 - V_2}\right)F_T. \quad (6.7)$$

For the second lens,

$$F_2\left(\frac{V_2 - V_1}{V_2}\right) = F_T$$

and

$$F_2 = -\left(\frac{V_2}{V_1 - V_2}\right)F_T. \quad (6.8)$$

EXAMPLE
Given two lenses, one having an index of refraction of 1.50 and an Abbe number of 60 and the other having an index of refraction of 1.60 and an Abbe number of 40, design an achromatic lens having a refracting power of –2.00 D.

$$F_1 = \left(\frac{60}{60-40}\right)(-2)$$
$$= \left(\frac{60}{40}\right)(-2) = -6.00 \text{ D.}$$
$$F_2 = -\left(\frac{40}{60-40}\right)(-2)$$
$$= \left(\frac{-40}{20}\right)(-2) = +4.00 \text{ D.}$$

The only use for achromatic doublets in ophthalmic lens design is for some high-powered lenses such as those used as aids for low vision. For ordinary ophthalmic lenses, doublets are excessively thick and heavy. Achromatic lenses correct only for longitudinal chromatic aberration and leave some lateral color uncorrected.

One possible reason that the eye tolerates longitudinal chromatic aberration is that the *eye itself* has about 1 D of longitudinal chromatic aberration. In addition, the eye is most sensitive (in photopic vision) to a wavelength of about 555 nm, with a decrease in sensitivity toward the blue and red regions. The accommodative responses made by the eye have been hypothesized to be based to some extent on the eye's chromatic aberration interval. The visual system seems to be well adapted to its own chromatic aberration and apparently adapts easily to the additional chromatic aberration caused by an ophthalmic lens. There are, however, two situations in which lateral chromatic aberration may be a problem:

1. As discussed in Chapter 1, Section 1.10, lenses with a low Abbe number may produce undesirable lateral chromatic aberration with peripheral gaze.
2. Wearers of fused bifocal lenses sometimes complain of seeing color fringes, particularly when flint segments are used. (This problem is discussed further in Chapter 8, Section 8.20.)

MONOCHROMATIC ABERRATIONS

The five monochromatic aberrations, as originally defined by Seidel, are spherical aberration, coma, oblique astigmatism, curvature of image, and distortion.

Spherical aberration occurs when a pencil of light is refracted by a large-aperture optical system, which occurs because different zones of the aperture have different focal lengths. Spherical aberration affects the sharpness of image points.

Coma occurs when oblique rays are refracted by a large-aperture optical system. Coma also affects the sharpness of image points.

Oblique astigmatism occurs when oblique rays are refracted by a small-aperture system and affects both sharpness of image points and image position. Even when oblique astigmatism is corrected, curvature of image is still present.

Curvature of image manifests itself as a curved image surface for a flat object surface, and primarily affects image position. However, if the curvature of the image surface does not match that of the screen on which the image is formed, peripheral portions of the image are blurred.

Distortion occurs when the magnification of an extended object varies with its distance from the optical axis. Distortion affects image shape and lateral position, but not image clarity.

The center of rotation of the moving eye and the pupil limit the bundle of rays received by the spectacle-lens–eye system, with the result that spherical aberration and coma are usually of little concern in lens design. As for the aberrations affecting narrow bundles of rays, only *oblique astigmatism* and *curvature of image* need to be considered in routine ophthalmic lens design. Distortion is a significant aberration only for high-powered lenses and for unusual cases of anisometropia.

either *positive* or *negative*. In positive spherical aberration (shown in Figure 6–7), peripheral rays have a shorter focal length than central rays; in negative spherical aberration, the central rays have the shorter focal length. Of the two types of aberration, positive spherical aberration is the most common. The three-dimensional surface that encloses the totality of the refracted rays is called a *caustic surface*. The caustic surface is a symmetrical, funnel-shaped figure with the small end of the funnel (called the *cusp*) located at the paraxial image.

Longitudinal (or *axial*) spherical aberration refers to the separation of the paraxial focus and the peripheral focus, in diopters, along the optic axis. *Lateral* (or *transverse*) spherical aberration is specified in terms of the diameter of the *confusion disc* at the paraxial focus—the confusion disc is the image formed on a screen placed at any point along the caustic surface.

Spherical aberration is a problem only for *large-aperture* optical systems. Longitudinal spherical aberration increases with the square of the aperture; lateral spherical aberration increases with the cube of the aperture. In addition to controlling the size of the aperture, spherical aberration may be controlled by varying the bend of the lens, that is, by manipulating the curvature of each of the two surfaces without changing the refracting power of the lens. As a general rule, spherical aberration is minimized when rays traverse the lens symmetrically, in which case the refraction is equally divided between the two surfaces.

Spherical aberration is not too important for ophthalmic lenses of moderate power because the eye uses only a small portion of the lens at any one time as a result of the limiting aperture of the pupil. However, for lenses of high power (+10.00 D or more, as required by aphakics), spherical aber-

6.8. Spherical Aberration

Spherical aberration occurs because each zone of a lens has its own focal length for rays originating on the optic axis, which vary from the optic axis to the edge of the lens, as shown in Figure 6–7. Normally, the deviating power of a lens increases toward the periphery. The increase is an inherent property of any lens (given by Prentice's rule) but in the case of spherical aberration the deviating power increases too rapidly, or not rapidly enough, to maintain a point focus for a point object. Spherical aberration may be

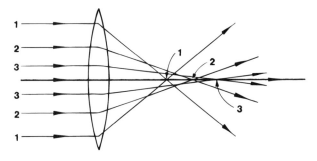

FIGURE 6–7. **Spherical aberration.**

ration can be serious. In high-powered lenses, spherical aberration can be controlled by the use of *aspheric surfaces*. An aspheric surface is an ellipsoid or parabolic surface that gradually flattens in curvature from the center to the edge. Aspheric lenses may be made of glass, but these lenses are very difficult to grind and are therefore very expensive. An easier way to manufacture an aspheric surface is to *mold* it, using a plastic material for the lens and a glass mold.

Without the use of an aspheric surface, a minimum of spherical aberration occurs when a *crossed* lens is used. This is a lens in which the front surface power is greater than the back surface power by a factor of 6, or

$$\frac{F_1}{F_2} = 6.$$

In the form of a plus lens, the crossed lens is a bi-convex lens. Although minimizing spherical aberration, such a lens allows considerable amounts of oblique astigmatism and distortion to occur.

As a practical matter, spherical aberration is considered in ophthalmic lens design only for high-powered convex lenses, for which plastic aspheric lenses are routinely used.

6.9. Coma

Coma, like spherical aberration, occurs because each zone of a lens has its own focal length. However, spherical aberration occurs for beams of light that are parallel to the optic axis of a lens; coma occurs for *oblique* beams (Figure 6–8). As a result, the image of a point object resembles a *comet*, or a teardrop. Another difference between spherical aberration and coma is that the imagery in spherical aberration has an axis of symmetry, which coincides with the optic axis or with the *chief ray* (the ray that passes through the center of the entrance pupil), but the imagery in coma is not symmetrical with respect to the optic axis or the chief ray.

Like spherical aberration, coma is a problem mainly for large-aperture optical systems and can be largely ignored in the design of spectacle lenses because of the limiting effect of the pupil. Factors that can be used to control coma, in addition to aperture size, are the form of the lens and the angle of obliquity.

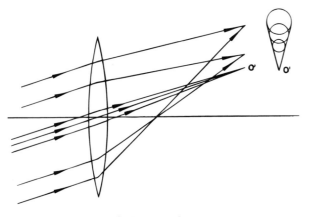

FIGURE 6–8.   **Coma.**

In an optical system for which spherical aberration is corrected, coma is corrected when, for all rays proceeding from an object point, the ratio of the sines of the slope angles (α and α'), of each pair of corresponding incident and emergent rays, is constant. This is shown by the expression

$$\frac{\sin \alpha}{\sin \alpha'} = \frac{y}{y'} = \text{constant}.$$

This relationship is known as *Abbe's sine condition*.

If an optical system is corrected for spherical aberration for a pair of conjugate points, M and M′, and the sine condition is satisfied for those points, an extra-axial object point, Q, lying close to the axis and located in a plane normal to the axis at M, produces an image, Q′, that is free from coma. The points M and M′ are called *aplanatic points*. Only one pair of aplanatic points exists for any optical system.

6.10. Oblique Astigmatism

Oblique astigmatism (also called *radial* astigmatism or *marginal* astigmatism) occurs when a narrow pencil of light from an object passes obliquely through a spherical surface. Rays of light do not form a point focus, but form the characteristic *interval of Sturm*, containing two line foci and the circle of least confusion, as if the surface were toric rather than spherical. The term oblique astigmatism is used to distinguish this type of astigmatism from the astigmatism produced by a cylindrical or toric lens for an object situated on the optic axis. The amount of astigmatism between the two focal lines is the *dioptric separation* of the two line foci. The size of the circle of least confusion and the corresponding lengths of the focal lines are determined by the amount of astigmatism and the size of the aperture.

The terminology necessary for describing this aberration can be understood by referring to Figure 6–9. The *tangential plane* (or median plane) is the plane containing the chief ray from the object point and the optic axis; the *tangential focus*, T (primary focus or meridional focus), is the focus formed by the rays in the tangential plane. The *sagittal plane* (equatorial plane) is the plane containing the chief ray from the object point that is also perpendicular to the tangential plane; the *sagittal focus*, S (equatorial or secondary focus), is the focus formed by the rays in the sagittal plane. The tangential focus lies in the sagittal plane, and the sagittal focus lies in the tangential plane. The amount of oblique astigmatism is equal to the dioptric separation between the tangential focus, T, and the sagittal focus, S.

As described in Section 6.11, when a lens forms an image of a plane object, the image lies along a curved surface, known as the *Petzval* surface, which is located at the secondary focal point of the lens. When oblique astigmatism is present, a *true* Petzval surface does not exist—it can exist *only* if oblique astigmatism has been eliminated. When oblique astigmatism exists, both the tangential (T) and the sagittal (S) foci fall on the *same side* of the theoretical Petzval surface, that is, they both may be in front of or behind the Petzval surface, but they can never straddle it.

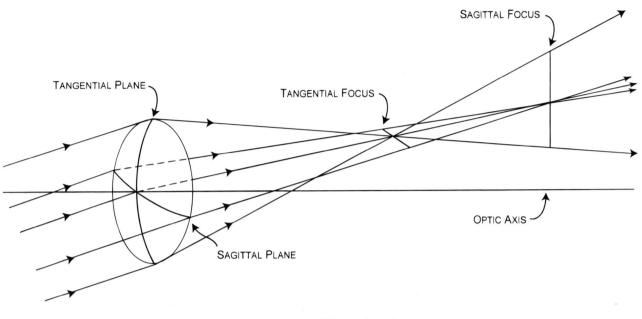

TANGENTIAL PLANE

TANGENTIAL FOCUS

SAGITTAL FOCUS

OPTIC AXIS

SAGITTAL PLANE

FIGURE 6–9. **Oblique astigmatism.**

The relationship between the tangential and sagittal surfaces in regard to the Petzval surface, P, is such that

$$\frac{\overline{PT}}{\overline{PS}} = \frac{3}{1}, \tag{6.9}$$

or, T is three times as far from P as is S (Figure 6–10), and

$$\overline{PS} = \frac{\overline{ST}}{2}.$$

Oblique astigmatism exists only for *point objects*, not for extended objects. However, an extended object may be considered to be made up of an infinite number of points, each of which is subject to oblique astigmatism. As shown in Figure 6–11, for an object made up of an infinite number of points, each point gives rise to both a tangential and a sagittal focus. If all tangential foci are considered together, they form a paraboloidal surface; in like manner, all sagittal foci, taken together, form a second paraboloidal surface. The curvature of the tangential surface is always steeper than that of the sagittal surface (Figure 6–11). The surface formed by the tangential foci has the appearance of a teacup and the surface formed by the sagittal foci has the appearance of a saucer, with the result that the diagram shown in Figure 6–11 is known as the *teacup and saucer diagram*. The teacup and saucer surfaces represent the loci of all tangential and sagittal images.

The two surfaces touch each other, on the optic axis, at the point conjugate to a point object on the optic axis. Between the two surfaces, one may construct a third surface, which represents the position of the circle of least confusion for each point object. For a spherical lens, the entire teacup and saucer configuration is symmetrical about the optic axis, with the result that these surfaces can be represented by sections in a plane including the optic axis (as shown in Figure 6–10).

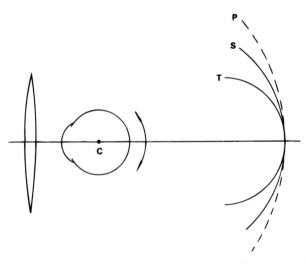

FIGURE 6–10. **The relationship between the tangential and sagittal image surfaces and the Petzval surface.**

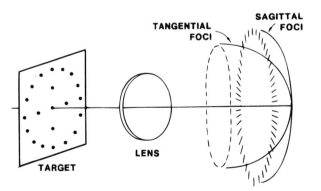

FIGURE 6–11. **The teacup and saucer diagram.**

It is possible to produce spherical lenses that are free from oblique astigmatism for a given position of the center of rotation of the eye. Jalie[2] derived the following expression for the back surface power, F_2, of a lens of power F for which there is no oblique astigmatism:

$$F_2 = \frac{F}{2} - 13.85 \pm \sqrt{30 - 2.87F - 0.182F^2}. \quad (6.10)$$

Jalie assumed that the viewing distance is infinity, that the center of rotation of the eye is located 27 mm behind the lens, and that the index of refraction of the lens is 1.523. The range of lens powers over which this equation is effective is approximately −23.00 to +7.25 D. Beyond these limits, spherical spectacle lenses cannot be made entirely free of oblique astigmatism, but one form of lens produces a *minimal* amount of oblique astigmatism (Figure 6–12). By differentiating Equation 6.10 and setting the differential coefficient equal to zero, we obtain

$$F_2 = \frac{F}{2} - \frac{L_2{'}(n^2 - 1)}{n + 2}.$$

If $n = 1.523$ and if $L_2{'}$ (the dioptric value of the distance from the lens to the center of rotation of the eye) = 37 D, the lens form required to minimize astigmatism is

$$F_2 = \frac{F}{2} - 13.85. \quad (6.11)$$

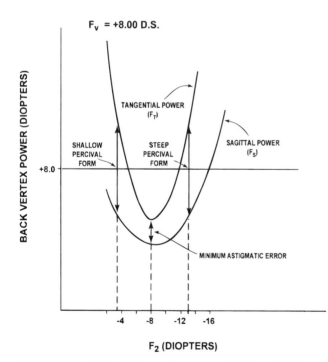

F_V = +8.00 D.S.

BACK VERTEX POWER (DIOPTERS)

TANGENTIAL POWER (F_T)

SHALLOW PERCIVAL FORM

STEEP PERCIVAL FORM

SAGITTAL POWER (F_S)

+8.0

MINIMUM ASTIGMATIC ERROR

-4   -8   -12   -16

F_2 (DIOPTERS)

FIGURE 6–12.   **Spherical lenses of powers greater than +7.00 D cannot be made point-focal (zero oblique astigmatism). The sagittal and tangential power curves do not intersect. As indicated for a +8.00-D lens, there is a form for which the oblique astigmatism is at a minimum. (Reprinted with permission from M. Katz, Distortion of Ophthalmic Lenses Calculated at the Farpoint Sphere.** *Optom. Vis. Science,* **Vol. 60, p. 951, © The American Academy of Optometry, 1983.)**

Thus, a +13.00-DS lens exhibits minimum oblique astigmatism if its back surface power is:

$$F_2 = \frac{13.00}{2} - 13.85.$$
$$F_2 = -7.35 \text{ D}.$$

There are *two* solutions for Equation 6.10: the positive root and the negative root. Therefore, there are two forms of lenses that are free of oblique astigmatism, *point-focal* lenses. If the positive root is used,

$$F_2 = \frac{F}{2} - 13.85 + \sqrt{30 - 2.87F - 0.182F^2}.$$

F_2 has a longer (or flatter) radius of curvature than if the negative root is used. If the negative root is used,

$$F_2 = \frac{F}{2} - 13.85 - \sqrt{30 - 2.87F - 0.182F^2}.$$

F_2 has a shorter (or steeper) radius of curvature than if the positive root is used.

The steeper lens form obtained by using the negative root is called the *Wollaston* form, named for William Wollaston, who in 1804 studied image formation experimentally by using different forms of lenses. Wollaston concluded that the best image for oblique rays is produced by the use of very steep surface powers.

The shallow lens form obtained by using the positive root is called the *Ostwalt* form, named for F. Ostwalt, of France, who in 1898 presented calculations for lenses that were free from oblique astigmatism and concluded that there were two lens forms that give zero astigmatism—a shallow form that was ultimately named for him and a deeper form similar to that of Wollaston.

Theoretically, for a lens of power F, there are two forms of the lens, the shallow Ostwalt form and the steeper Wollaston form, each of which produces zero oblique astigmatism. The Wollaston form not only eliminates oblique astigmatism but also minimizes *distortion* (see Section 6.12). However, the Wollaston form is more expensive, is difficult to manufacture, is less desirable cosmetically because of its bulbous appearance, and is more difficult to mount, support, and retain in a frame. The Ostwalt form, therefore, is used as a basis for the design of modern ophthalmic lenses.

If, within the range of lens powers over which oblique astigmatism is zero, both the Ostwalt and Wollaston forms are plotted, an ellipse is generated, which is known as *Tscherning's ellipse* (Figure 6–13). In 1904, M. Tscherning presented equations providing the theoretical basis for the treatment of oblique astigmatism.

THE TSCHERNING ELLIPSE. Tscherning's ellipse is the locus of points showing the relationship between the power of a surface (either front or back) and the power of the lens for which oblique astigmatism is eliminated. A unique Tscherning's ellipse is based on specific assumptions of the lens designer, such as (1) the fixation distance, (2) the angle of view, (3) the stop distance (the distance from the back pole of the lens to the center of rotation of the eye), (4) the index of refraction of the lens, and (5) the thickness of the lens. As assumptions are altered, the ellipse expands and shrinks, and

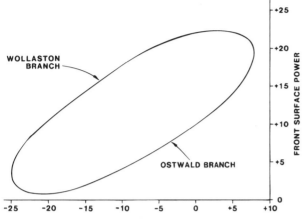

FIGURE 6–13. **Tscherning's ellipse, plotting both the Ostwalt and Wollaston forms of zero oblique astigmatism lenses.**

FIGURE 6–14. **The influence of stop distance on the form of a +4.00 DS lens for the correction of oblique astigmatism. The use of a stop distance of 30.0 mm instead of 23.5 mm flattens the back surface power from approximately –7.25 to –6.00 D.**

moves to a slightly different position. For each set of assumptions the ellipse changes in location and form; hence, constructing a *family of ellipses* is possible.

For ophthalmic lenses, two assumptions alter the Tscherning ellipse in a significant way. If the stop distance is increased, the form of the lens becomes *shallower* (Figure 6–14). If the fixation distance is reduced, as in near vision, the lens form again becomes *shallower*. If other assumptions remain constant, a change in fixation from far vision to near vision requires that a lens must be made flatter by about 2.00 D if zero oblique astigmatism is desired.

6.11. Curvature of Image

An ophthalmic lens does not form a plane image for a plane object; it forms a *curved* image, as shown in Figure 6–15. The curvature of the image is a function of the correcting lens, and the image surface is known as *Petzval's surface*. The radius of curvature of the image surface was shown by Petzval and Coddington[3] to be equal to the index of refraction of the lens times the secondary focal length of the lens,

$$r_{PS} = -nf'. \qquad (6.12)$$

The surface of the image formed by the eye, like the surface of the image formed by the lens, is also a *curved* surface. The function of an ophthalmic lens is to form an image at the *far point* of the eye—as the eye rotates, a spherical surface, known as the *far-point sphere*, is traced out (Figure 6–16). The center of curvature of the far-point sphere is assumed to be a point, the *center of rotation* of the eye, located approximately 27 mm behind the spectacle plane. Ideally, the image formed by an ophthalmic lens, for a moving eye, is formed on the far-point sphere of the eye. However, the aberration of curvature of image is absent only when the *image surface* (Petzval's surface) corresponds to that of the *far-point sphere*. As shown in Figure 6–16, the radius of curvature of the far-point sphere (for either a myopic eye or a hyperopic eye) is given by

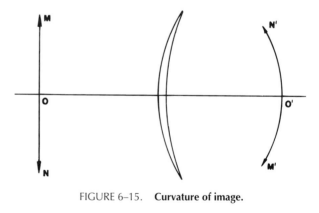

FIGURE 6–15. **Curvature of image.**

$$r_{FPS} = 0.027 - f'. \qquad (6.13)$$

Therefore, the image surface corresponds to the far-point sphere only when

$$r_{FPS} = r_{PS},$$

or when

$$0.027 - f' = -nf'. \qquad (6.14)$$

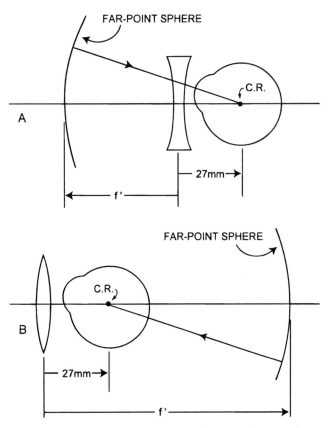

FIGURE 6–16.   **The far-point sphere. A, for a myopic eye; B, for a hyperopic eye. C.R. = center of rotation.**

By rearranging terms, we can solve for f':

$$f' - nf' = 0.027$$

$$f' = \frac{0.027}{1 - n}.$$

For a lens having an index of refraction of 1.523, the image surface and the far-point sphere coincide when

$$f' = \frac{0.027}{-0.523} = -0.0516 \text{ m}$$

$$F = -19.37 \text{ D}.$$

For any lens whose power is *other than* –19.37 D (assuming a center of rotation distance of 27 mm), in the absence of oblique astigmatism, little can be done to cause the Petzval surface of the lens to correspond to the far-point sphere of the eye (although for a given power of lens, using a lens having a lower index of refraction will reduce the radius of curvature of the Petzval surface and make it correspond more closely to the far-point sphere). The following examples show the relationship between the far-point sphere and the Petzval surface for commonly used lens powers.

EXAMPLE 1

Given a +2.00-D sphere, located at a distance of 27 mm in front of the center of rotation of the eye. How does the radius of curvature of the image surface compare to that of the far-point sphere of the eye?

As shown in Figure 6–17, the far-point sphere of the eye and the secondary focal plane of the +2.00 D sphere are located 500 mm behind the spectacle plane (A). The radius of curvature of the far-point sphere is therefore

$$r_{FPS} = 27 - 500 = -473 \text{ mm},$$

and the radius of curvature of the image surface is

$$r = \frac{n_d - 1}{}$$

Thus, the image surface is *flatter* than the far-point sphere of the eye that the lens is designed to correct.

EXAMPLE 2

Given a –2.00 D sphere, located at a distance of 27 mm from the center of rotation of the eye. How does the radius of curvature of the image surface compare to that of the far-point sphere of the eye?

The far-point sphere and the secondary focal plane of the –2.00 D sphere are located 500 mm in front of the spectacle plane, as shown in Figure 6–17B. The radius of curvature of the far-point sphere is therefore

$$r_{FPS} = 27 - (-500) = 527 \text{ mm},$$

and the radius of curvature of the image surface is

$$r_{PS} = -1.523(-500) = 761.5 \text{ mm}.$$

Again, the image surface is flatter than the far-point sphere.

In which of the cases does the *greater problem* occur? Figure 6–17 shows that when the hyperopic eye rotates into a secondary position, the lens *undercorrects* the hyperopia (because the focal length is too long); when the myopic eye rotates into a secondary position, the lens likewise *undercorrects* the myopia. Although the error is slightly greater for the hyperopic eye than that for the myopic eye, the hyperope has the advantage that vision can be cleared by accommodating slightly, whereas the myope has the disadvantage that accommodating only makes matters worse. This problem can be solved by slightly *overcorrecting* the myopic eye, so that a small amount of accommodation must be used for straight-ahead vision; but when the eye rotates to a secondary or tertiary position, vision clears without the need for accommodation.

Other than to slightly overcorrect the myopic eye, we have no method of controlling curvature of image when oblique astigmatism is absent. The far-point sphere, because it is a property of the eye, cannot be changed; the image surface, because it is a property of the correcting lens, can be altered only slightly by a change in the index of refraction of the lens material, but cannot be altered by a change in the form of (bending) the lens. Only if oblique astigmatism is permitted to exist in the spectacle lens can curvature of image be controlled (see discussion in Section 6.14).

If we wish to steepen the image surface of a single lens, the radius of curvature of the Petzval surface must be as short as possible, which for a given lens requires a low refractive index. If two lenses can be used, one plus lens and one minus lens (similar to an achromatic doublet), curvature of image will be eliminated when

$$n_1 f_1' + n_2 f_2' = 0.$$

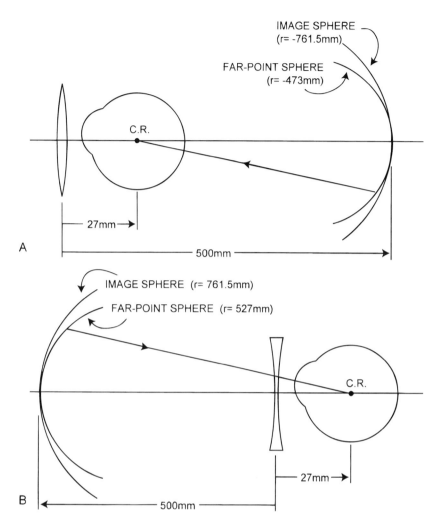

FAR-POINT SPHERE
(r= -473mm)

IMAGE SPHERE
(r= -761.5mm)

C.R.

27mm →

← 500mm →

A

IMAGE SPHERE (r= 761.5mm)

FAR-POINT SPHERE (r= 527mm)

C.R.

27mm →

← 500mm →

B

FIGURE 6–17. **Relationship between the image surface and the far-point sphere. A, for a 2.00-D hyperope; B, for a 2.00-D myope. C.R. = center of rotation.**

However, from a strictly practical point of view, a change in the index of refraction or use of a doublet would seldom, if ever, be seriously considered for an ophthalmic lens.

6.12. Distortion

Distortion is not concerned with sharpness of an image but with the ability of the optical system to reproduce faithfully an image of the geometric shape of the object. Distortion occurs when the magnification of an extended image varies with the distance of the corresponding object from the optical axis. When the ratio of the image size (y') to the object size (y) has a constant value for all object sizes, no distortion exists and the condition of *orthoscopy* is achieved. If, however, the ratio of image size to object size varies for different object sizes, distortion (rather than orthoscopy) is present. Distortion occurs as *barrel* distortion or as *pincushion* distortion (Figure 6–18). Barrel distortion occurs if the image size to object size ratio decreases with an increase in object size (compare A with B), and pin-

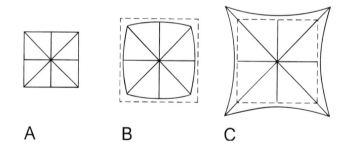

A   B   C

FIGURE 6–18. **Distortion. A, square object; B, barrel distortion; C, pincushion distortion.**

cushion distortion occurs if the image size to object size ratio increases with an increase in object size (compare A with C).

Spectacle lenses, especially those of high power, produce distortion. For plus spectacle lenses, the virtual image suffers *pincushion* distortion; for minus spectacle lenses, the virtual image suffers *barrel* distortion.

When formed by a centered, or *coaxial*, spherical optical system, distortion has radial symmetry about the opti-

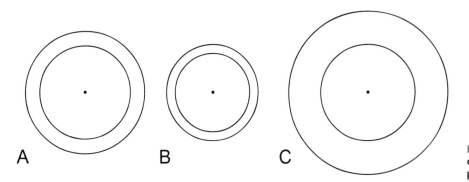

FIGURE 6–19.   Distortion. A, object, two concentric circles; B, barrel distortion; C, pincushion distortion.

cal axis. Pincushion and barrel distortion are examples of symmetrical distortion formed when an object is *square* in shape. However, a *circular* object, having its center on the optical axis, is imaged as a circle. In this special case, distortion does not alter the shape of the image. The geometric condition for distortion-free reproduction is that the distance between any two points on the image bears a constant ratio to the distance between two corresponding points on the object. For example, if an object consisting of two concentric circles is affected by distortion, the ratio of the respective diameters of the circles making up the object are different from the corresponding ratio of the diameters of the circles making up the image. Thus, in Figure 6–19, the ratio of the diameters of the object is 1.43 to 1.0 (A), and the ratio of the respective diameters of the image is 1.23 to 1.0 (B), so barrel distortion is present. In Figure 6–19C, the ratio of the respective diameters is 1.73 to 1.0, so pincushion distortion is present. Hence, the images in Figure 6–19B and C are not distortion-free reproductions of the object (A), even though the respective images are true circles.

If an optical system is not centered, distortion may not be symmetrical. A *prism* produces asymmetrical distortion, as shown in Figure 6–20. Because the optical elements of the human eye are not centered, the distortion of the retinal image may be asymmetrical.

A *chief ray* (or *principal ray*) of a pencil of light is one that passes through the center of an aperture. The chief ray from each point on an extended object forms an angle of incidence (α) and an angle of refraction (α') with the optical axis. When $\tan \alpha' / \tan \alpha$ is a constant for every chief ray, the image is uniformly magnified throughout the field of view, and the image is free of distortion, a condition known as fulfilling the *tangent condition* for orthoscopy. The constancy of $\tan \alpha' / \tan \alpha$ for all corresponding points of the image and the object is the criterion for geometric congruence of the figures.

The positions of the *stops* in an optical system greatly influence the amount and type of distortion. If an aperture stop is placed with its center coincident with the optical center of a thin convex lens (Figure 6–21), no distortion occurs. However, if a stop is placed behind a thin convex lens (Figure 6–22), the real image manifests pincushion distortion (A). If the stop is placed in front of the lens, barrel distortion is produced (B). Distortion is

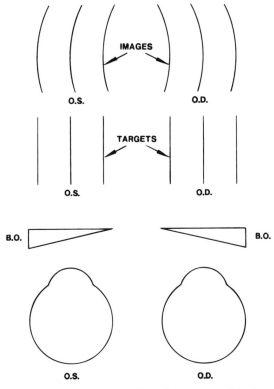

FIGURE 6–20.   Asymmetrical distortion, produced by base-out prisms.

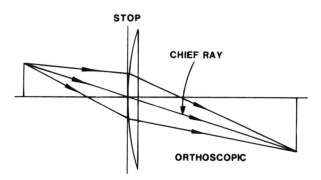

FIGURE 6–21.   No distortion occurs when the center of an aperture stop coincides with the optical center of a thin convex lens; the condition is known as orthoscopy.

FIGURE 6–22.   **A, pincushion distortion caused by a stop placed behind a plus lens. B, barrel distortion caused by a stop placed in front of a plus lens.**

often reduced in complex optical systems by separation of the optical components of the system and by proper placement of the stops.

As with spherical aberration and coma, distortion is a problem mainly for lenses of high power. Distortion tends to falsify the positions of objects and cause vertical lines to wave as the line of sight intersects different zones of the lens. The situation in which distortion most often causes a problem occurs with the newly aphakic patient—an individual who has just begun to wear strong plus lenses after cataract surgery. The patient experiences severe pincushion distortion and eventually learns that the effects of distortion (such as doorways appearing to be convex toward the center) can be minimized by looking straight ahead through the centers of the lenses.

Distortion is largely ignored in the design of ophthalmic lenses. Although distortion can be minimized or even eliminated by using very steep back curves (the Wollaston form, as discussed in Section 6.10), such lenses are difficult to manufacture and are cosmetically unacceptable. However, even moderately steep back surfaces of the Ostwalt form (–3.00 or –4.00 D) are of some help in controlling distortion in high-powered plus lenses, and the practice of using aspheric surfaces (to eliminate spherical aberration) in these lenses is also helpful.

PRINCIPLES OF LENS DESIGN

6.13. Requirements of Lens Design

The *far point* of the eye has been defined (Chapter 5) as the point conjugate to the fovea with accommodation relaxed. As the eye moves in various directions of gaze, it rotates about a fixed point, the *center of rotation*. The fovea and the far point also rotate with the eye; the far point generates a surface concentric with the center of rotation, called the *far-point sphere* (described in Section 6.11 and shown in Figure 6–16). For a sharp image of a distant object point to be formed on the fovea for all directions of gaze, the image formed by the spectacle lens must be a point image falling on the far-point sphere. For an object to be seen clearly, all rays entering the eye from a point object must be focused on the fovea. Hence, the chief ray must also pass through the center of rotation of the eye.

Although the pupil of the eye actually moves around the center of rotation for all directions of gaze, the light behaves as if the eye had a *fixed stop* the size of the pupil, situated at the center of rotation of the eye. With this concept, the problem of lens design is greatly simplified because the optical system of the eye can be ignored—the lens designer simply *replaces* the optical system of the eye with the far-point sphere and a stop aperture located at the center of rotation.

If a patient's eye is refracted at a known vertex distance and if a lens of the correct back vertex power is fitted at that vertex distance, the prescription will be correct when the patient looks along the optic axis of the lens. As the eye rotates

behind the lens, so that the line of sight passes through different portions of the lens, the prescription should be correct for oblique angles of gaze. However, the radius of curvature of the back surface of an ophthalmic lens is usually longer than the radius of the arc generated by the motion of the cornea (Figure 6–23), which results in lenses with different base curves having different vertex distances for identical viewing angles, and makes difficult comparison of

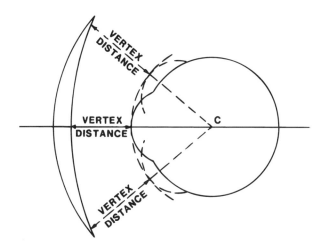

FIGURE 6–23.   **Variation in vertex distance with movement of the eye.**

the performance of one lens to that of another. For example, a patient who requires a +3.00 DS prescription at a vertex distance of 13 mm measured along the optic axis of a lens will require a correction of +3.00 D at 13 mm in front of the cornea, regardless of head or eye position (that is, regardless of where the visual axis passes through the lens).

To avoid the problem of differing lens powers for differing positions of the visual axis, calculations are referred to a theoretical spherical surface, known as the *vertex sphere* (Figure 6–24). As the eye turns to look in various directions of gaze, each point on the vertex sphere is equidistant from the cornea. The vertex sphere is tangent to the back pole of the lens, and its center of curvature is located at the center of rotation of the eye. One of the objects of lens design is to provide an accurate correction over this theoretical surface. An important property of the vertex sphere is that it remains in the same position regardless of changes in *lens form* as long as the lens is always placed at the same vertex distance. The vertex sphere provides a reference point for a given angle of view from which the tangential and sagittal powers can be compared for different lens forms.

The task of the lens designer, therefore, is to design a lens, placed at a specified distance in front of the center of rotation of the eye, with its optic axis passing through the center of rotation so that narrow pencils of light (passing through both peripheral and central portions of the lens) are refracted in such a manner that they pass through the stop position at the center of rotation and converge on (for a positive lens) or diverge from (for a negative lens) the far-point sphere of the eye.

6.14. Lens Design Variables

An ophthalmic lens designer appears to have available the following variables:

1. The number of lenses per aperture
2. The index of refraction
3. Lens thickness
4. Vertex distance
5. Lens form

However, examination of each variable shows some are *fixed* in ophthalmic lens design or are not easily subject to variation in any practical manner.

1. *Number of Lenses.* Because of weight and appearance, a single lens is routinely used. Doublets are almost never used.

2. *Index of Refraction.* The index of refraction is not considered a design variable because once a particular ophthalmic material is selected for a lens series, the index of refraction is a standard number. Ophthalmic materials with high indices of refraction are selected not for design considerations but to reduce the thickness of the lens. However, the use of a lens material with a substantially different index of refraction requires an alteration in the design to maintain off-axis performance (Figure 6–25).

3. *Lens Thickness.* Because of factors such as workability, stability, safety, appearance, and weight, thickness is not usually considered a variable. For a given power, thickness may, however, be varied within rather narrow limits.

4. *Vertex Distance.* This variable also supports only minor variations. Too great a vertex distance severely limits the field of view of a lens and is unsightly; extremely short vertex distances are impractical because of human facial structure.

5. *Lens Form.* The radius of curvature of the front surface, r_1, or that of the back surface, r_2, may be varied. Once a value has been set for either the front or the back surface radius of curvature (for a lens of a given back vertex power), the value for the other radius of curvature is fixed. Radius of curvature (in terms of the surface powers, F_1 and F_2) can be varied within rather wide limits. Lens form, therefore, is a variable that lens designers may use to minimize aberrations. Fortunately, the aberrations of oblique astigmatism and curvature of image can be controlled by proper choice of lens form.

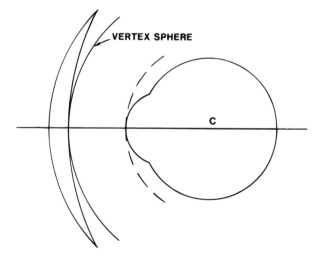

FIGURE 6–24.   **The vertex sphere. Each point on the vertex sphere is equidistant from the cornea, as the eye rotates.**

FIGURE 6–25.   **The variation in Tscherning's ellipse with two different indices of refraction.**

The lens designer, therefore, essentially has only one variable—lens form (bending)—to control lens aberrations. However, with only one degree of freedom, it is impossible to control *all* aberrations. Spectacle lenses suffer from both chromatic and monochromatic aberrations, but these aberrations are not all equally detrimental. *Chromatic aberration* is usually of little importance and is mostly ignored. Because the eye itself suffers from chromatic aberration, adaptation to this aberration very likely occurs. In addition, the eye has its greatest sensitivity in the central portion of the visible spectrum; the extremes of the visible spectrum are relatively ineffective. Correction by a doublet results in both a heavy and an unattractive lens. *Spherical aberration* and *coma* are aperture-dependent aberrations; because of the small effective aperture at the center of rotation of the eye, these aberrations have relatively small effects in comparison with those of the other monochromatic aberrations. *Distortion* is a problem only for high-powered lenses and for large amounts of anisometropia. Because distortion can be controlled only by severe bending of the lens, it is ignored except in unusual circumstances.

The aberrations of greatest importance in the design of ophthalmic lenses are *oblique astigmatism* and *curvature of image*. Of the two, oblique astigmatism is usually of greater concern. It is mainly controlled by varying the form of the lens. In the process, curvature of image can also be modified.

With only one degree of freedom, the lens designer may address the correction of either oblique astigmatism or curvature of image, or may make a compromise between the two. *Corrected-curve* and *best-form* are adjectives used to describe a lens that is designed to control oblique astigmatism, curvature of image, or both, for oblique directions of view through the lens. A corrected-curve lens should have a rationale underlying its design. For lenses of identical power, different lens forms arise from different philosophical concepts regarding the intent of the design. Each manufacturer should clearly state its lens design philosophy so that the optometrist may intelligently select the lens form best suited to a particular patient.

Two schools of thought exist in the design of ophthalmic lenses. One approach is to concentrate solely on the reduction of oblique astigmatism and to ignore the residual curvature of image error. Lenses made on the basis of this approach are known as *point-focal* lenses. On the other hand, if primary consideration is given to reduction of curvature of image and allowing a residual amount of oblique astigmatism to exist, the lens design conforms to Percival's design philosophy. (Percival, an English ophthalmologist, believed that the correction of curvature of image was more important than the elimination of oblique astigmatism.)

The lens designer is not faced with an arbitrary choice between the point-focal and the Percival principles of corrections. There is room for compromise. For example, a designer could set an arbitrary limit for the amount of the uncorrected oblique astigmatism and use this latitude to reduce the mean oblique (curvature of image) error. Although neither oblique astigmatism nor mean oblique error is reduced to zero, both errors may fall beneath noticeable physiologic levels. Figure 6–26 illustrates the alternatives open to the lens designer.

FIGURE 6–26.   Sagittal (F_S) and tangential (F_T) powers at 30° obliquity for a +4.00 DS as a function of second surface power, F_2. Point-focal or zero oblique astigmatism forms occur at the two intersections of the curves. The Percival forms, giving a mean oblique power of zero, occur where the tangential and sagittal powers symmetrically straddle the vertex power. (Reprinted with permission from M. Katz, Distortion of Ophthalmic Lenses Calculated at the Farpoint Sphere. *Optom. Vis. Science*, Vol. 60, p. 951, © The American Academy of Optometry, 1983.)

Although lens designers hold different views as to which aberration should be maximally corrected for optimum performance, most seem to favor the correction of oblique astigmatism and have only a secondary interest in curvature of image error. As stated in Section 6.11, oblique astigmatism can be eliminated with the point image of a point object falling on a curved surface, known as the Petzval surface. The ideal lens design produces a point image of a distant object on the far-point sphere. The discrepancy between the Petzval surface and the far-point sphere determines the amount of *curvature of image error*, often called the *power error*. Basically, oblique astigmatism is an astigmatic error, and curvature of image is a spherical error. The radius of curvature of the Petzval surface is equal to $-nf'$, and the radius of curvature of the far-point sphere is equal to $0.027 -f'$ (assuming a distance of 27 mm from the back vertex of the lens to the center of rotation of the eye), so the Petzval surface and the far-point sphere coincide only when

$$0.027 - f' = -nf',$$

when

$$f' = \frac{0.027}{1 - n},$$

or when

$F = -19.37$ D (assuming an index of refraction of 1.523).

Thus, only when ametropia approaches 19.37 D of myopia will the far-point sphere and the Petzval surface coincide. Figure 6–17 indicates that the dioptric difference between the Petzval surface and the far-point sphere at a particular angle of rotation of the eye is not only a function of the difference between the radius of the Petzval surface and the radius of the far-point sphere, but is also a function of the angle of rotation of the eye. For other lens powers for which oblique astigmatism is eliminated, images of object points fall on the Petzval surface but the Petzval surface does not coincide with the far-point sphere.

For corrected hyperopia, the Petzval surface is always *flatter* (having a longer radius of curvature) than the far-point sphere, so *undercorrection* of the hyperopia occurs. If accommodation is used, the Petzval surface may be made to coincide with the far-point sphere for various angles of gaze. For corrected myopia, the Petzval surface is again *flatter* than the far-point sphere, and, again, *undercorrection* occurs. If the myopia is properly corrected, relaxation of additional accommodation is not possible, with the result that objects seen in oblique directions of gaze (through peripheral portions of the lens) are blurred. A slight overcorrection of the patient's myopia, however, although requiring a small amount of accommodation for axial objects, allows objects in oblique directions to be seen clearly.

In the absence of oblique astigmatism, curvature of image error is the dioptric difference separating the Petzval surface and the far-point sphere. On the other hand, if oblique astigmatism is present, the *amount* of oblique astigmatism is indicated by the dioptric separation between the tangential and sagittal foci, that is,

$$\text{oblique astigmatism} = F_T - F_S. \quad (6.15)$$

The algebraic mean of the tangential and the sagittal powers, that is,

$$\frac{F_T + F_S}{2} \quad (6.16)$$

is called the *mean oblique power*, and determines the dioptric position of the circle of least confusion, which lies at the dioptric midpoint between the tangential and sagittal foci for an oblique pencil of rays. The difference between the mean oblique power and the back vertex power, that is,

$$\frac{F_T + F_S}{2} - F_V \quad (6.17)$$

is known as the *mean oblique error*, or the *power error*.

If the mean oblique error is zero, the circle of least confusion (for the tangential and sagittal images) falls on the far point sphere. This satisfies the Percival design philosophy. If the circle of least confusion (for the tangential and sagittal images) falls on the far-point sphere, the mean oblique error, or *power error*, is zero. This also satisfies the Percival design philosophy.

The lens form needed to eliminate oblique astigmatism for distance vision is not the same as that needed for near vision. Most lens designers who follow the point-focal design method tend to select the form needed for *distance* vision. The form necessary to eliminate oblique astigmatism (point-focal form) for *near* vision is 2.00-D flatter than the form needed for distance vision. The Percival form needed to bring the mean oblique error to zero, for distance vision, is somewhat flatter than the point-focal form for distance vision. In fact, the Percival form for *distance* vision is essentially free of oblique astigmatism for *near* vision.

6.15. Lens Design Assumptions

When the eye turns behind a stationary spectacle lens, the fovea turns with it, but the pencil of light forming the foveal image traverses different zones of the spectacle lens. The designer's role is to design a lens so that the performance of the lens in these different zones is as satisfactory as possible. First, the designer must formulate a design philosophy. Because there is no single *best-form* lens of a given power that eliminates both oblique astigmatism and curvature of image error simultaneously, the principle of design must be articulated.

The designer must make assumptions about how the lens will be used and worn. If the conditions under which the lens is used and worn match the assumptions made by the designer, the lens will perform as intended. Most lens designers make the following classic assumptions:

1. The center of rotation of the eye is a fixed point with respect to the cornea.
2. The optic axis of the correcting lens passes through the center of rotation of the eye.
3. The foveal chief ray passes through the center of rotation of the eye.

On the basis of these assumptions, the optics of the eye can be ignored except for the eye's center of rotation and the far-point sphere. The center of rotation is considered to be the stop in the system, through which all rays must pass.

Assumptions for which there is less agreement include:

1. *The Viewing Distance.* Different base curves are required for distance vision and near vision. This principle applies to both point-focal designs and zero mean oblique error (Percival) designs. As a general rule, the closer the viewing distance, the shallower the lens form.

2. *Angle of Obliquity.* The amount of oblique astigmatism increases as the square of the distance of the object point from the optic axis. For example, oblique power errors at 15° of ocular rotation are only 25% of the oblique power errors for 30° of ocular rotation. The most common choice for the angle of obliquity is 30°. The greater the angle of obliquity, the flatter the base curve must be.

3. *The Stop Distance.* The stop distance is the distance from the back pole of the spectacle lens to the center of rotation of the eye and is made up of the vertex distance plus the distance from the cornea to the center of rotation. The magnitude of the stop distance has become increasingly controversial. Early lens designers used 25 mm as the stop distance, but 27 mm has become a typical value. Generally, myopes are expected to have larger stop distances than hyperopes. As lenses have increased in size, the vertex distance component of the stop distance has in-

FIGURE 6–27.   A surfacing chart. This chart allows the practitioner to compare series of lenses available from different manufacturers. (Reprinted with permission from Vision-Ease Corp., St. Cloud, MN.)

creased. As the stop distance increases, the lens form must be shallower (see Figure 6–14).

4. *Lens Thickness.* Lens thickness is usually ignored in approximate expressions for calculating the extent of an aberration. When it is taken into account, none of the aberrations is significantly affected.

6.16. The Base Curve of a Lens

Lens form is usually discussed in terms of the base curve of the lens in question. The term *base curve* has been given many meanings and is often loosely and incorrectly used. When used in connection with ophthalmic lens design, the term base curve refers to a standard curvature ground onto a lens for a grouping of powers. This definition has two meanings: (1) A lens designer may specify a +6.00-D base curve for every lens in a series of lenses. With this system, there would be only one base curve for the whole series. (2) A designer may specify a different base curve for each lens in the series and thus have, in effect, an almost infinite number of base curves. In practice, the concept of base curve usually means a compromise between the use of a single base curve for all lenses and a different base curve for each lens. For example, a –5.50-D base curve may be used for lenses between powers of +2.00 and +3.00 D, and so forth.

A corrected-curve lens *series* is made up of a group of base curves, each used over a range of prescription powers. The base curve can be designated in terms of the refracting power of either the *front* or the *back* surface of the lens. A small number of front surface base curves results in a large number of back surface powers, whereas a small number of back surface base curves results in a large number of front surface powers. The number of base curves available for a lens series provides an index of the precision of the design. However, when the number of base curves of two or more corrected-curve lens series are compared, the base curves must refer to the *same surface* (front or back) of the lens. The number of base curves, in itself, does not provide insight into the philosophy of the lens design or the quality of the manufactured product.

Because several lenses are grouped together in a lens series, a means of indicating their relationships must be available along with the intended use of the semifinished blanks and grinding instructions for local prescription laborato-

ries. To meet this need, the manufacturer provides the laboratory with a surfacing chart (Figure 6–27). The surfacing chart (1) provides information regarding the *surface power* of the particular manufacturer's lenses, which allows the practitioner to make comparisons between lenses available from different manufacturers; and (2) furnishes surfacing instructions, so that local optical laboratories can select semifinished blanks and surface the lenses according to the designer's intent.

Lens manufacturers supply lenses to optical laboratories as (1) *finished uncut lenses,* with both surfaces finished, ready to be cut, edged, and mounted in the frame (unless the manufacturing practice is known, a finished lens provides no clue as to whether the front or back curve is the base curve) and as (2) *semifinished lenses* that have a finished side and an unfinished side, with the base curve on the finished side. The location of the base curve (whether the manufacturer has finished the front or the back side of the lens) differs for different types of lenses. For *uncorrected spheres* (those for which there has been no attempt to control oblique astigmatism), the base curve for a plus lens is on the *back* side of the lens; for a minus lens, the base curve is on the *front* of the lens. Standard base curves for these lenses are –6.00 D for plus lenses and +6.00 D for minus lenses. *Uncorrected sphero-cylinders* are always made in front toric form, that is, the sphere is ground on the back side, and the base curve is the flattest of the two curves on the front side of the lens.

The base curve is somewhat different for *corrected* lenses (those for which oblique astigmatism or curvature of image, or both, have been controlled). For corrected *spheres,* the base curve is usually on the front for both plus and minus lenses. Exceptions occur for some higher powers of lenses. For corrected *sphero-cylinders,* the toric curve may be on the front surface (positive toric) or on the back surface (negative toric). If the lens is made in positive toric form, the base curve is the flattest curvature on the front surface; but in the negative toric form, the base curve is the spherical front surface. There are distinct advantages to *back-toric* lenses, as discussed later in the chapter.

All *multifocal* lenses have the base curve ground on the side of the lens that provides the additional power for near vision. This is true of fused, one-piece, and progressive addition multifocals. All toric multifocals are negative torics (except for the back-surface one-piece multifocal lens) and therefore have both the spherical surface (the base curve) and the added power for near vision on the front side of the lens.

HISTORY AND EVOLUTION OF LENS DESIGN

6.17. Spherical Lenses

The earliest ophthalmic lenses were bi-convex in form; bi-concave lenses were developed later. Both these lenses were popular because they were easy to manufacture. The surface powers for bi-convex and bi-concave lenses are weaker than that for any other lens form, and both sides

of these lenses have the same curvature. As lens-manufacturing skills increased, "flat" lenses were produced: a plus lens having a flat back surface and a minus lens having a flat front surface.

In 1804, William Wollaston, an English physician and chemist, proposed a convex-concave (meniscus) form of lens and established its superiority over the plano-spherical and equi-sided bi-convex and bi-concave forms by investigating the image formation produced by different forms of lenses. Wollaston did not provide the theoretical proof of the superiority of this lens but demonstrated its performance experimentally. His more deeply curved lens form gave a wider field of vision. Wollaston called the lenses *periscopic*, "to-look-around," lenses. He concluded that the best form of spectacle lens was one designed so that a small oblique pencil of light made equal angles with the two surfaces of the lens. Theoretically, the Wollaston design was a sound one, and a patent was issued for the periscopic lens in 1804. However, because of the deep curvatures required, the lenses were difficult to manufacture.

In 1874 Rodenstock, in Germany, introduced lenses that approached the periscopic concept of Wollaston. In 1867 the German firm of Nitsche and Gunther introduced the 1.25-D uniform-surface lens, commonly referred to as the periscopic lens. In this series, a plus lens had a –1.25 D back surface, and a minus lens had a +1.25 D front surface. This series of periscopic lenses was a standard lens for many years. Nitsche and Gunther later offered another landmark lens, the 6.00 D base curve lens, and the term *meniscus*, meaning "moon-shaped," was adopted for these lenses. For plus spherical lenses, the back surface had a power of –6.00 D, and minus spherical lenses had a front surface power of +6.00 D. For lenses not designed to control aberrations (noncorrected lenses), the 6.00 D uniform lenses, still referred to as meniscus lenses, continue to be used.

In 1898 F. Ostwalt, a French oculist, published the results of calculations for a series of spherical lenses designed to eliminate oblique astigmatism. His calculations produced lenses of much shallower design than those of Wollaston. In the period 1904–1908, Tscherning, who first realized the significance of the center of rotation of the eye as a reference point in lens design, demonstrated that for an extended range of lens powers (from approximately +7.00 to –22.00 D), oblique astigmatism could be eliminated by either of two forms of bent lenses, the shallower Ostwalt form and the deeper Wollaston form. Further, Tscherning found that if the surface powers of both forms are plotted graphically, they form an *ellipse*. As described in Section 6.8 and shown in Figure 6–13, this is known as *Tscherning's ellipse*. Tscherning's calculations applied only to infinitely thin lenses and to the elimination of oblique astigmatism for paraxial rays. Although lenses of the Wollaston form produce less distortion than those of the Ostwalt form, the Ostwalt form results in a shallower lens, and these lenses are both easier to produce and cosmetically superior. For these reasons, modern lenses conform to the Ostwalt form of the Tscherning ellipse.

In 1908, Moritz von Rohr, extending the work of Allvar Gullstrand, began research in spectacle lens design with the intent of eliminating oblique astigmatism. He chose the rigorous, tedious method of trigonometric ray tracing to evaluate the performance of the lenses. Von Rohr made the following assumptions: (1) the primary thrust was to eliminate oblique astigmatism; (2) the distance from the back pole of the lens to the center of rotation of the eye (the stop distance) was 25 mm; (3) the viewing angle was 35° for plus lenses and 30° for minus lenses; (4) the viewing distance

was infinity; (5) each lens had a specific thickness; and (6) sphero-cylindrical lenses would be manufactured in plus toric form.

Zeiss Optical Company patented von Rohr's lens design as the *Punktal* (point-forming) lens in 1911 and started production in 1913. Each individual lens power was ground with an optimal curvature, which resulted in the need for several thousand separate surface curvatures. Because each lens of the Punktal series had its own surface powers, about 15,000 uncut lenses were necessary to service most prescriptions. The cost of such a lens inventory was prohibitive; consequently, many optical laboratories failed to carry the full range of uncut lenses. Unfortunately, special factory orders and ensuing delays were common. These lenses were not widely used in the United States, but were well received in Europe. Spectacle lens correction as created and implemented by von Rohr provided a classic foundation for lens design for many years. Von Rohr is also credited with creating the *back vertex system* of specifying ophthalmic lens power, as well as the concept of *vertex refraction*.

In 1947 the Punktal lens series was recomputed by Wolfgang Roos. Although continuing to emphasize correction of oblique astigmatism, Roos decided its correction should be for both near distances and at infinity. Lens sizes had increased significantly since von Rohr's calculations. Roos extended the range of correction for oblique astigmatism beyond the viewing angle of 30°. Setting a tolerance of 0.20 D of oblique astigmatism, the new Punktal lenses provided correction of oblique astigmatism for distances from infinity to 25 cm and for lens diameters of as large as 50 mm. However, he attached more importance to the correction for near objects than for distant objects. This adaptation of the design, for larger angles of obliquity and for viewing distances nearer than infinity, produced lenses that were shallower in form than the original Punktal lenses. However, by increasing the tolerance for oblique astigmatism, Roos greatly decreased the number of lens blanks required for the new lens series.

Currently, Punktal lenses by Zeiss are made in both positive toric form and negative toric form. Positive toric form lenses are used for most plus lenses and low-powered minus lenses; negative toric lenses are used for strong minus lenses. In the low-powered plus lenses and weak minus lenses in which the cylindrical component exceeds 4.00 D, the lenses are available in either positive toric form or negative toric form. The transition range is designed to provide uniform construction in cases of anisometropia, in which magnification properties and esthetic considerations become important.

In 1919, Edgar Tillyer patented a lens design in which both oblique astigmatism and curvature of image (power error) were considered. American Optical Company made these lenses available to the profession in 1926 under the trade name Tillyer. The calculations for the Tillyer lens series were based on a viewing angle of 30°, a distance from the back surface of the lens to the center of rotation of 27 mm, and vision for objects at infinity.

Because oblique astigmatism and power error cannot be reduced to zero with the same lens design, Tillyer decided to let oblique astigmatism become as large as 0.12 D for weak prescriptions and as much as 0.25 D for strong prescriptions, as long as the power error could be reduced. He also decided to permit both aberrations to reach these tolerance levels if the number of base curves could be reduced. He discovered that he could maintain the tolerance levels with a single base curve that satisfied a range of prescriptions. Thus, Tillyer laid the groundwork for a "stepped," or "clustered," base-curve series for corrected-curve lenses. Because of the consideration given to power error, Tillyer lenses were *flatter* than Punktal lenses. For spherical powers ranging from +7.00 to –20.00 D and for cylinders as much as 6.00 D, 19 base curves were used. For powers of +7.00 to –5.00 D, the Tillyer lenses were made in positive toric form with the base curve as the flatter curve on the front surface. For lenses of –5.00 to –20.00 D, the toric surface was placed on the back and the base curve was the spherical curve on the front surface.

In 1928, Bausch & Lomb Optical Company introduced the Orthogon lens. The Orthogon lens was designed by Wilbur Rayton, who modified the Punktal calculations as a way to group lenses together on a common base curve. The fundamental principle in the Orthogon lens design, like the Punktal design from which it was derived, was the correction of oblique astigmatism. No correction of curvature of image was incorporated into the design. Calculations were based on a distance from the back surface to the center of rotation of 25 mm, a viewing angle of 30°, and vision for objects at infinity. In most cases, oblique astigmatism was around 0.05 D but was permitted to increase to 0.25 D in rare instances. The Orthogon lenses were made in positive toric form with the base curve usually the flatter curve on the front of the lens. However, for lenses of +6.00 to +8.00 D, the base curve was on the back of the lens. Orthogon single-vision lenses are supplied in uncut and semifinished lenses in prescriptions from +8.00 to –12.00 D and use 12 base curves. The Orthogon lens was slightly *steeper* than the Tillyer lens.

The Widesite lens, a product of Shuron Optical Company, was designed on the basis of 14 base curves. All lenses are made in positive toric form. For semifinished spherocylindrical lenses, the front surfaces were finished in five base curves: +5.50, +6.50, +7.00, +8.00, and +9.00 D. For semifinished spheres the back surfaces were ground on nine base curves: –5.00, –5.25, –5.75, –6.50, –7.00, –7.75, –8.75, –9.25, and –12.00 D. Finished lenses were supplied with the same base curves as semifinished lenses. While primarily correcting for oblique astigmatism, correction was limited to 5% of the axial power of the lens.

In 1920 the Kurova corrected-curve lens was introduced by Continental Optical Company. The lens was probably the earliest corrected-curve lens made in this country, although the first lenses were not based on a complete lens design analysis. In 1925 F. E. Duckwall redesigned the lenses. The lens calculations were based on a distance from the back surface of the lens to the center of rotation of 25 mm, a viewing angle of 30°, and vision for objects at infinity. The goal in the Kurova lens design was to reduce oblique astigmatism to insignificant levels and, at the same time, to minimize power error (curvature of image error). In order of importance, errors were listed as marginal astigmatism first, plus power error next, and minus power error last. The Kurova lens series was made in positive toric form with the base curve as the flatter curve on the front surface. The lenses were made in both finished and semifinished form, with 39 base curves ranging from +2.50 to +12.50 D.

In 1950 the Normalsite corrected-curve series was introduced by the Titmus Optical Company. The lens was designed by Foster Klingaman, who based his calculations on a stop distance of 27 mm, a viewing angle of 30°, and an object distance of 13 feet. The Normalsite lens was the first American lens to correct for an object distance closer than infinity. Primary consideration was given to the correction of oblique astigmatism at the intermediate distance of 13 feet, and secondary consideration was given to the curvature of image error, also at 13 feet. Because near object distances require flatter lens forms than infinite object distances and because consideration of curvature of image error also requires flatter lens forms, the Normalsite lenses were flatter than most other lenses on the market. For lenses having powers from +7.00 to –8.00 D, the lens was produced with a positive toric surface with the base curve as the shallower front surface curve. For lenses from –8.25 to –13.00 D, the lenses were made in negative toric form, with the base curve as the spherical curve on the front surface.

In early 1964 Univis Lens Company, primarily known for multifocal products, introduced the Best-Form lens, a negative toric lens. The lens was subsequently updated and renamed the Uni-Form lens. The lens designer was E. W. Bechtold. His calculations were based on a stop distance of 27 mm, a viewing angle of 30°, and a viewing distance of infinity. The lens had negative toric construction, with the base curve as the spherical curve on the front surface. Primary attention was given to the correction of oblique astigmatism. The performance of Uni-Form lenses was determined by modulation transfer function (MTF) testing, which involves the ratio of the contrast of the image to the contrast of the object. Uni-Form lenses were discontinued in 1971.

Soon after the introduction of the Best-Form lens in 1964, American Optical Company marketed a negative toric corrected-curve lens called the Tillyer Masterpiece lens. This lens was designed by J. K. Davis, H. H. Fernald, and A. W. Rayner. With the availability of high-speed computing equipment, calculations were made for (1) stop distances of 27 to 33 mm (which include 90% of the population), (2) viewing angles of 20°, 30°, and 40° from the optical axis, (3) object distances of infinity and 30, 16, and 13 inches, and (4) ray plots for each principal meridian and for meridians 45 degrees from the principal meridians. Aberrations considered were oblique astigmatism, curvature of image, and lateral chromatic aberration. A single blur index was developed mathematically, in which the contribution of each aberration to the blur was summed, which produced an index of blur for each possible design of the lens. The lens design with the smallest blur index theoretically provided the best image. Figure 6–28 shows a plot of a +4.00-D lens with 18 different curves and displays the blur index and the oblique astigmatism for different angles of view, object distances, and stop distances. The base curve selected must be a compromise. Visual inspection indicates that the range of –4.00

FIGURE 6–28. **Plot showing the blur index and oblique astigmatism for a +4.00 D lens. The blur index is shown with broken lines, and astigmatism is shown with solid lines. (Reprinted with permission from J. K. Davis, H. G. Fernald, and A. W. Rayner,** *The Tillyer Masterpiece Lens, a Technical Discussion,* **American Optical Corp., 1964.)**

to –4.25 D is the best compromise. In practice, computer programs, with priorities set by the lens designer, indicate the best compromise.

Consideration of longer stop distances, object distances closer than infinity, and power errors resulted in a lens noticeably shallower (1.50 to 2.00 D) than the original positive toric Tillyer lens. The lens was not an unqualified success. Patients who used their lenses mainly for distance vision reported that when they looked through the peripheral portions of the flatter lenses, images were not as sharp

as those produced with the steeper lens design. Because the detail that the eye must resolve for near vision is not as fine as the detail required for distance vision, it is more important to generate a lens form that strictly controls off-axis aberrations for distant objects than to compromise for near vision. Subsequently, the lens was redesigned, resulting in a *steeper lens.* The second generation of Masterpiece lenses was called the Masterpiece II lens.

After Shuron Optical and Continental Optical companies merged, Shuron's positive toric Widesite lens was integrated with Continental's positive toric Kurova series to form a single Kurova positive toric series. In 1966 the Shuron-Continental Division of Textron, Inc. introduced a negative toric series, the Kurova Shursite. The calculations for the Shursite lens were based on stop distances of 26.5 mm (for a power of +8.00 D) to 31.00 mm (for a power of –8.00 D), depending on lens power; viewing angles of 20°, 30°, and 40°; and object distances of infinity and 14 inches. Selection of base curves was made on the basis of a compromise between the correction of oblique astigmatism, power error, and lateral chromatic aberration. The lens is manufactured in negative toric form, with the base curve as the spherical curve on the front surface. Twenty base curves range from +0.50 to +12.00 D. The Shursite lens bendings fall roughly midway between the steeper Uni-Form lens and the original, shallower, Tillyer Masterpiece lens. The bendings of the Shursite negative toric lenses do not depart significantly from those of Shuron-Continental's Kurova positive toric series.

6.18. Sphero-Cylindrical Lens Design

A high percentage of lens prescriptions incorporate a cylindrical component for the correction of astigmatism. Bannon and Walsh[4] found, in a study of 200 patients, that 83% of their patients had a sufficient amount of astigmatism to warrant its correction. Lenses for the correction of astigmatism possess two principal meridians that parallel the principal meridians of the eye. The power of the lens is minimal in one principal meridian and maximal in the other. A lens that corrects astigmatism is customarily made up of a spherical component and a cylindrical component, in much the same way that the correction obtained by the use of a refractor consists of a spherical element and a cylindrical element.

In practice, the surfaces of lenses used for the correction of astigmatism are surfaces of revolution (see Chapter 2). Most lenses for the correction of astigmatism have a spherical surface on one side and a toric surface on the other, with the sum of the surface powers in each principal meridian fixed to render the image of the lens/eye system stigmatic for axial vision.

A sphero-cylindrical lens has *two* powers. Light from an object point on the optical axis incident on a sphero-cylindrical lens forms an astigmatic pencil after refraction and passes in succession through two focal lines. To correct the eye for axial gaze, the two astigmatic focal lines must fall on the respective far points for the two principal meridians of the eye. When the eye rotates to view objects not located on the optical axis, each far point generates a corresponding *far-point sphere*. To form on the retina a point image for a point object for all directions of gaze, the astigmatic focal lines formed by the lens should, after refraction, fall on the respective far-point spheres.

The sphero-cylindrical lens is subject to the same aberrations as is the spherical lens. As the eye looks obliquely through peripheral portions of a lens, the aberrations of oblique astigmatism and curvature of image are superimposed on the astigmatic pencil produced by the lens, which

results in removal of the line foci from their ideal positions on the respective far-point spheres. Hence, the astigmatic effect for rays passing through peripheral portions of the lens differs from that along the optical axis of the lens. The discrepancy between the image surfaces formed by the line foci and their respective far-point spheres varies with different directions of gaze. Thus, the teacup and saucer figure associated with oblique astigmatism generated by a spherical lens becomes a much more complex figure that defies simple conceptual description.

To provide the same effective power of the astigmatic lens over the entire lens, the same method as that used in dealing with a spherical lens is available, that is, bending the lens. Because the lens has a spherical surface on one side and a toric surface on the other, it is not possible to cause both image surfaces to coincide with their corresponding far-point spheres. Although equalizing the amount of astigmatism in each of the principal meridians for a given angle of view is possible, the amount of astigmatism may differ from the intended astigmatic correction (the correction present along the optical axis). When the cylinder component is small, the form suitable for the spherical component is often used. For larger cylindrical components, the powers of the two principal meridians are averaged, which results in a compromise in performance for each principal meridian.

6.19. Negative versus Positive Toric Lenses

Although all corrected-curve sphero-cylindrical lenses were originally designed as *positive* toric lenses, almost all have now been redesigned as *negative* torics. One advantage of a negative toric lens is that most multifocal lenses are negative torics (having the bifocal addition on the front). If, during the pre-presbyopic years, an individual wears negative toric lenses, adaptation to a different lens form is not necessary when multifocal lenses are first worn.

However, a more important advantage of negative toric lenses has to do with *spectacle magnification*. Spectacle magnification is given by the formula

$$SM = \left(\frac{1}{1 - F_1 \frac{t}{n}}\right)\left(\frac{1}{1 - hF_V}\right), \quad (6.18)$$

where F_1 = front surface power, t = thickness, n = the index of refraction, h = the distance from the back pole of the lens to the entrance pupil of the eye, and F_V = back vertex power of the lens. The first member of the right-hand side of the equation relates to the form of the lens and is called the *shape factor*; the second member relates to the power of the lens and is called the *power factor*.

For a positive toric lens, there are two values of F_1 and two values of F_V. Therefore, the power of the front surface, F_1, contributes to the magnification difference between the two meridians. However, for a negative toric lens, F_1 has the same value for both meridians, with the result that the meridional magnification is less than that for a positive toric lens.

In addition to the optical advantages of negative toric lenses, these lenses can be made more attractive than positive toric lenses. Negative toric lenses with a significant cylindrical component can be edged with the bevel placed at a constant distance from the spherical front surface so that the thick edges of the most minus meridian are hidden, either within the frame or behind the frame. Such a lens is also easier to mount. Because the bevel follows the spherical contour of the front surface, the entire extent of the bevel lies in a single plane, which makes the lens easier to mount (and retain) in the frame. The first manufacturer to mass-produce a negative toric single-vision lens was the American Optical Company, with its Tillyer Masterpiece lens of 1964. The Shuron-Continental Kurova Shursite minus cylinder negative toric lens was introduced in 1966.

6.20. Aspheric Lens Designs

In a broad sense, *aspheric* means "*not spherical.*" By this definition, aspheric surfaces include toric surfaces. However, in ophthalmic optics the term *aspheric* describes a surface that is axially or rotationally symmetrical and is formed by the rotation of a portion of a parabola and an ellipse, or a hyperbola. Because toric surfaces have circular cross-sections in both principal meridians, they are described as nonspherical as distinct from aspheric.

The history of aspheric surfaces began in the early part of this century. Moritz von Rohr of Zeiss Optical Company, in a notable patent, first described an aspheric lens in detail. Then, on the basis of Gullstrand's earlier work, Zeiss commercially produced in 1909 an aspheric back surface lens, called the Katral lens, for the correction of aphakia. In 1958 an American ophthalmologist, David Volk, was successful in producing for aphakia an excellent aspheric lens in glass, called the Volk Conoid Lens. In the early 1970s Robert Welsh, an ophthalmologist, introduced the Welsh 4-Drop Lens for aphakia. This lens consisted of four blended spherical zones beyond the spherical central area. This category of lenses became known as *zonal aspheric lenses.*

In 1976, Davis and Fernald patented a series of aspheric ophthalmic lenses. The design concept was not based on customary methods of manipulation of the form of the lens, but instead preselected a bending for power, which subsequently corrected off-axis performance by making one of the lens surfaces aspheric. The Davis/Fernald patent is significant in lens design, because it describes a method of determining the asphericity required to provide good off-axis performance in a lens that would produce poor off-axis performance if it were constructed with spherical surfaces. On publication of the patent, lens designers directed their attention to these types of flatter, thinner forms, which are in common use today.

In 1980 Whitney, Reilly, and Young patented the Ful-Vue aspheric blended lenticular lens for American Optical Company. The advantage of this lens was the large diameter (66 mm) available. Mo Jalie of England, in 1980, published a patent directed toward lenses of lower power that delivered good cosmetic appearance and good off-axis op-

tical performance and that used very flat lenses with one hyperboloidal surface.

Until the 1980s, aspherical surfaces were reserved for high plus prescriptions that fell beyond the upper limit of the Tscherning Ellipse, that is, above +7.50 D. Although lenses beyond this limit cannot be made entirely free of oblique astigmatism with spherical surfaces, as described in Section 6.10, there is a form of lens with spherical surfaces that produces a *minimum* amount of oblique astigmatism. By using aspheric surfaces for lenses above +7.50 D, oblique astigmatism may be controlled.

How is oblique astigmatism reduced by aspheric surfaces? With most aspheric surfaces used for ophthalmic lenses, the curvature extending radially or tangentially in all directions from the center changes progressively, and the curvature in the opposite meridian (circumferentially) also changes progressively, but the change is much less rapid than it is in the radial direction. The power change along the radial or tangential direction is about three times as great as the change in the circumferential direction.[5] Thus, all aspheric surfaces are inherently astigmatic away from the center. The inherent astigmatism of aspheric surfaces is used to balance the oblique astigmatism caused by gazing obliquely through the lens.

With the acceptance of CR-39 and similar plastic materials for spectacle lenses, the replication of aspheric surfaces by plastic molding or casting reduced the cost of producing aspheric surfaces. Furthermore, with the advent of computer-assisted design and computer numerically controlled grinding techniques, it became possible to manufacture surfaces of almost any complexity. An interest in improving the cosmetic appearance of lenses and reducing the weight, "bulginess," and thickness (usually in large spectacles) provided the impetus for extending the use of aspheric surfaces to lens powers less than +7.50 D and also to minus lenses.

The rationale underlying the design of modern, thin, low-power aspherics is based on a two-stage process. First, the lens is made much flatter in form by using a flatter base curve, which reduces the bulge forward from the frame. An examination of an accurate sagitta table demonstrates that the sagittae are not strictly proportional to surface powers but increase at a faster rate than the surface power (Table 6–1). For example, the sagitta of a lens surface of 1.00 D, index 1.523, with a diameter of 70 mm, is 1.18 mm; the sagitta of a surface of 10.00 D, with the same index and diameter, is 13.44 mm. Therefore, steeply curved lenses tend to be thicker than flatter lenses with other factors such as power, index of refraction, lens diameter, and edge thickness held constant. For example, the following two CR-39 lenses, index 1.50, are made with a power of +4.00 D, a diameter of 70 mm, and an edge thickness of 1.0 mm. Lens A, which has a back surface power of –4.75 D and a front surface power of +8.45 D is 6.5 mm thick. Lens B, which has a back surface power of –1.50 D and a front surface power of +5.38 D, is only 6.0 mm thick. Thus, lens B with the flatter design is 0.5 mm thinner than the more steeply formed lens A.

However, the change to the flatter form increases the off-axis power errors beyond that of the steeper best-form design. The second stage of the process is to provide aspheric surfaces. By appropriate aspherization of the lens surfaces, it is possible to further improve the cosmetic appearance, reduce

TABLE 6-1
Sagittae of Lens Surfaces (for n = 1.523)

Surface Power (D)	Lens Diameter (mm)						
	40	44	48	52	56	60	70
1	0.38	0.46	0.55	0.65	0.75	0.86	1.18
2	0.77	0.93	1.10	1.29	1.50	1.73	2.40
3	1.15	1.39	1.66	1.95	2.26	2.60	3.52
4	1.54	1.86	2.22	2.61	3.03	3.49	4.75
5	1.93	2.34	2.79	3.28	3.82	4.39	6.03
6	2.33	2.82	3.37	3.97	4.62	5.33	7.33
7	2.73	3.31	3.96	4.67	5.44	6.29	8.71
8	3.13	3.81	4.56	5.39	6.30	7.29	10.16
9	3.55	4.33	5.19	6.14	7.19	8.34	11.72
10	3.98	4.86	5.84	6.92	8.13	9.46	13.44
11	4.42	5.40	6.50	7.74	9.12	10.66	15.40
12	4.86	5.96	7.20	8.60	10.18	11.97	17.61
13	5.33	6.55	7.94	9.53	11.34	13.43	20.43
14	5.81	7.17	8.73	10.53	12.63	15.10	24.31
15	6.31	7.82	9.57	11.64	14.09	17.10	31.82

thickness and weight, and reduce off-axis errors to the level obtained with best-form lenses with spherical surfaces.

Invariably, the front surface of the lens is made aspheric and the back surface is reserved for the cylinder component if present. The asphericity of the front surface is selected to correct off-axis aberrations. For plus lenses, the aspheric front surface flattens toward the periphery in the form of an oblate ellipse (Figure 6–29), with the aspheric surface reducing the sagittal depth and the lens thickness (A). For minus lenses, the aspheric front surface steepens from the center toward the edge in the form of a prolate ellipse, which produces thinner edges (B). Thus, these lenses can be made thinner for the same aperture or have a wider aperture for the same thickness. Additional reduction in thickness may be obtained by using high-index materials. However, many high-index materials have a low Abbe number, with the result that the increased chromatic aberration may compromise visual performance, especially for high-powered lenses. Because most high-index materials are new, complications may arise in tinting, coating, and processing; as these lenses age, long-term factors such as discoloration and durability cannot yet be predicted.

For minus lenses, an additional consideration is the minimum center thickness required for a lens to pass the drop-ball test. For example, CR-39 plastic lenses normally require a 2.0-mm center thickness to pass the drop-ball test; polycarbonate and some other plastic materials can pass the drop-ball test with a center thickness of only 1.5 mm.

Two additional benefits accompany aspheric lens design: (1) the magnification of the eye and surrounding structures, as seen by an observer, is reduced; and (2) the spectacle magnification for the patient is similarly reduced.

The benefits of aspheric design are most apparent and appreciated with high plus lenses. The flatter, thinner, lighter lenses and decreased magnification are readily apparent. However, in minus prescriptions, the improvements are more subtle because the asphericity is not as pronounced as that with plus lens prescriptions—minus lenses are already made on flatter base curves.

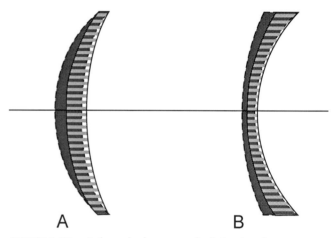

FIGURE 6–29.   **A, for a plus lens, an aspheric front surface causes a decrease in center thickness; B, for a minus lens, an aspheric front surface causes a decrease in edge thickness.**

When aspheric lenses are used, off-axis power errors caused by improper fitting, such as tilt and decentration, are larger than those for lenses with spherical surfaces. The number of errors can be as high as twice that occurring in lenses with spherical surfaces and can be expected to lower visual performance.[6] A front aspherical surface is spherical only in the areas immediately surrounding the vertex. Careful fitting is necessary to ensure that the optic axis of the aspherical surface passes through the center of rotation of the eye. To achieve this effect, the following design considerations must be met:

1. The vertex of the surface must be positioned horizontally by using monocular (split) interpupillary distances as determined with a corneal reflection pupillometer. Most manufacturers of aspherics premark the front vertex position.

2. If prism is required, the lenses should not be decentered to obtain the prism; any prismatic effect should be achieved by working prism on the back surface (to ensure that the first condition is not violated).

3. The vertex of the front surface must be dropped 1 mm from the center of the pupil, with the eyes in the primary position, for every 2 degrees of pantoscopic tilt.

Some patients accustomed to spherical lens designs may experience adaptation symptoms, especially if the lenses are of high power. Problems could originate from inadequate patient education as to what to expect, improper fitting procedures, changes in the magnification properties, and changes in the amount and location of reflected images from the lens surfaces and back surface eyelid touch.

Unfortunately, many manufacturers of aspheric lenses do not give a complete description of the topography of the aspheric surfaces that they use. Therefore, it is difficult to assess scientifically the optical performance of specific designs or make comparisons among various designs. Assessment is further complicated because a lens gauge cannot be used by the practitioner to measure the nature of the asphericity. Moving the lens gauge across the front surface may indicate that the surface is aspheric if the surface power varies with the movement, but it is not an accurate measurement of asphericity.

Failure to identify the nature of an aspheric surface without sophisticated laboratory equipment can create a problem if a lens is to be duplicated. This problem could be solved if manufacturers of aspheric lenses brandmarked their lenses as most manufacturers of progressive addition lenses currently do.

Aspheric lenses should be considered as an alternative to spherical lenses for patients who wear prescriptions greater than ±4.00 D because this level of lens power affects important optical, weight, and cosmetic characteristics. Presently, aspheric lenses cost appreciably more than spherical lenses, and cost considerations may slow the growth of aspheric lenses, especially in the lower-power ranges in which the benefits are not readily apparent. Table 6–2 lists representative plastic aspheric single-vision lenses. Aspheric lenses are discussed further in Chapter 11.

TABLE 6–2
Optical Properties of Representative Plastic Aspheric Single Vision Lenses

Manufacturer/Supplier	Lens Name	Material	Rx Range
Optima	Hyperindex 166 Aspheric	1.66 index Hard Resin	−10.00 to +8.00 DS
Optima	Hyperindex 1.60	1.60 index Hard Resin	Plano to −14.25 DS +2.25 to +10.00 DS
Rodenstock	Cosmolit 1.6	1.60 index Hard Resin	−10.00 to +12.00 DS
Seiko	Super 16 Diacoat Mx	1.60 index Hard Resin	−10.00 to +6.00 DS
Gentex	Profile	1.586 index Polycarbonate	−10.00 to +8.00 DS
Sola	ASL	1.586 index	−10.00 to +6.00 DS
Vision-Ease	Versa-Lite Asphereyes	1.586 index Polycarbonate	−8.00 to +3.00 DS
X-Cel	High-X Aspire	1.57 index Hard Resin	−11.50 to +9.50 DS
Signet Armorlite	TrimLine Aspheric	1.56 index Hard Resin	−10.00 to +9.50 DS
Sola	ASL	1.54 index Spectralite	−12.00 to +6.00 DS
Sola	ASL	1.537 index Spectralite Transitions*	−12.00 to +8.00 DS
American Optical	Aspherite	1.498 index Hard resin	−12.00 to +8.00 DS
Orcolite	Focalite	1.498 index Hard resin	+0.25 to +8.00 DS
Signet Armorlite	Trimline	1.498 index Hard Resin	−8.00 to +8.00 DS
Rodenstock	Cosmolit 1.50 Aspheric	1.498 index Hard Resin	−10.00 to +12.00 DS
Silor	Hyperol Natural Plus	1.498 index Hard Resin	+2.00 to +9.00 DS
Zeiss	Claret Hyperal	1.498 index Hard Resin	+2.25 to +7.00 DS

* Photochromic

THE OPTOMETRIST'S ROLE IN LENS DESIGN

The optometrist who places an order for eyewear and dispenses the eyewear to the patient is ultimately responsible for the performance of the lenses. Before 1972, most single-vision spectacle lenses were mass-produced as uncut lenses. The manufacturers of such lenses selected the objectives of lens design and developed a series of lenses to achieve these objectives (described in Section 6.17). Manufacturers provided information to optometrists to aquaint them with the advantages and uniqueness of their particular lens design. Optometrists were encouraged to order lenses by trade name. The major manufacturers of lenses were also manufacturers of ophthalmic equipment and operated branch ophthalmic laboratories throughout the U.S. The manufacturers, therefore, designed the lenses and sold the optometrist examination equipment, and the manufacturer's local laboratory supplied the finished glasses. The responsibility for the performance of the lenses, then, rested solely on the manufacturer, with the result that the optometrist learned, by experience, where quality and service could be obtained.

The ANSI Z80.1-1995 is a *specification* standard in which the laboratory tries to meet the specifications laid down by the optometrist. The laboratory does not exercise any judgment or create the design; it merely adheres to the specifications provided by the optometrist. Design is handled by the manufacturer by determining the number of base curves available (the more, the better), and by the optometrist who now has the responsibility to ensure that the lens provides a quality image.

The optical laboratory now has the prerogative of selecting the base curve for a lens unless the base curve has been specified by the practitioner who ordered the lens. Although most laboratories are likely to continue to supply lenses that minimize oblique astigmatism and curvature of image, it is possible that, in filling a given prescription, the laboratory may not have in stock either a corrected-curve uncut lens or a semifinished lens from which a proper corrected-curve lens can be made. Further, it is difficult to insert deeply curved plus lenses into large frames; thus, the laboratory may resort to shallower lens forms when plus lenses are ordered.

6.21. Changes in the Optical Industry and in ANSI Standards

In recent years, the optical industry has undergone many changes. Because of financial reasons, the major lens manufacturers no longer maintain branch optical laboratories. Lens product identification and product loyalty have diminished greatly. Other factors, also, have affected the optometrist's relationship with optical laboratories. The proliferation of larger lens sizes has made it difficult and costly for a laboratory to maintain an adequate stock of uncut and semifinished lenses for a large variety of corrected-curve lenses. There has been a switch to negative toric lenses that laboratories finish from semifinished lenses. Tolerances are lower for laboratory-processed semifinished lenses than they are for stock lenses provided by the manufacturer.

A significant change affecting lens design occurred when the American National Standards Institute (ANSI) Z80.1-1972 Standard for ophthalmic lenses was revised in 1979. Unless an optometrist chose a criterion other than the correction of oblique astigmatism and curvature of image, and requested this choice in the order to the optical laboratory, the heretofore existing 1972 ANSI Standard required the laboratory to supply a lens with a base curve that would limit the unwanted cylinder and sphere power at certain points along the meridians of maximal and minimal power. These points, designated by ANSI as points A and B, were selected so that they each subtended an angle of 30 degrees with the optic axis of the lens, as measured from the center of rotation of the eye. By selecting the base curve to meet the 1972 ANSI Standard, the optical laboratory determined the basis of lens design. The ANSI Z80.1-1979 Standard and its successors, the Z80.1-1987 and the Z80.1-1995 Standards, do not require that ophthalmic lenses meet any specific tolerance for off-axis performance.

6.22. Base Curve Specification

The practitioner should become more involved in lens design than has been necessary in the past. When ordering lenses for a patient, the optometrist can provide the appropriate base curve by using the following procedures:

1. The optometrist should use only those laboratories that use semifinished lens blanks from reputable lens manufacturers and adhere to the base curve selection charts provided by the manufacturers.
2. The practitioner can acquire base curve selection charts from manufacturers and specify base curves to optical laboratories.

The optometrist should be well informed concerning ophthalmic lens design, and should obtain from lens manufacturers accurate and specific information concerning the optical performance of their lenses. Fry,[7,8] in a series of papers, summarized what an optometrist should know about the characteristics of lenses to keep them relatively free from oblique astigmatism and curvature of image. In another series of papers, Davis[9-11] attempted to help the practitioner identify the properties of lenses designed to have superior performance.

Fry[12] has also proposed that the spherical equivalent of each lens can be computed and, as seen in Table 6–3 and Figure 6–30 (both reproduced from Fry's paper) diagrams can be used for selecting the base curve on the spherical front side of a given lens. The laboratory should be allowed a tolerance of ±0.75 D in base curve selections, as specified in the ANSI Z80.1-1995 Standard.

On occasion, an optometrist may wish to order base curves other than those provided on uncut stock or semifinished

TABLE 6–3
Base Curves for Spheres and Back Toric Glass Lenses (Index = 1.523)

Base Curve	Ranges of Power for Spherical Equivalent*	
	Lower Limit	Upper Limit
+12.50	+6.399	—
+10.50	+4.387	+6.399
+8.50	+1.446	+4.387
+6.50	–2.106	+1.446
+4.50	–5.880	–2.106
+2.50	–10.503	–5.880
+0.50	—	–10.503

*As described by Fry, the spherical equivalent (the algebraic sum of the sphere and one-half the cylinder) is first computed, and this table (or Figure 6–30) can be used for selecting a lens with a given base curve on the front surface. In the case of anisometropia, the base curve for the lens with the stronger power is selected first, and the same base curve is used for the weaker lens.

SOURCE: Adapted from G. A. Fry, The Optometrist's New Role in the Use of Corrected-Curve Lenses. *J. Am. Optom. Assoc.* Vol. 50, p. 562, 1979.

FIGURE 6–30. **Diagram for use in selecting the base curve (spherical front curve), proposed by G. A. Fry. (Reprinted with permission from G. A. Fry, The Optometrist's New Role in the Use of Corrected-Curve Lenses.** *J. Am. Optom. Assoc.,* **Vol. 50, p. 562, 1979.)**

lenses. Surfacing charts are available from manufacturers and list the base curves for each power range. Specific information, such as the ideal curves for certain stop and object distances and tolerances for astigmatism and power errors, should be acquired to assist in evaluating various curvatures and in ordering special base curves when needed.

The optometrist can determine two principal variables influencing lens design calculations: lens *stop distance* and *object distance*. Normally, the lens designer makes assumptions concerning these variables. The more nearly these assumptions are met when the lenses are worn, the better the performance of the lenses.

The *stop distance* is the sum of the vertex distance and the distance from the cornea to the eye's center of rotation. The practitioner can approximate the stop distance by measuring the vertex distance and estimating the center of rotation distance. To obtain the vertex distance, eyewire distance should be measured with the selected frame in place and the sagittal distance of the lens should be added to that sum. For example, with a vertical lens dimension of 42 mm, the

sagittal distance is approximately 0.75 mm for every 2.00 D of minus back surface power. The center of rotation distance can also be estimated because it is related to the axial length of the eye. If the average dioptric value of the corneal curvature is added to the mean spherical refractive error, and then 42.50 D is subtracted from the result, the value of the axial ametropia is obtained. For example, if a patient's keratometer findings are 43.00 D at 180° combined with 44.00 D at 90°, and the spherical refractive error is –4.00 D, one first adds the mean keratometer finding (43.50 D) to –4.00 D, which is 39.50; subtracting 42.50 from this result, one finds the value of the patient's axial ametropia is –3.00 D. The center of rotation distance is about 15 mm for an average emmetropic eye. This value changes approximately 0.15 mm for each diopter of axial ametropia. Thus, the center of rotation distance increases with axial myopia and decreases with axial hyperopia. For the example given above, the center of rotation distance is 15 mm + 3 (0.15 mm) = 15.45 mm.

When the actual lens stop distance is greater than that assumed by the lens designer, a flatter base curve provides better lens performance. The base curve should be specified as approximately 0.25 D flatter or steeper for each millimeter that the stop distance is longer or shorter than the value anticipated by the designer. The minimum significant change in base curve is approximately 0.50 D.

The patient's preferred viewing distance can also be used as a basis for changing the base curve. A long viewing distance generally requires a steeper base curve than does a short viewing distance. If lenses are prescribed or used primarily for one distance, the practitioner should consider this fact when selecting a base curve.

Because oblique astigmatism cannot be completely eliminated in both principal meridians of a toric lens with a spherical surface in one side and a toric surface on the other, stock lens design tends to balance the residual astigmatic error for the two principal meridians; however, a lens can be designed to improve the performance in one principal meridian at the expense of the other. If one principal meridian is frequently used more than the other, the curves should be selected according to the prescription in the meridian of greatest interest.

All lenses function best when the optic axis passes through the eye's center of rotation (the sighting center). *Pantoscopic tilt* brings the bottom of the lens closer to the cheeks and consequently tilts the optic axis of the lens. For the optic axis to pass through the center of rotation, the pole of the lens must be dropped 1 mm below the center of the pupil for every 2 degrees of pantoscopic tilt, as discussed in Section 2.20. By keeping these variables in mind, the practitioner can provide patients with well-designed lenses that will provide optimum performance.

References

1. Southall, J. P. C. *Mirrors, Prisms and Lenses,* 3rd edition. Macmillan, New York, pp. 545–550, 1933.
2. Jalie, M. *The Principles of Ophthalmic Lenses,* 3rd edition. Association of Dispensing Opticians, London, pp. 410–411, 1977.

3. Southall, J. P. C. *Mirrors, Prisms and Lenses*, 3rd edition. Macmillan, New York, pp. 538–540, 1933.

4. Bannon, R. E., and Walsh, R. On Astigmatism, Part IV. *Am. J. Optom. Arch. Am. Acad. Optom.*, Vol. 22, pp. 263–277, 1945.

5. Davis, J. K. Aspheric Lenses: What's Possible and What Isn't. *Rev. Optom.*, Vol. 115, pp. 68–74, 1978.

6. Atchison, D. A., and Tame, S. A. Sensitivity of Off-Axis Performance of Aspheric Spectacle Lenses to Tilt and Decentration. *Ophthalmol. Physiol. Opt.*, Vol. 53, pp. 322–326, 1993.

7. Fry, G. A. Computation of Unwanted Sphere and Cylinder in the Periphery of a Spectacle Lens. *Am. J. Optom. Physiol. Optics*, Vol. 54, pp. 606–616, 1977.

8. Fry, G. A. Choosing the Base Curve for an Ophthalmic Lens. *Am. J. Optom. Physiol. Optics*, Vol. 55, pp. 238–248, 1978.

9. Davis, J. K. Corrected-Curve Lenses and Lens Quality. *Am. J. Optom. Arch. Amer. Acad. Optom.*, Vol. 39, pp. 135–148, 1962.

10. Davis, J. K., Fernald, H. G., and Rayner, A. W. An Analysis of Ophthalmic Lens Design. *Am. J. Optom. Arch. Am. Acad. Optom.*, Vol. 44, pp. 400–421, 1964.

11. Davis, J. K. Stock Lenses and Custom Design. *Am. J. Optom. Arch. Am. Acad. Optom.*, Vol. 44, pp. 776–800, 1967.

12. Fry, G. A. The Optometrist's New Role in the Use of Corrected-Curve Lenses. *J. Am. Optom. Assoc.*, Vol. 50, pp. 561–562, 1979.

Questions

1. A thin prism of refracting angle 8° is made of glass for which the refractive indices are d line = 1.50, C line = 1.48, and F line = 1.53. What is the dispersive power of the glass?

2. A thin prism of refracting angle 4° is made of glass for which the refractive indices are d line = 1.50, C line = 1.48, and F line = 1.53. What is the Abbe value of the glass?

3. What is the amount of longitudinal chromatic aberration of a +6.00 D crown glass lens with an Abbe value of 65?

4. A thin prism of refracting angle 8° is made of glass for which the refractive indices are d line = 1.50, C line = 1.48, F line = 1.53. What is the chromatic aberration of the prism?

5. A +5.00 D lens has indices of 1.52, 1.53, and 1.54, for the C, d, and F Fraunhofer lines, respectively. What is the amount of the longitudinal chromatic aberration?

6. It is required to make an achromatic lens of +5.00 D, using crown glass of index 1.50 with an Abbe value of 70, and flint glass for which the index is 1.60, with an Abbe value of 40. What are the powers of the crown and flint lenses, respectively?

7. It is required to make an achromatic prism of 3 prism diopters, using a crown glass for which the index of refraction = 1.52, dispersive power = 1/60, and a flint glass for which the index of refraction = 1.61, dispersive power = 1/38. Find the powers of the prism components.

8. The equivalent focal length of a positive achromatic doublet (composed of two lenses with zero separation) is 24 cm. If the converging crown glass lens has a focal length of 18 cm, what is the focal length of the diverging flint glass lens?

9. A cemented achromatic lens of +2.00 D is made of crown glass (index of refraction, 1.5; Abbe number, 60) and flint glass (index of refraction, 1.6; Abbe number, 40). The exposed (uncemented) surface of the flint glass has a power of −1.60 D. The curvatures of the cemented surfaces are equal. What is the power of the exposed (uncemented) surface of the crown glass?

10. When looking 30 degrees from the center of a +7.00 D lens, the sagittal focal power is +6.88 D and the tangential focal power is +7.48 D. What is the curvature of field or power error?

11. When looking up 30 degrees from the center of a −9.00-D lens at a cross formed of horizontal and vertical lines, the sagittal focal power is −8.90 D and the amount of oblique astigmatism is −0.36 D. What is the amount of blur expressed in diopters of the horizontal lines on the cross?

12. A +3.00 D lens (index, 1.523) is prescribed. Assume the lens is located 27 mm from the center of rotation. What is the radius of curvature of the Petzval surface?

13. A −3.00 D lens (index, 1.523) is prescribed. Assume the lens is located 27 mm from the center of rotation. What is the radius of the far-point sphere?

14. A lens of index 1.50 is designed to eliminate marginal astigmatism. If the lens is worn 25 mm in front of the center of rotation of the eye, at what power will the Petzval surface and the far-point sphere coincide?

CHAPTER SEVEN

Absorptive Lenses and Lens Coatings

The human eye has evolved in the presence of solar radiation, which includes not only the visible spectrum, extending from approximately 400 to 700 nm, but also the neighboring ultraviolet (UV) and infrared (IR) regions of the spectrum. Radiation in both the UV and IR regions has been found to have harmful effects on the ocular tissues; fortunately, these effects can be controlled, to a great extent, if absorptive lenses are worn.

Lenses made of clear ophthalmic crown glass or clear CR-39 plastic transmit only about 92% of incident visible light, as a result of the loss by reflection at the front and back surfaces; because of the absorption of some UV and IR radiation, the lenses transmit somewhat smaller amounts of radiation in these regions of the spectrum. Absorption in the UV and IR regions (or even in the visible spectrum) can, however, be increased by the addition of absorbers to the batch of glass or plastic.

There are several types of absorptive lenses, such as lenses designed for general wear, which absorb the spectrum evenly; lenses designed to selectively absorb UV or IR radiation, or both; and lenses designed to selectively absorb bands of radiation within the visible spectrum. In addition, there are lenses (called *photochromic* lenses) that have the property of varying the absorption of radiation on the basis of the ambient illumination level; that is, they increase absorption in high levels of illumination and decrease absorption in lower levels of illumination.

Lens reflections may present a problem for the wearer of the lenses and for an observer. From the wearer's point of view, reflections from the lens surfaces may be annoying and can be minimized by the use of an antireflective coating. Reflections annoying to the observer include the rings seen near the edges of minus lenses. There are several methods for minimizing the reflections.

EFFECTS OF RADIATION ON THE EYE

7.1. The Nature of Light

Radiation is a physical term defining the transfer of energy through space, from an emitter or radiator to a receiver. When light is emitted by a source and is subsequently absorbed by a receptor, a net transfer of energy occurs. The sun is a radiator, producing energy that radiates through space in all directions. The sun's radiation is called *electromagnetic* radiation because it consists of an oscillatory electric field and an oscillatory magnetic field and which are perpendicular to one another and to the direction of propagation of the radiation. At any point along the path of propagation, the oscillations of the electric and magnetic fields are synchronized with each other: Their maxima and minima occur simultaneously. These forces oscillate about their positions in a transverse direction, akin to the movement of a cork bobbing from ripples on the surface of a body of water. The electromagnetic fields do not move in the direction of propagation. On the contrary, it is the *wave* that advances.

In a vacuum, all electromagnetic energy travels at a velocity of 10^{10} meters per second (186,000 miles/sec). However, it is slowed down in any medium other than a vacuum. The velocity of light in any medium, X, is an indication of the *optical denseness*, or *refractive index*, of the medium, as expressed in the following formula:

$$\text{refractive index of medium X} = \frac{\text{velocity of light in a vacuum}}{\text{velocity of light in medium X}} \quad (7.1)$$

or

$$\text{velocity of light in medium X} = \frac{\text{velocity of light in a vacuum}}{\text{refractive index of medium X}}$$

Thus, when light travels from a vacuum to another medium, the index of refraction of that medium is the factor by which the velocity of light is *reduced* in that medium. Not only is the velocity reduced in various media, light is also absorbed differentially in various media. Historically, the nature of light has been closely studied and debated. Although the nature of light is still not clearly understood, electromagnetic radiation has been shown to possess both *particlelike* and *wavelike* characteristics. According to the particle theory, radiant energy consists of discrete units of energy, called *quanta*, or *photons*. The particle theory accounts for the interchange of energy between radiation and matter, for emission and absorption of radiation, and for the photoelectric effect. Conversely, the wave theory is used to explain the phenomena of refraction, reflection, interference, and polarization. These theories are used interchangeably, one theory explaining some observations or phenomena, and the other theory explaining others. The two theories, therefore, complement rather than compete with each other.

Light traveling through a transparent medium is more easily represented as *waves*; interactions occurring between light and matter can be more readily explained by considering light as if it were made up of *particles*. The wavelike property of radiant energy allows light to be described in terms of standard wave motion parameters (Figure 7–1). If two points on adjacent waves have the same displacement and position, the points are said to be *in phase*. Examples of pairs of points that are in phase are adjacent maxima (crests), adjacent minima (troughs), or alternate zeros. The distance between any two points in phase of adjacent waves, in a vacuum, is referred to as the *wavelength* (λ). The wavelength is generally specified in *nanometers* (nm) (formerly called millimicrons); a nanometer is equal to 10^{-9} m. If a point on a wave moves in such a manner that it retraces its path at regular intervals of time, its motion is described as *periodic*. Each vibration is called a *cycle*, and the number of cycles of a particular wave train emitted from, passing through, or arriving at a given point is termed the *frequency*. Hence,

$$\text{frequency} = \frac{\text{velocity in a vacuum}}{\text{wavelength in a vacuum}}. \quad (7.2)$$

The frequency of a wavefront is a more fundamental attribute than is velocity or wavelength. Frequency is a property of the emitting source and remains constant regardless of the medium through which the radiation may travel. It is apparent from Equation 7.2 that the wavelength is always directly proportional to the velocity; when one is reduced by a factor of n (refractive index), the other is reduced by the same factor.

In quantum theory, each photon has associated with it a *quantum* of energy, whose magnitude is directly proportional to the frequency with which the emission occurs. Therefore, because the energy (momentum) of a photon is directly proportional to its frequency, and because the frequency is inversely related to the wavelength, the shorter wavelengths of electromagnetic radiation possess higher

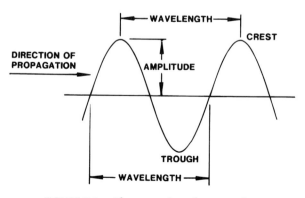

FIGURE 7–1.   **The parameters of wave motion.**

energy, or momentum, per photon than do the longer wavelengths of radiation.

The components of the electromagnetic radiations form a continuous range of radiations differing in frequency and, therefore, also differing in wavelength. The range is called the *electromagnetic spectrum*. The electromagnetic spectrum has been divided arbitrarily into regions depending on wavelength. The enormous range of electromagnetic radiation (Figure 7–2) extends from the very short cosmic rays (as short as 10^{-13} m) through gamma rays, x-rays, UV radiation, visible light, IR radiation, and radio rays (as long as 10^6 m).

7.2. The Optical Spectrum

Although the sun is the source of most of the electromagnetic radiation occurring naturally in the atmosphere, on the surface of the earth we are subjected to only a small portion of the sun's radiation because much of it is filtered out by water particles, ozone, oxygen, and carbon dioxide. Oxygen and the ozone layer remove the deadly short-wavelength (shorter than 280 nm) UV radiation, and water and carbon dioxide decrease the amount of IR radiation at the earth's surface (most IR radiation above 3000 nm is filtered out by the earth's atmosphere). Thus, we are regularly exposed to some UV radi-

FIGURE 7–2.   **The electromagnetic spectrum. (Reprinted with permission from D. Pitts, *J. Am. Optom. Assoc.*, Vol. 52, p. 12, 1981.)**

ation, the visible spectrum, and the IR portion of the electromagnetic spectrum. Although exposure to radiation bordering on the visible spectrum does not cause the sensation of vision, these bands of radiation can exert harmful effects on the eyes.

UV radiation extends approximately from 10 to 380 nm. Because certain bands of UV radiation are associated with particular biological effects, the UV spectrum is arbitrarily subdivided into three bands: UV-A extends from 380 to 320 nm, UV-B from 320 to 290 nm, and UV-C from 290 to 200 nm. Sometimes, because of their positions relative to the visible spectrum, UV-A is called *near UV*, UV-B is called *middle UV*, and UV-C is called *far UV*. In this context, the term *optical spectrum* (or *optical radiation*) is used to encompass the UV, visible, and infrared ranges of the spectrum.

Light may be defined as a form of electromagnetic radiant energy that is capable of stimulating our retinal photoreceptors, and causing the sensation of vision. The visible spectrum, extending from approximately 380 to 760 nm, occupies a narrow band of the total electromagnetic spectrum. There are no sharp cutoffs at the upper and lower limits, so it is difficult to determine the range of wavelengths included in the visible spectrum with any degree of certainty. The range varies with the level of illumination, the clarity of the crystalline lens of the eye, and other factors relative to the observer. Within the specified boundaries, radiation reaching the retina acts as a physical stimulus to produce electrical impulses that are conducted via the optic nerve to the occipital cortex of the brain, which provides the sensation of vision, even color vision! Color vision is a mental process: The rays of light are not colored. The response of the eye is not uniform within the visible spectrum, the *luminous efficiency*, or *luminosity*, of light varying with wavelength. If we plot the average luminosity as a function of the wavelength, we generate the photopic *luminosity curve*, shown in Figure 7–3.

If we consider an *octave* to be a doubling of the frequency (as in music), the visible spectrum consists of only 1 octave of a total of 60 octaves in the electromagnetic spectrum. The IR spectrum extends from 760 to 10^6 nm, or 1 mm. The IR spectrum is also divided into three portions: IR-A extends from 760 to 1400 nm, IR-B extends from 1400 to 3000 nm, and IR-C extends from 3000 nm to 1 mm. Although the visible spectrum occupies only 1 octave, UV radiation occupies almost 4 octaves and IR radiation occupies slightly more than 7 octaves. The divisions of UV and IR spectra are summarized in Table 7–1.

In addition to the electromagnetic radiation produced by the sun, manufactured radiation sources emit UV, visible, and IR radiation. Many manufactured sources of radiation have beneficial uses, but they may also be sources of potential hazard if not used properly.

7.3. Classification of Radiation Effects

Draper's law states that for radiation to have an effect on a substance through which it travels, it must be *absorbed* by the substance. Radiation has *no* effect (beneficial or deleterious) on a substance through which it is completely trans-

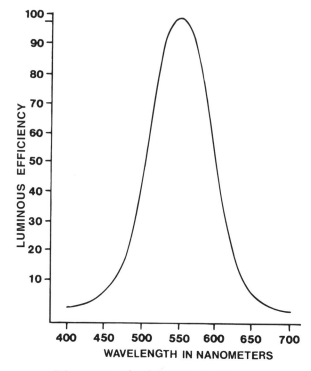

FIGURE 7–3.   **The photopic luminosity curve.**

TABLE 7–1
Divisions of the Ultraviolet and Infrared Spectra

	Ultraviolet (nm)	Infrared (nm)
A (near)	380–320	760–1400
B (middle)	320–290	1400–3000
C (far)	290–200	3000–1,000,000

mitted or by which it is completely reflected. For example, radiation in the region of the visible spectrum causes the sensation of vision because it is absorbed by the photopigments of the retina. The effects of radiation take two forms: ionizing and nonionizing.

Ionizing Radiation

Ionizing radiation is caused by the disintegration of atoms with the release of subatomic particles or rays. This radiation carries energy levels so high that it exceeds the binding energy of the electrons of the irradiated substance and causes ejection of electrons from various orbits of the atom; this leaves the atom with a positive electric charge, known as an ion. Ionizing radiation can occur as a natural phenomenon or can be produced artificially. Ionizing radiation travels as particles (alpha and beta) or as waves such as x-rays and gamma rays, which are a part of the electromagnetic spectrum.

Ionizing radiation is the atomic equivalent of a "bull in the china shop." When ionizing radiation penetrates living tissue, it wreaks havoc on the atoms and molecules in its path and sets off a chain of events that can destroy living cells or make them function abnormally. People employed in occupations such as nuclear physics, radiology, uranium mining, and engineering are at risk from ionizing radiation. Most ionizing radiation passes through the eye, but a small amount is absorbed. The damage depends on the exposure time, concentration, and the type of radiation. In general, low-penetrating radiation such as beta particles requires more exposure than does highly penetrating radiation such as gamma rays and x-rays. Ionizing radiation may have a direct or indirect effect on ocular tissues. A direct effect may produce cellular anomalies or death. Indirect effects can result in damage to the blood vessels and thus restrict the blood supply to the tissues.

Ionizing radiation can affect nearly all ocular tissues. Of the ocular tissues, the conjunctiva, cornea, and lens are the most vulnerable.[1] At low levels, the conjunctival vessels become engorged and the cornea loses its normal luster. Heavier doses result in exfoliation of the epithelial cells, corneal ulcers, and keratitis.

The most common effect of ionizing radiation is the formation of cataracts. Cataract development follows a latent period of several months or years. The younger the person, the shorter the latent period and the greater the lens damage. High levels of ionizing radiation can result in retinal damage and degeneration[2]; extremely high levels can result in sudden blindness.

Nonionizing Radiation

If the energy transmitted by the radiation is lower than the binding energy of the electrons of the irradiated material, the atom is raised to a higher energy level and is said to be in an excited state. Molecules in an excited state have different chemical and physical properties than do molecules in the resting, or ground, state. Most forms of electromagnetic radiation are nonionizing, such as radio waves, heat, and light. However, in the classification of the effects of radiation which follows, the discussion is limited to the effects of *optical radiation*, previously defined as the UV, visible, and IR ranges of the spectrum.

When radiation is absorbed by an ocular tissue, various effects are produced by the transfer of radiant energy to the molecules and atoms of the absorbing tissue. The absorbed energy can affect the visual apparatus in the following ways:

1. *The Thermal Effect.* This is a heating effect, brought about by the absorption of radiant energy by the molecule, which raises the molecule from the resting state to an excited state. A return to the resting state can occur by the dissipation of heat arising from molecular collision. Solar retinopathy, caused by looking directly at a solar eclipse, is an example of a thermal lesion.

2. *The Photochemical Effect.* When radiant energy is absorbed, the molecule that absorbs it may decompose or chemically react to produce a unique chemical product. This is the effect that, in the visible spectrum, produces a chemical reaction in the retina initiating the sensation of vision. However, harmful photochemical effects can occur with other ocular tissues, such as photokeratitis produced by excessive absorption of UV radiation by the cornea.

3. *Photoluminescence (fluorescence).* Fluorescence is the phenomenon in which radiant energy of one wavelength is absorbed and radiant energy of a different wavelength (usually longer) is emitted, as described by *Stoke's law.* Thus, the emitted radiation has a lower energy level than the absorbed radiation. The crystalline lens is capable of visible fluorescence when illuminated by UV light.

7.4. Concentration of Radiant Energy by the Eye

Absorption of radiant energy by a specific tissue depends on its molecular structure and its chemical composition. However, the amount of damage arising from radiant energy absorption is proportional to the radiant energy absorbed per unit of mass or volume. As radiant energy passes through the eye, it is attenuated in a number of ways: (1) absorption by the (apparently transparent) ocular media, (2) scattering within the eye, (3) reflection by the various optical interfaces, and (4) loss caused by the aberrations of the eye's optical system. Most absorptive losses occur in the anterior structures of the eye. Offsetting attenuation is the concentration of energy brought about by the focusing effects of the cornea and the lens.

The concentration of radiant energy within the eye also depends on the size of the pupil and the angular extent of the source. With increasing pupil size, the illumination on the retina increases by the square of the pupillary radius, as shown in Figure 7–4. For a point source of high intensity, refraction by the eye's optical system concentrates the energy on the retina (A) and causes tissue damage, but has little effect on the cornea and the lens. An example of this type of damage is *solar retinopathy*, which can occur after exposure to a solar eclipse. For extended sources, the radiant energy is sharply concentrated in the lens, as shown in Figure 7–4B, but

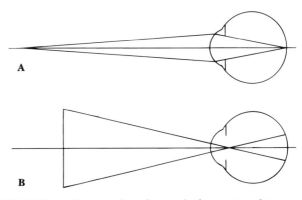

FIGURE 7–4.   **Concentration of energy in the eye. A, point source; B, extended source.**

widely distributed on the retina. The possibility of a source of radiation causing damage to ocular tissues depends both on the *intensity* and on the *angular size* of the source of the radiation. Although a small source of low-intensity radiation is usually harmless to the retina, an extended source (such as a desert or a body of water) of the same intensity may provide a dangerous concentration of radiant energy in the lens.

7.5. Absorption of Radiation by the Ocular Tissues

The *tear layer* absorbs only a small amount of radiation. It absorbs UV radiation below about 290 nm and IR radiation above about 3000 nm and, therefore, transmits radiation from approximately 290 to 3000 nm.

The *cornea*, like the tear layer, absorbs UV radiation below about 290 nm and IR radiation above 3000 nm. However, the cornea has *partial* transmission for UV in the range of 290 to 315 nm and for IR in the range of 1000 to 3000 nm. The cornea, therefore, has relatively high transmission in the range extending from about 315 to 1000 nm, which includes the longer UV wavelengths, all the visible spectrum, and the shorter IR wavelengths. The transmission of the cornea (particularly for the shorter wavelengths) decreases markedly with age.

The *aqueous humor* absorbs very little radiation, with the result that any radiation that is transmitted by the cornea is also transmitted by the aqueous humor, and passes to the iris and the lens.

In the *iris*, the uveal pigment absorbs radiation and converts it into heat. This conversion can be accompanied by a marked contraction of the pupil, probably because of the release of histamine.

The *lens*, like the cornea, has variable absorption properties, depending on age. The lens of a child absorbs UV radiation below about 310 nm and IR radiation beyond 2500 nm, and thus transmits UV radiation between about 310 and 380 nm, all the visible spectrum, and IR radiation up to 2500 nm. The lens of an older adult, on the other hand, absorbs almost all radiation below about 375 nm and therefore transmits very little UV radiation. However, there is no change in the absorption of IR radiation with increasing age.

The *vitreous* mainly absorbs radiation below 290 nm and above 1600 nm and therefore transmits to the retina radiation in the range from 290 to 1600 nm. However, as the crystalline lens absorbs more UV radiation with increasing age, the amount of UV radiation available to the vitreous gradually decreases.

The radiation received by the *retina* is the radiation transmitted by the vitreous. Although UV radiation received by the retina decreases in amount with age, IR radiation does not decrease in amount—94% of IR radiation of 770 nm reaches the retina, then falls to 90% at 900 nm and to a very low level beyond 1500 nm.

The *eye as a whole* absorbs and transmits about the same amount of visible radiation as it would if it were a layer of water approximately 1 inch thick. Transmission of radiation by the ocular media is summarized in Table 7–2.

TABLE 7–2
Transmission of Radiation by the Ocular Media

	Ultraviolet (nm)	Visible (nm)	Infrared (nm)
Tear layer	290–380	380–760	760–3000
Cornea	290–380*	380–760	760–3000*
Aqueous	290–380*	380–760	760–3000*
Lens (child)	310–380*	380–760	760–2500*
Lens (older adult)	375–380*	380–760*	760–2500*
Vitreous	290–380*	380–760	760–1600*

*There is *partial* transmission for some wavelengths in the indicated range.

7.6. Effects of Ultraviolet Radiation

UV radiation can have harmful effects on the conjunctiva and cornea by causing photophthalmia and the development of pterygia, pingueculae, and band-shaped keratopathy; it can affect the lens and cause cataracts, and it can affect the retina and cause macular degeneration.

Photophthalmia

The primary effect resulting from absorption of UV radiation of 300 nm and below is *photochemical* damage to the corneal epithelium. This is known as *photophthalmia, photokeratitis*, or *photoconjunctivitis*. Because the corneal epithelium absorbs most UV radiation, corneal damage is confined to this layer. These effects occur after a latent period, which may vary from 30 minutes to 24 hours, the length of time depending on the intensity of exposure. In addition, the photochemical effect tends to be a *cumulative* effect. Repeated exposures, with intermissions equivalent to a single long exposure as long as the intermissions are sufficiently short (24 hr or less), keep physiologic healing from occurring.

In acute photokeratitis, the patient experiences the sensation of a foreign body, photophobia, lacrimation, blepharospasm, redness, and edema. The clinical picture is also seen in *snowblindness*, which occurs with long exposure to UV radiation reflected from large areas of snow. *Welder's flash* (*welder's keratitis*) is a similar condition experienced by arc welders who strike an arc before they lower their protective helmet.

Photokeratitis is self-limiting; the acute symptoms disappear within 24 to 48 hours. The corneal rehabilitation is remarkably rapid. Permanent damage is rare, and occurs only with extremely high-intensity exposure.

Pterygia, Pingueculae, and Band-Shaped Keratopathy

Repeated, long-continued exposure to UV radiation is widely thought to be a causative factor in the development of pterygia, pingueculae, and nodular band-shaped keratopathies. *Pterygia* are growths of vascular and connective tissue into the epithelium of the bulbar conjunctiva and the cornea. A significantly high incidence of pterygia is found among outdoor workers who are exposed to UV radiation.[3] However, a much greater effect can be ascribed to physical trauma such as wind and dust.

Pingueculae are small, yellowish elevated concretions of bulbar conjunctiva. They have long been associated with continued exposure to solar radiation.[4] Microtrauma from windborne particles may also play a role in pingueculae.

Eyes affected with nodular *band-shaped keratopathy* have white or cream-colored opacities between the epithelium and Bowman's layer, which are distributed symmetrically in the interpalpebral portions of the two corneas. The terms *spheroid degeneration* and *climatic droplet keratopathy* are also used for this condition.[5] The association of UV radiation with band-shaped keratopathies is more firmly established than it is with pterygia or pingueculae. The prevalence of this condition peaks sharply in limited geographic areas; in the United States the incidence is very low.

Cataract

The crystalline lens is continuously exposed to near UV radiation (transmitted by the tear layer, cornea, and aqueous) in the 290- to 380-nm range. One of the cumulative effects of the radiation is the formation of lens pigments that cause an increasing yellow coloration of the lens nucleus. The deepening coloration further increases the absorption of UV radiation in the 290- to 380-nm range, as well as the absorption of visible light. The pigments are mainly produced in the nucleus and lead to a decrease in the light transmission of the lens as one grows older.

Although only small amounts of UV radiation reach the lens, the cumulative effects of exposure to UV over a period of many years may be responsible for producing lens opacities, in particular, the brown or *brunescent* cataract of the nucleus. The avascular lens, with its inefficient metabolic system, is vulnerable, apparently because its repair mechanisms are not as well developed as those of the cornea or the retina.

Recent epidemiologic studies of the incidence of cataracts in various geographic and climactic regions support a relationship between sunlight and nuclear senile cataracts.[6–9] Specifically, UV-B (290–320 nm) has been implicated as the causative factor, on the basis of biochemical, photochemical, and physiologic studies.[10–13] Both the UV-absorbing pigments in the lens and the fluorescence of the lens increase with age, and fluorescent substances in the lens may be responsible for other changes, such as darkening of the lens, which leads to the brunescent (brown) form of senile cataract.[14–15] Environmental, nutritional, and genetic factors are also known to play a role in the etiology of cataracts, but epidemiologic and experimental data suggest that UV radiation is an important factor.

In an epidemiologic study of 838 watermen who worked in Chesapeake Bay, Taylor et al.[16] found that high cumulative levels of exposure to UV-B (290–320 nm) significantly increased the risk of cortical cataract. However, cumulative levels of exposure to UV-B were not associated with increased risk of nuclear cataract, and exposure to UV-A (320–400 nm) was not associated with increased risk of either cortical or nuclear cataract. The mean age of the watermen was 53.0 years, and 140 were older than 70 years. Cumulative exposure was calculated on the basis of the yearly ocular exposure to UV radiation for each subject for each year of life beyond the age of 15. Of the 838 subjects, 111 (13%) had cortical opacities, 229 (27%) had nuclear opacities, and 14 (2%) had posterior subcapsular cataracts. Taylor et al.[16] concluded that a hat with a brim and close-fitting sunglasses with UV-B absorbing lenses should be worn at times of maximal exposure to sunlight.

Fluorescence

The phenomenon of photoluminescence (fluorescence) occurs when a substance absorbs radiation of one wavelength and emits radiation of a different (usually longer) wavelength. Visible fluorescence of the lens has been noted for more than 100 years. When radiant energy is absorbed, the absorbing molecules are raised to more active, more excited states—*fluorescence* is a mechanism of deactivation through the emission of photons.

The fluorescence of the ocular lens is a well-known phenomenon. If an ultraviolet light source (a "black light," such as that used to evaluate the fit of a contact lens) is held in front of the eye, the lens fluoresces with an eerie, greenish yellow color. A source of 370 to 390 nm is most effective for its production. The amount of fluorescence of the lens increases slowly with increasing age. The absorption of UV light by the ocular lens has been linked to the formation of fluorescent material within the lens. As the amount of this material, called *fluorogens*, increases with time, there is a parallel increase in the yellowish color of the lens. This may be one of the factors associated with the aging of the lens.

Retina

In the normal eye, the retina is shielded from much of the UV radiation (as described above) by the filtering action of the cornea and the lens. Under ambient solar radiation, the small amount of UV radiation reaching the retina is not likely to cause any serious retinal damage. Nevertheless, it is possible that repeated exposure for a period of years may lead to some degree of damage because of a slow, cumulative effect.

When the lens has been removed because of cataract, the aphakic eye is subjected to UV radiation in the range of 320 to 380 nm, which had previously been filtered out by the lens.[17] In addition, the amount of *visible* radiation increases in aphakia. The absorption of UV radiation by the pigment epithelium of the retina and by the choroid enhances the potential for photochemical and thermal damage. Ham et al.,[18] working with aphakic monkeys, found that in the absence of the lens there was sufficient UV-A radiation in the environment to damage the retina. Cystoid macular edema is a well-known complication of cataract surgery and may be caused by the increased amount of UV-A and visible radiation reaching the retina of the aphakic eye.

In the 1992 Charles Prentice Award Lecture, "Optometry and the Preservation of Visual Health," Young[19] cited many studies indicating that UV radiation causes retinal damage. In one study,[20] patients who regularly wore sunglasses typically showed less age-related damage to retinal cones; in another study,[21] individuals with intraocular lenses that absorbed UV in one eye but not in the other suffered a decline in sensitivity of short-wavelength-sensitive cones in the unprotected eye; in yet another study,[22] there was a decrease in age-related macular degeneration in myopic patients who had worn spectacles since childhood, apparently because of reduced ocular UV exposure during their first 25 years of life.

Ultraviolet and Photosensitization

Radiant energy is transmitted as discrete units called photons, the energy of which is wavelength-dependent. The first step in the photobiological process involves the absorption of a molecule (called a *chromaphore*) of one of these photons. When absorption occurs, the molecule leaves its ground state and becomes electronically excited. The excited molecule may return to the ground state through various mechanisms such as fluorescence, phosphorescence, heat, or photoproduct formation.

When the pathway for energy dissipation does not return the starting molecule to its original ground state, the molecule has been structurally reorganized—a photochemical reaction has occurred. Photochemical reactions involve changes *only* in the molecules that absorb the radiation. The alteration in one molecule as a result of absorption of photons in other molecules is a *photosensitized* reaction. The absorbing molecule is referred to as a *photosensitizer.*

Photosensitization is the enhanced reaction to normally harmless radiation (particularly UV-A and visible) that are induced by the presence of a chemical photosensitizer. The photosensitizer may be present by oral ingestion, direct application to the skin, or may be endogenous with the occurrence of a metabolite. Although most photosensitizing reactions occur in the skin, some occur in the eye and internal organs under special circumstances.

Photosensitization reactions are classified as *phototoxic* or *photoallergic*, with clinical overlap between the two. Phototoxic reactions are immediate, erythematous, localized, and short-lived. Photoallergic reactions, activating the immune system, are delayed, eczematous, persistent, and widespread. Although both phototoxic and photoallergic reactions may produce acute, short-term effects, the long-term implications of photoallergic reactions are more serious.

The production of photoproducts is not necessarily harmful to the cell, and some are even beneficial. Long-term injuries may be avoided through cellular and repair mechanisms. The bleaching and regeneration of rhodopsin

is an example of a beneficial photochemical reaction, as is the production of vitamin D in the skin.

The list of photosensitization chemicals includes not only pharmaceutical compounds used in routine health-care procedures, but also chemicals used for industrial and agricultural purposes. Photosensitizers include topical and oral medications such as analgesics (naproxen), antibacterial agents (tetracyclines, sulfanilamides), tranquilizers (phenothiazines), diuretics (chlorthiazides), antifungals (griseofulvin), antimalarial agents (chloroquine), oral contraceptives (estrogens), and photochemotherapeutic agents (psoralens).

Oral psoralens are specifically used as photosensitizers in combination with UV-A radiation to treat psoriasis and vitiligo. The term PUVA (psoralens UVA) is used to describe this treatment. During PUVA treatment and during the entire period of photosensitization, eye protection from UV radiation is essential, even indoors.

Clinicians should be informed of the photosensitizing characteristics of particular medications. Patients who are given medications that are known, or suspected, to be ocular photosensitizers should be given protective eyewear that filters out the radiation effective in producing the reaction. In this regard, aphakic and pseudophakic patients should be given special attention.

7.7. Effects of Visible Radiation

Because they are transparent, the cornea, aqueous, lens, and vitreous all transmit most radiation in the visible spectrum (380 to 760 nm). The absorption of these wavelengths by the photoreceptors of the retina initiates the photochemical and neural processes that cause the sensation of *vision*. Because human eyes have become adapted to the visual environment in which they have evolved, normal levels of visible light resulting from ambient solar radiation are not ordinarily considered to be hazardous. However, unusually high levels of radiation within the visible spectrum (whether solar or artificial radiation) can cause both photochemical and thermal injury to the retina. The visible wavelengths are not only transmitted by the cornea and lens but are focused on the retina so that the radiation per unit area reaching the retina is markedly higher than that reaching the cornea. If the offending source emits both visible and near IR radiation, much of the visible radiation and a smaller but significant amount of the IR radiation is transmitted to the retina and absorbed by the photoreceptors, retinal pigment epithelium, and choroid. The short-wavelength end of the visible spectrum (where the energy level is high) tends to produce photochemical damage; the longer wavelengths of the visible spectrum tend to produce both photochemical and thermal damage; IR radiation produces only thermal damage.

Even at levels that are not capable of producing retinopathy, prolonged absorption of visible radiation may have undesirable functional effects. Although the normal *dark adaptation* process requires from 30 to 40 minutes, exposure to strong sunlight for 3 or 4 hours or longer so thoroughly bleaches the retinal photopigments that a significantly longer dark-adaptation time is required for a period of 24 hours or longer after exposure.[23] In a situation in which viewing requirements are critical (for example, driving home at dusk after a day at the beach) filtering lenses should be worn during the day to preserve the retina's ability to adapt to low illumination levels at night.

Violet and Blue Radiation

In recent years, not only UV radiation but also violet and blue radiation have been implicated in the etiology of age-related macular degeneration, which is the leading cause of blindness for people older than age 65 in the United States.[24] Although age-related macular degeneration is an important cause of blindness, its pathogenesis is poorly understood. Increasing evidence implicates chronic light exposure as a major factor. Long-term exposure to low levels of UV and visible radiation has been shown to cause damage to the photoreceptor—especially the cones—and to the retinal pigment epithelium.[25,26] Because the retina is vulnerable to damage from radiation between 400 and 500 nm, Young[27] proposed that protective eyewear should absorb 90% of the radiation in this region of the spectrum.

Solar Retinopathy

Also known as "eclipse blindness," solar retinopathy is caused by staring at the sun, even for very short periods of time, without suitable eye protection. The refracting power of the cornea and lens greatly increase the total amount of radiant energy striking the retina per unit area compared with that per unit striking the cornea. In solar retinitis, the patient usually notices a small, dense, central scotoma, a loss of visual acuity, chromatopsia (colored tinges), and metamorphopsia (distortion of perceived images). Many cases of solar retinopathy tend to occur after an eclipse of the sun, despite widely disseminated warnings against direct observation of a solar eclipse.

Opinions on the cause of retinopathy associated with sungazing have undergone modification in recent times; previously, thermal insult from focused IR radiation was considered to be the spectral source. However, Ham et al.[28] attributed the damage primarily to photochemical trauma in the outer segments of the photoreceptor after exposure of the retina to high energy, short wavelengths of the visible spectrum (400–500 nm). These wavelengths are enormously more hazardous to the retina than the low-energy portion (500–700 nm). Because the transition occurs at the border between the perceived colors of green and blue, the phenomenon is known as the *blue light hazard.*

If exposure is intense for a long period of time, thermal injury to the retinal pigment epithelium—the result of absorption of long-wavelength visible light and IR radiation—may occur simultaneously with the photochemical changes.

7.8. Effects of Infrared Radiation

Wavelengths longer than 3000 nm do not reach the earth's surface because they are absorbed by water and carbon dioxide in the atmosphere. Even for wavelengths shorter than 3000 nm, photon energy decreases with increasing wavelength, with the result that the region of IR radiation involved in ocular damage extends only from 780 to 2000 nm. Most radiation beyond 1400 nm is absorbed by the tears and the cornea. At the present time, there is little evidence that absorption of ambient solar IR radiation is damaging to the ocular tissues. However, artificial sources of high-intensity IR radiation, such as carbon, tungsten, and xenon arc lamps, photoflood lamps, and some laser sources, produce levels of IR radiation significantly higher than corresponding radiation obtained from the sun.

If the eye is subjected to high-intensity sources of IR radiation, absorption of the radiation can cause rotational and vibrational changes in the molecules and produce a thermal lesion. The hazardous effect of elevated temperature on tissue is the loss of conformation, that is, a change in the very delicate spatial structure of biomolecules, a process known as *denaturation.*

Temperature increases produce loss of function in globular proteins such as enzymes, and the loss of function in such proteins, associated with conformational changes, constitutes the thermal cell damage that may lead to cell death and necrosis. Although photochemical damage from UV radiation occurs only after a latent period, thermal damage from infrared radiation occurs immediately. Thermal lesions can be manifested in the *cornea* as coagulation and lead to opacification; in the *iris* as congestion, depigmentation, and atrophy caused by the absorption of IR radiation by the iris pigment; in the *lens* as exfoliation of the lens capsule, coagulation of protein, and the production of cataract; and in the *retina* as a necrotic burn.

The potential for the development of cataract from IR radiation has long been known in workers, such as glass-blowers and blast furnace operators, who are exposed to high levels of heat radiation. As mentioned previously, radiation from an extended source, when undergoing refraction by the cornea and the anterior lens surface, is concentrated in the posterior region of the lens and then distributed in the lens and over a wide area of the retina. Concentration of radiation from an extended source produces thermal effects that, during a period of years, may cause, initially, an anterior subcapsular cataract, and a posterior subcapsular cataract may subsequently develop.

Anterior lenticular lesions are often found adjacent to thermal lesions of the iris after exposure to IR radiation. The IR radiation is absorbed by the pigmented epithelium of the iris, is converted to heat, and is then transmitted to adjacent tissues.

A retinal burn occurs when the eye is exposed to a point-like source of IR radiation of high intensity, such as the sun. Eclipse blindness (sun blindness) arises as a result of observing an eclipse of the sun without adequate ocular protection. The IR radiation is absorbed by the pigment epithelium of the retina and by the choroid and causes a thermal lesion involving both these tissues. The lesion often occurs in the *macular* area.

7.9. Other Forms of Radiation

Although the effects of ultraviolet, visible, and infrared radiation have been the focus thus far, this does not imply that other regions of the electromagnetic radiation spectrum are harmless. Long-wavelength microwaves and diathermy as well as ionizing radiation such as x-rays and gamma rays are known to produce adverse effects on the eyes and on other living tissues. However, these sources are usually present only in special installations, and systems of protection are normally present for such installations. The basic protection principle involves *prevention* of propagation of the radiation by some form of shielding.

7.10. Recommended Levels of Retinal Illumination

For a given level of ambient illumination, the amount of illumination reaching the retina is controlled by the pupil. Pupil sizes vary in diameter from about 2 mm in very bright illumination to about 8 mm in low illumination; the variations in pupil diameter change the irradiance of the retina by a factor of 1 mm^2 compared to 4 mm^2, or 16 times. However, the wide range of illumination under which the retina is capable of functioning is more a result of *retinal adaptation* than of variation in pupil size. The retina is capable of adapting its sensitivity by a factor of 100,000 from the lowest to the highest illumination levels.

Although the eye is capable of functioning in such an incredibly wide range of illumination levels, high levels of illumination *can* cause discomfort. According to Richards,[29] an ideal level of illumination is 400 footlamberts (ftL). This level of illumination would occur on a typical summer day if one were reading under the shade of a big tree. However, on a bright summer day without the shade tree, the level of illumination is much higher than 400 ftL. For example, on a bright, sunny Texas day in the middle of July, the illumination level can reach 10,000 ftL. This exceeds the "comfortable" 400-footlambert level by a factor of 10,000 to 400, or 25 to 1, and would require a filter with a transmittance of 1 to 25, or 4%. Even with a more typical illumination level of 5000 footlamberts, the comfort level is exceeded by a factor of 12.5 to 1 and would require a filter with a transmittance of 8%.

Thus, undesirable effects result from excessive levels of illumination, not only in the UV and IR regions, but in the visible region of the spectrum. Although most patients who request sunglasses or other tinted lenses do so because of visual discomfort, it is important for these lenses to be designed to control UV and IR radiation as well as visible light.

Glare

The term *glare* refers to the presence of one or more areas in the field of vision that are of sufficient brightness to cause an unpleasant sensation, a temporary blurring of vision, or a feeling of ocular fatigue. Glare can be classified as veiling (disability) glare, discomfort glare, and specular reflection glare. These classifications are not mutually exclusive, and their effects can be additive.

Veiling or disability glare arises from stray light falling on the retina, usually from scatter by the media of the eye. The light that is scattered falls as a patch of veiling illuminance on the fovea and reduces the contrast of the retinal image and thereby reduces visibility and visual performance. When a person is in a visual environment in which there are extended light sources (sky, sand, brightly illuminated walls, etc.) the reflected images are large in angular subtense. This leads to veiling glare, which contributes to reduction in contrasts observed in the visual field.

Discomfort glare occurs when the illumination in a part of the visual field is much greater than the level of illumination for which the retina is adapted. An extreme case of glare often occurs during night driving—the retina is adapted to a very low level of illumination, but the headlights of an oncoming car emit a level of illumination that is sufficiently greater than the level of adaptation and causes extreme discomfort. Discomfort glare occurs when the ratio between the highest level of illumination in the visual field and the background illumination exceeds a ratio of 3 to 1. The importance of background illumination, to avoid glare, was emphasized in the early days of television. In viewing television, discomfort is likely to occur if the level of illumination of the television screen exceeds three times that of the background. In this situation, glare can be avoided by having a low level of illumination (rather than complete darkness) in the room.

Specular reflection glare occurs when patches of bright light are reflected from smooth, shiny surfaces into the eye. Typical reflecting surfaces include expanses of water, snowfields, roadways, and plate glass. Reflections are not only annoying but interfere with visibility, at times seriously.

Many people think they need sunglasses to protect their eyes from discomfort caused by glare. Tinted lenses or other filters are, unfortunately, of little help in controlling disability or discomfort glare. If a "hot spot" in the visual field is ten times as bright as the background illumination, the use of a filter with 50% transmittance (or any other percentage of transmittance) is not helpful—*everything* in the visual field, both the hot spot and the background, are reduced by the same percentage. However, light-polarizing lenses (see Section 7.14) are useful in controlling specular reflection glare because they have the property of filtering out polarized reflected light.

_____ ABSORPTIVE LENSES _____

7.11. Reflection, Absorption, and Transmission

When light is incident on a lens, some light is reflected by each of the lens surfaces, some is absorbed by the lens, and the remainder is transmitted. As shown in Figure 7–5, the percentage of transmitted light is found by calculating the percentage of light lost by reflection at the front surface, the percentage lost by absorption, and the percentage lost by reflection at the back surface.

The amount of light *reflected* by a lens surface, in air, is given by the Fresnel equation

$$I_R = \frac{(n' - n)^2}{(n' + n)^2}(I). \qquad (7.3)$$

For clear ophthalmic crown glass with an index of refraction of 1.523, the light lost by reflection at the front surface is

$$\frac{(0.523)^2}{(2.523)^2} = \frac{0.2735}{6.3655}$$
$$= 0.043 = 4.3\%.$$

Because clear ophthalmic crown glass absorbs no light, the percentage of incident (entering) light remaining when the light reaches the back surface of the lens is

$$100 - 4.3 = 95.7\%,$$

the light lost by reflection at the back surface of the lens is

$$(0.957)\frac{(0.523)^2}{(2.523)^2}$$
$$= 0.041 = 4.1\%,$$

and the light transmitted by the lens is

$$100 - 4.3 - 4.1 = 91.6\%.$$

For a plastic lens (made of CR-39) with an index of refraction of 1.498, the light loss at the front surface is

$$\frac{(0.498)^2}{(2.498)^2} = \frac{0.248}{6.240}$$
$$= 0.040 = 4.0\%,$$

and the light loss at the back surface is

$$(0.96)(0.40)$$
$$= 0.038 = 3.8\%.$$

The light transmitted by the lens, assuming that no light is absorbed, is

$$100 - 4.0 - 3.8 = 92.2\%,$$

or about 0.6% higher than that transmitted by an ophthalmic crown glass lens.

The amount of light *absorbed* by a lens is given by *Lambert's law* of absorption, which states that for an absorptive material such as a tinted lens layers of equal thickness absorb equal quantities (or percentages) of light regardless of the intensity of the light. Figure 7–6 shows a lens divided into several layers of equal thickness. The intensity of light incident on the front surface (the first layer or unit) of the lens is designated as I; the intensity continuing past the front surface is designated as I_0 (equal to $I - R$). As it passes through the first layer, the light is transmitted by the amount indicated by a factor, q, the *transmittance factor*. For example, if $q = 0.5$ per unit, the intensity of light leaving the first unit is 0.5 of the intensity at the front surface of the lens (after reflection). If we call the second layer of the lens I_1, the third I_2, and so forth,

$$I_1 = I_0(q)$$
$$I_2 = I_1(q) = I_0(q)^2$$
$$I_3 = I_2(q) = I_0(q)^3$$

and

$$I^x = I_0(q)^x. \qquad (7.4)$$

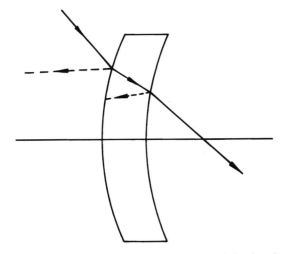

FIGURE 7–5.   **Reflection, absorption, and transmission by a lens.**

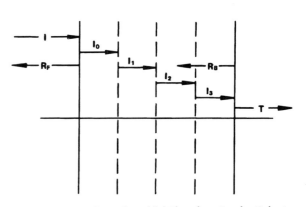

FIGURE 7–6.   **Absorption of light by a lens (Lambert's law).**

The total transmission of the lens, T, is then

$$T = I_x - R_B,$$

With R_B designating the light lost by reflection at the back surface of the lens.

EXAMPLE

Given an ophthalmic lens, 6 mm thick, having a transmission factor, q, of 0.8 per 2 mm of thickness, and an index of refraction of 1.523, what is the transmission, T, of this lens? The light lost by reflection at the front surface is

$$R_F = \frac{(0.523)^2}{(2.523)^2} = 0.043.$$

The intensity of light entering the first layer of the lens, after reflection, is

$$I_0 = I - R_F$$
$$= 1 - 0.043$$
$$= 0.957.$$

The total amount of light transmitted to the back surface after losses by absorption is

$$I_3 = I_0(q^3)$$
$$= 0.957(0.8^3)$$
$$= 0.957(0.512)$$
$$= 0.49.$$

The light reflected by the back surface, R_B, is

$$R_B = (0.49)\frac{(0.523)^2}{(2.253)^2}$$
$$= (0.49)(0.043)$$
$$= 0.021$$

and the total transmission, T, of the lens is equal to

$$T = I_3 - R_B$$
$$= 0.49 - 0.021$$
$$= 0.469 = 46.9\%.$$

7.12. Opacity

Additional terms that are used in connection with absorptive lenses are *opacity* and *density*. Opacity is defined as the reciprocal of transmission,

$$O = \frac{1}{T}. \tag{7.5}$$

For the lens in the above example, with a transmission of 46.9%,

$$O = \frac{1}{0.469} = 2.13.$$

If light passes through a number of lenses, one after another, the *ultimate transmission* is found by multiplying the separate transmissions of each of the lenses,

$$T_U = (T_1)(T_2)(T_3)\cdots,$$

and the *ultimate opacity* is found by multiplying the separate opacities of the lenses,

$$O_U = (O_1)(O_2)(O_3)\cdots.$$

EXAMPLE

An automobile driver wears a tinted lens with a transmission of 80% and looks through a windshield with a transmission of 70%. What are (1) the ultimate transmission and (2) the ultimate opacity of the windshield–lens combination?

(1) The ultimate transmission is equal to

$$T_U = (T_1)(T_2)$$
$$= (0.80)(0.70)$$
$$= 0.56 = 56\%.$$

(2) The ultimate opacity is equal to

$$O = (O_1)(O_2)$$
$$= \left(\frac{1}{0.80}\right)\left(\frac{1}{0.70}\right)$$
$$= (1.25)(1.43) = 1.79.$$

7.13. Density

In solving problems concerning the transmission of light by a lens, it is convenient to translate the transmission into the optical *density* of the material. The use of the concept of density is convenient because if the density is stated for a given thickness of material, the density may be found for any other thickness by the use of proportion. Once the transmission of a material is known, the density may be found by use of the relationship

$$\text{density} = \log_{10} \text{opacity}$$
$$= \log \frac{1}{T}$$
$$= \log 1 - \log T$$
$$= 0.0 - \log T.$$

$$\text{density} = -\log T. \tag{7.6}$$

The calculation of the transmission of a given lens, when losses by reflection are considered, is mathematically simplified when transmission is stated in terms of density. Because the transmission of a medium is the ratio of transmitted light to incident light, the transmission of each surface can be expressed as a density. Hence, for a simple lens, the total density of the lens may be considered to consist of the two *surface densities* and a *media density*. The density of the front surface of the lens is designated by

$$D_s = \log \frac{1}{I_0}, \tag{7.7}$$

where

$$I_0 = I - R_1.$$

The media density is the density per unit thickness, (log $1/q$), multiplied by the number of units, (x), with the result that

$$\text{media density} = (x)(D/\text{unit}).$$

Since the total density of a lens is the sum of the densities of the parts, then the total density is given by the expression

$$D = 2 \text{ surface densities} + (\text{number of units})(\text{density per unit})$$

$$D = 2D_s + (x)(D/\text{unit}). \qquad (7.8)$$

EXAMPLE 1
A lens 2 mm thick has a refractive index of 1.523 and a total transmission of 30%. If a transmission of 50% is desired, what must be the thickness of the lens?

The density of the 2-mm-thick lens is found by the formula

$$D = -\log T$$
$$= -\log 0.3$$
$$= -(-0.523) = 0.523.$$

The reflection from the front surface is found by

$$R_1 = \left(\frac{n' - n}{n' + n}\right)^2 = \left(\frac{0.523}{2.523}\right)^2$$
$$= 0.043 = 4.3\%.$$

The transmission, T, of the front surface is given by

$$T = I - R_1 = 100 - 4.3 = 95.7\%.$$

The front surface density is equal to

$$D_s = -\log T = -\log 0.957$$
$$= -(-0.0191) = 0.0191.$$

The two surface densities (front and back) are equal to

$$2(0.0191) = 0.0382.$$

The total density of the lens is given by the relationship

$$0.523 = 2D_s + D_{med}.$$

Therefore,

$$D_{med} = 0.523 - 0.0382 = 0.4848.$$

Since the lens is 2 mm thick, the density per millimeter of thickness is

$$\frac{0.4848}{2} = 0.2424.$$

The density of a lens with a transmission of 50% is

$$D = -\log T = -\log 0.5 = -(-0.301) = 0.301.$$
$$D = 2D_s + (\text{number of units})(D/\text{unit})$$
$$0.301 = 0.0382 + (\text{number of units})(0.2424),$$

or

$$(0.2424)(\text{number of units}) = 0.301 - 0.0382$$
$$= 0.2628.$$

and,

$$(\text{number of units}) = \frac{0.2628}{0.2424} = 1.08.$$

The thickness of the lens is therefore equal to 1.08 mm.

EXAMPLE 2
If the above lens is made 3.5 mm thick, what would be its transmission?

$$\text{Total density} = 2D_s + (\text{number of units})(D/\text{unit})$$
$$= 0.382 + (3.5)(0.2424)$$
$$= 0.0382 + 0.8484$$
$$= 0.8866.$$

Therefore, the density of this lens, if made in a thickness of 3.5 mm, would be 0.8866.

$$\log T = -D = -0.8866.$$
The antilog of $-0.8866 = 0.1298$,

and the transmission of the lens is therefore 12.98%.

7.14. Methods of Manufacturing Absorptive Lenses

An *absorptive lens* is one that is used for the specific purpose of reducing the amount of transmitted light or radiant energy; thus it acts as a *filter*. Absorptive lenses are sometimes referred to as *tinted* or *colored* lenses because they are not usually clear and colorless, as are lenses made of white ophthalmic crown glass. The absorption may be *uniform* (or neutral), absorbing visible light of all wavelengths, or *selective*, absorbing some wavelengths more than others.

Presently, the major forms of absorptive lenses produced by lens manufacturers are: (1) tinted solid glass lenses, (2) glass lenses with surface coatings, (3) tinted plastic lenses, (4) photochromic lenses, and (5) polarizing lenses.

Tinted Solid Glass Lenses

The principal ingredients of white ophthalmic crown glass are silica, soda, and lime, to which small amounts of potassium, aluminum, and barium oxides are added to provide the desired physical and chemical properties. To produce a tinted lens, one or more *metals* or *metallic oxides* are introduced into the basic batch at the start of the process. The spectral transmission characteristics of the finished lenses are controlled by the quantities of these metals and metallic oxides present at the initial batch stage. The concentration of metals and metallic oxides incorporated to produce colors in lenses is less than 1% (even for dense colors). The elements most commonly used and the colors they produce are:

iron	green
manganese	pink
cobalt	blue
cerium	pinkish brown
nickel	brown
uranium	yellow
chromium	green
gold	red
silver	yellow
didymium	pink
vanadium	pale green

The color imparted by the addition of an absorptive substance is of no particular significance, merely an incidental by-product. The color of the lens does not indicate the specific absorptive characteristics of the lens for the UV or IR regions of the spectrum. The apparent color of a lens depends on those portions of the visible spectrum that are transmitted—if a lens transmits more of the green portion of the visible spectrum than it does of the blue, the lens appears to be green by transmitted light. When we speak of the color of a filter, we mean the apparent color of a "standard white" object seen through it. This apparent color is useful for determining the general effect on the visible portion of the spectrum. If the transmission is *uniform* across the visible spectrum, the lens appears to be a *neutral gray*, and any colors viewed through it are not appreciably changed. However, the overall *brightness* of the scene appears to decrease. If the transmission over the visible spectrum is not uniform, but *selective*, the lens appears to have a distinct color, and the color of any object viewed through the lens may be altered.

Different absorptive substances may produce lenses of similar color, but the spectral transmission curves for the lenses differ. When one is provided with a spectral transmission curve for a lens, it is not possible to determine the color of the lens. Although the spectral transmission curve of a lens is the major consideration, the color of the lens is useful for identification purposes and may have important psychological and cosmetic ramifications. In addition, the *depth* of the color provides a general indication of the level of transmission of the visible spectrum.

Solid glass tinted lenses were the earliest absorptive lenses to be produced. These lenses have many advantages compared with other methods of producing absorptive lenses—they may be produced in large quantities at low cost, the transmission is affected very little by surface scratching, there is an absence of the reflections that are associated with surface coatings, and no special equipment is needed for surfacing and finishing the lenses. Disadvantages include a variation in transmission from center to edge (for lenses of high power), a variation in transmission from one eye to the other for patients with large amounts of anisometropia, the permanence of the tint (it cannot be removed), and the large inventory of semifinished lenses required to service a wide range of prescriptions.

Glass Lenses with Surface Coatings

A lens is tinted by depositing a thin metallic oxide on the surface of the lens. The coating is deposited on the lens by an evaporation process conducted under a vacuum at high temperatures. Because of the high temperature required, the vacuum coating process cannot be used with plastic lenses.

The density of the coated lens depends on the thickness of the metallic oxide coating. Because the index of refraction of the metallic oxides is higher than the index of refraction of the underlying glass, the amount of light reflected from the absorptive coating is greater than the amount reflected from the uncoated front surface of the glass (the coating is deposited on the *back* surface of the glass). To reduce the amount of light reflected by the coating, an antireflective coating of magnesium fluoride is placed on the metallic oxide coating. When the lens is thoroughly cleaned and the coating properly applied, the resulting hardness is equal to that of ophthalmic crown glass. The coating has high resistance to wear and to chemical interaction. If the coating is applied uniformly across the surface of the lens, the transmission of light is uniform from edge to edge.

Metallic coatings may also be applied to solid glass tinted lenses in the following circumstances: (1) to darken a lens that the patient believes is too light; (2) to minimize, by the application of a metallic oxide coating on either the front or back surface of the lens, the variation in transmission of light from the center of a lens to its edge, which can occur in a solid glass tinted lens of high power and which can cause unsatisfactory performance or appearance.

Tinted Plastic Lenses

Plastic lenses cannot be surface coated by evaporation because they would be deformed by the high temperature required. Consequently, plastic lenses are tinted by dipping them in a solution containing the appropriate organic dye. The resulting density depends on the nature of the dye and the length of time the lens is immersed in the solution. To achieve a particular tint and transmission, the lens may be dipped into several different tinted solutions. Because the dye penetrates the surface layer of the lens to a uniform depth, the lenses are of uniform density regardless of variation in thickness from the center to the edge. If the tint is too dark, or for any reason needs to be changed, some tint can be removed by dipping the lens in a bleaching solution.

The color of dyed plastic lenses is not as stable as color in glass lenses. Most dyed plastic lenses fade with time, but some fade more rapidly than others. Proportionately lighter tints fade more than do darker tints. (To avoid legal pitfalls, the optometrist should request from the supplier not only the transmittance characteristics but the fading rate.) Different plastic materials—including CR-39 from various sources and even lenses from the same supplier but from a different manufacturing batch—absorb dyes at dissimilar rates. Lenses that are molded or cast may absorb tint at a different rate than those with ground and polished surfaces. As a lens ages, it again changes—a patient's old lens may not tint the same color as a new one.

Photochromic Lenses

In 1964 Corning, Inc. introduced glass lenses that were *photochromic*, that is, lenses that darken when exposed to long-wavelength UV radiation. Photochromic glass, with an index of refraction of 1.523, contains microscopic crystals of silver halide. On absorption of long-wavelength UV radiation, the silver halide crystals decompose into silver and halogen atoms and the lens becomes darker. The rigid matrix of the glass holds the silver and halogen in close proximity and, on removal of the activating UV radiation, the silver and halogen atoms recombine into silver halide crystals, with the result that the lens becomes lighter. The darkening rate depends on temperature; the lower the temperature, the faster and deeper the amount of darkening. Hence, the degree of darkening depends on a number of factors, such as the intensity of the radiation, the length of exposure, and the ambient temperature. The rate of *fading* depends on the composition of the glass, the temperature (thermal bleaching—the higher the temperature, the faster the fading), and exposure to wavelengths longer than those used for darkening (optical bleaching). In general, lenses darken faster than they fade. The cycle of darkening and fading is apparently inexhaustible. Photochromic lenses are discussed further in Section 7.21.

Polarizing Lenses

Electromagnetic radiation is transmitted by a process exhibiting both particlelike and wavelike behavior. Wavelike behavior is useful for explaining the phenomenon of polarization (Figure 7–7). Ordinarily, a light beam is composed of many *wave trains*, each with its plane of vibration oriented in a random direction, but always at right angles to the direction of propagation. An end-on view of the wave can be represented diagrammatically, as shown in Figure 7–7A. The beam of light is circularly symmetrical and is said to be *unpolarized*. Some types of crystals, such as quartz, tourmaline, and calcite, have the property of either partially or totally suppressing the vibrations in a particular direction. When the vibration is partially suppressed in a particular direction, the beam is not circularly symmetrical and the wave train is said to be *partially polarized* (Figure 7–7B). When the vibration is restricted to a single plane, the transmitted light is said to be *plane polarized*, or *linearly polarized* (Figure 7–7C).

When direct sunlight (which is unpolarized) is specularly reflected by particles or surface materials, it becomes partially or completely polarized, depending on the angle of incidence and the nature of the reflecting material. Materials that best polarize light by reflectance are generally nonconductors, called *dielectrics*, such as glass, pavement, sand, and snow. The light reflected from a dielectric surface is completely polarized at a specific angle of inci-

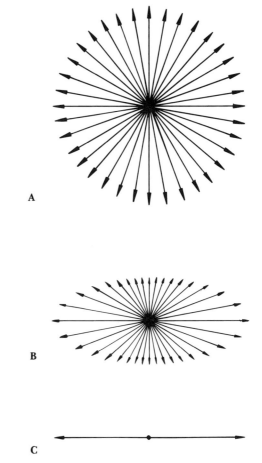

FIGURE 7–7.   **Polarization of light. A, end-on view of an unpolarized beam; B, a partially polarized beam; C, a plane-polarized, or linearly polarized, beam.**

dence (*Brewster's angle*), a point at which the angle between the associated refracted and reflected rays at the surface is 90°. This occurs when the tangent of the angle of incidence is equal to the index of refraction of the medium to which the light is incident, that is,

$$\tan i \ = n.$$

For specularly reflected light from ophthalmic crown glass of refractive index 1.523, Brewster's angle is about 57°; for water, with an index of 1.333, Brewster's angle is about 53°.

The plane of polarization (vibration) of the reflected light is parallel to the reflecting surface or perpendicular to the plane of the incident light, as shown in Figure 7–8. Hence, for a horizontal reflecting surface, the plane of polarization is horizontal. Specularly reflected light is highly localized, is intense, and appears to be *white* in color when reflected from a mirrorlike surface. Because of the veiling glare, specularly reflected light provides no useful information about the color, texture, or other properties of the underlying surface. In effect, it *obscures* the surface and, if intense, may be visually uncomfortable. When the angle of incidence is near Brewster's angle, the reflected light is strongly polarized but, at adjacent angles, the reflected light

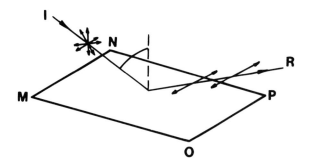

FIGURE 7–8.   **The plane of polarization of reflected light is parallel to the reflecting surface.**

consists of both polarized and unpolarized light (partial polarization). If a polarizing lens (called an *analyzer*) with its plane of polarization in the vertical meridian is placed in the path of a beam of light reflected from a horizontal surface, it absorbs the reflected polarized light. The elimination of specularly reflected horizontally polarized light improves visual acuity by reestablishing the natural balance of light intensities and restores fidelity to the surface color.

Polarizing filters are made by heating and stretching a thin sheet of polyvinyl alcohol to about four times its original length. The stretching aligns the molecular structure into long chains parallel to the direction of stretch. The sheet is then passed through a weak iodine solution, and the iodine molecules diffuse into the polyvinyl layer and attach themselves to the chains of long molecules, which thereby creates a polarizing filter. The thin polarizing sheet is then laminated between two layers of coated cellulose acetate butyrate and is pressed to the desired curvature. For glass lenses, the polarizing material is laminated between two layers of glass, which may be tinted and surfaced to any desired power.

The transmission of light from a polarized lens depends on both the degree of plane polarization and the absorptive nature of the laminated material. Standard polarized sunglasses are uniform-density lenses from the center to the edge because the tinted layer has a uniform thickness. Special additives in the tint coating increase the absorption of UV radiation. The unaided eye does not usually distinguish between polarized and unpolarized light. However, if a diffuse blue background is viewed through a rotating plane polarizer, a yellowish, double-ended, brushlike figure is seen, originating from the point of fixation, on the blue background. The brushes rotate with the plane of vibration of the polarizer. This phenomenon, known as *Haidinger's brushes*, is thought to be caused by the double-refraction effect of the radial nerve fibers of Henle surrounding the fovea. The double-refraction effect is used in the diagnosis of amblyopia and strabismus to detect eccentric fixation.

Polarizing lenses offer distinct advantages to fishermen who experience glare from the surface of the water, to motorists who find the reflected glare from highway surfaces annoying, and to skiers faced with large expanses of snow. The permanent, physiologic effects (if any) of polarized light on the eye are unknown.

7.15. Categories of Absorptive Lenses and Specification of Transmission

Absorptive lenses may be arbitrarily considered in terms of the following categories:

1. Lenses designed for general wear, which absorb the spectrum evenly and absorb little more UV radiation, visible light, or IR radiation than that absorbed by clear ophthalmic crown glass.
2. Lenses that selectively absorb UV radiation and transmit the visible spectrum more or less evenly.
3. Lenses designed for outdoor use, commonly called sunglasses, with low-average transmittance.
4. Lenses that selectively absorb portions of the visible spectrum in a nonuniform manner.
5. Lenses whose absorption characteristics vary with the level and type of illumination (photochromic lenses).
6. Miscellaneous absorptive lenses.
7. Lenses designed for occupational use, which selectively absorb particular wavelengths or have high absorption.

Specification of Transmission

The transmission properties of a lens are illustrated by means of a spectral transmittance curve, such as those shown in Figures 7–9 and 7–10. A spectral transmittance curve shows the percentage of transmission for all the visible spectrum and for portions of the UV and IR wavelengths. These curves depict the amount of radiant energy transmitted as a percentage of the radiant energy entering the lens, as a function of wavelength. The single percentage number given for a particular lens refers to the area under the curve within the visible spectrum.

Manufacturers' transmission data (such as those shown in Figure 7–9) are based on a lens thickness of 2 mm. For thicker or thinner lenses, the transmission is lower or higher, respectively. This should be kept in mind by the

FIGURE 7–9.   **Spectral transmittance curves for general wear lenses, Vision-Ease Pink.** (Reprinted with permission from D. G. Pitts and B. Maslovitz, unpublished data.)

FIGURE 7–10.   Spectral transmittance curves for ophthalmic crown glass lenses: clear ophthalmic crown and sunglasses gray #3, green #3, and tan #3. (Modified from Pitts, D. G. Sunglasses for Ocular Protection. In D. G. Pitts and R. N. Kleinstein, Eds., *Environmental Vision: Interaction of the Eye, Vision and the Environment.* Butterworth–Heinemann, Boston, 1993.)

practitioner prescribing or recommending absorptive lenses. For example, a hyperope whose lenses may have an average thickness of 4 mm will have almost twice the loss of light transmission for a given tint as will a myope or low hyperope whose lenses are only about 2 mm thick.

7.16. General-Wear Lenses Absorbing the Spectrum Evenly

Lenses in this category are very lightly tinted and absorb little or no more UV, visible, or IR radiation than does clear ophthalmic glass. These tints are known as "indoor" or as "cosmetic" tints. Because transmission across the spectrum is fairly uniform for these lenses, color values of objects are changed very little. Representative transmission curves of lenses in this category, shown in Figure 7–9, are remarkably similar, falling very close to one another. Some lenses contain ingredients, such as cerium oxide, that render them slightly more absorptive for short wavelengths than is light crown glass. The lenses in this category are so similar in appearance that it is often difficult to distinguish one manufacturer's lens from that of another, especially under the low illumination levels found in an examination room, or even to determine whether the lens has a tint at all. (One method of detecting a very light tint is to place the pair of glasses on a white sheet of paper; another is to remove one lens from the frame—if the lens is viewed through its edge, a distinct color may be seen.) When such a lens is being replaced, replacing *both* lenses is wise because the color differences are so subtle. However, if only one lens is ordered, it is a good idea to send the glasses to the laboratory so that color and density of tint can be matched.

The value of lightly tinted lenses has long been debated; some optometrists prescribe them on a fairly regular basis

and others prescribe them only with great reluctance. Even though such a lens transmits almost as much light as clear crown glass, many wearers are convinced that the lenses make their vision more comfortable and that the tint is beneficial. The origin of the reported vision comfort is not clearly understood. Perhaps the effects measurable at any one moment are small, but the comfortable feeling represents the sum of the effects during continuous wear. Knoll[30] suggested that one factor might be the attenuation of the intensity of reflected images, especially those reflected images formed after multiple traverses through the lens.

Clinical Note. If a patient has been wearing lightly tinted lenses and likes them, it is usually best *not* to arbitrarily remove the tint. When a new prescription is ordered, the tint should be duplicated as nearly as possible.

Patients who frequently ask for light tints for general wear include (1) lightly pigmented individuals, such as albinos; (2) patients with high refractive errors, especially aphakics and myopes; (3) patients who work under conditions of poorly designed artificial illumination, or with video display terminals (see Chapter 8); (4) patients who are not in good general health; (5) patients who have neurasthenic or neurotic tendencies.

Patients who work under conditions of poorly designed illumination usually report glare that interferes with vision and produces discomfort. When the visual environment includes extended light sources such as large windows or brightly illuminated walls, reflected images have a large angular subtense, which can produce veiling glare and can lead to a reduction of contrast in the visual field. The patient may conclude that *fluorescent lighting* is the cause of the problem—some practitioners routinely prescribe a pinkish-brown tint for patients who work under fluorescent lighting.

Lightly tinted lenses are often considered to have a definite *cosmetic* value, because some of the "glassiness" of the lenses is removed by tinting. When used with fused bifocal lenses, the tint tends to camouflage the bifocal segment. Lenses available include the Vision-Ease Pink (Vision Ease Company) lenses (Figure 7–9). The lightest of these lenses has an average transmission (throughout the visible spectrum) of approximately 88%, only 4% less than that of clear crown glass. Optical companies also make darker lenses in this group, such as Vision-Ease Pink #2 and Pink #3 (Figure 7–9).

For general-purpose wear, especially when the lenses will be used for *night driving*, only the lightest of tints should be used. For some patients, these lenses may be "habit forming"—once having worn such a tint, the patient may request a *darker* tint. The patient may wish to use the darker tint for both general wear and as a substitute for sunglass lenses. However, any fixed tinted lens (i.e., not photochromic) that gives significant reduction of illumination outdoors is *too dark* for inside use and for nighttime wear.

Most roadways are poorly illuminated at night, and the introduction of a lens tint can further reduce illumination. The natural illumination of the stars and the moon provide light for determining the outline of the roadbed and the contours of the surrounding landscape essential for country driving. The wearing of darkly tinted lenses (often combined with a tinted windshield) can create an illuminated field that is greatly restricted and confined to the paths of the headlight beams. Even a small reduction in the illumination available for night driving can decrease the *seeing distance* (the distance at which a nonilluminated object can be seen) in front of the vehicle. If the seeing distance is less than the braking or stopping distance for a particular speed, a person may drive into a stalled or slowly moving vehicle.

One method of maximizing the transmission of an absorptive lens that will be used for night driving is to place an antireflective coating on a lens with one of the lightest general-wear tints. The increase in transmission caused by the coating will be sufficient to offset the loss from absorption by the tint, with the result that the lens will have a transmission level equal to that of clear crown glass. The coating also has the additional advantage of appreciably reducing the intensity of light reflected by the lens surfaces.

If a patient is uncomfortable in outdoor illumination, the lightest of the general-wear tints is not likely to be helpful. Because darker general-wear tints cause problems with inadequate illumination for indoor wear and for night driving, a separate pair of glasses may be prescribed. An alternative would be a pair of glasses with photochromic lenses.

The darker shades of neutral density tints (#2 and #3 tints) may be useful for photophobia associated with albinism or for pathologic conditions affecting the cornea, conjunctiva, or iris. The transmission curves of the darker tints often differ significantly from those of the lighter tints. They absorb disproportionately more radiation in the short-wavelength visible region and therefore tend to take on a reddish-brown color.

7.17. Lenses That Selectively Absorb UV Radiation but Uniformly Transmit the Visible Spectrum

As noted in Section 7.6, exposure of the cornea to UV radiation can cause photokeratitis. Wavelengths shorter than 290 nm primarily affect the corneal epithelium; wavelengths in the 290- to 315-nm range cause damage to the corneal stroma, Descemet's membrane, and the endothelium; they can also produce secondary uveitis.[31] UV radiation is thought to be responsible for various forms of retinal pathology including cystoid macular edema.

Protection from solar and artificially produced near UV radiation is recommended for individuals who are repeatedly subjected to UV radiation during occupational, medical, or recreational activities. Pitts[32] pointed out that exposure to UV radiation under normal living conditions can be considered safe because the eyes are protected by the eyebrows (eyes are set below and behind the eyebrows and recessed in the orbits). Furthermore, because the line of sight is ordinarily not directed toward the sun, the energy of the UV radiation reaching the eyes is attenuated by atmospheric absorption and scattering. However, in

environments in which the nominal intensities of near UV radiation are exceeded, protection should be provided for the potential hazards of UV exposure. The amount of UV radiation increases with increasing altitude, with the result that outdoor activities such as skiing and mountain climbing can greatly increase the level of UV exposure. Solar reflections from large expanses of snow, water, or sand contain significant amounts of UV radiation. Although the most common source of UV radiation is sunlight, a host of artificial light sources used in manufacturing and in health-related activities emit potentially hazardous levels of UV radiation. These sources include fluorescent lamps, mercury discharge lamps, lasers, and welding arcs.

To prevent possible ocular damage and to minimize discomfort and the loss of visual function, eye protection from UV radiation should be provided for certain individuals. UV-absorbing lenses should be prescribed for any patient who encounters excessive exposure to UV radiation in industrial, health-care, or recreational activities. Protection from UV radiation should also be provided for patients taking photosensitizing pharmaceuticals (as described above). Furthermore, because the retina of the aphakic eye is subjected to increased levels of UV and visible radiation, the aphakic patient should wear lenses that absorb UV radiation and significantly reduce visible radiation, especially at the blue end of the visible spectrum.

Ocular protection from UV radiation can be provided by means of absorptive or reflective filters. Absorptive filters are manufactured by adding substances to the lens material; reflective filters are designed by coating the lens with the appropriate reflecting material. Pitts[32] has recommended that a UV filter should absorb all radiation to 380 nm. The absorption characteristics of clear spectacle lenses differ slightly from one manufacturer to another and differ for different materials (i.e., glass vs. plastic). As shown in Figure 7–10, clear ophthalmic crown glass transmits UV radiation beginning at a wavelength of approximately 300 nm and the transmission rises rapidly for longer UV wavelengths. However, the plastic material CR-39 (Figure 7–11) transmits UV radiation from only about 350 nm upward and this transmission also rises rapidly for longer UV wavelengths.

Polycarbonate (see Chapter 1) is a plastic material with very high impact resistance and is available in normal prescription powers. Hard coatings are necessary to protect the relatively soft surface. Recently, a coating has been formulated to incorporate special UV absorbers that screen out all UV radiation below 380 nm (Figure 7–12). Thus, the coated polycarbonate lens is not only virtually indestructible and resistant to surface abrasion but also provides adequate protection from UV radiation. Most clear, high-index, hard resin lenses (n = 1.60) have a cutoff of about 380 nm for UV radiation (Figure 7–13).

Neither glass nor the more commonly used CR-39 plastic provides adequate absorption of all UV radiation (i.e., up to 380 nm). However, many products have been introduced for this purpose. A lens manufacturer should supply a spectral transmission curve for a lens allegedly designed to eliminate UV radiation; the specific absorption and transmission prop-

FIGURE 7–11. Spectral transmittance curves of CR-39 ophthalmic lenses: clear CR-39 and CR-39 sunlenses gray #3, green #3, and brown #3. (Modified from Pitts, D. G. Sunglasses for Ocular Protection. In D. G. Pitts and R. N. Kleinstein, Eds., *Environmental Vision: Interaction of the Eye, Vision and the Environment.* Butterworth–Heinemann, Boston, 1993.)

FIGURE 7–12. Spectral transmittance curves of polycarbonate ophthalmic lenses: clear polycarbonate and polycarbonate sunlenses gray #3, green #3, and tan #3. (Modified from Pitts, D. G. Sunglasses for Ocular Protection. In D. G. Pitts and R. N. Kleinstein, Eds., *Environmental Vision: Interaction of the Eye, Vision and the Environment,* Butterworth–Heinemann, Boston, 1993.)

erties of a lens *cannot* be determined by the *color* of the lens. Tints that fail to eliminate UV radiation adequately can cause harm. For example, if the lowered transmission in the visible spectrum causes the pupil to dilate behind a tinted lens, higher levels of UV radiation will reach the crystalline lens than the levels that would exist if the patient wore an *untinted* lens and the pupil had been in its normal, undilated state.

FIGURE 7–13. Spectral transmittance curves of high index (1.60) polyurethane plastics: clear polyurethane plastic and polyurethane sunlenses gray #3, green #3, and brown #3. (Reprinted with permission from D. Pitts, unpublished data.)

CR-39 Plastic Lenses

Several CR-39 plastic lenses containing UV absorbers are currently available. These include the UV-400 (Optical Radiation Corp.), which eliminates all radiation shorter than 400 nm; the Vision-Ease Lite-Gard UV (Figure 7–14), which absorbs 95% of all radiation in the 250 to 400 nm range; the UVS lens by Silor Optical, which absorbs 94% to 96% of the radiation below the 400 nm level; and the Recreational Innovations NoIR lenses #111 and #112 (NoIR Medical Technologies), shown in Figure 7–15, which absorb all radiation below 400 nm.

Glass Lenses

Glass lenses that transmit less than 5% of UV radiation below 400 nm include American Optical's Hazemaster, the Vision-Ease Yellow (Figure 7–16), and Bausch & Lomb's Kalichrome. These are all *yellow* lenses and have been promoted both as shooting lenses and as night-driving lenses (see Section 7.19).

The *Spectra Shield Human II* (Spectra-Shield Corp.) lens is a unique glass lens coated with 28 layers of dielectric material on the concave surface of the lens. It is designed to reflect all UV radiation below 400 nm and all IR radiation above 700 nm.

Photochromic lenses from Corning, Inc., such as *Photogray II, Photogray Extra, Photobrown Extra, Photosun II, Photogray Extra-16, Photobrown Extra-16, Photogray Thin and Dark,* and *Photobrown Thin and Dark,* transmit *no* UV radiation in the range of 290 to 315 nm (UV-B) in the fully darkened state and transmit less than 4% in the range of 315 to 380 nm (UV-A) (see Section 7.20).

FIGURE 7–14.   Spectral transmittance curves for Vision-Ease (clear CR-39) and Lite-Gard UV lenses. (Reprinted with permission from D. Pitts and B. Maslovitz, unpublished data.)

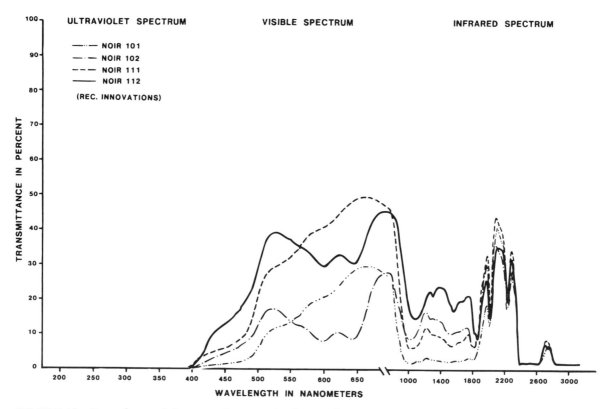

FIGURE 7–15.   Spectral transmission curves for Recreational Innovations NoIR #101, #102, #111, #112. (Reprinted with permission from D. Pitts and B. Maslovitz, unpublished data.)

FIGURE 7–16. Spectral transmission curves for Vision-Ease Blue and Striking Yellow. (Reprinted with permission from D. Pitts and B. Maslovitz, unpublished data.)

7.18. Lenses Designed for Outdoor Use

Most lenses in this category absorb sufficient radiation in the visible spectrum to be considered as *sunglass* lenses. The American Bureau of Standards has defined a sunglass lens as one that transmits less than 67% of incident light. This is an arbitrary definition—for sufficient protection for bright daylight conditions, transmission should be about 10% to 20%. Some lenses in this category are listed in Table 7–3; their transmission curves are shown in various figures in the chapter, as indicated in Table 7–3. Most lenses are not sufficiently dark to wear in conditions of extremely high illumination. As noted previously, exposure to 10,000 ftL (equal to 34,260 cd/m²) of illumination would require a lens with absorption levels of about 4%. The only lenses that are close to this range are the Gray #3 glass lens (Figure 7–10), the Gray #3 CR-39 lens (Figure 7–11), the Gray #3 and Brown #3 hard resin 1.60 lenses, the Recreational Innovations NoIR #102 lens (Figure 7–15), the Gray Polarized line of lenses (plane of polarization 180°, Figure 7–17), and Recreational Innovations NoIR #107, #108, and #109 lenses (Figure 7–18).

Luria[33] conducted a study to determine which neutral filter was most preferred for bright sunlight in summer and winter. In summer, when the light level was about 14,000 cd/m², the preferred optical density of the filter was 1.0 (transmission, 10%). In the winter, against a bright snowy background, the light levels were 17,000 to 27,500 cd/m², and the preferred optical density was 1.3 (transmission of

4.8%). In both cases, the light level was reduced with the preferred filter to about 1000 to 1400 cd/m² at the eye. The optical density most preferred ranged from 1.05 to 1.60 (transmission, 8.9 to 2.5%). The preferred optical densities reported by Luria are considerably darker than the density of most sunglasses that are currently available commercially. Luria's study confirms the observation of Richards[29] that 400 ftL (1370 cd/m²) is the optimal level for comfortable vision.

None of the lenses in this category should be used as *general-wear* lenses. Their transmission is *much too low* for safe use in night driving, and if darkly tinted lenses are used for *indoor* wear, the eyes become adapted to such a low level of illumination that the lenses tend to lose their effectiveness for outdoor wear.

Ultraviolet Absorption

Although all lenses designed for outdoor use have excellent absorption in the 200- to 300-nm portion of the UV region, some have inadequate absorption in the longer 300- to 400-nm range. In Table 7–3, the only lenses having less than 5% transmittance in this range are the Green #3 and Tan #3 glass lenses (Figure 7–10); the Gray #3, Green #3, and Brown #3 CR-39 lenses (Figure 7–11); the Gray #3, Green #3, and Brown #3 polycarbonate lenses (Figure 7–12); the Gray #3, Green #3, and Brown #3 high-index 1.60 hard resin lenses (Figure 7–13); Recreational Innovations NoIR #101, #111,

TABLE 7–3
Representative Absorptive Lenses

Color	Lens Name	Material	Transmission Curve Illustrated
Green	Green #3	Glass	Figure 7–10
		CR-39	Figure 7–11
		Polycarbonate	Figure 7–12
		Hard Resin	Figure 7–13
	Recreational Innovations NoIR #107, #108, #109	Plastic	Figure 7–18
Gray	Gray #3	Glass	Figure 7–10
		CR-39	Figure 7–11
		Polycarbonate	Figure 7–12
		Hard Resin	Figure 7–13
	Gray	Polarized	Figure 7–17
Brown or Tan	Tan #3	Glass	Figure 7–10
	Brown #3	CR-39	Figure 7–11
		Polycarbonate	Figure 7–12
		Hard Resin	Figure 7–13
	Recreational Innovations NoIR #101, #102, #111, #112	Plastic	Figure 7–15
Pink	Vision-Ease Pink	Glass	Figure 7–9
Yellow	Vision-Ease Yellow	Glass	Figure 7–16
Blue	Vision-Ease Blue	Glass	Figure 7–16
Pale bluish green	Vision-Ease Unisol (Therminon)	Glass	Figure 7–19

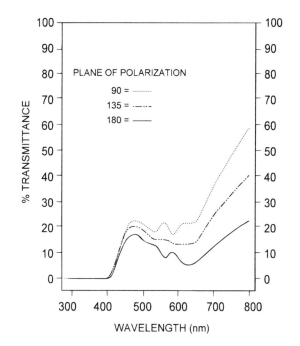

FIGURE 7–17. **Spectral transmittance curves of a gray polarized lens. Most polarized lenses are mounted in the spectacle frame to absorb sunlight reflected from horizontal surfaces such as water, concrete, glass, and roadways. Sunlight incident on horizontal surfaces is reflected plane-polarized and parallel to the plane of the surface (horizontally). The sun-glass lens designed to absorb light reflected from horizontal surfaces transmits vertically polarized light but absorbs horizontally polarized light. This graph demonstrates that the percentage of transmittance and color of transmitted light varies with the plane of polarization. (Reprinted with permission from D. Pitts, unpublished data.)**

and #112 lenses (Figure 7–15); and NoIR #107, #108, and #109 lenses (Figure 7–18). The Gray #3 glass lens (Figure 7–10) transmits more than 20% in this range.

Infrared Absorption

Some lenses listed in Table 7–3 have good absorption in the IR region of the spectrum. For example, lenses having less than 15% transmittance in the range of 700 to 1500 nm are the Gray #3, Green #3, and Tan #3 glass lenses (Figure 7–10), Recreational Innovations NoIR #101, #102, #111, and #112 lenses (Figure 7–15), and Recreational Innovations NoIR #107, #108, and #109 lenses (Figure 7–18). However, several plastic tinted lenses, such as CR-39 (Figure 7–11), polycarbonate (Figure 7–12), high-index 1.60 hard resin (Figure 7–13), and polarized lenses (Figure 7–17), have high transmittances in the IR region.

Pitts et al.[34] showed that the level of exposure to IR radiation required to cause ocular damage is quite high compared with the level of exposure to UV radiation required for ocular damage to occur. On the other hand, Clark[35] asserted that lenses having high IR transmission can be hazardous—because the reduced visible light transmission causes the pupil to dilate (as noted also in the discussion of UV radiation), the retina may actually receive *more* IR radiation than it would if an absorptive lens were not worn. In another paper, Clark[36] concluded that there is no advantage for *colored* absorptive lenses, and that absorptive lenses should be neutral gray. However, of the presently available lenses, only the *dark green* lenses consistently reduce transmission in the IR region of the spectrum.

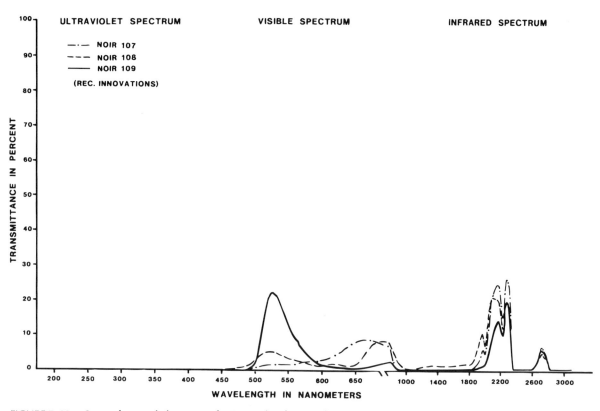

FIGURE 7–18.   Spectral transmission curves for Recreational Innovations NoIR #107, #108, and #109. (Reprinted with permission from D. Pitts and B. Maslovitz, unpublished data.)

7.19. Lenses That Selectively Absorb Portions of the Visible Spectrum

Although not commonly used, lenses that selectively absorb portions of the visible spectrum are available. These lenses are yellow, blue, and bluish green. The yellow lenses include the American Optical Hazemaster, the Vision-Ease Yellow (Figure 7–16), and the Bausch & Lomb Kalichrome. The blue lenses include the Vision-Ease Blue (Figure 7–16); the bluish green lenses include the Vision-Ease Unisol (Therminon) lenses (Figure 7–19).

The Hazemaster, Vision-Ease Yellow, and Kalichrome absorb almost *all* illumination below 500 nm and, therefore, greatly reduce the *scattering* of light (scattering is mainly caused by the wavelengths in the blue end of the spectrum). Because the retina is most sensitive to radiation of 555 nm, it has been suggested that lenses having high relative transmission at or near this wavelength aid visual acuity at night. Consequently, yellow lenses have been promoted as "night-driving lenses."

Colors have different subjective effects on different observers. For some people, yellow glasses create a brighter environment and a sense of seeing better, even though the lenses obviously absorb some light and, therefore, reduce the brightness of the environment. Wright[37] attributes this observation to the association of yellow color with sunlight

and, hence, with a high level of illumination. Other observers find yellow glasses disquieting and uncomfortable and report that they see better without them.

Because short-wavelength radiation is scattered more by fog and haze than is long-wavelength radiation, yellow light should reduce the scattering effects of fog and haze. Theoretically, yellow light should also reduce the chromatic aberration of the eye. However, because the retina has a decreased sensitivity to short-wavelength radiation, yellow lenses are not as helpful in reducing the effects of chromatic aberration of the eye as they are in applications in photography. In fact, at low levels of illumination, when maximal sensitivity of the eye shifts from 555 to 510 nm, yellow glasses can have a negative effect on vision because of the decreased sensitivity of the eye for the longer wavelengths.

A number of researchers have studied the effect of yellow lenses on visual performance, and the results of these studies have been negative. Luckiesh and Holladay[38] found that yellow light does not provide an advantage in foggy or misty weather. Richards[39] found a small but statistically significant loss of vision occurring with yellow lenses. According to Blackwell,[40] yellow driving glasses reduce visual detection distances by 33% compared with wearing no glasses. Davey[41] found that glare-recovery time was 29% longer with yellow glasses than without. Often, there is barely sufficient illumination for night driving, and the loss of illumination when

FIGURE 7–19.   Spectral transmission curve for Vision-Ease Unisol (Therminon). (Reprinted with permission from D. Pitts and B. Maslovitz, unpublished data.)

yellow lenses are worn is potentially dangerous. Expert opinion advises that *yellow lenses should not be worn for night driving.*

Yellow lenses have also been recommended for hunting and skeet shooting because scattered light may create a problem in these activities. Bierman[42] tested the shooting ability of 50 men, with and without yellow lenses. Most were not better marksmen with the yellow lenses, and many were worse. Interestingly, for the 19 men who liked the yellow lenses, scores were higher with the lenses than without them; for the 26 men who disliked the lenses, scores were higher without the lenses. These lenses should therefore be prescribed for shooting only when, for a given patient, they have proven to be beneficial.

The Vision-Ease Blue lens (Figure 7–16) is used strictly for cosmetic purposes. The pale bluish green Vision-Ease Unisol (Therminon) lenses (Figure 7–19) have almost the same transmittance as crown glass in the visible spectrum but have a gradual reduction in transmittance in the IR region. These lenses are claimed to be *cool* lenses, and their use has been proposed for patients whose eyes are constantly exposed to highly reflective white surfaces and for cooks and others who must work in environments in which there is an excessive amount of IR radiation. Some wearers of these lenses tend to become "hooked" on the lenses and are unhappy if the practitioner unknowingly switches them to another pale tint or to clear lenses.

One of the earliest absorptive lenses to be introduced was the Crookes series of glass lenses, developed by Sir

William Crookes. These are smoke-colored lenses that absorb all UV radiation below 350 nm and are unique in that they have additional absorption bands in the yellow region of the visible spectrum. The absorption bands result from the incorporation of didymium (a mixture of the elements neodymium and praseodymium) and cerium oxide. The spectral transmission curve of the Hoya Crookes A #2 lens is shown in Figure 7–20.

Recently, Schott Glass Technologies has introduced Amethyst Contrast Enhancement Glass (ACE) that has the effect of heightening the ability of the wearer to discriminate colors toward the ends of the visible spectrum, that is, to enhance perception of the red and blue tones (Figure 7–21). Enhancement of the visual sensitivity to the end colors of the visible spectrum is achieved by selective repression of the central colors of green and yellow. ACE glass uses rare earth oxides such as didymium in its composition as narrow band absorbers.

ACE glass has a refractive index of 1.560, an Abbe number of 49.2, and a density of 2.91 g/cm³. It is available in both plano and single vision prescription form. Although it has a relatively low luminous transmittance of 38 percent, it is not recommended for sunglass use unless a UV filtering coating is applied. ACE is recommended for specialty applications in leisure and occupational activities such as hunting, target and trap shooting, bird watching and for comfort in viewing video display terminals (see also Chapter 8).

FIGURE 7–20.   Spectral transmission curve for Hoya Crookes A #2. Note the absorption bands in the yellow region of the spectrum. (Reprinted with permission from D. Pitts and B. Maslovitz, unpublished data.)

FIGURE 7–21.   **Spectral transmittance for Amethyst Contrast Enhancement Glass (ACE). (Reprinted with permission from Schott Glass Technologies, Inc.)**

7.20. Photochromic Lenses

Lenses made of photochromic glass have the remarkable property of darkening when exposed to sunlight and reverting to their original state in the absence of sunlight. The photochromic properties of these lenses are caused by very minute *silver halide* crystals that are precipitated from the homogeneous melt during initial cooling or during subsequent reheating at temperatures between the annealing and softening points for a long enough period of time for the crystals to grow to optimal size.

The photochromic process is basically the same as the photolytic dissociation of silver halide into silver and halogen that occurs with silver halide photographic material; the difference is that the photographic process is *irreversible*, but the photochromic process occurring in glass can be reversed. In photography, the host matrix permits the halogen to diffuse away from the original crystal site and the halogens are no longer available for recombination when irradiation ceases. Hence, after suitable chemical treatment, a permanent photographic image is formed by the stable silver particles. Photochromic glass, on the other hand, is impervious, chemically inert, and rigid. These characteristics prevent loss of the halogen by diffusion and exclude atmospheric oxygen and moisture, which might cause side reactions. Thus, the released halogens are confined to the immediate vicinity of the crystal site and a recombination of silver and halogen can take place after active irradiation ceases. The recombination process is enhanced by exposure to heat (thermal bleaching) or visible radiation of relatively long wavelength (optical bleaching).

In both photographic film and photochromic glasses, silver ions and electrons resulting from the dissociation of silver halide regroup to form opaque silver colloids (specks) of appreciable size. The opaque silver colloids are the entities that absorb *visible* light in much the same manner as any metal and that cause the photochromic glass to appear dark. When the activating light is removed, the silver colloids in the glass begin to split apart into silver ions. They recombine with the halide ions that are still trapped within the molecular structure of the glass and again form light-sensitive silver halide microcrystals.

A major factor in determining speeds of response, range of densities, and base colors of photochromic glass is the mixture of the host glass material. Corning, Inc. describes its host photochromic glass as *alkali borosilicate* crown glass; Chance-Pilkington Ltd. (England) labels its photochromic host glass as an *alumino-phosphate* glass.

There are three manufacturers of wide-range, swift-acting photochromic glass in the Western world: Corning, Inc., Chance-Pilkington, and Deutsche Spezialglas AG (Desag). Confusion exists in marketing trade names of photochromic glass. For example, Corning glasses are marketed under Corning's registered names but are also sold under Rodenstock and Hoya glass trade names. Both Zeiss and Rodenstock use the same Desag photochromic glass but sell it under different brand names. Chance-Pilkington Ltd. markets its own photochromic glass but has issued a license for the production of its glass in the United States by Schott Optical. Bausch & Lomb uses both Corning and Chance-Pilkington photochromic glasses.

The wavelength that induces darkening depends on the chemical composition of the glass. Glasses containing only silver chloride are sensitive to wavelengths from approximately 300 to 400 nm with optimal activation about 350 nm.[43] The longer wavelength limit of spectral sensitivity for darkening is *higher* for glasses containing heavier halogens such as silver bromide (as high as 550 nm) or silver iodide (as high as 650 nm).[44] The addition of other sensitizers in trace quantities enhances the sensitivity and photochromic darkening. These include the oxides of arsenic, antimony, tin, and copper. Copper oxide is an especially effective sensitizer and is believed to enter the silver halide crystals as a cuprous ion.

Crystal *size* and *spacing* determine the resolution and transparency in the unactivated state. Silver halide crystals are 50 to 100 Å in diameter, and the average spacing is from 500 to 1000 Å.[43] In general, glasses with crystals less than 50 Å in diameter are not photochromic. Above 300 Å, the glass becomes translucent. For particles with an average diameter of 100 Å and an average spacing of 600 Å between particles, the concentration is about 4×10^{15} particles per cubic centimeter.[43]

Photochromic glasses differ from organic photochromic materials in that they are immune to fatigue or deterioration of their photochromic performance with extended use. Because they are trapped within the glass, the microcrystals are available for cycles of darkening and fading in the lens indefinitely. However, new photochromic lenses need to go through a "breaking-in" period. Exposure of the glass to sunlight for several full darkening-fading cycles is necessary before the normal operating performance can be reached. If a pair of glasses with these lenses is not used for long periods of time, the breaking-in cycles must be repeated.

The first photochromic lens produced commercially in the United States was the Bestlite lens, introduced by Corning in 1965. The Bestlite lens was superseded by the Photogray lens in 1968; the Photogray lens had increased darkening with sunlight exposure and a more uniform spectral recovery. In 1971 Corning introduced the Photosun lens. In sunlight it darkened to a transmittance of 25% but

faded to a transmittance of only 68% overnight. Corning's second generation of lenses includes the Photogray Extra lens (1978) and the Photobrown Extra lens (1981). These lenses differ from the original Photogray lens in both darkening and fading more quickly. Within 60 seconds in sunlight, the Photogray Extra darkens to 22% transmittance and the Photobrown Extra darkens to 24% transmittance. When removed from activating radiation for 5 minutes, the Photogray Extra fades to 62% transmittance and the Photobrown Extra fades to 64% transmittance. Overnight, the Photogray Extra fades to 87% transmittance and the Photobrown Extra fades to 86% transmittance.

Both Photogray Extra and Photobrown Extra respond more to visible light than do other Corning photochromic glasses. Each darkens slightly in a brightly lighted room. Photogray Extra and Photobrown Extra are available in both one-piece and fused multifocal construction. The segment used in fused multifocal construction is made of clear glass; therefore, when the lens is fully darkened, the segment area is lighter than the distance portion of the lens.

The optical and physical properties of Photogray Extra and Photobrown Extra are similar to those of other Corning photochromic lenses. The index of refraction is 1.523, the same as ophthalmic crown glass. However, the specific gravity of Photogray Extra and Photobrown Extra is less than that of other Corning photochromic glass and ophthalmic crown glass. Photogray Extra and Photobrown Extra weigh 2.41 g/cc compared to 2.54 g/cc for ophthalmic crown glass.

Photosun II was introduced in 1983. It is darker in both the faded and the darkened states than other Corning photochromic lenses. The transmittance is 41% in the faded state and 12% in the darkened state. After 1 minute of exposure to direct sunlight, it darkens to 16% transmittance; within 1 hour, it reaches its maximal darkness of 12%. In the fading process, Photosun II lightens to 29% transmittance within 5 minutes. Overnight, it will fade to 41% transmittance.

The Photogray II was introduced in 1984 as a second-generation replacement for the Photogray lens. Fully faded, the Photogray II offers the highest transmission of any Corning photochromic lens, transmitting 87% of incident visible light. When fully darkened, this lens transmits 42% of visible light. It will darken to 85% of its range within the first 60 seconds of activation, and within 1 hour it will reach its maximal darkness of 42% transmission. Photogray II lenses fade the fastest of any current Corning photochromic lens, recovering 70% of the fully faded transmittance in the first 5 minutes after being removed from sunlight and then fading overnight to 87% transmittance.

In 1990 Corning introduced two high-index glass photochromic lenses, Photogray Extra-16 (PGX-16) and Photobrown Extra-16 (PBX-16). Each lens has a refractive index of 1.6005, an Abbe number of 42, and a density of 2.73 g/cc. The Photogray Extra-16 has a transmittance of 83% in the faded state and 22% in the darkened state; the Photobrown Extra-16 has a transmittance of 83% in the faded state and 30% in the darkened state.

The proliferation of thinner high-index plastic lens designs has made the weight of glass lenses an issue. In 1994 Corning developed Photogray Thin and Dark and Photobrown Thin and Dark lenses. These lenses have a standard refractive index of 1.523 and are packed with silver halide microcrystals (5 quadrillion/cc). The lenses are designed to be ground to a 1.50-mm center thickness in *plano* and *minus* prescriptions. By making the ion exchange in chem-tempering more efficient, the lenses have approximately the same impact resistance as Photogray Extra and Photobrown Extra lenses 2.0 mm thick. The Photogray Thin and Dark has a transmittance of 86% in the faded state and 16% in the darkened state; the Photobrown Thin and Dark has a transmittance of 85% in the faded state and 15% when darkened.

Transmittance curves for current Corning photochromic lenses are shown in Figures 7–22 through 7–29. The transmittance ranges of available Corning photochromic lenses are compared in Figure 7–30.

Although many factors influence the transmittance of a specific photochromic glass, the principal factors are

1. Intensity of the incident radiation
2. Wavelength of the incident radiation
3. Temperature of the glass
4. Thickness of the glass

FIGURE 7–22. Spectral transmittance curves for Corning Photogray Extra, in faded and darkened states. (Reprinted with permission from Corning, Inc.)

FIGURE 7–24. Spectral transmittance curves for Corning Photosun II, in faded and darkened states. (Reprinted with permission from Corning, Inc.)

FIGURE 7–23. Spectral transmittance curves for Corning Photobrown Extra, in faded and darkened states. (Reprinted with permission from Corning, Inc.)

FIGURE 7–25. Spectral transmittance curves for Corning Photogray II, in faded and darkened states. (Reprinted with permission from Corning, Inc.)

FIGURE 7–26. Spectral transmittance for Corning Photogray Extra-16. (Reprinted with permission from Corning, Inc.)

FIGURE 7–28. Spectral transmittance for Corning Photobrown Extra-16. (Reprinted with permission from Corning, Inc.)

FIGURE 7–27. Spectral transmittance for Corning Photogray Thin and Dark. (Reprinted with permission from Corning, Inc.)

FIGURE 7–29. Spectral transmittance for Corning Photobrown Thin and Dark. (Reprinted with permission from Corning, Inc.)

5. Previous heat treatment
6. Exposure history

At controlled temperatures, the transmittance decreases as the intensity of the sunlight increases. When the transmittance of a photochromic lens is recorded over an entire day, it shows a characteristic pattern of decreasing transmittance beginning at dawn, continuing to decrease until saturation is achieved, then beginning to fade before sunset and continuing to fade until the next morning. On overcast or cloudy days, the lenses are as dark as they are in full sunlight. The

closer the wavelength of incident radiation is to the optimal wavelength for activation, the darker the lens becomes.

As a general rule, photochromic lenses are also temperature dependent—the lenses are *darker* in cool temperatures and *lighter* in warm temperatures. The rate of fading in darkness increases with the temperature (thermal bleaching). However, the darkening rate is relatively insensitive to temperature.

The silver halide microcrystals are distributed uniformly throughout the glass. However, photochromic glass can be uniformly activated throughout its total depth only if suffi-

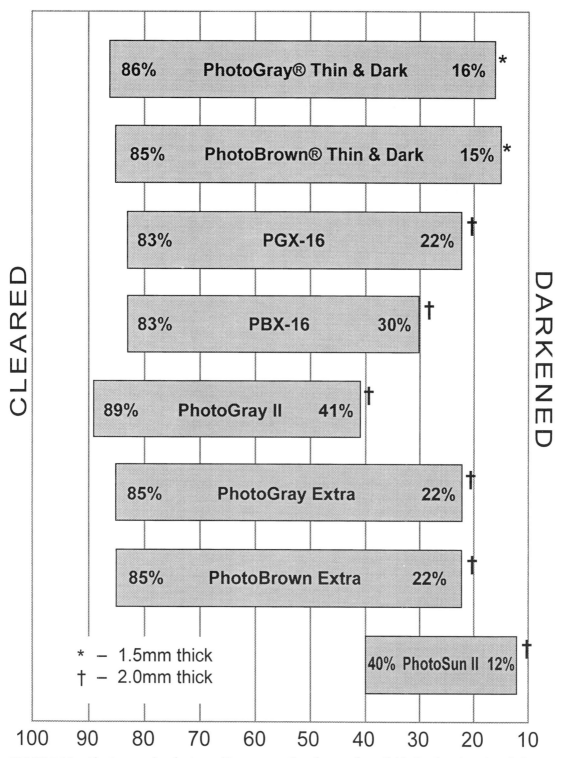

FIGURE 7–30.   **Chart comparing the transmittance properties of currently available Corning photochromic lenses. (Reprinted with permission from Corning, Inc.)**

cient energy intensity is applied. Intense darkening occurs near the incident surface and, with increasing depth, the glass becomes more transparent, depending on the exposure energy. The predominance of surface darkening means that the lenses function essentially as *uniform-density* lenses (see Section 7.24). Although the greatest darkening occurs near the exposed surface of the glass, some darkening occurs at deeper levels. Therefore, thicker lenses may darken somewhat more than thinner ones, and thicker lenses take longer to fade to the near-clear state.

Although photochromic lenses may be toughened by either chem-tempering or air-tempering, Corning recommends *chem-tempering*. Lenses that have been chem-tempered usually exhibit greater impact resistance than air-tempered lenses at the same thickness. Air-tempering produces a lens that is darker at high temperatures, retains more tint in the overnight faded state, and fades more slowly than a chem-tempered lens. Chemically tempered lenses fade more rapidly than air-tempered lenses and have a wider range of transmittance between the fully faded and darkened states.

Up to a point, both the degree and speed of darkening increase with the number of darkening and fading cycles a photochromic lens undergoes. People who spend a large amount of time outdoors generally have darker lenses in the fully activated state than people who spend only a moderate amount of time outdoors. All photochromic lenses darken faster than they fade. For example, Photogray Extra lenses darken in sunlight to 22% transmittance in 60 seconds but fade to only 62% transmittance in 5 minutes. The fading process for Corning photochromic lenses may be speeded up and the residual tint reduced quickly by holding the lenses under warm, running tap water for 30 seconds. Although not needed routinely, this procedure is useful on occasions when it is desirable to reach maximal fading very quickly.

The darkening of photochromic lenses is triggered mainly by long UV radiation and short visible radiation. Automobile windshields and side windows absorb and reflect much activating UV radiation and thereby reduce the amount of UV radiation reaching the photochromic lenses. Hence, the lenses do not darken completely when worn while a person drives an automobile; people who drive during daylight hours may be disappointed by the performance of the lenses.

Replacement of a broken photochromic lens can sometimes present a problem because after replacement one lens may be darker than the other or the two lenses may not darken or lighten at the same rate. In replacing one lens, it is recommended that the original lens be chemically tempered in the same bath as the new lens. If tempering the original lens along with the new lens is not feasible, the original lens may be placed in boiling water or in an oven at 212°F (100°C) for at least 1 hour.

When antireflective or tinted *coating* is applied to photochromic lenses, it must be applied within a critical temperature range of approximately 230°C to 375°C. Temperature controls in this range are critical to the performance of the photochromic lenses. Therefore, the time, temperature, and cooling must be closely controlled. Any mismatch in color or transmittance that arises from the coating operation can usually be corrected by placing the lenses in a 400°C to 425°C oven for approximately 25 minutes and then allowing the lenses to cool at room temperature.

Any coating that absorbs near UV radiation should be applied only to the *back* surface of the lens. Otherwise, the coating may reduce the photochromic action that causes the lens to darken on exposure to sunlight. An antireflection coating produces little change in the behavior of photochromic lenses, apart from the slightly higher transmission, as expected.[45]

Although many people believe that a single pair of photochromic lenses can act as a substitute for two pairs of glasses (sunglasses for daytime outdoor wear and clear glasses for indoor and after-dark wear), the wearing of *any* photochromic lens for night driving is questionable. Even the lightest of these tints (such as Photogray II, Photogray Extra, or Photobrown Extra) fades to a transmittance of only 89%, 85%, or 85% respectively; this level is reached only after *overnight* fading. However, the wearing of Photosun II lenses for night driving is absolutely unacceptable, because these lenses fade to a transmittance of only 40%.

Corning Glare Control Lenses

In 1981 the Medical Optics Department of Corning introduced the CPF 550S lens. In 1983 Corning followed with two more lenses, CPF 511-S and CPF 527-S. In 1989 two more lenses were added: one lighter, the CPF 450, and one darker, the CPF 550-XD (Extra Dark). The numerical product designations of 450, 511, 527, and 550 refer to the spectral cutoff characteristics (in nanometers) of the lenses.

The CPF 511 and CPF 527 lenses are produced with a multilayer coating called the *Design Series*. The spectral cutoffs remain the same, but overall transmittance is reduced. These special lenses are intended to relieve the symptoms of glare discomfort, reduced visual acuity associated with certain eye disorders, or both. The lenses eliminate virtually all UV energy and the blue end of the visible spectrum. The lenses were not intended as a treatment or cure for ocular disorders but were developed to reduce some side effects associated with the disorders. Patients who have the following conditions are likely candidates for the CPF lenses: developing cataracts, aphakia and pseudophakia, diabetic retinopathy, macular degeneration, corneal dystrophies, retinitis pigmentosa, optic atrophy, albinism, aniridia, and glaucoma. Patients who have one or more of the following symptoms may also find the CPF filters helpful: reduced vision because of light scattering, sensitivity to glare, severe photophobia, reduced vision because of loss of contrast, and prolonged adaptation time.

The CPF lenses are produced by subjecting surface-treated Photogray Extra photochromic lenses to carefully controlled temperatures in a hydrogen oven. This process modifies the surface structures of the silver halide crystals, the mechanism of photochromicity in glass materials, to induce blue-light filtering to the required wavelength while preserving the photochromic effects. Table 7–4 lists the properties and the spectral transmittance curves for each of the five lenses (in the darkened and lightened states) shown in Figure 7–31.

The lenses are available only from Corning Medical Optics Department and can be obtained in plano power and by prescription (single vision, bifocals, trifocals, and aphakic lenticular). It is recommended that the lenses be mounted in a Corning side-shield frame, but they can be mounted into most frames. Because the lenses absorb blue light, it may be difficult for some people wearing these lenses to identify traffic signals and warning signs. The lenses should therefore be worn with caution when a person drives. CPF lenses should not be worn at night. The lenses can be chemically tempered.

Lynch and Brilliant[46] conducted an evaluation of the CPF 550 lens on 16 patients with retinitis pigmentosa. The CPF lenses improved scores of visual acuity in most subjects by one-fourth line of letters as tested by Snellen charts. Contrast sensitivity and adaptation time were not improved, but the subjects reported a decreased sensitivity to glare.

TABLE 7–4
Corning Glare Control Lens Characteristics

Lens Type	Visible Light Cutoff (nm)	Transmittance in Darkened State (%)	Transmittance in Faded State (%)	Ultraviolet Absorption (%)	
				UV-B	UV-A
CPF 450	450	18	73	100	97
CPF 511-S	511	12	47	100	99
CPF 511-DN	511	10	34	100	99
CPF 527-S	527	9	34	100	98
CPF 527-DN	527	8	26	100	99
CPF 550-S	550	5	20	100	99
CPF 550-XD	550	3	8	100	99

FIGURE 7–31.   **Spectral transmittance curves for Corning Glare Control lenses in darkened and faded states. (Reprinted with permission from Corning, Inc.)**

Parker and Miller,[47] using a forced-choice method, provided CPF lenses to 70 patients from a low-vision clinic. The patients selected were those who had been diagnosed as suffering from disease of the eye, ocular effects of systemic disease associated with light sensitivity, or who complained of light sensitivity associated with aging of the eye. Improvements in visual acuity scores of one-half line of letters on Snellen charts was found in 15 patients (21%); 54 patients (77%) reported improved vision; 5 patients (7%) found no change; 11 patients (16%) rejected the lenses. Of the 11 patients who rejected the CPF lenses, all but one had age-related macular degeneration.

Plastic Photochromic Lenses

The first plastic photochromic lens to be manufactured in the United States was American Optical's Photolite lens, introduced in 1982. The lens was manufactured not by a dye-pot process but by chemical impregnation. The darkening phase of the lens was very temperature-sensitive: the cooler the temperature, the darker the lens. The lens fully darkened to 45% transmittance and faded to 90% transmittance. However, after 2 years, the activated transmittance decreased to half the original change, from 45% to 67% transmittance in the fully darkened state. The Photolite lens is no longer available.

Transitions Optical was established in the United States by Pittsburg Plate Glass (PPG) industries—the original manufacturer of the CR-39 monomer—and Essilor International to produce and market a plastic photochromic material. In 1990 Transitions Optical introduced the Transitions lens. Rather than using silver halide crystals, this lens owes its darkening and lightening characteristics to the presence of organic molecular groups, *indolino spirorazines* (ISN). This photochromic material is allowed to penetrate the lens surface to a depth of 100 to 150 microns. The marriage of this chemistry is not to CR-39 as in previous lenses but to a special CR-300 series developed by PPG especially for this product.

When activated by UV radiation in sunlight, the colorless ISN molecules are ruptured and change to a different structure. The altered form absorbs visible radiation, darkens, and thus reduces the amount of light that penetrates the lens. When the lens is removed from sunlight, the chemical reaction reverses and the lens returns to its clear state. Wearers of these lenses found that they failed to darken as much or as quickly as glass photochromic lenses, particularly in warm weather.

In 1992 the Transitions lens was replaced by the Transitions Plus lens, which darkened faster and deeper than the original Transitions lens. The new product was the result of a newly patented ISN formula as well as a new resin, CR-307. At 70°F, the faded transmittance is 84% and, in the darkened state, the transmittance is 25%. After a short period of time, the Transitions Plus lens was renamed Transitions. Compared with glass photochromic lenses whose darkening properties are maintained and even enhanced over time, Transitions lenses gradually lose their darkening ability with time. The photoreactive response decreases 25% after 300 hours of use—approximately 2 years. Transitions lenses have a factory-applied, scratch-resistant coating. Antireflective coatings are not recommended because they diminish the amount of UV radiation needed to activate the ISN compound. The lens accepts a back surface

TABLE 7–5
Characteristics of Representative Glass and Plastic Photochromic Lenses

Manufacturer or Supplier	Lens Name	Abbe Number	Specific Gravity	Transmission (approximate %)	
				Dark	Faded
Glass; index 1.523					
Corning	Photogray II	57	2.41	41	89
Corning	Photosun II	57	2.41	12	41
Corning	Photogray Extra	57	2.41	22	85
Corning	Photobrown Extra	57	2.41	22	85
Corning	Photogray Thin and Dark*	57	2.38	16	86
Corning	Photobrown Thin and Dark*	57	2.38	15	85
Pilkington	Reactolite (gray)	57	2.42	16	90
Pilkington	Reactolite (brown)	57	2.42	16	90
Rodenstock	Colormatic S (gray)	58	2.55	15	75
Rodenstock	Colormatic SB (brown)	58	2.55	15	75
Zeiss	Umbramatic SR (gray)	57	2.41	25	85
Zeiss	Umbramatic SB (brown)	57	2.41	25	85
Glass; index 1.60					
Corning	Photogray Extra-16	42	2.73	22	85
Corning	Photobrown Extra-16	42	2.73	22	85
Rodenstock	Colormatic 1.6 (brown)	43	2.76	30	88
Schott	HC Photosolar	42.5	2.75	27	89
Zeiss	Umbramatic SL (brown)	43	2.75	30	85
Plastic; index 1.50					
Transitions Optical	Transitions (gray)	59	1.31	25	83
Rodenstock	Colormatic (gray-blue)	58	1.32	35	78
Plastic; high-index					
Sola (1.537)	Spectralite Transitions (gray)	47	1.21	25	83
Seiko (1.55)	Changers (gray)	45	1.21	28	86

*1.50 mm thick

tint, but custom tinting may produce unpredictable and unattractive results.

In the fall of 1995, Seiko Optical Products introduced *Changers,* the newest plastic photochromic lens. The Changers lens differs from the Transitions lens in that the photochromic molecules are distributed throughout the lens rather than imbibed only into the surface. When faded, the transmittance is 86%; in the darkened state, the transmittance is 28%.

The Changers lens is composed of a high-index (1.55) monomer with an aspheric front surface. The lenses have a factory applied scratch-resistant coating; and antireflection coating and tinting are available. As with glass photochromic lenses, Changers must undergo a break-in period of 6 or 7 darkening/fading cycles before reaching optimal performance.

Transitions and Changers lenses are described as comfort tints because they do darken sufficiently outdoors so as to be used as sunglasses. Both lenses undergo degradation in photochromic performance with use by failing to darken fully. In order to darken, plastic photochromic lenses rely on reorganization of organic molecules and structural transformation, a process that includes some non-reversible reactions which produce a finite fatigue life. Data concerning representative glass and plastic photochromic lenses are given in Table 7–5.

The Corlon Lens

In 1982 Corning introduced a new type of lens, called the *Corlon* lens, which combined both glass and plastic. The Corlon lens is made of two layers. The front (convex) layer is a thin glass lens of white crown glass or photochromatic glass (Photogray Extra); the back layer is a very thin layer of special polyurethane plastic bonded to the glass lens (Figure 7–32). The glass layer has a central thickness of about 1.3 mm (in minus power prescriptions) in white crown glass and a center thickness of 1.5 mm in photochromic material. The polyurethane layer is only 0.4 mm thick.

Corning discontinued the manufacture of the Corlon lens because delamination often occurred during surfacing and edging operations.

Younger Protective Lens Series Filter Lenses

In 1984, Younger optics introduced a series of four CR-39 plastic lenses designed to selectively filter out UV and visible blue radiation. These lenses are known as the Protective Lens Series (PLS). They are not photochromic lenses, nor are they tinted (dyed, and therefore having the dye present only at the surface), but are manufactured in such a way that the protective additives are present throughout the lens material and therefore cannot be bleached or removed. The PLS filter lenses cut off virtually all UV and blue visible radiation below the wavelengths designated by the product name. For example, the pale yellow PLS 400 lens eliminates all radiation shorter than 400 nm; the orange-amber PLS 530 lens blocks out 95% to 97% of UV and blue radiation as long as 530 nm; the brown PLS 540 lens blocks 95% to 97% of the UV and blue radiation as long as 540 nm; and the red PLS 550 lens blocks out 95% to 97% of UV and visible light radiation as long as 550 nm. The natural color of any PLS lens can be changed by the use of a cosmetic tint with standard tinting methods, and does not affect the performance of the lens.

The manufacturer recommends these lenses for protection against UV and visible blue radiation because Ham et al.[28] suggested that short-wavelength radiation (including both UV and blue) can be hazardous. The lenses are also recommended for patients with pathologic conditions such as cataracts, corneal dystrophies, macular degeneration, and retinitis pigmentosa.

7.21. Miscellaneous Absorptive Lenses

Absorptive lenses falling in the miscellaneous category include uniform-density lenses, gradient-density lenses, and cosmetic tints.

Uniform-Density Lenses

As already pointed out, when an absorptive lens is made of a glass having a through-and-through tint, the amount of light absorbed is a function of lens thickness (Figure 7–33) and therefore varies from the center to the edge of the lens—a high minus lens is noticeably lighter at the center; a high plus lens is noticeably darker at the center; and a lens containing a cylinder has a lighter streak, corresponding to the meridian of the minus cylinder axis, running across the lens. These problems can be avoided if a thin layer of tinted glass is fused to the clear lens. The tinted glass is fused to the *flatter* surface of the lens (Figure 7–34), usually the back surface of a plus lens (A) or the front surface of a minus lens (B). Such a lens is known as a *uniform-density* lens.

The problem of nonuniform density does not occur with dyed plastic lenses, with photochromic lenses, or with coated lenses. In the case of *dyed plastic* lenses, the dye penetrates the lens surface uniformly throughout the surface and therefore causes a tint of uniform density. With *photochromic* lenses, the darkening involves mainly the silver halide crystals on or near the surface (as discussed in Section 7.20), resulting in a uniform appearance. *Coated* lenses also have a uniform-density appearance because the coating is applied uniformly over the lens surface.

Gradient-Density Lenses

A gradient-density lens is designed so that light transmission gradually increases from the top to the bottom of the lens. Such a lens may be made either by coating a glass lens or by dyeing a plastic lens.

PHOTOCHROMIC OR CLEAR LAYER   **POLYURETHANE LAYER (0.4 mm THICK)**

FIGURE 7–32. **The Corlon lens.**

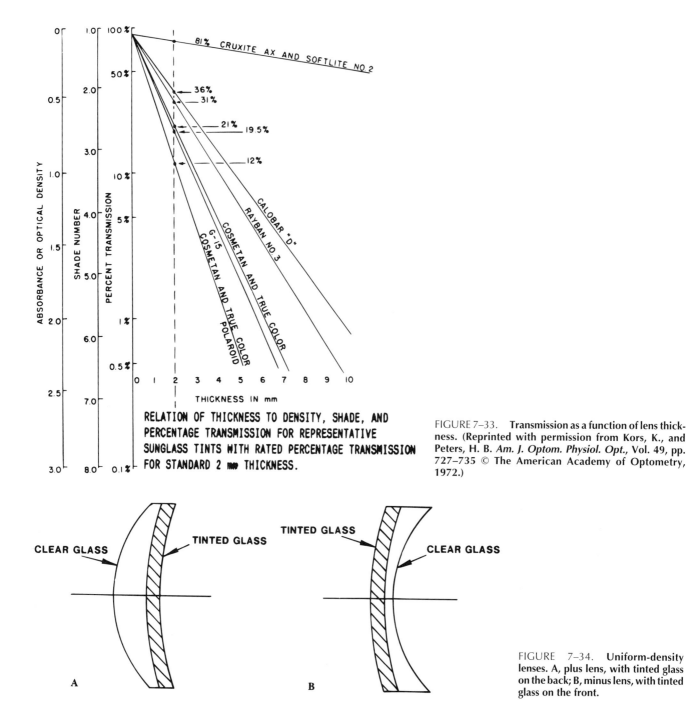

RELATION OF THICKNESS TO DENSITY, SHADE, AND
PERCENTAGE TRANSMISSION FOR REPRESENTATIVE
SUNGLASS TINTS WITH RATED PERCENTAGE TRANSMISSION
FOR STANDARD 2 mm THICKNESS.

FIGURE 7–33.   **Transmission as a function of lens thickness.** (Reprinted with permission from Kors, K., and Peters, H. B. *Am. J. Optom. Physiol. Opt.*, Vol. 49, pp. 727–735 © The American Academy of Optometry, 1972.)

FIGURE   7–34.   **Uniform-density lenses. A, plus lens, with tinted glass on the back; B, minus lens, with tinted glass on the front.**

Fashion Lenses

Plastic lenses differ from glass lenses in that they can easily be tinted by the ophthalmic dispenser using a dyeing process. One factor in the increasing popularity of plastic lenses, beginning in the 1970s, was the availability of the tinting process. Although these dyed lenses are intended strictly as *fashion* lenses, they can be responsible for some of the same problems already described for photochromic lenses: (1) if the lenses are heavily dyed, they may be too dark to use for night driving and (2) there is a tendency for many of these tints to have high trans-

mittances in the IR region, with the result that they should not be used as sunglass lenses. Transmittance curves for some tinted plastic fashion lenses are shown in Figure 7–35.

7.22. Lens Thickness and Transmittance

As discussed in Section 7.11, when a prescription glass lens is made in an absorptive material, a variation in transmission across the lens occurs because of the variation in thick-

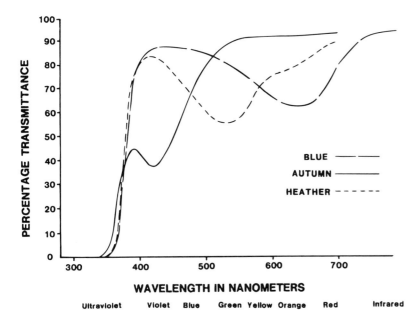

FIGURE 7-35. **Spectral transmission curves for American Optical Tintolite tinted CR-39 (fashion) lenses.** (Reprinted with permission from *Guide to Coatings, Dyes, Tints, Hues, Shades*, American Optical Corp., 1969.)

ness. Normally, absorptive lenses are rated in terms of transmission for a lens of a constant thickness of 2 mm. However, the difference between a rated transmission for a 2-mm-thick lens and the actual transmission, at various points on a lens of high power, can be large. In addition, many patients find the variation in density across the lens cosmetically unattractive because it draws attention to the high power of the lens. Because tint identification by the practitioner is made on the basis of samples that are approximately 2 mm thick, tint recognition and identification become more difficult with large variations in thickness.

A high plus lens made from absorptive glass has lower actual transmittance than the rated transmittance, and the transmission increases from the center to the edge of the lens. A high minus lens may have approximately the rated transmittance at the center of the lens with a decrease in transmission toward the edge. Figure 7–33 illustrates the transmission as a function of lens thickness. For a lens of a given diameter, center thickness or edge thickness may be estimated as shown in Figure 7–33 and Table 7–6. Using these sources, the center-to-edge transmission of a particular prescription can be estimated. The same sources are also useful if one wishes to order a lens with particular transmission at the center or the edge of the lens.

As the visual axis passes through various areas of a strong absorptive lens, the eye must adapt to different levels of brightness. If an individual is adapted to a certain brightness level, the question arises as to how much this level can be changed instantly without impairing visual performance or requiring a significant period of adaptation. Davis and Fernald[48] believe that a ±0.25- to ±0.50-log unit difference in illumination appears reasonable. The 0.25-log unit difference means a change in percentage transmission of approximately 1.8 times; a 0.50-log unit difference means a change in percentage transmission of approximately 3.2 times.

For lenses having a cylindrical component, the two principal meridians behave differently, so both meridians must be considered. For strong absorptive prescriptions, con-

stant adaptation activity is required because various zones of the lens are used. Fatigue or impaired visual performance is likely to result. The solution for the problem of variations in transmission across a lens is to provide lenses designed to provide essentially uniform transmission across the entire lens—such lenses are known as *uniform-density* lenses and are discussed in Section 7.21.

When an anisometropic patient wears absorptive lenses, the transmittance of one lens (the more minus or less plus lens) is greater than that of the other lens. The resulting difference in retinal illumination for the two eyes can cause spatial distortions in the presence of a moving object. In 1922 Pulfrich demonstrated that if a filter is held in front of one eye of a normally sighted subject, a pendulum swinging in the frontal plane is perceived as moving in an elliptical path. The classic explanation for this phenomenon is that there are differential arrival times (latency differences) at the visual cortex for the neural impulses for the two eyes.

Hall[49] found that depth perception was diminished when the binocular visibility relationship is altered and concluded that balanced binocular visibility is essential to good depth perception. Hence, binocularity may be compromised when a person wears two lenses that vary significantly in transmission. A discrepancy or a perceptual conflict between stereoscopic and monocular clues to spatial arrangements may result in ophthalmic vertigo and difficulties in orientation.[50] When a person wearing two such lenses drives an automobile, the apparent displacements of moving objects may constitute a hazard.

For occupational use, the luminous transmittance of lenses with shade numbers 1.5 to 3.0 (61.1%–13.9% transmittance) must be within 10% of each other. For shade numbers 4.0 to 14.0 (transmittance 5.18%–0.0027%) the luminous transmittance of a pair of lenses should be within 20% of each other. Following these guidelines, the transmittance of a pair of sunglass lenses should be within 20% of each other. Lenses may be matched by alteration of thickness, by the use of coatings, or by use of uniform-density lenses.

TABLE 7–6
Chart for Estimating Thickness for Various Lens Diameters*

	Diameter Power (mm)								
	58	56	54	52	50	48	46	44	42
+7.00	7.1	6.7	6.2	5.8	5.4	5.0	4.6	4.3	4.0
+6.50	6.7	6.3	5.8	5.4	5.1	4.7	4.4	4.1	3.8
+6.00	6.1	5.8	5.4	5.0	4.7	4.4	4.1	3.8	3.5
+5.50	5.7	5.4	5.0	4.7	4.4	4.1	3.8	3.6	3.3
+5.00	5.3	5.0	4.7	4.4	4.2	3.9	3.6	3.4	3.1
+4.50	4.9	4.6	4.3	4.1	3.8	3.6	3.3	3.1	3.0
+4.00	4.4	4.2	4.0	3.7	3.5	3.3	3.1	2.9	2.8
+3.50	4.0	3.8	3.6	3.4	3.2	3.0	2.9	2.8	2.7
+3.00	3.5	3.3	3.2	3.0	2.9	2.8	2.8	2.7	2.6
+2.50	3.1	3.0	2.8	2.8	2.7	2.6	2.6	2.5	2.5
+2.00	2.8	2.7	2.5	2.5	2.5	2.5	2.5	2.4	2.4
+1.50	2.6	2.6	2.3	2.3	2.3	2.3	2.3	2.3	2.3
+1.00	2.4	2.3	2.1	2.1	2.1	2.1	2.1	2.1	2.1
+0.50	2.2	2.1	2.0	2.0	2.0	2.0	2.0	2.0	2.0

*Assumes edge thickness minimum of 1.0 mm and average of center thickness and edge thickness minimum of 2.0 mm.
SOURCE: Adapted from Davis, J. K., and Fernald, H. G. *Am. J. Optom. Arch. Am. Acad. Optom.,* Vol. 46, No. 8, p. 574, 1969.

7.23. Prescribing Absorptive Lenses

With the large number of absorptive lenses available, it is almost impossible for the optometrist to be familiar with all of them. Furthermore, the task of selecting absorptive lenses is complicated because lens composition, color, and cost are not suitable criteria for predicting the amount of near UV, visible, or near IR radiation that a specific lens will transmit. Although dark-appearing tints generally filter out more visible spectrum than do the lighter tints, differences occur among lenses that appear to be the same. Generally, plastic lenses (CR-39) filter more near UV radiation than do glass lenses, but exceptions occur. Within a range of similar dark tints, there is no way to predict by appearance which lenses effectively filter significant quantities of near UV or near IR radiation. Effective filtering in a specific region of the spectrum is no guarantee of effective absorption in another region of the spectrum.

An alarming number of *nonprescription* sunglasses have been found to transmit bands of UV radiation—to have ultraviolet "windows."[51] Studies suggest that an inappropriately large number of tinted lenses transmit large amounts of UV radiation as well as visible and IR radiation.[52] Lenses that attenuate visible radiation much more than they attenuate UV radiation may be harmful on two counts. First, wearing lenses that attenuate visible radiation while transmitting much UV radiation enables the eye to function in a high-intensity environment for longer periods of time than it could without the filter and, thereby, increases the exposure to UV radiation. Second, the attenuation of the visible radiation by the filter causes the pupil of the eye to dilate, which in turn causes the incident radiation on the lens to be reduced by a greater amount than the reduction in retinal illumination. If the UV radiation is not appreciably reduced, the dilated pupil may pass more UV radiation with the lens than it does when *no lens* is worn.

Patients are subjected to a wide range of wavelengths and intensities of illumination in their work and in recreational activities. The optometrist must have available a range of absorptive lenses that are suitable for the environment in which

the wearer works or intends to use the glasses. To prescribe intelligently and to explain to the patient why a lens is recommended, the optometrist must be fully aware of the transmission properties of lenses available for use. Other characteristics such as the lens composition (glass or plastic), method of obtaining the tint (solid or coating, fixed or variable tint), durability, and appearance should also be considered when recommending a particular lens. Many patients are particularly interested in the cosmetic appearance of the lenses and tend to select sunglasses on the basis of appearance. Because color affects different people differently, the subjective reaction to the appearance of the environment as seen through the lenses is also an important consideration.

Tints may be demonstrated by having plano lenses glazed *binocularly*, in plastic spectacle fronts. If feasible, the patient should be given the opportunity to assess the color and density of an absorptive lens in a natural sunlight environment. Allowance must be made for differences in the thickness of the sample and the finished prescription lenses.

Patients often depend on eye practitioners to advise them about the *need* for absorptive lenses and about the color or shade to be worn. To assist practitioners in determining whether absorptive lenses are needed, an instrument known as the Alpascope (Alpa Corp.) was developed. The Alpascope target consists of two parallel bars of light. Beginning with a low level of illumination as the patient views the target, the illumination level is gradually increased until the patient reports that the two bars of light have fused into one. The lower the level of illumination required for the two bars to fuse, the greater the patient's sensitivity to light. In a study conducted by Becnel et al.,[53] an extremely high correlation was found between Alpascope findings and the patient's complaint (or lack of complaint) regarding sensitivity to light. Although the use of such an instrument may provide the practitioner with information that is helpful in advising the patient, the results of this study indicate that the patient's own complaint (or lack of complaint) concerning light sensitivity usually provides sufficient evidence, that is, patients' complaints of light sensitivity should be taken seriously.

In advising a patient about absorptive lenses, the practitioner should question the patient about sensitivity to light and about the activities and levels of illumination for which the lenses are to be used. For outdoor activities in bright daylight, most patients who are sensitive to light benefit most from lenses having transmittances in the 10% to 20% range. On the other hand, older patients who have small pupils (and perhaps early crystalline lens opacities) require a somewhat *lighter* than average tint.

Although the transmittance of the lighter, indoor tints (Vision-Ease Pink #1 and others) is very little less than that of clear crown glass, some patients have worn such lenses for several years and are completely convinced that the lenses provide greater visual comfort than clear lenses. Experience shows that in these cases it is wise to *continue* the use of the tinted lenses. However, if a medium-dark shade is worn, the practitioner should probably recommend switching to the next lighter shade.

7.24. Summary of Recommendations

Absorption of Ultraviolet Radiation

There is abundant and consistent evidence that direct photochemical or UV radiation can cause damage to the cornea, the lens, and the retina. The best and simplest treatment for direct UV photochemical damage to ocular tissues is prevention by eliminating or reducing the entry of UV radiation into the eye. All types of ophthalmic lens materials, including spectacles, contact lenses, and intraocular lens implants, should be required to include UV protection to at least 380 nm. Because exposure to UV radiation is cumulative, early and regular use of UV protection can prevent, reduce, or delay UV effects during an ever-increasing life span. No known benefits are gained by exposing any part of the eye to UV radiation; it is potentially harmful to every part of the eye.

UV protection can be incorporated into nearly all optical materials currently in use; building in protection is inexpensive and does not interfere with vision. Many patients are at high risk from UV exposure, and the recommendations for UV protection apply even more forcefully to these patients. Aphakic and pseudophakic patients, even if only one ocular lens has been removed, should be provided with lenses that filter all UV radiation shorter than 400 nm for both clear lenses used indoors and sunglasses used outdoors. Patients under treatment with photosensitizing medications such as psoralens or phenothiazines should be provided with UV protection to prevent photoinduced damage to the eye. UV-absorbing lenses should be used by patients who encounter indoor exposure to high levels of UV radiation from industrial, therapeutic, or cosmetic light sources.

Sunglasses

Pitts[54] stated that the optimal sunglass lens should have the following characteristics: (1) it should protect the eyes from excess ambient luminance, (2) it should eliminate the portions of the spectrum that are hazardous to the eyes, (3) it should maintain optimal dark adaptation and night vision, (4) it should require minimum care, and (5) it should provide adequate impact resistance.

Sunglass lenses should be prescribed to give the best possible seeing under the conditions of use. As mentioned earlier, according to Richards,[29] an ideal level of luminance is 400 ftL (1370 cd/m²), the level of luminance under the shade of a big tree on a sunny summer day. Davis[55] noted that the luminance comfort zone is 350 to 2000 cd/m².

The luminance reflected by light-colored pavement and open fields on a typical summer day is about 7000 cd/m². A 20% filter reduces this level to 1400 cd/m². However, the luminance from sunny snowfields and bright beaches averages about 15,000 cd/m². For winter sports and, especially, at high altitudes, the luminance may exceed 15,000 cd/m². An 8% to 10% filter brings the scene into the comfort zone. For a person who spends long periods of time near bright sand or on snowfields at high altitudes where the air is clear, sunglasses with a transmittance of approximately 5% may be appropriate. However, these lenses should not be used for driving because they blacken shady roadside areas, especially when the wearer enters the shade from a bright open scene. The American National Standards Institute (ANSI) Z980.3-1986 Sunglass Standard recommends that lenses having less than 8% transmittance *not* be used for driving, even during daylight hours.

If a lens is too dark, obliquely incident light from behind may strike the back surface of the lens and be reflected into the eye. For ophthalmic crown glass, the intensity of the reflected image is 4.3% of the incident light and may be equal to the intensity of the transmitted image, or be even higher if the lens is made of a high-index material. An antireflective coating on the back surface of the lens greatly reduces the intensity of such images.

In addition to reducing the ambient radiation to a comfortable level, *all* sunglasses should cut off UV radiation at 400 nm and have relatively low transmittance in the blue end of the visible spectrum, but still allow differentiation of red and green (such as traffic signal lights). Effective sunglasses should also be large enough to provide adequate fields of view, but the frame and temples should not be so thick that peripheral vision is unduly restricted, especially when the glasses are worn for driving an automobile. The frame should be adjusted so that it is comfortable and should be designed to fit closely to block UV light that may enter from the sides or top; however, there must be enough space to give sufficient ventilation to reduce fogging.

Protection from solar radiation can also be enhanced if a person wears a hat or cap with a wide brim when outdoors, especially during the hours of 10:00 A.M. to 3:00 P.M.

7.25. Standards for Absorptive Lenses

The current ANSI Standard for sunglass lenses is designated as ANSI Z80.3-1986, for ophthalmic nonprescription sunglasses and fashion eyewear.[56] The Standard was developed with input from representatives of optometry, ophthalmology, and the ophthalmic lens industry. The Z80.3 Standard places sunglasses and fashion eyewear into three categories on the basis of their intended primary function:

1. *General Purpose (attenuation of light).* This category includes lenses that have 8% to 40% transmittance in the visible range, with a level of UV-A not greater than the transmittance in the visible range and a UV-B level not greater than one-half the transmittance in the visible range or in excess of 5%.

2. *Cosmetic Use.* This category includes lenses having more than 40% transmittance in the visible range. The UV-A level must not be greater than the amount of the visible range and the UV-B level must not be greater than one-half the amount of the visible range nor exceed 30% transmittance.

3. *Special Purpose (skiing, mountain climbing, beach).* The *minimal* transmittance for the visible spectrum is 3%. The UV-A level permitted is one-half the amount of the visible spectrum, and the UV-B level can be no greater than 1%.

Lenses having a luminous transmittance less than 8% are not recommended for driving. The Standards state that near IR (790–1400 nm) transmittance limits are not required because there is no evidence of need.

The ophthalmic profession, the scientific community, and the public press have questioned the efficacy of the 1986 Sunglass Standard. Members of the ophthalmic professions have criticized the Standard for not having a category for the complete elimination of UV radiation—this could easily be done inexpensively by the use of modern plastic materials—and for not specifying a limitation of short-wavelength (violet and blue) visible radiation. Many authorities have proposed that all ophthalmic lenses eliminate 100% of UV radiation; Young[27] suggested that ophthalmic lenses also eliminate 90% of visible radiation between 400 and 500 nm. In late 1993, the National Society for the Prevention of Blindness, the American Optometric Association, and the American Academy of Ophthalmology issued a joint statement recommending that sunglasses used outdoors in the bright sun should absorb 99% to 100% of the full UV spectrum to 400 nm.[57]

The ANSI Z80.3 Committee recently completed a revision of the Z80.3-1986 Standard; publication is scheduled for the spring of 1996 (Daniel Torgersen, Optical Laboratories Association, personal communication, January 1996.). The Food and Drug Administration (FDA) is also considering a ruling defining acceptable UV transmittance levels for nonprescription sunglasses. It is important to note that ANSI standards are only recommendations; FDA regulations have the force of law. [It seems ironic that the current controversy focuses on nonprescription absorptive lenses, and yet no standards exist for prescription absorptive lenses, except for lenses intended for industrial purposes. The ANSI Z280.1-1995 Standard states that lens manufacturers who claim specific UV-attenuating properties must state the average transmittance between 290 and 315 nm (UV-B) and between 315 and 380 nm (UV-A). Apparently, in prescribing absorptive lenses, optometrists and ophthalmologists are expected to use their own informed judgment.]

7.26. Absorptive Lenses Designed for Occupational Use

Protective glasses for industrial workers must protect the wearer from potential mechanical and chemical injury and also from possible radiant energy damage. Specially designed absorptive lenses are available for a number of occupations, such as blast furnace operation, glassblowing, and welding. Current standards[58] require that an absorptive lens for industrial workers must almost completely absorb both the UV and IR radiation from harmful sources. Consequently, absorption is high for both the blue and red regions of the visible spectrum, with maximal transmittance in the bluish green or greenish yellow regions of the spectrum (with the result that these lenses are bluish green or greenish yellow in color).

The proper function of an absorptive lens designed for industrial use involves not only the protection of the wearer from UV and IR radiation but also the reduction of the radiation in the visible spectrum to a comfortable level so that the industrial operation can be performed as efficiently as possible. The luminous transmittance of a filter determines its appropriateness for a particular industrial task.

Welding lenses are available in two general categories: Class I, for general-purpose use; and Class II, for operations producing high radiant flux at the wavelengths of the sodium lines (589.3 nm). Class II lenses are similar to Class I lenses in reducing UV and IR radiation but differ from Class I lenses in that they contain *didymium*, which reduces the transmittance in the 589.3-nm region to a relatively low value. The high absorption of welding glasses for the UV and IR regions of the spectrum provides protection from any source of radiant energy that may be encountered in an industrial environment, as long as the proper density is used. Because individual needs may differ, the appropriate density for a particular operation may be personally selected on a trial basis for optimal results. Within reasonable limits, the industrial worker should choose the density that seems suitable for his or her eyes and for the nature of the welding process.

The luminous transmission of a welding lens is specified in terms of a *shade number*. Shade numbers increase with increasing absorption (decreasing transmission). The relationship between optical density, luminous transmittance, and shade number is given by the following equations:
As discussed in Section 7.13,

$$\text{optical density} = \log_{10}\frac{1}{T} = -\log_{10}T$$

where T (transmittance) is expressed as a decimal.
Once optical density is known, the shade number is calculated by the following equation:

$$\text{shade number} = \frac{7}{3}(\text{optical density}) + 1.$$

or

$$\text{optical density} = \frac{3}{7}(\text{shade number} - 1),$$

Shade numbers run in discrete steps from 1.5 to 14. Tolerances in transmittances permit each transmittance value to fall within a particular shade number. The shade numbers and percentage transmittances are as follows:

Shade Number	Percentage Transmission
1.5	61.1
1.7	50.1
2.0	37.3
2.5	22.8
3.0	13.9
4.0	5.18
5.0	1.93
6.0	0.72
7.0	0.27
8.0	0.10
9.0	0.037
10.0	0.0139
11.0	0.0052
12.0	0.0019
13.0	0.00072
14.0	0.00027

An inspection of a shade number and its corresponding percentage transmission reveals that if a given shade number is altered by 7.0, the percentage transmission changes by a factor of 1000. For example, if a lens of shade number 2.0 is exchanged for a lens of shade number 9.0, the transmission decreases from 37.3% to 0.037%; if a lens of shade number 14 is exchanged for a lens of shade number 7.0, the transmission changes from 0.00027% to 0.27%. In each of the above examples, the optical density changes by 3.0.

Lenses having shade numbers from 1.5 to 3.0 are useful for people who are exposed to strong light from cutting and welding operations but who do not perform these operations themselves. Shade number 4 is intended for the same use as shade numbers 1.5 to 3.0, but for conditions involving greater luminous flux. Shade number 5 is intended for persons who do light gas cutting and welding and light electronic spot welding. Shade numbers 6 and 7 are intended for persons who do gas cutting, medium gas welding, and arc welding to 30 amperes. Shade number 8 is intended for persons who do heavy gas welding and arc welding and cutting using more than 30 amperes but not exceeding 75 amperes. Shade numbers 9 through 14 are quite dark, and are used for persons who do arc welding and cutting that exceeds 75 amperes.

Trade names for welding lenses include Arc-Ban (Bausch & Lomb) (Figure 7–36), Cescoweld by Chicago Eye Shield (Figure 7–37), Filterweld by American Optical (Figure 7–38), and Willson-Weld by Willson Products (Figure 7–39). For shade numbers 1.5 to 3.0, the ANSI Z87.1 1989 Standard[58] specifies that the luminous transmittances of a pair of lenses must be within 10% of each other. For shade numbers 4.0 through 14.0, luminous transmittances of a pair of lenses must be within 20% of each other.

FIGURE 7–36.   Spectral transmission curves for Bausch & Lomb Arc-Ban welding lenses. The arrow on each transmission curve points to the appropriate scale. (Reprinted from R. Stair, *Spectral Transmission Properties and Use of Eye Protective Glass*, National Bureau of Standards Circular No. 471, 1948.)

FIGURE 7–37.   Spectral transmission curves for Chicago Eye Shield Co. Cescoweld welding lenses. The arrow on each transmission curve points to the appropriate scale. (Reprinted from R. Stair, *Spectral Transmission Properties and Use of Eye Protective Glass*, National Bureau of Standards Circular No. 471, 1948.)

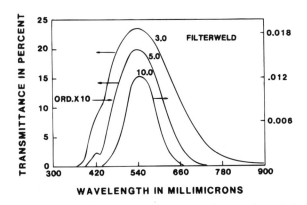

FIGURE 7–38.   Spectral transmission curves for American Optical Filterweld welding lenses. The arrow on each transmission curve points to the appropriate scale. (Reprinted from R. Stair, *Spectral Transmission Properties and Use of Eye Protective Glass*, National Bureau of Standards Circular No. 471, 1948.)

FIGURE 7–39.   **Spectral transmission curves for Willson Products Willson-Weld welding lenses. The arrow on each transmission curve points to the appropriate scale. (Reprinted from R. Stair, Spectral Transmission Properties and Use of Eye Protective Glass, National Bureau of Standards Circular No. 471, 1948.)**

LENS REFLECTIONS AND COATINGS

7.27. Reflections from Spectacle Lens Surfaces

When light reaches the boundary between two transparent media having different indices of refraction, most light is refracted, but a small amount is reflected. Reflected light may be troublesome to the wearer of spectacle lenses because it can produce ghost images, falsification of image position, haze, and loss of contrast. In addition, reflected light can be annoying to observers because it may obscure the wearer's eye with a veiling glare and accentuate that glasses are being worn. Reflected images may become troublesome to a spectacle wearer under the following conditions:

1. The reflected image is located near a fixated object;
2. The reflected image is sufficiently intense to stand out from its background;
3. The reflected image is in focus or capable of being made clear by accommodation.

For light of normal or nearly normal incidence, the intensity of light reflected from a surface separating two media of different indices is given, as shown in Section 7.11, by Fresnel's equation:

$$I_R = \frac{\left(n' - n\right)^2}{\left(n' + n\right)^2}(I).$$

Also, as shown in Section 7.11, for ophthalmic crown glass having an index of refraction of 1.523, surrounded by air, the intensity of light lost by reflection from the first surface is 4.3% of the original intensity; if we assume that no light is lost by absorption, the loss by reflection from the back surface of the lens is 4.1%, with the result that the intensity of the transmitted beam is 91.6% of the intensity entering the lens.

By inspection of Fresnel's equation, we may conclude the following:

1. The intensity of the reflected beam is unaffected by the direction of the incident light, that is, whether it traverses from air to glass or from glass to air.
2. The intensity of the reflected beam increases as the index of refraction increases. Hence, the reflection intensity is greater for lenses made with high-index glass (such as High-Lite) than for lenses made with ophthalmic crown glass or with CR-39 plastic.
3. Because the index of refraction increases toward the blue end of the spectrum, the reflected image contains more blue light than red light. Therefore, the reflected image may appear slightly bluish in color and the transmitted light, deficient in blue, may appear slightly yellowish.

7.28. Types of Surface Reflections

The surfaces that are primarily involved in forming reflected images are the front and back surfaces of the spectacle lens and the front surface of the wearer's cornea. Although these reflecting surfaces may participate in the formation of an infinite number of reflected images, which may or may not enter the eye, only a few images have any significance. In Figure 7–40, five common sources of spectacle lens reflections are shown. They may be described as follows:

1. *Image Formed by Light Coming from Behind the Spectacle Lens and Reflected by the Back Surface of the Lens into the Eye* (Figure 7–40A). An image formed by reflection from the back surface of the lens has the highest intensity of any possible spectacle lens reflection. As already shown, for crown glass having an index of refraction of 1.523, the reflection has an intensity of 4.3% of the intensity of the incident light. When lens sizes were small, this type of reflection was seldom a problem, but with the larger lens sizes now in use, it may prove to be a problem for some wearers. For example, when the face is strongly illuminated, reflected images of

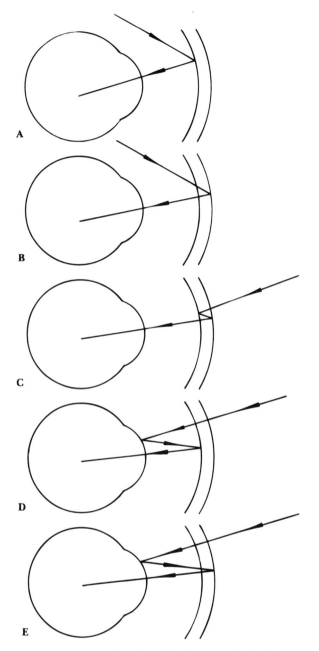

FIGURE 7–40. **Types of surface reflections. Note that in A and B the light is incident on the back surface of the lens; in C, D, and E the light is incident on the front surface of the lens.**

flected from the back surface of the lens, is ordinarily troublesome to the wearer.

3. *Image Formed by a Light Source in Front of the Lens, Formed by Two Internal Reflections Initially by the Back Surface and Then by the Front Surface of the Lens and into the Eye.* This is a less intense reflection than the two described above. It is often referred to as the double internal reflection ghost image (Figure 7–40C). If we assume no loss of light by absorption, the intensity of this image for ophthalmic crown glass is only 0.17% of the intensity of the incident light. Though of relatively low intensity, this reflected image is one of the most troublesome of the ghost images arising from a light source in front of the eye. Every lens presents ghost images of this type, but for most powers of lenses the images are not in focus, and the intensity is so low that the images are not seen. However, if there is a small, bright source of light against a dark background, as, for example, a street light at night or lights in a darkened theater, the ghost image may be sufficiently bright to be noticeable.

For weak minus lenses, the images of bright objects peripheral to the wearer's line of sight are reflected *toward the center* of the lens. For example, bright overhead lights are reflected downward, and the ghost image is formed between the source and the center of the lens. When the wearer moves his or her head, the ghost image moves in the same direction. On the other hand, for the wearer of a plus lens, the ghost images are displaced farther from the optical center of the lens, so they usually cause little or no trouble. However, if the wearer looks at a light source directly through the optical center of the lens, the ghost image is superimposed on the source and is not seen.

The position and intensity of this ghost image are essentially independent of the base curve of the lens, so changing the base curve will prove to be of no help. Changing the pantoscopic tilt of the lens also has little effect on the ghost image. For lenses of low minus power, with the same power for both eyes, and if the source of annoyance is in one direction only, the lenses can be decentered or can be ordered with prism so that the optical center of the lens is moved toward the source forming the reflected image. For example, if overhead lights are a source of annoyance to a patient, the optical centers of the lenses can be raised, or base-down prism power can be ordered, so that the ghost image lies farther away from the patient's line of sight.

4. *Image Formed when Light Passes through the Lens, Is Reflected by the Cornea, and Is Reflected into the Eye by the Back Surface of the Lens.* This reflected image is illustrated in Figure 7–40D. If no loss of light occurs by absorption, the intensity of the reflected image is 0.09% of that of the incident light. If the front surface of the cornea has a radius of curvature of 8 mm, the catoptric (reflecting) power of the cornea is about –250.00 D, with the result that the cornea forms an image of the real source at a distance of 4 mm behind the apex of the cornea. This small image becomes a source of reflection at the back surface of the lens, and hence is reflected back into the eye. There are several solutions to the problem: The position of the ghost image can be displaced by angling the lens, or a sharp image can be thrown out of focus by changing the lens form (base curve) or by changing the vertex distance.

the eye or the adnexa may be seen by the wearer. Fortunately, the concave back surfaces used for most ophthalmic lenses tend to limit the directions from which incident light may be reflected into the eye. Fitting the lens as close to the eye as possible and slightly "face-forming" the frame tends to reduce the likelihood of reflections entering the eye.

2. *Image Formed by Light Coming from Behind the Lens, Undergoing Internal Reflection by the Front Surface, and Refracted by the Back Surface into the Eye.* This reflection, shown in Figure 7–40B, is somewhat less intense than the reflection described above. For clear ophthalmic crown glass, the intensity of this image is 3.94% of that of the incident light. Neither of these two types of images, formed by light re-

5. *Image Formed by Light Reflected from the Cornea and Then Internally Reflected by the Front Surface of the Lens and into the Eye* (Figure 7–40E). As with ghost image number 4, the cornea forms an image of a real source approximately 4 mm behind the vertex of the cornea, which then becomes a source of reflection at the front surface of the lens. The intensity of this ghost image for ophthalmic crown glass is 0.08% of that of the incident light. This type of ghost image may be displaced by angling the frame, by changing lens form, or by changing vertex distance.

6. *Other Reflections.* The wearer of a flat-top bifocal or trifocal lens may be subjected to ghost images and flare caused by reflections from the segment top. The manufacturer may address this potential problem by angling the top of the segment and by placing an absorptive coating on the top of the segment before the segment is fused into the carrier lens. The coating absorbs the light that would normally participate in the ghost image or create flare.

7.29. Methods of Controlling Surface Reflections

The methods available for minimizing the annoyance of surface reflections are base curve selection, alteration of pantoscopic tilt, changing the vertex distance, selection of small lens sizes, patient education and counseling, and the use of antireflective coatings.

Base Curve Selection

Depending on the source of the reflection, the location, size, and clarity of reflections may be altered by using a steeper or flatter base curve than would normally be used. However, the change in the base curve must usually be large to correct the problem, and making such a base-curve change would compromise the advantages of corrected-curve lens construction. The use of a special base curve requires grinding a custom lens, which would add to the cost of the patients' lenses. Unless the source of the reflection has been analyzed correctly, a change in base curve may not achieve the desired result. For these reasons, base curves are seldom changed as a way to minimize reflections. However, by choosing the flattest base curve that is consistent with acceptable optical performance, the object field of view of the two reflecting surfaces of the lens is reduced, which thereby reduces the potential number of reflected images visible to the wearer or to an observer facing the wearer.

Alteration of Pantoscopic Tilt

When a constantly recurring reflection is determined to be produced by a given light source, a change in pantoscopic tilt of the lens has the effect of rotating the object fields of view of the reflecting surfaces away from troublesome light sources (such as artificial lights or outdoor lighting coming through windows). However, the resultant object field may

prove to contain new light sources, with the result that little may be gained.

Changing the Vertex Distance

A change in the vertex distance may have the advantage of focusing the ghost image in a different plane. However, the vertex distance of a lens can be altered only to a limited extent. Both from the optical and cosmetic points of view, this alteration is practical only within no more than 2 or 3 mm in either direction. Alteration of vertex distance is particularly difficult for frames with fixed nose pads.

Selection of Small Lens Sizes

Selection of a smaller lens size than usual also reduces the object fields of view of the two reflecting surfaces of the lens by reducing the area available for reflection.

Patient Education and Counseling

When a patient complains of the presence of ghost images, he or she may need only to be informed that the reflected images are normal occurrences. If basic information is provided about the nature and origin of the ghost images, the patient may accept them and learn to ignore them.

7.30. Antireflective Coatings

If the methods discussed above (particularly alteration of the pantoscopic tilt and patient education) do not provide relief from reflected images, an antireflective coating should be placed on *both* surfaces of the lens. Although an antireflective coating does not completely eliminate the ghost images caused by reflection, it can reduce their intensity enough so that they will not be bothersome to the wearer or to an observer.

According to the principle of *interference*, whenever two waves of equal intensity or amplitude produced by a monochromatic source are superimposed, neutralization (cancellation) occurs if the path difference is an odd number of half wavelengths, and *reinforcement* occurs if the path difference is equal to an even number of half wavelengths. In addition, when light is reflected from a surface with an index of refraction higher than the index of the medium in which the light has previously traveled, a phase change of 180 degrees takes place. When the reflecting surface has a lower index of refraction than the incident medium, no phase change occurs.

When a transparent coating is applied to the surface of an ophthalmic lens, two reflection waves occur, one from the front surface of the coating and one from the interface between the coating and the glass. According to the principles of interference, the two reflection waves cancel one another if two conditions are met: (1) the *amplitude* condition requires that the two reflection waves must be of equal amplitude; (2) the *path* condition requires that the two re-flection waves be one-half wavelength out of phase. Examination of the amplitude condition tells the index of refraction of the coating; the path condition reveals the proper thickness of the coating.

To satisfy the amplitude condition, the intensity of the reflection from the air–coating interface, R_1, must be equal to the intensity of the reflection from the coating–glass interface, R_2. Using Fresnel's equation, where n_c specifies the index of refraction of the coating and n_g specifies the index of refraction of the glass,

$$R_1 = \left(\frac{n_c - 1}{n_c + 1}\right)^2 = R_2 = \left(\frac{n_g - n_c}{n_g + n_c}\right)^2,$$

or

$$\left(\frac{n_c - 1}{n_c + 1}\right) = \left(\frac{n_g - n_c}{n_g + n_c}\right),$$

and

$$(n_c + 1)(n_g - n_c) = (n_c - 1)(n_g + n_c)$$

or

$$n_c n_g + n_g - n_c^2 - n_c = n_c n_g - n_g + n_c^2 - n_c$$
$$2n_g = 2n_c^2,$$

and therefore

$$n_c = \sqrt{n_g}.$$

Thus, to satisfy the amplitude condition, the index of refraction of the coating should be equal to the square root of the index of refraction of the glass. When applied to ophthalmic crown glass ($n = 1.523$) the index of refraction of the coating should be

$$\sqrt{1.523} = 1.234.$$

In addition to having the ideal index of refraction, the coating must have good adhesive properties, it must be sufficiently hard, and it must be insoluble in water. Of the known materials having an index of refraction of 1.234, all are either too soft or are too soluble in water. A compromise material must therefore be accepted to obtain a sufficiently hard coating that is water resistant. *Magnesium fluoride* has the optimal combination of optical and physical properties and is used almost universally for antireflective coatings of glass lenses. Its refractive index, approximately 1.38, is too high to completely satisfy the amplitude condition when applied to ophthalmic crown glass. This causes an incomplete neutralization of reflections, with the result that the reflectance of a surface cannot be reduced to zero for any wavelength. The ideal glass to use with magnesium fluoride would have an index of refraction of 1.38^2, or 1.904. Therefore, more efficient results are obtained when magnesium fluoride is applied to glasses with a high index of refraction. When applied to High-Lite glass, which has an index of 1.70, the intensity of the reflections is reduced from 6.8% of the incident light (for ophthalmic crown glass) to 0.30% of the incident light.

To satisfy the *path* condition, the two reflected waves must be out of phase by one-half wavelength at the point of interference. Because the wave reflected from the coating–glass interface traverses the coating *twice*, the wave will be one-half wavelength out of phase with the reflected wave at the air–coating interface if the coating is made with an *optical thickness* of *one-quarter wavelength*. If two wavefronts are out of phase by any *odd* number of wavelengths, and if the wavefronts are generated by any coating with an optical thickness of the same odd number of quarter wavelengths, the path condition is satisfied. However, the minimum optical thickness (one-quarter wavelength) produces the highest quality coating and is the thickness that is usually applied.

It is important to distinguish between *optical* thickness and *physical* (actual) thickness. The optical thickness is the product of the physical thickness and the index of refraction of the coating. Hence, the optical thickness is $\lambda/4$, and the physical thickness is $\lambda/4n$.

The stipulation that the optical path difference should be one-half wavelength is correct for only one particular wavelength of monochromatic light. Although the eye is sensitive to a wide range of wavelengths, the path condition can be satisfied only for monochromatic light. The wavelength generally selected is 555 nm, the wavelength of maximal visibility. The reflection for this wavelength is essentially eliminated, but reflections gradually increase toward the red and violet ends of the spectrum. The combination of red and violet reflected light causes the lens surface to appear to have a *purplish* or *magenta* color. Early workers noted that the magenta color resembled the bloom of ripened fruit, and the coating process was spoken of as "blooming" the lenses. The magenta color of a coated lens is so unique that, during the coating process, the color is used to assess the *thickness* of the coating. If the coating is too thin, the lens surface has a pale straw-colored or amber appearance; if the coating is too thick, the surface has a pale blue appearance.

To produce antireflective coatings that are effective for more than one wavelength requires the application of multilayer or broad-band coating material. The refractive index and the optimal thickness of each layer are chosen so that the combination of the amplitudes of all waves reflected from boundaries sums to zero across many wavelengths. Although a camera lens may have as many as seven or more layers of an antireflective coating, multicoated ophthalmic lenses are given only three or four layers. The Zeiss Super ET and the Hoya 99 Multicoat lenses (Figure 7–41) are examples of multicoated glass ophthalmic lenses.

7.31. Optical Principles of Antireflective Coatings

The optical principles involved in antireflective coatings may be understood with the help of Figure 7–42. In this diagram, N_g represents an ophthalmic crown glass lens and N_c represents a coating of one-quarter wavelength applied to the lens. AP and BO are parallel rays, in air, incident on the surface, XX′, of the coating. All angles of incidence, re-

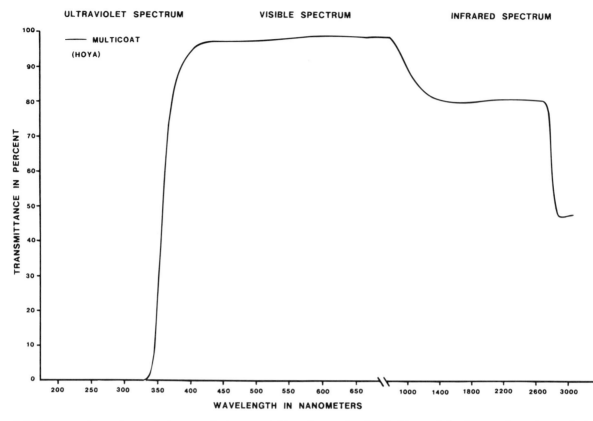

ULTRAVIOLET SPECTRUM   VISIBLE SPECTRUM   INFRARED SPECTRUM

FIGURE 7–41.   **Spectral transmission curve for Hoya 99 Multicoat lenses. (Reprinted with permission from D. Pitts and B. Maslovitz, unpublished data.)**

fraction, and reflection are considered to be very small. Some of the incident light designated by AP (solid line) as well as by BO (dashed line) is *reflected* in directions PM and ON, and some is *refracted* in directions PK and OL. When ray APK reaches the boundary, YY′, between the coating and the glass, some light is reflected in the direction KO, and some is refracted in the direction KQ. At point O on the surface of the coating, a portion of the light is reflected internally in the direction OL, and a portion is refracted in the direction ON.

Inspection of the diagram indicates that ray APKO has traveled a distance PKO *farther* than has ray BO. Because the angles of incidence and refraction are very small, and because the coating has an optical thickness of one-quarter wavelength, ray APKO has traveled *one-half wavelength* farther than has ray BO at arrival at point O. Because the index N_c is greater than that of N_a (air), and because N_g is greater than N_c, there is a change in phase of 180° in the reflected ray KO at K and in the reflected ray ON at O. Therefore, as a result of the phase changes in the reflected rays at K and O and the difference in path lengths of APKO and BO, the reflected ray ON (dashed) and the refracted ray ON (solid) are out of phase by 180 degrees at point O, and neutralization (cancellation) occurs.

The use of an antireflective coating results not only in the attenuation of bothersome reflections but also in an increase in the *transmission* of the lens. Figure 7–42 shows that at point O the refracted ray (dashed line) and the internally reflected ray (solid line) are *in phase*, with the result that reinforcement occurs, which increases the transmission of the lens.

As pointed out by Knoll,[30] *tinted* glass lenses often reduce the intensity of reflected images. The effect of a tinted lens on each type of reflection depends on the number of times the reflected light traverses the lens before it enters the eye. How many times the light involved in producing each type of reflection traverses the lens is given below (see also Figure 7–40):

Type of Reflection	Number of Times Traversed
A	0
B	2
C	3
D	1
E	3

When multiple traverses occur, the effective transmittance can be found by raising the nominal transmission to a power equal to the number of traverses. For example, if the nominal transmittance for a medium of a tinted lens is 90%, the effective transmittance after two traverses is 81% and after three traverses is 72.9%. Therefore, for a lens medium having a nominal transmission of 90%, image B in Figure 7–40 is reduced to 81%, image C and image E are each reduced to 73%, and image D has a transmission of 90% of the intensity produced when an untinted lens is used. Even a lightly tinted lens with an absorbance of only 4% per 2 mm of lens thickness is effective in reducing the C- or E-type reflection by about 12%; a slightly darker tint with an ab-

FIGURE 7–42. **Optical principles of an antireflective coating.**

sorbance of 8% per 2 mm of thickness reduces the intensity of the reflections by 22%.

7.32. Production of Antireflective Coatings

Glass

The first step in the production of a magnesium fluoride coating is a thorough cleaning of the lens to be coated. The lens is then placed in a bell-shaped chamber in which a vacuum is created to remove all air that might interfere with the deposition of magnesium fluoride. The lens is heated to about 300°C, which contributes to the hardness of the coating. Magnesium fluoride pellets are then heated to about 2500°C to produce vaporization. As the magnesium fluoride evaporates, it is deposited on the surface of the lens. During the deposition, an operator observes the color of the light reflected from a test lens of high refractive index. The eye is particularly sensitive to the development of the characteristic magenta color, so this method of thickness control is satisfactory. However, the eye may be replaced by a photoelectric cell screened by a green filter transmitting light of wavelength 555 nm. The output of the photoelectric cell diminishes as the coating thickens and reaches a minimum when the correct thickness is achieved.

Plastic

The principal difference in the processing of CR-39 plastic and glass lenses for an antireflection coating is the temperature to which lenses are heated during the coating process: CR-39 lenses are heated to less than 100°C; glass lenses must be heated to a temperature as high as 300°C. If CR-39 material is heated to a temperature exceeding

100°C (before, during, or after deposition of the coating), the material may lose its form stability and optical characteristics.

Plastic lenses must be prepared by careful cleaning and must be baked for at least 2 hours before coating to remove water vapor and volatile organic compounds. The coating process is then carried out in a vacuum environment with use of electron beam evaporation sources and microprocessor-controlled monitoring techniques. A single, thin coating placed directly on a plastic lens surface is seldom hard and durable enough to withstand the severe conditions ophthalmic lenses usually encounter. Because plastic lenses cannot withstand the high temperature (250–300°C) required to attain a sufficiently hard coating with magnesium fluoride, sodium dioxide (quartz) is generally used as a substitute. However, the refractive index of quartz (1.46 to 1.48) is too close to the refractive index of CR-39 (1.50) to achieve an effective reduction in reflection with only a quartz coat.

More efficient reduction of reflection is obtained by artificially increasing the refractive index of the substrate by applying a relatively thin, high-index film before the deposition of the low-index quartz film. The high refractive index coatings used are generally oxides of titanium, tantalum, zirconium, hafnium, praseodymium, and aluminum, or a mixture thereof.

Multilayer or broad-band antireflection coatings are applied to both plastic and glass lenses. Multilayer and broadband coatings produce a residual reflection color that is different from the traditional magenta color of single-layer coating—multilayer coatings are violet or gold and broadband coatings are typically green or blue.

Hydrophobic Coatings

Antireflective coatings are relatively soft and tend to scratch easily. In addition, they tend to display greasy marks and smudges and require careful cleaning. It is a paradox that the better and more effective the coating (i.e., the greater the transmittance), the greater the chance it will show smudges and marks. Because the lenses reflect so little light, any marked or smudged area produces an increase in reflection and thus becomes more visible. The lens does not become more "dirty" because of the coating, as all lenses at times have marks or smudges on the surface; the antireflection-coated lens simply exhibits marks more noticeably.

To increase the hardness of the coating and to make the marks less obvious and the surfaces easier to clean, *hydrophobic* coatings have been recently developed. The *hydrophobic coating* is a special layer of silicon coating over the top layer of antireflection coating. The silicon deposits a smooth, flexible, and microscopically thin coating that has no effect on the antireflection properties. The hydrophobic coating causes water and grease to form smaller droplets, which thus have a smaller area of contact with the lens surface. Therefore, they cannot adhere well and can be removed relatively easily.

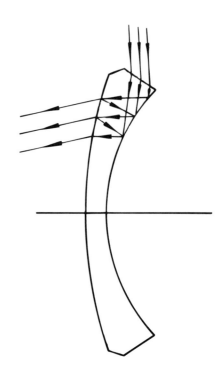

FIGURE 7–43.   **The multiple-ring effect.**

7.33. Reflections Annoying to the Observer

Some reflections from the surface of an ophthalmic lens are not noticed by the lens wearer but are annoying or distracting to an observer. These reflections cause the lenses to produce "flashes" of light that come and go with the movement of the wearer's head. The reflections enhance the "glassiness" of the appearance of the lenses and call attention to the lenses rather than to the eyes. They conceal the eyes from the observer, which makes eye contact difficult. Eyes are highly expressive aids to communication, and wearing spectacles can impair this form of communication. This is detrimental enough in daily personal contacts with individuals or with small groups of people, but for entertainers, teachers, ministers, and others who wear glasses when appearing before large audiences, reflections can add a serious impediment to effective communication. Spectacle wearers who must appear before television or movie cameras or before press photographers are subject to brilliant light sources that increase the number and intensity of these reflections. An antireflective coating provides a distinct improvement in the appearance of the lenses and gives cleaner, fresher, and warmer appearance to the wearer's eyes. In this image-conscious age, in which spectacles can detract from one's overall appearance, antireflective coatings are of particular benefit to those whose appearance receives careful scrutiny by the public.

The Multiple-Ring Effect

In addition to the reflections formed by the surfaces of the lenses, the *edges* of the lenses are responsible for the multiple rings seen just inside the edges of high minus lenses

(Figure 7–43). These are true images of the edge of the lens and are caused by internal reflections that begin at the lens edge and reflect their way toward the center of the lens until they strike the surface at an angle that permits refraction by the lens surface and into the eye of the observer. This process is then repeated, and multiple ring reflections may be seen. The rings are more pronounced for oblique angles than for straight-ahead viewing. The ring reflections also depend on such factors as the power of the lens, the curvatures of the surfaces, and the angle and distribution of the bevel. These reflections are the same color as the edge of the lens.

An antireflective surface coating is helpful in attenuating the intensity of the multiple-ring effect for straight-ahead viewing or for viewing at moderately oblique angles but is less helpful for extremely oblique angles of view. However, various forms of *edge treatment* can be helpful in this regard. *Edge coating* makes the rings less noticeable by reducing the granularity of the edge. *Painting* the edge a neutral gray color also tends to make the rings less noticeable. A third method of edge treatment is the use of a *semitransparent* edge. Such an edge can be produced by using an edging wheel that results in a fine, semitransparent grain rather than a coarse white grain on the beveled lens edge. The same effect can be achieved, for a plastic lens, by slightly *buffing* the edge. Another effective procedure for a plastic lens is to tint (dye) the lens after it has been edged. The tint can be so light that the transmission of the lens is affected very little for straight-ahead viewing. The dyeing procedure is effective because the dye penetrates a short distance beyond the lens surface. For multiple reflections, the reflected beam within the lens traverses the thin, dyed zone several times at an oblique angle. The reflected beam is thus significantly attenuated.

One of the most effective ways of coping with the multiple-ring effect involves the use of the hide-a-bevel edge treatment. As shown in Figure 7–44, this edge treatment consists of a flat edge with a small, narrow bevel protruding from the flat edge. With such an edge, there is a smaller area of ground glass from which reflections can arise, and the angle the flat edge makes with the lens surfaces is such that the rays tend to be reflected so that they do not enter the observer's eye.

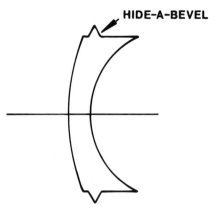

FIGURE 7–44.   **Hide-a-bevel edge treatment.**

References

1. North R. V. *Work and the Eye.* Oxford University Press, New York, p. 75, 1993.
2. Cibis, P. A., Newell, W. K., and Eichel, B. Ocular Effects Produced by High Intensity X-Radiaton. *Arch. Ophthalmol.,* Vol. 53, pp. 652–663, 1955.
3. Mackenzie, F., Hirst, L., Batislutta, D., and Green, A. Risk Analysis in the Development of Pterygia. *Ophthalmology,* Vol. 99, pp. 644–650, 1992.
4. Klintworth, G. K. Chronic Acute Keratopathy—A Condition Associated with Elastosis (Pinguecula) and Typified by Characteristic Extra-cellular Concretions. *Am. J. Pathol.,* Vol. 67, pp. 327–348, 1972.
5. Anderson, T., and Fuglsang, H. Droplet Degeneration in North Cameroon, Prevalence and Clinical Appearance. *Br. J. Ophthalmol.,* Vol. 60, pp. 256–262, 1976.
6. Hiller, R., Gracometti, L., and Yuen, K. Sunlight and Cataract, an Epidemiological Investigation. *Am. J. Epidemiol.,* Vol. 105, pp. 450–459, 1977.
7. Hollows, F., and Moran, D. Cataract—The Ultraviolet Risk Factor. *Lancet,* pp. 1249–1250, 1981.
8. Zigman, S. The Role of Sunlight in Human Cataract Formation. *Surv. Ophthalmol.,* Vol. 27, pp. 317–326, 1983.
9. Taylor, H. The Environment and the Lens. *Br. J. Ophthalmol.,* Vol. 64, pp. 304–310, 1980.
10. Buckingham, R. H., and Pirie, A. The Effect of Light on Lens Proteins in Vitro. *Exp. Eye Res.,* Vol. 14, pp. 297–299, 1972.
11. Van Heyningen, R. What Happens to the Human Lens in Cataract? *Sci. Am.,* Vol. 233, pp. 70–81, 1976.
12. Lerman, S. *Radiant Energy and the Eye.* Macmillan, New York, pp. 131–186, 1980.
13. Parrish, J., Anderson, R., Urback, F., and Pitts, D. *Biological Effects of Ultraviolet Radiation with Emphasis on Human Responses to Longwave Ultraviolet.* Plenum Press, New York, pp. 177–219, 1978.
14. Lerman, S. Lens Fluorescence in Aging and Cataract Formation. *Doc. Ophthalmol. Proc. Series 8,* pp. 241–260, 1976.
15. Lerman, S., and Borkman, R. A Molecular Model of Lens Aging, Nuclear and Cortical Cataract Formation. *Metabol. Pediatr. Ophthalmol.,* Vol. 3, pp. 27–35, 1979.
16. Taylor, R. H., West, S. K., Rosenthal, F. S., et al. Effect of Ultraviolet Radiation on Cataract Formation. *New Engl. J. Med.,* Vol. 319, pp. 1429–1433, 1988.
17. Boettner, E., and Wolter, J. Transmission of the Ocular Media. *Invest. Ophthalmol.,* Vol. 1, pp. 766–783, 1962.

18. Ham, W., Mueller, H., Ruffolo, J., Guerry, D. III, and Guerry, R. K. Action Spectrum for Retinal Injury from Near UV Radiation in the Aphakic Monkey. *Am. J. Ophthalmol.,* Vol. 93, pp. 299–306, 1982.
19. Young, R. W. The Charles F. Prentice Medal Award Lecture, 1992: Optometry and the Preservation of Visual Health. *Optom. Vis. Sci.,* Vol. 70, pp. 255–262, 1993.
20. Werner, J. S., and Steele, V. G. Sensitivity of Human Foveal Color Mechanisms throughout the Life Span. *J. Opt. Soc. Am. A,* Vol. 5, pp. 2122–2130, 1988.
21. Werner, J. S., Steele, V. G., and Ploff, D. S. Loss of Human Photoreceptor Sensitivity Associated with Chronic Exposure to Ultraviolet Radiation. *Ophthalmology,* Vol. 96, pp. 1552–1559, 1989.
22. Weiter, J. Phototoxic Changes in the Retina. In D. Miller, Ed., *Clinical Light Damage to the Eye.* Springer-Verlag, New York, pp. 79–125, 1986.
23. Hecht, S., Hendley, C. D., Ross, S., and Richmond, P. M. The Effect of Exposure to Sunlight on Night Vision. *Am. J. Ophthalmol.,* Vol. 31, p. 1533, 1948.
24. Kahn, H. A., and Moorhead, H. B. *Statistics on Blindness in the Model Reporting Area.* Department of Health, Education, and Welfare. Publication No. (NIH) 73-427, 1969–1970.
25. Heriot, W. J. Light and Retinal Pigment Epithelium: The Link in Senile Macular Degeneration. In J. Cromly-Dillon, E. S. Rosen, and J. Marsall, Eds., *Hazards of Light, Myths and Realities.* Pergamon Press, New York, pp. 187–196, 1986.
26. Mainster, M. A. Light and Macular Degeneration: A Biophysical and Clinical Perspective. *Eye,* Vol. 1, pp. 304–310, 1987.
27. Young, R. W. The Family of Sunlight-related Eye Diseases. *Optom. Vis. Sci.,* Vol. 71, pp. 125–144, 1994.
28. Ham, W., Mueller, H., and Sliney, D. Retinal Sensitivity and Damage from Short Wavelength Light. *Nature,* Vol. 260, pp. 153–155, 1976.
29. Richards, O. W. Sunglasses for Eye Protection. *Am. J. Optom. Arch. Amer. Acad. Optom.,* Vol. 48, pp. 200–203, 1971.
30. Knoll, H. Ophthalmic Lens Reflections. *Optom. Weekly,* Vol. 53, No. 31, pp. 517–518, 1962.
31. Pitts, D. G., and Cullen, A. P. *Ocular Ultraviolet Effects from 295 nm to 400 nm in the Rabbit Eye.* DHEW (NIOSH), Publication No. 75-175, 1977.
32. Pitts, D. Threat of Ultraviolet Radiation to the Eye—How to Protect Against It. *J. Am. Optom. Assoc.,* Vol. 52, pp. 949–957, 1981.
33. Luria, S. M. Preferred Density of Sunglasses. *Am. J. Optom. Physiol. Opt.,* Vol. 61, pp. 379–402, 1984.
34. Pitts, D. C., Cullen, A. P., and Dayhaw-Barker, P. Determination of Ocular Thresholds for Infrared Radiation Cataractogenesis. DHHS (NIOSH) Publ. No. 80-121, 1980.

35. Clark, B. A. J. Infrared Transmission Limits for Sunglasses. *Austr. J. Optom.*, Vol. 52, pp. 167–186, 1969.

36. Clark, B. A. J. Color in Sunglass Lenses. *Am. J. Optom. Arch. Amer. Acad. Optom.*, Vol. 46, pp. 825–840, 1969.

37. Wright, W. D. *Photometry and the Eye*. The Hatton Press, London, p. 127, 1949.

38. Luckiesh, M., and Holladay, L. L. Penetration of Fog by Light from Sodium and Tungsten Lamps. *J. Opt. Soc. Am.*, Vol. 31, pp. 528–530, 1941.

39. Richards, O. W. Yellow Glasses Fail to Improve Seeing at Night-Driving Luminances. *Highway Res. Abstr.*, Vol. 23, pp. 32–36, 1953.

40. Blackwell, H. R. The Effect of Tinted Optical Media upon Visual Efficiency at Low Luminances. *J. Opt. Soc. Am.*, Vol. 43, p. 815, 1953.

41. Davey, J. B. Seeing Times with Yellow Driving Glasses. *Optician*, Vol. 136, p. 651, 1959.

42. Bierman, E. O. Tinted Lenses in Shooting. *Am. J. Ophthalmol.*, Vol. 35, pp. 859–860, 1952.

43. Megla, G. K. Optical Properties and Application of Photochromic Glass. *Appl. Optics*, Vol. 5, No. 6, pp. 945–960, 1966.

44. Armistead, W. H., and Stookey, S. D. Photochromic Silicate Glasses Sensitized by Silver Halide. *Science*, Vol. 144, pp. 150–154, 1964.

45. Douthwaite, W. A., and Elliott, P. A Comparison of Photogray Glass with Surface Tints. *Optician*, Vol. 162, pp. 15–16, 1971.

46. Lynch, D. M., and Brilliant, R. An evaluation of the Corning CPF 550 Lens. *Optom. Monthly*, Vol. 75, pp. 36–42, 1984.

47. Parker, E., and Miller, G. Photochromic Lenses for the Relief of Photophobia. *Optician*, Vol. 208, pp. 24–28, 1994.

48. Davis, J. K., and Fernald, H. G. Prescription Sunglasses. *Am. J. Optom. Arch. Amer. Acad. Optom.*, Vol. 46, No. 8, pp. 572–577, 1969.

49. Hall, R. M. Theoretical and Practical Considerations of the Pulfrich Phenomenon. *Am. J. Optom. Arch. Amer. Acad. Optom.*, Vol. 15, No. 2, pp. 31–46, 1928.

50. Lederer, J. Anisopia. *Australas. J. Optom.*, Vol. 40, No. 1, pp. 13–38, 1957.

51. Anderson, W. J., and Gebel, R. K. H. Ultraviolet Windows in Commercial Sunglasses. *Appl. Optics*, Vol. 16, pp. 515–517, 1977.

52. Borgwardt, B., Fishman, G. A., and Vander Meulen, D. Spectral Transmission Characteristics of Tinted Lenses. *Arch. Ophthalmol.*, Vol. 99, pp. 293–297, 1981.

53. Becnel, L., Fruge, P., and Coullard, G. Validation Studies of the Alpascope. *J. Tex. Optom. Assoc.*, Vol. 24, pp. 7–12, Oct. 1968.

54. Pitts, D. G. Sunglasses for Ocular Protection. In D. G. Pitts and R. N. Kleinstein, Eds., *Environmental Vision: Interaction of the Eye, Vision, and the Environment*. Butterworth-Heinemann, Boston, pp. 299–311, 1993.

55. Davis, J. K. Prescribing for Visibility. *Probl. Optom.*, Vol. 2, pp. 131–155, 1990.

56. *American National Standard for Ophthalmics: Nonprescription Sunglasses and Fashion Eyewear Requirements, Z80.3-1986.* American National Standards Institute, Inc., New York, 1986.

57. NSPB, AAO, AOA Issue Statement on Maximum UV Protection. *Vision Monday*, Vol. 7, p. 10, 1993.

58. *American National Standard Practice for Occupational and Educational Eye and Face Protection, Z87.1-1989.* American National Standards Institute, Inc., New York, 1989.

Questions

1. A lens is made of glass with an index of 1.69. What is the index of refraction for the ideal antireflection coating for the lens?

2. An ideal antireflection coating is to be placed on glass that has a refractive index of 1.621. What is the minimal physical thickness of the coating required for light of wavelength 590 nm?

3. What is the percentage of perpendicularly incident light reflected from a *surface* between air and glass with a refractive index of 1.62?

4. Assuming there is no absorption, what is the percentage of perpendicularly incident light transmitted by a lens of index 1.70?

5. What is the total amount of light transmitted through a clear lens of index 1.50 coated on both sides with a substance of index 1.30?

6. A lens is 4 mm thick at its center. The index of refraction is 1.50. The transmission factor is 0.5 per mm. Ignoring reflection, what is the transmission at its center?

7. A lens is 3 mm thick at its center. The index of refraction is 1.50. The transmission factor is 0.2 per mm. Ignoring reflection, what is the density at its center?

8. A lens is 2 mm thick at its center. The index of refraction is 1.50. The transmission factor is 0.2 per mm. Ignoring reflection, what is the opacity at its center?

9. What would be the combined optical density of two absorptive lenses each having a light transmission of 20%?

10. A lens having a transmission of 50% is placed next to a lens having a transmission of 20%. What is the transmission of the combination?

11. A +4.00 D lens is 5.6 mm thick at its pole. The index of the glass is 1.5 and the transmission factor is 0.5 per mm. Assuming no loss of light by reflection, at what distance from the pole is there 25% transmission?

12. A spectacle or crown lens of index of refraction of 1.523 has a total transmission of 50% for a thickness of 2 mm. What is the total transmission for a lens of this material made 5.0 mm thick?

13. An ophthalmic crown lens with an index of refraction of 1.523 has a transmission of 15% for a thickness of 2.2 mm. What is the transmission for a lens of this material made 3.6 mm thick?

14. A tinted contact lens of index 1.49 has a transmission of 20% at a thickness of 1.0 mm. When the lens is made with a center thickness of 0.2 mm, what is the total transmission?

15. A welder decides that, when welding, the proper illumination occurs when he places a shade number 8 and a shade number 3 together. If he wished to replace the two lenses by a single lens, what would be the shade number of the single lens?

16. What would be the luminous transmission of a welding lens with a shade number of 8.0?

17. A glass filter of index 1.523, which is 1 mm thick, transmits 80% of the incident light on it. If a transmission of 50% is desired, what would be the thickness of a single glass filter of the same material?

18. A −10.00 D tinted lens is 1 mm thick at its center. The index of refraction is 1.50. The transmission factor is 0.5 per mm. Assuming no loss by reflection,
    (a) plot a graph illustrating transmission as a function of its thickness.

(b) plot a graph illustrating transmission as a function of the *distance (h) from the optical center.*

19. A ghost image is formed by reflections on a clear ophthalmic crown lens in the following manner: The light source is behind the head and the light is refracted at the back surface but reflected at the front surface toward the back surface, where it undergoes refraction toward the eye. What is the final intensity on the cornea compared to the 100% source of intensity?

20. A patient wears lenses of refractive index 1.50 with a back surface power of –3.00 D. Light from a bright source located behind the head at a great distance is reflected from the back surface into the eye. The patient can see the reflected image clearly without accommodating. What is the power of the correction lens?

21. A patient wears lenses of index 1.50 with a back surface power –11.00 D. When the outer canthus is brightly illuminated, the patient can see a reflected image of the outer canthus from the back surface of the lens without accommodating. The outer canthus lies 20 mm from the back surface of the lens. What is the power of the correction lens?

22. A 6-mm-thick lens with a refractive index of 1.523 has a total transmission of 49.62%. If the lens is made 4 mm thick, the total transmission is 60.9%. If the lens is made 1.0 mm thick, what is its total transmission?

CHAPTER EIGHT

Multifocal Lenses

The crystalline lens continues to grow throughout life. As additional layers of lens fibers are laid down underneath the lens capsule, the older layers of fibers are trapped in the nucleus of the lens where they become compressed and gradually lose their elasticity. The loss of elasticity of the lens nucleus is responsible for the gradual loss of the ciliary muscle's ability to bring about an increase in the vergence of light when accommodation is attempted. The near point of accommodation therefore gradually recedes with age, so that by about the age of 45 years it becomes difficult, if not impossible, for most people to see clearly for near-vision tasks without the assistance of plus lens power in addition to any lens power required for distance vision. Although the near-vision add may be supplied in the form of a pair of glasses for close work only, most people who require lenses for distance vision find it more convenient to wear only one pair of glasses with two or more focal powers. Early multifocal lenses provided only two focal powers, but later developments provided trifocal lenses, occupational multifocal lenses, and progressive addition lenses.

This chapter discusses the physical characteristics of multifocal lenses, beginning with the history and development of these lenses, and then discusses the physical characteristics, manufacturing processes, optical design principles, performance characteristics, and the clinical application of multifocal lenses. The chapter concludes with a discussion of invisible bifocals and progressive addition lenses.

_____PHYSICAL CHARACTERISTICS_____

8.1. History and Development of Multifocal Lenses

Benjamin Franklin is credited with the invention of the bifocal lens. In a letter written in 1785 to a friend, Franklin commented that he had formerly worn two pairs of spectacles, one for distance vision and one for reading, but because he found the arrangement sometimes inconvenient, he had the lenses cut in half, and had half of each kind mounted in the same frame (Figure 8–1). Franklin's bifocal lens was similar in appearance to the Executive one-piece bifocal that is available today, a lens with a dividing line across its width.

Franklin's bifocal had excellent optical properties with sharp imagery over the entire reading field. Because the distance-vision and reading portions were separate lenses, the optical centers could be placed at the same level as the dividing line or could be separated, as desired. Because both parts of the lens were made of the same material, there was little difference in the chromatic aberration of the two portions. However, the Franklin bifocal suffered from two disadvantages. First, the dividing line produced annoying reflections, it tended to collect dust and dirt, and it was conspicuous and unsightly. Second, the two portions of the lens were held in position by the eyewire of the frame, which was a weak structure that could easily come apart.

The next bifocal lens was the Solid Upcurve bifocal, invented by Isaac Schnaitmann of Philadelphia in 1837. This was the first commercially successful, one-piece bifocal lens. Starting with a lens ground for the wearer's reading prescription, the lens was made by grinding a flatter curvature on the upper portion of the back surface of the lens, which reduced the plus power sufficiently for distance vision (Figure 8–2). The desirable attributes of this lens included invisibility, structural strength, little chromatic aberration, and a wide field of view for reading. However, there were serious disadvantages. Because of the limited choice of surface powers, significant amounts of aberration were usually present in the distance portion, which restricted the field of vision. In addition, the resurfacing of the upper portion of the back surface moved the optical center of the distance portion of the lens below its

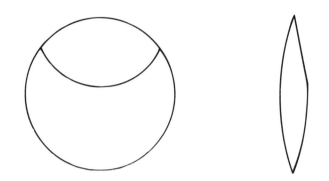

FIGURE 8–2. **The Solid Upcurve bifocal, showing base-down prismatic effect in the distance portion.**

original position. Consequently, the distance portion contained a strong base-down prismatic effect. The combination of aberrations and strong prismatic effects in the distance portion produced intolerable optical results.

In 1888 (more than 100 years after Franklin's invention of the bifocal lens) August Morck reinvented the Franklin bifocal in a modified form. Called the Perfection bifocal, this lens had a curved dividing line and the two pieces of glass had beveled edges, which made the lens more stable in its frame (Figure 8–3). The lens performed much like the Franklin bifocal, but the distance-vision portion was larger than the near-vision portion. It also had most of the disadvantages of the Franklin bifocal: a conspicuous dividing line that tended to collect dust and dirt and a difficult and expensive manufacturing process.

Morck also invented the Cemented bifocal and filed a patent for it in 1888 (Figure 8–4). A thin glass wafer with the same index of refraction as the major lens was cemented to the back surface of the major lens. The adhesive used was Canada balsam, which has an index of refraction essentially the same as that of glass. The front surface of the wafer had the same curvature as the back surface of the major lens; hence, no power change occurred between the back surface of the major lens and the front surface of the wafer. The back surface of the wafer was made less concave than the back surface of the major lens, and the power of the addition was simply the difference in power between

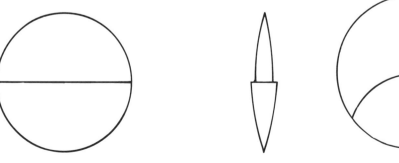

FIGURE 8–1. **Benjamin Franklin's bifocal.**

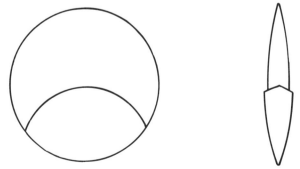

FIGURE 8–3. **The Perfection bifocal.**

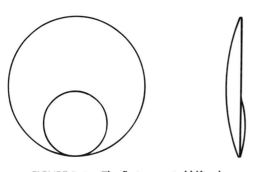

FIGURE 8–4. **The first cemented bifocal.**

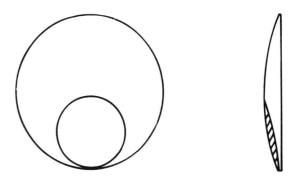

FIGURE 8–6. **The fused Kryptok bifocal.**

the back surface of the major lens and the back surface of the wafer.

This lens was satisfactory both optically and cosmetically, and was widely used into the twentieth century. However, its defects became well-known. The shoulder around the dividing line collected dirt; the adherence of the wafer was affected by changes in temperature; the cement had a tendency to darken with use; and the wafer had a tendency to fall off. Cemented bifocals are still used occasionally for special purposes such as a temporary bifocal, an experimental correction, or for a bifocal used as a low-vision aid. Epoxy resin (Araldite) is now used as a cement.

The next step in the development of the bifocal lens was made by John Borsch who, in 1899, invented the Cemented Kryptok bifocal. Borsch ground a countersink curve in the form of a depression in the front surface of the lens, then cemented a wafer made of flint glass ($n = 1.67$) into the countersink area, and covered the surface of the entire lens with a thin meniscus of glass cemented into place (Figure 8–5). The name *Kryptok* was derived from the Greek word meaning "hidden." This was the first bifocal lens in which the reading addition was created by using a material with a higher index of refraction than that of the major lens. This lens was difficult to manufacture because six surfaces had to be ground and polished. The cover plate was thin and fragile, the cemented surfaces tended to darken, and the lens easily came apart.

In 1908 John Borsch, Jr., developed the first *fused* bifocal lens, which was also called a Kryptok lens (Figure 8–6). In making this lens, a flint bifocal segment in the form of a button was fused under high temperature into a countersink

area in the front surface of the major lens; hence, a cover glass was not needed. After the segment button was fused to the major lens, the same curvature was ground on the entire front surface of the lens. The front surface curvature was spherical, because a toric front surface would have produced a different cylindrical power in the distance portion than that in the near-vision portion of the lens. Hence, any cylindrical component had to be ground on the back surface of the lens. The Kryptok bifocal was the precursor of all modern fused bifocal lenses and is still in use today.

The Kryptok provided many advantages over the earlier bifocals. The segment edges did not collect dust and dirt; the segment did not fall out, become discolored, or chip; and the segment was relatively invisible. Lenses could be produced in large quantities on a commercial scale at low cost. The shortcomings of this lens were the result of the use of two kinds of glass and the temperature (600°C–700°C) required for fusing the segment to the major lens. To prevent strain from developing along the fused surface, the coefficients of expansion of the two glasses must be matched from the fusing temperature to room temperature, and high-speed polishing of the surfaces to be fused often produces tension on the surfaces. During heating for fusion, the tension may be released, which produces an irregular, undulating surface.

When competitively priced forms of this lens are made, the surfaces to be fused are deliberately not matched in curvature—the surface of the button is left somewhat *steeper* than that of the countersink curve to allow air bubbles to escape during the fusing process. This procedure tends to produce a fused surface that is not perfectly spherical after the fusing is completed. If the fusing temperature is not rigidly controlled and becomes too high, the countersink surface of the major lens collapses and becomes distorted. If the temperature rises too high, the flint and crown glasses mix along the lines of fusion and form an alloy layer that produces a hazy image.

An additional problem with the Kryptok bifocal is that *transverse chromatic aberration* is often a problem. The reading portion, consisting of two optical elements with different indices of refraction, is in the form of a *doublet*. For a doublet to be achromatic, the dioptric powers of the two elements must be opposite in sign and the Abbe (V) values must be in the same ratio as the dioptric powers (Figure 8–7). To be achromatic, a doublet with a resul-

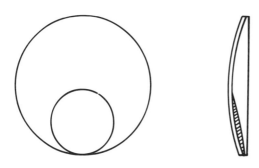

FIGURE 8–5. **The Cemented Kryptok bifocal.**

tant *positive* refractive power consists of a convex element made of crown glass and a concave element made of a higher index (flint) glass. Such a doublet is shown in Figure 8–7A. However, a Kryptok bifocal with a positive resultant refractive power has a form just the *opposite* of the form required for an achromatic lens—it has a convex element of flint glass and a concave element of crown glass (Figure 8–7B).

The reading portion of a Kryptok bifocal has a positive resultant power whenever (1) the power of the distance portion is positive or (2) the power of the distance portion is negative but weaker than the power of the addition. In these instances, noticeable amounts of chromatic aberration may be present, with the result that the wearer may complain of seeing color fringes around objects; in addition, the chromatism may reduce the depth of focus at the reading point.

For a doublet with a resultant *minus* power to be achromatic, it must consist of a concave crown glass and a convex glass of higher index of refraction. This is indeed the case for any Kryptok bifocal lens in which the minus power of the distance portion of the lens is higher than the plus power of the add; thus, for such lenses, chromatic aberration is not likely to present a problem.

An important improvement in the design of fused bifocals was made by Henry Courmettes, a French national living in New York. In 1915, Courmettes patented the idea of fusing into a major lens a button (segment) that was made of two kinds of glass. The upper portion of the button was identical in index of refraction to that of the major lens, but the lower portion had a higher index of refraction. The two pieces of glass were ground so that they had perfectly flat edges, which produced a straight dividing line after they had been fused along the flat edges. As shown in Figure 8–8, the composite button was subsequently fused into the

countersink depression of the major lens. After the fused composite button was ground and polished, the upper half of the button could no longer be seen because it was made of glass having the same index as the major lens. Only the boundary between the crown glass and the higher index glass in the lower part of the composite button remained visible. All fused straight-top bifocals and trifocals now in use were designed with the Courmettes process by other manufacturers after 1915 (Figure 8–9).

The first straight-top bifocal to be patented was the B (bar) segment, shown in Figure 8–9A. It was designed by two Englishmen, W. Watson and G. Culver, and was patented in 1931. In an unusual development, four men (Clement, Price, M. H. Stanley, and V. Hancock) working independently almost simultaneously filed substantially identical patent applications for the D-style segment (which looks like a capital "D" lying on its back) shown in Figure 8–9B. The patent was finally issued to M. H. Stanley in 1933. The R (ribbon) segment was developed by Jack Silverman and patented in 1932. The R-Compensated series of lenses (designed for the compensation of vertical prismatic effects at near vision and consisting of 7 segments designated R-4 through R-10) was patented by Silverman in 1933.

Many other designs of fused bifocals, using the basic Courmettes process, have been developed since 1915, but only a few have actually been manufactured. Modifications of the D-style have included the Panoptik, with rounded corners, designed by James Hammond, and the curved-top version, called the Widesite, designed by Price. These two lenses are shown in Figure 8–10.

The first *one-piece* bifocal to have commercial success was the Solid Upcurve bifocal (described above) introduced in 1837. During the next 70 years, many patents were issued for other one-piece bifocals, but none was

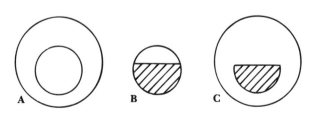

FIGURE 8–7.   **A, an achromatic doublet, consisting of a convex crown glass element and a concave flint glass element; B, a Kryptok bifocal, with a reading portion consisting of a concave crown glass element and a convex flint glass element.**

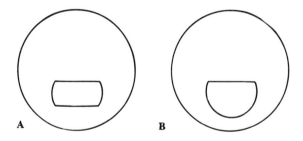

FIGURE 8–9.   **A, the first straight-top fused bifocal with a B segment; B, the D-style straight-top fused bifocal.**

FIGURE 8–8.   **The Courmettes fusing process. A, major lens with countersink curve; B, button made of two kinds of glass; C, the finished straight-top bifocal lens.**

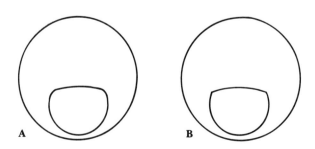

FIGURE 8–10.   **Modified straight-top fused bifocals. A, the Panoptik; B, the Widesite.**

produced successfully on a commercial basis. In 1910 Charles Conner, an optician from Indianapolis, succeeded in producing a bifocal ground from a single piece of glass with a uniform index of refraction. Connor called his lens the Ultex bifocal. Patents were granted to Conner for both the lens and the grinding process. In 1910 the One Piece Bifocal Company, predecessor of the Continental Optical Company, was organized to manufacture the Ultex bifocal.

For the Ultex lens, the additional plus power for the reading segment is obtained by a change in curvature, usually on the back surface. On a large lens blank, the back surface is ground in the form of a saucer having a round disk at the center (which forms the near-vision portion of the lens) and a steeper or more concave curvature at the periphery (which forms the distance-vision portion). This lens is shown in Figure 8–11. Although it is possible to grind a one-piece segment of any size, certain stock diameters are produced. For example, the Ultex A is ground with a central disk 38 mm in diameter (Figure 8–12). After it is ground the blank is cut into two lenses, each having a segment height of 19 mm (Figure 8–12A). If a segment height larger than 19 mm is required, only one lens (with a segment height of 32 mm) is cut from the blank. The Ultex AA, also called the AL (Figure 8–12B), is made in this manner. Segments as small as 22 mm round (the Ultex B) can be produced. The Ultex-style bifocal is currently available in the A, AA (or AL), and B segments.

The next step in the development of the one-piece bifocal took place almost 50 years later when, in 1954, the Americal Optical Company developed the Executive bifocal. The front surface of this lens has a more convex cur-

vature in the lower portion than it has in the upper portion, which creates a ledge that one can easily feel; the lens has a straight dividing line across its width (Figure 8–13). The Executive-style bifocal has proven to be a popular lens and is now manufactured by several companies under a variety of trade names.

The invention of the *trifocal* lens (Figure 8–14) can be traced to an English inventor, John Isaac Hawkins. In 1826 Hawkins, at age 54, published a description of a pair of trifocal lenses that he had designed for his own use. The trifocals were made of three separate pieces of glass, and Hawkins provided detailed specifications for their manufacture. The first commercially available fused trifocal was the round-top trifocal (Figure 8–14A), which was developed simultaneously, but independently, by several individuals. The developers of this lens were L. W. Bugbee, Clement, J. Hammond, V. Hancock, and Price; a patent was issued to V. Hancock in 1932. The first straight-top fused trifocal (Figure 8–14B) was developed by V. Hancock in 1936. Shortly after the development of the Ultex bifocal in 1910, Conner developed the curved-top Ultex trifocal (Figure 8–14C); and in 1954 American Optical designed the Executive trifocal (Figure 8–14D) to accompany its Executive bifocal.

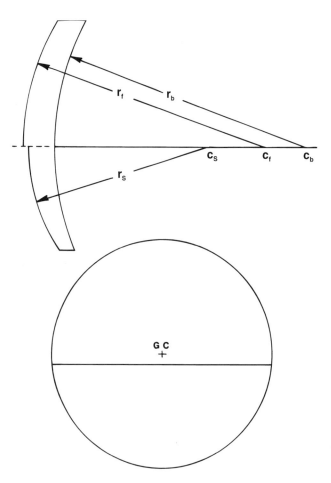

FIGURE 8–13.   **The Executive one-piece straight-top bifocal. GC = geometric center.**

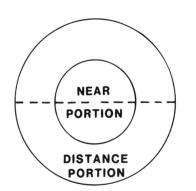

FIGURE 8–11.   **Large lens blank used for grinding the Ultex one-piece bifocal, which results in two lenses.**

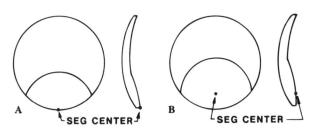

FIGURE 8–12.   **Ultex one-piece bifocals. A, Ultex A; B, Ultex AL.**

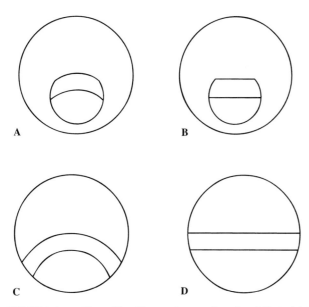

FIGURE 8–14.   **Glass trifocal lenses. A, curved-top fused; B, straight-top fused; C, Ultex one-piece; D, Executive-type one-piece.**

8.2. Fused Bifocal Lenses

Fused bifocal lenses are currently available in a large variety of segment styles, all of which can be categorized as round segments, straight-top segments, or modified straight-top segments. All fused bifocal segments, whether round, straight-top, modified straight-top, or ribbon segments, have the bifocal segment located on the *front* surface of the lens. Because the segment side of the lens must have a spherical surface, a fused bifocal lens requiring a cylinder must be made in a negative toric form.

Round Segments

The original Kryptok bifocal is the least expensive bifocal available because it does not have a corrected-curve lens, and it has a flint segment with a small Abbe value, which often results in a large amount of chromatic aberration. The word *Kryptok* is no longer protected by a patent, so the lens can be manufactured by any company. In the past, the Kryptok lens was available in many segment sizes, but it is now available only as a 22-mm segment.

In addition to the Kryptok, each manufacturer has developed a round segment bifocal, using the company's particular corrected curves. All these lenses use barium crown glass (rather than flint glass) in the segment. Because of its high Abbe number, barium crown glass has no more chromatic aberration than ophthalmic crown glass. Segments of these bifocals are routinely 22 mm in diameter, with the segment optical center (Figure 8–15) located at the geometric center of the segment (11 mm below the segment top) in the uncut form (A). Lenses in this category are the Sola RS and the Vision-Ease CRF. Representative round fused bifocals are listed in Table 8–1.

Straight-Top Segments

Undoubtedly, the most commonly used bifocal is the straight-top fused bifocal, first developed by the Univis Lens Company of Dayton, Ohio. As already described, the original Univis Sentinel D was made by fusing together a truncated, round, high-index segment and a small crown glass segment, with the resulting segment fused into the countersink area. The upper edge of the straight-top segment is located 6 mm below the 22-mm circle, with the result that the segment center is located 5 mm below the segment top (Figure 8–15B).

When the Univis patent expired, other lens manufacturers introduced straight-top bifocal lenses. These lenses are now available in a 22 × 16-mm segment, a 25 × 17.5-mm segment, a 28 × 19-mm segment, and a 35 × 22.5-mm segment. In all these lenses, the segment center is located approximately 5 mm below the segment top. Representative straight-top fused bifocals are listed in Table 8–1.

Modified Straight-Top Segments

After the successful introduction of the Univis D bifocal, other manufacturers developed modified forms of the straight-top bifocal. The earliest of these lenses were the

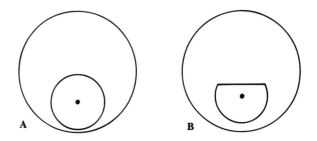

FIGURE 8–15.   **Location of segment optical centers. A, round fused segment; B, straight-top segment.**

TABLE 8–1
Representative Glass Fused Bifocals

Shape	Name (Co.)	Segment Size
Round	Kryptok	22
	CFR (Lantz)	22, 25
	RS (Sola)	22
	CFR (Vision-Ease)	22, 25
	CFR (X-Cel)	22, 25
Straight-top	FT (Vision-Ease)	22, 28, 35
	D (X-Cel)	22, 25, 28, 35
	Kote-Line (Lantz)	25, 28, 35
	FT (Sola)	25, 28, 35
Modified	22-C (Vision-Ease)	22 × 16
Straight-top	25-C (Vision-Ease)	25 × 17.5
	28-C (Vision-Ease)	28 × 19
	P-24 (Vision-Ease)	24 × 16.5
Ribbon	R-14 (Vision-Ease)	22 × 14
Segments	B-9 (Vision-Ease)	22 × 9
	Ribbon Seg (X-Cel)	22 × 14
	Ribbon Seg (X-Cel)	22 × 9

Bausch & Lomb Panoptik and the Shuron Widesite, already mentioned and illustrated in Figure 8–10. The Panoptik bifocal had a 22 × 14.5-mm segment with slightly rounded corners and the Widesite had a slightly curved top. Recently, Vision-Ease introduced the Vision-Ease P bifocal, similar in shape to the Panoptik; Vision-Ease also manufactures the Vision-Ease C, similar in shape to the Widesite. The Vision-Ease C bifocal is available in 22-, 25-, and 28-mm widths. See Table 8–1 for a list of representative modified straight-top bifocals.

Ribbon Segments

The ribbon segment is essentially a straight-top segment with the lower part cut off (as shown in Figure 8–9A) and is designed so that the wearer will have distance vision both below and above the segment. These lenses are available in 22 × 14-mm segments as the Vision-Ease R and the X-Cel Ribbon Seg. The ribbon segment is also available in a 22 × 9-mm segment, manufactured as the Vision-Ease B and the X-Cel Ribbon Seg. See Table 8–1 for a list of representative ribbon segment bifocals.

8.3. One-Piece Bifocal Lenses

One-piece bifocal lenses are available in both round and straight-top styles. For some round one-piece bifocals, the segment is located on the *back* surface of the lens; if a cylindrical correction is needed, it must be ground on the front surface. However, for one-piece bifocals in which the segment is on the front surface, a negative toric form is used (as with fused bifocals).

Round Segments

The original Ultex A and AL, described in Section 8.1, have large, round segments, the lower parts of which have been cut off. These segments are sometimes referred to as *hemispheric* segments. Both the A and AL segments are 38 to 40 mm in diameter; in uncut form, the A is 19 to 20 mm high and the AL is 30 to 35 mm high. The Philtex One-Piece A and the Philtex One-Piece AL are available with the segment on either the front or back surfaces of the lens. The Phillips Lens Company produces a 22-mm round one-piece bifocal called the B Style. The segment is located on the back surface; therefore the cylinder is placed on the front surface, in plus cylinder form.

Important Note. On casual inspection, the rarely encountered one-piece B Style bifocal closely resembles the frequently used 22-mm round fused bifocal. If a lens has a cylindrical component, it is important to distinguish these lenses from each other when one duplicates a pair of lenses or replaces a single lens because the one-piece B Style bifocal is constructed in plus cylinder form, and the 22-mm round fused bifocal is made in minus cylinder form. The one-piece B Style bifocal can be identified by using a lens gauge on the back surface or by feeling the change in curvature from the segment to the major lens.

Straight-Top Segments

In addition to the Executive lenses, straight-top one-piece bifocals are now available—the Sola BiLine, X-Cel E-Style, and the Vision-Ease Bifield. The standard height in uncut form for all these segments is 25 mm, with the exception of the X-Cel E-Style High-Seg, which is 29 mm high. Representative one-piece bifocals are listed in Table 8–2.

TABLE 8–2
Representative Glass One-Piece Bifocals

Shape	Name (Co.)	Segment Size
Round	Philtex One-Piece B, Style CC; segment on back surface (Phillips Lens Co.)	22
Hemispheric	Philtex One-Piece A, Style CC; segment on back surface (Phillips Lens Co.)	38 × 19
	Philtex One-Piece A, Style CX; segment on front surface (Phillips Lens Co.)	40 × 19
	Philtex One-Piece AL, Style CC; segment on back surface (Phillips Lens Co.)	38 × 30
	Philtex One-Piece AL, Style CX; segment on front surface (Phillips Lens Co.)	40 × 35
	Plus Base Ultex; segment on front surface (Vision-Ease)	40 × 20
	Ultex A; segment on front surface (X-Cel)	40 × 19
Straight-top	Executive (American Optical)	25
	Bi-Line (Sola)	25
	Bifield (Vision-Ease)	25
	E-Style (X-Cel)	25
	E-Style High Seg (X-Cel)	29

8.4. Double-Segment Bifocals

A double-segment bifocal lens has two segments, one below eye level and the other above eye level; the lens is intended for use by electricians, painters, and others whose occupations require close work above eye level. Most lenses are of the straight-top variety and are available in both fused and one-piece styles. In almost all these lenses, the separation between the upper and lower segments is 13 mm.

The first double-segment bifocal introduced was the Univis Double D, which was available in 22-mm and 25-mm segment widths. Vision-Ease and X-Cel make 22-mm, 25-mm, and 28-mm double straight-top bifocals. American Optical makes the Executive in double bifocal form; X-Cel makes the E-Style Double Segment (a one-piece bifocal similar in appearance to the Double-D Executive); Vision-Ease and X-Cel make double round fused segments.

In most double bifocals, the power of the addition in the upper segment is equal to that of the addition in the lower segment. The exception is the Tillyer Double Executive, in which the upper segment has approximately two-thirds the power of the lower segment. For example, for a lower segment power of +1.50 D add, the upper segment has an addition of +1.00 D, and for a lower segment having an add of +2.50 D, the upper add is +1.75 D. Representative double-segment bifocals are shown in Figure 8–16 and are listed in Table 8–3.

8.5. Minus Add Bifocal

The *minus add* bifocal is a lens designed predominantly for close work, but it has a relatively small distance-vision window at the top. Although not widely used, this lens should be considered for a presbyope, such as a barber or postal clerk, whose occupation requires a large field for near-vision work. The first lens of this kind was the Solid Upcurve bifocal, described in Section 8.1. A minus add lens is currently available in an Ultex-style one-piece form called the Rede-Rite bifocal. Instead of the segment top being located at the upper edge of the wearer's lower eyelid (as in most bifocal fitting), this lens usually has the top of the segment located above the center of the pupil.

Additional methods of obtaining an unusually large reading field include use of a 29-mm-high straight-top one-piece (Executive-style) bifocal, or the use of an Ultex AL bifocal, which can be as high as 35 mm. Even the standard Executive-style bifocal can be fitted as high as 25 mm; for most wearers, this fit puts the segment top well above the center of the pupil. See Figure 8–17 and Table 8–4 for representative minus add lenses.

8.6. Trifocal Lenses

A presbyope who requires a near addition of +1.75 D or more is likely to have difficulty seeing at arm's length

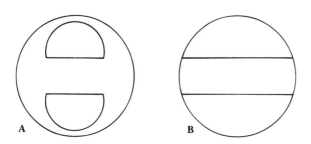

FIGURE 8–16.   **Double-segment bifocals. A, fused Double-D; B, Double Executive bifocal.**

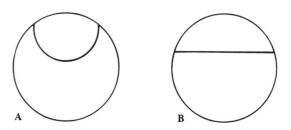

FIGURE 8–17.   **Minus add bifocals. A, Ultex Rede-Rite bifocal; B, 29-mm-high Executive bifocal.**

TABLE 8–3
Representative Glass Double-Segment Bifocals

Name (Co.)	Segment Separation	Segment Width
Executive Double (American Optical)	14	—
E-Style Double Seg (Excel)	14	—
Dual FT-35 (Lantz)	16	35
Kote Line Dual FT (Lantz)	13	25, 28
Dual D (Vision-Ease)	13	22, 25, 28
Maximum DD 35 (Vision-Ease)	15	35
Double-Seg Flat Top (X-Cel)	13	25, 28, 35
Double CFR 22 round (Vision-Ease)	13	22
Double Seg round (X-Cel)	13	22, 25

TABLE 8–4
Representative Glass Bifocals, One-Piece Rede-Rite Style: Minus Add in Upper Portion

Name (Co.)	Segment Size
Philtex One-Piece A, Style CC, Rede-Rite; segment on back surface (Phillips Lens Co.)	38 × 19
Philtex One-Piece A, Style CX, Rede-Rite; segment on front surface (Phillips Lens Co.)	40 × 19
Philtex One-Piece AL, Style CC, Rede-Rite; segment on back surface (Phillips Lens Co.)	38 × 30
Philtex One-Piece AL, Style CX, Rede-Rite; segment on front surface (Phillips Lens Co.)	40 × 35

through *either* the distance-vision portion or the near-vision portion of his bifocal lenses. For arm's length vision, the near point of accommodation through the *distance* portion of the lens is beyond the object of regard, and through the *near* portion of the lens, the far point of accommodation is too close for the object of regard. Clear vision at arm's length, however, can be provided by the use of a trifocal lens. First introduced by Univis as Continuous Vision lenses, trifocal lenses have an intermediate segment located just above the near segment (as described in Section 8.1) with a power normally one-half that of the reading addition.

In the original Univis Continuous Vision lens, the height of the intermediate segment was 6 mm; later, an 8-mm "occupational" segment was introduced. At the present time, almost all trifocals have an intermediate segment 7 mm high. Trifocal lenses are available in straight-top styles, in both fused and one-piece forms. Round (hemispheric) trifocals are made with one-piece construction only. Representative trifocal lenses are illustrated in Figure 8–14 and are listed in Tables 8–5 and 8–6.

8.7. Quadrifocals

Quadrifocals are useful for patients who not only require the intermediate-vision range of a trifocal lens but also perform much close work above eye level. All current quadrifocals are straight-top fused construction. Some patients report that these lenses restrict their field of view for nonoccupational uses such as driving. Representative quadrifocals are listed in Table 8–7.

TABLE 8–5
Representative Glass Fused Trifocals

Name (Co.)	Segment Size
6 × 22 Ribbon Seg (Vision-Ease)	6 × 22
FT 6 × 22 (Vision-Ease)	6 × 22
FT 6 × 28 (Vision-Ease)	6 × 28
FT 7 × 23 (Vision-Ease)	7 × 23
7 × 24 C Style (Vision-Ease)	7 × 24
Kote-Line (Lantz)	7 × 25
FTT 7 × 25 (Sola)	7 × 25
FT 7 × 25 mm (Vision-Ease)	7 × 25
FT 7 × 25 (X-Cel)	7 × 25
Kote-Line (Lantz)	7 × 28
FTT 7 × 28 (Sola)	7 × 28
FT 7 × 28 (Vision-Ease)	7 × 28
FT 7 × 28 (X-Cel)	7 × 28
Kote-Line (Lantz)	7 × 35
FTT 7 × 35 (Sola)	7 × 35
FT 7 × 35 (Vision-Ease)	7 × 35
FT 7 × 35 (X-Cel)	7 × 35
FT 8 × 25 (Vision-Ease)	8 × 25
FT 10 × 25 (Vision-Ease)	10 × 25
FT 10 × 28 (Vision-Ease)	10 × 28
FT 10 × 35 (Vision-Ease)	10 × 35

TABLE 8–6
Representative Glass One-Piece Trifocals

Name (Co.)	Segment Size
Philtex One-Piece AL, Style CX; segment on front surface (Phillips Lens Co.)	7–8 × 28
Philtex One-Piece A, Style CX; segment on back surface (Phillips Lens Co.)	7.5–8.5 × 32
Philtex One-Piece X, Style CC; segment on back surface (Phillips Lens Co.)	7.5–8.5 × 32
Executive (American Optical)	7 × —
Trifield (Vision-Ease)	7 × —
E-Style (X-Cel)	7 × —

TABLE 8–7
Representative Glass Quadrifocals

Manufacturer	Style	Size		Segment Separation
		Top	Bottom	
Lantz	Straight-top	25	7 × 25	10
		28	7 × 28	10
		35	7 × 35	13
Vision-Ease	Straight-top	25	7 × 25	13
		28	7 × 28	13
X-Cel	Straight-top	25	7 × 25	13
		28	7 × 28	13
		35	7 × 35	15

8.8. Plastic Multifocal Lenses

In recent years, plastic multifocal lenses have taken an increasing share of the ophthalmic lens market. As demand has increased, additional styles have become available. At the present time, all plastic multifocals are of *one-piece* construction. The multifocal segment is usually located on the front side of the lens. The lenses are produced either in the finished form, with both sides finished, or in the semifinished form, with only the front side molded by the manufacturer. When only the front surface has been finished, the laboratory used by the practitioner must finish the back surface to the required prescription.

The traditional *thermosetting* plastic (such as CR-39) multifocals include those having round segments, which are available in 22-, 24-, 25-, 28-, and 35-mm diameters. Straight-top segments are available in 22-, 25-, 28-, and 35-mm widths. Full-field Executive-style bifocals are made available by several manufacturers.

A wide variety of thermosetting plastic *trifocals* are also available. The most common types are the straight-top, round-bottom trifocals, available in 7 × 22-mm, 7 × 28-mm, and 8 × 35-mm segments. In addition, the Executive-style trifocal is available with a 7-mm intermediate segment. An increasing range of polycarbonate *thermoplastic* multifocals is also available. Polycarbonate bifocals are available in straight-top 25-, 28-, and 35-mm widths and with the Executive-style segment. Polycarbonate lenses are also available in straight-top 7 × 28-mm-wide trifocals.

Several manufacturers have recently introduced bifocals of high-index plastic material which ranges in refractive index from 1.54 to 1.60. Presently, high-index plastic bifocals are of the straight-top construction in 28- and 35-mm widths; a 7 × 28-mm-wide trifocal is also available in high-index plastic material. Representative plastic bifocals, double bifocals, and trifocals are listed in Tables 8–8, 8–9, and 8–10.

8.9. Occupational Multifocals

The prescription/spectacle design that meets the general visual requirements of presbyopes does not usually suffice for special occupational tasks. In recent years, great interest and concern has focused on the visual requirements of

video display terminals (VDT) operators. The rapid trend to computerization has introduced VDTs into millions of offices, work stations, and homes. Many VDT operators experience a variety of eye-related symptoms associated with their work. This result is not unexpected because an examination of the VDT work station reveals that VDT operators are required to use their eyes in ways they have not previously used them.

Presbyopia and improper correction of presbyopia for VDT use are frequent causes of symptoms.[1] An inappropriate prescription and lens design for VDT visual function causes the user to tilt his or her head backward and to lean forward toward the VDT, which produces poor vision and muscle pain, especially in the neck, shoulders, and back. The goal in prescribing for the visual needs of VDT operators is to ensure that the prescription provides (1) focusing for the proper working distance, (2) comfortable head and eye positions, (3) a sufficiently wide field of view to reduce excessive eye and head movements, and (4) illumination and glare control. Not all VDT operators use VDTs in the

TABLE 8–8
Representative Plastic Bifocals

Material	Index	Style	Manufacturer	Segment Size
CR-39	1.498	Round	Silor	22, 24, 25
			Aire-o-Lite	22, 25, 28
			Signet Armorlite	22, 24
			Sola	22, 24, 40
			Vision-Ease	22, 25, 40
			X-Cel	22
			Younger	22, 40
			American Optical	24
			Phillips Lens Co.	26
CR-39	1.498	Straight-top	Signet Armorlite	22, 25, 28, 35
			Vision-Ease	22, 25, 28, 35
			American Optical	22, 28
			Silor	25, 28, 35
			X-Cel	25, 28, 35
			Younger	25, 28, 35, 45
CR-39	1.498	Modified Straight-top	Vision-Ease	25, 28
			Rodenstock	28, 40
CR-39	1.498	Executive-style	American Optical	—
			Orcolite	—
			Signet Armorlite	—
			Silor	—
Spectralite	1.537	Straight-top	Sola	28
High-Index	1.55	Straight-top	Younger	28, 35
High-Index	1.56	Straight-top	Signet Armorlite	28, 35
			Vision-Ease	28, 35
			Younger	28, 35
High-Index	1.57	Straight-top	X-Cel	28, 35
Polycarbonate	1.586	Straight-top	Aire-o-Lite	25, 28, 35
			Vision-Ease	25, 28, 35
			Gentex	28, 35
			Orcolite	25, 28, 35
		Executive-style	Gentex	—
High-Index	1.60	Straight-top	Optima	28
			Silor	28

TABLE 8–9
Representative Plastic Double-Segment Bifocals

Material	Style	Manufacturer	Segment/Size Top/Bottom	Segment Separation
CR-39	Double Round	Aire-o-Lite	25/25	14
CR-39	Double Straight-top	Sola	25/28	15
		Vision-Ease	25/25	13
		Vision-Ease	35/35	15
		X-Cel	28/28	14
		Younger	28/28	14
CR-39	Double	American Optical	—	14
Executive-style	Orcolite	—	—	14
	X-Cel	—	—	14

TABLE 8–10
Representative Plastic Trifocals

Material	Index	Style	Manufacturer	Size
CR-39	1.498	Straight-top	Orcolite	7 × 25, 7 × 28, 8 × 35
			Signet Armorlite	7 × 25, 7 × 28, 7 × 35
			Silor	7 × 25, 7 × 28, 8 × 35
			Sola	7 × 25, 7 × 28, 8 × 35
			Vision-Ease	7 × 25, 7 × 28, 8 × 35
			X-Cel	7 × 25, 7 × 28, 8 × 35
			Younger	7 × 28
CR-39	1.498	Modified Straight-top	Rodenstock	10 × 40
CR-39	1.498	Executive-style	American Optical	7 × —
			Orcolite	7 × —
			Signet Armorlite	7 × —
			Sola	7 × —
			X-Cel	7 × —
CR-39	1.498	Hemisphere	Aire-o-Lite	7 × 22
			Younger Ultex	8 × 32
Spectralite	1.537	Straight-top	Sola	8 × 35
High-Index	1.56	Straight-top	Signet Armorlite	7 × 28
			Vision-Ease	7 × 28
High-Index	1.57	Straight-top	X-Cel	7 × 28
Polycarbonate	1.586	Straight-top	Gentex	7 × 28
			Orcolite	7 × 28
			Vision-Ease	7 × 28

same manner. Prescribing for the presbyopic VDT user requires crucial considerations such as

1. Distance from the eyes to the screen
2. Distance from the eyes to the source document being typed (if possible, the document should be located close to the screen and at the same distance as the screen from the eyes)
3. Distance from the eyes to the keyboard
4. Position of the screen in relation to eye level (if possible, the center of the screen should be 10–20 degrees below eye level)
5. Reduction of overt glare or reflections from the screen

For early presbyopia, the prescription of +0.50 to +0.75 D add made in single-vision form may provide a suitable solution. This prescription provides a wide field of view;

its disadvantage is that distance vision is slightly blurred. For advanced presbyopes, bifocals that incorporate the lens power for the screen distance in the top of the lenses and the near-vision power in the segment (set low for reading) may work well. To eliminate diffuse reflections, a neutral-density filter with an antireflective coating is effective; for specular reflections, neutral-density filters with an antireflective coating and *dense-mesh filters* (filters with a greater proportion of strand-to-pore area) are equally effective.[2]

Many special trifocals have been designed to assist in work-related visual performance. These lenses are characterized by having an intermediate-range segment with a large vertical dimension; most also provide a generous lateral field of view (Figure 8–18). The power of the intermediate addition is usually higher than the conventional 50% of the near addition and runs from 60% to 74%.

The cathode ray tube (CRT) trifocal was designed specifically for VDT operators (Figure 8–18A). The vertical dimension of the intermediate segment is 14 mm and provides a generous vertical field of view. This lens is suitable for any occupation that requires a high percentage of work done at an intermediate distance.

The ED, FD, and F/D trifocals (Figures 8–18B, 8–18C) are Executive-style lenses incorporating a straight-top near segment. This kind of lens has the advantage that the intermediate field extends both above and below the near segment and on either side of that segment. The KCB and CRT DataLite trifocals are straight-top trifocals that are 10 mm × 35-mm wide (Figure 8–18D), 12 × 35-mm wide (Figure 8–18E) and 14 × 35-mm wide (Figure 8–18F). The EPD trifocal (Figure 8–18G) is 14 × 35 mm wide and is the only *glass* trifocal in the group. The Rodenstock curved-top trifocal has a 10 × 40-mm wide segment (Figure 8–18H).

In a study by Barresi and Rosenthal,[3] New York office workers who reported job-related vision problems received job evaluations and eye examinations and were provided with occupational glasses as appropriate. Frequent VDT users (those who spend more than two-thirds of the work day using a VDT) reported higher symptom prevalence and severity than did non-VDT users for headaches, back and neck ache, eyestrain, blurred near vision, eye irritation, and double vision. A high proportion (71.27%) reported that eye problems at work reduced their work efficiency or accuracy. Occupational eyeglasses were prescribed for 76.8% of the 775 study subjects. The occupational glasses differed from the subjects' regular glasses in the following manner:

Change in lens power	44.7%
Change in segment height	33.9%
Tint provided	24.2%
Change in lens style (from single-vision to multifocals)	12.6%

In a follow-up survey, 93.8% of the respondents who had received occupational eyeglasses reported improved comfort and resolution of symptoms; 82.2% reported improved quality or efficiency in their work.

Conventional bifocals, trifocals, and progressive addition lenses that are not modified for a VDT-work distance may be usable, but they may also contribute to patients' complaints about visual discomfort and neck, shoulder, and back pain. Occupational progressive addition lenses are discussed in Section 8.31.

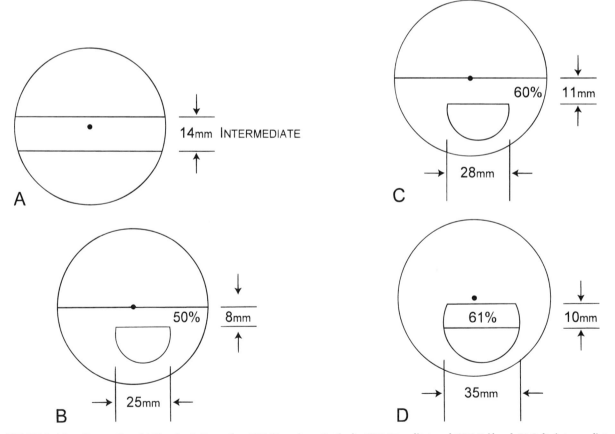

FIGURE 8–18. **Occupational trifocals. A, Executive CRT (American Optical), CRT (Orcolite) and CRT Trifocal (X-Cel); intermediate addition varies with power of near add; CR-39. B, ED Tri (Sola) Executive-style lens with straight-top segment; CR-39. C, FD (Orcolite) and F/D Trifocal (X-Cel) Executive-style lens with straight-top segment; CR-39. D, KCB, 10 × 35 (X-Cel) straight-top trifocal; CR-39. E, KCB, 12 × 35 (X-Cel); CR-39. F, CRT DataLite, 14 × 35 (Vision-Ease) straight-top trifocal; CR-39. G, EDP, 14 × 35 (Lantz) straight-top trifocal; glass. H, C style, 10 × 40 (Rodenstock) curved-top trifocal; CR-39.**

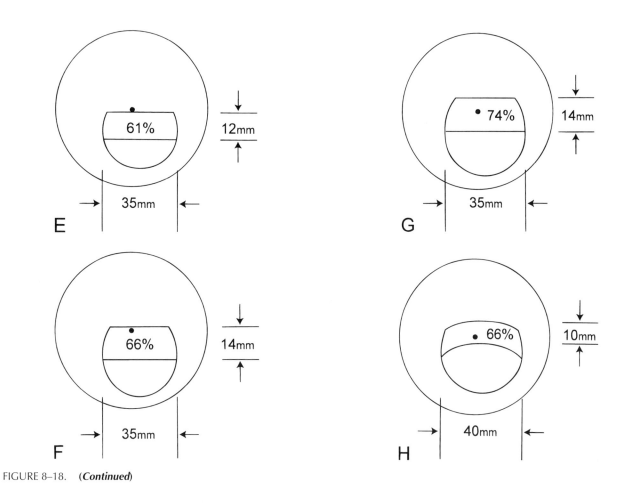

FIGURE 8–18.   (*Continued*)

MANUFACTURING PROCESSES FOR MULTIFOCAL LENSES

8.10. Glass Multifocals

Glass multifocal lenses are manufactured by using the processes of both fused and one-piece construction. These processes are illustrated in Figures 8–19 through 8–22.

Fused Multifocals

Fused multifocal lenses (Figure 8–19) are constructed of two or more separate pieces of glass fused together at a high temperature. A blank is selected for the major portion of the lens, and the concave side is ground to match the curvature of the fusing slab on which it rests. This prevents sagging of the blank's convex surface during fusion and prevents changes in curvature of the countersink surface. A countersink or depression curve is then ground and polished over the reading portion usually on the convex surface of the major lens. The curvature,

depth, and position of the countersink must be precisely determined to provide a segment with the desired amount of power in the reading addition. The countersink is usually made slightly larger than the diameter of the finished segment.

The segment button is made of a single piece of glass for *round* bifocals, of two truncated pieces of glass for *straight-*

FIGURE 8–19.   **Manufacturing process for a round fused bifocal lens such as the Kryptok.**

top bifocals, and of three truncated pieces for *ribbon* bifocals and *straight-top* trifocals. For round fused bifocals, the segments are usually made of barium crown glass or flint glass, both of which have higher indices of refraction than that of the major lens. For straight-top bifocals, the upper part of the segment button has the same composition and index of refraction as the major lens, but the lower portion is barium crown glass (Figure 8–20). For trifocals, the upper portion of the segment button is identical to the major lens, the intermediate portion has a higher index of refraction than the major lens, and the lower portion has a still higher index. For ribbon segments, the upper and lower portions are identical to the major lens, and the middle portion has a higher index than that of the major lens.

If the segment button is composed of more than one piece of glass, the truncated pieces are fused along their thin edges to form a composite segment button. Some manufacturers coat the truncated edges with pigmented coatings before fusion to help reduce the reflections from the segment line. The segment button is then ground and polished to precisely match the curvature of the countersink surface. The segment button and countersink surfaces of the major lens are meticulously cleaned and then assembled for fusing. The assembled blank then goes to the furnace room where it is heated until fusion occurs and is then slowly annealed and cooled to room temperature.

For the front surface, a generator is used to remove excess glass from the protruding button, to obtain the desired front surface curvature, and to reduce the segment to its approximate finished size. The front surface is then finely ground, smoothed, and polished to a precise finish. A final inspection verifies the accuracy of the procedures. The curvature placed on the front surface is always spherical; if a cylinder is required, it is placed on the back surface, in negative toric form. (If the front surface were made toric, there would be a difference in the cylinder power in the distance and near portions because of the difference in refractive indices, and for larger cylinders, a toric front surface would alter the *shape* of the segment.)

Once the front surface has been finished, the blank is in the *semifinished* form, which is the common form supplied to optical prescription laboratories. The back surface is then finished by the laboratory to the requirements of the prescription. Because the front surface on a semifinished blank is *fixed*, the curvature of the surface is often referred to as the *base curve*. When the front surface of a *straight-top* fused multifocal lens is completed, the ophthalmic crown glass portion of the segment becomes indistinguishable

from the major lens. As described for the Courmettes design, the segment blends into the major lens because it has the same index of refraction as that of the major lens. The border between the major lens and the higher-index portion of the major lens is visible because of the difference in the *reflectivity* of the two types of glass.

One-Piece Glass Multifocals

One-piece glass multifocal lenses are made from a single, homogeneous piece of glass, usually ophthalmic crown glass with an index of refraction of 1.523 and an Abbe value near 59. The increase in plus power in the reading portion is provided by a change of curvature on either the front or the back surface of the lens. Ingenious machinery has been designed to achieve the desired accuracy.

Round, or Ultex-style, one-piece bifocals are made by starting with a rough blank in the form of a large, saucer-shaped disk molded to the approximate curves to be ground (Figure 8–21). The molded saucers are then ground and polished on the surface opposite the segment side to aid final inspection of the dividing line between the distance and near portions of the lens. The blanks are then prepared for the segment side to be ground. The surface containing the segment is ground by using special abrasive wheels having two adjoining curves that grind the peripheral (distance) and the central (reading) areas on the same surface. The difference in curvature between these two areas determines the power of the bifocal addition. The abrasive wheel used for trifocals has three curves, each cutting its own area automatically. Thus, as it rotates about its center, the abrasive wheel simultaneously cuts the two fields of a bifocal lens or the three fields of a trifocal lens.

Each area on the front surface is then finely ground, smoothed, and polished. When the segment is placed on the back surface of the lens, the segment area has a longer radius of curvature (less minus power) than that of the distance portion. However, when the segment is on the front surface, the segment has a shorter radius (more plus power) than that of the distance portion. If any cylinder is needed, it is ground on the side opposite the segment. The base curve is the surface power of the distance area on the segment side of the lens.

The production of *straight-top*, or Executive-style, one-piece multifocal lenses is initiated by mounting molded blanks on a truncated sphere (Figure 8–22). A rotating-cup tool generates and polishes the reading segment surface as

FIGURE 8–20. **Manufacturing process for a straight-top fused bifocal lens.**

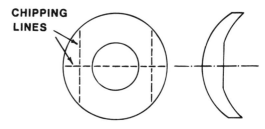

FIGURE 8–21. **Manufacturing process for an Ultex-style one-piece bifocal lens.**

FIGURE 8–22.   **Manufacturing process for an Executive one-piece bifocal lens. (Modified from J. Davis. A Study of Lens Construction and Use. *Int. Ophthalmol. Clin.*, Vol. 11, No. 1, p. 234, 1971.)**

the block and the mounted lens rotate in a circular path around a fixed axis of revolution. Because the generating and polishing tool is restricted to the lower portion of the front surface of the lens, a straight dividing line is created between the distance and reading portions of the lens. The reading area has a shorter radius (more plus power) than the distance area. Cylindrical power is ground on the back surface, with the base curve of the lens designated as the front surface power for the distance portion of the lens.

8.11. Plastic Multifocals

Most plastic multifocal lenses in the United States are made of CR-39 (thermosetting) or polycarbonate (thermoplastic) material. Lenses made from these two materials are manufactured by somewhat different methods.

Thermosetting multifocal lenses are commonly made by pouring liquid monomer, to which a suitable catalyst has been added, into casting molds. When the liquid is heated, polymerization takes place. To obtain precise lens curvatures and smooth surfaces, the casting molds are usually made of glass, with their highly polished mold surfaces—

surfaces polished more meticulously than the glass surfaces of spectacle lenses.

The process of manufacturing the segment surface of such a mold is unusual. First, the surface of the distance portion is generated on an ophthalmic crown glass blank that then undergoes chemical tempering. Ordinarily, toughening is done after a lens is completed, but if the lens were toughened after the reading surface had been finished, the distance surface would likely become distorted. After the distance surface is polished, the depressed segment surface is cut and polished. The mold retains the properties of a toughened lens because the toughened layer extends beyond the depressed segment surface.

For economic reasons, molds usually are not made for lens prescriptions that fall outside the normal range of use. For these prescriptions, a cast CR-39 blank is individually surfaced by conventional methods. To make semifinished blanks, the surface containing the segment (usually the front surface) is cast and the second surface is cut and polished at the prescription laboratory by methods similar to those used in finishing glass lenses. For thermosetting lenses that are finished by the manufacturer, *both* surfaces of the lens are cast.

Thermoplastic polycarbonate lenses are made by a process known as *injection molding*. First, the solid material is melted down and injected into a steel mold at a temperature of approximately 400°C. During the injection process, the polycarbonate assumes, under pressure, the same configuration as the highly polished steel mold. The mold squeezes the lens to prevent shrinkage and to ensure accuracy of the surfaces. Each lens-forming cycle requires approximately 90 to 130 seconds. The lenses are then inspected and sent through a coating machine. The surfaces of polycarbonate material are soft and are usually susceptible to scratches—far more so than the surfaces of CR-39 material. Therefore, all polycarbonate lenses are coated with an *organosilicon* material, which greatly increases the surface hardness. Although the first coatings used on polycarbonate lenses could not be tinted, the coatings currently in use may be tinted.

OPTICAL PRINCIPLES OF MULTIFOCAL LENS DESIGN

8.12. Powers of the Distance and Reading Portions

The total (resultant) refracting power in the reading portion of a bifocal lens consists of the power of the distance prescription combined with the power of the bifocal addition (*add*), as shown in the following examples:

Power of distance portion: +1.00 DS –0.50 DC x 180.
Power of reading addition: +2.00 DS.
Power of reading portion: +3.00 DS –0.50 DC x 180.

The formula for a bifocal lens is written so as to represent the formula for the distance portion of the lens combined

with the power of the reading addition, As shown below (for the right lens):

OD +1.00 DS –0.50 DC x 180, +2.00 D add.

When this formula appears without further instructions in a lens prescription, the prescription may be filled with a bifocal lens or with two single-vision lenses, one for distance vision and one for near vision. The power of the lens for near - vision corresponds to the power of the near portion of the bifocal prescription. When one writes an order for a pair of lenses, the power of the distance portion is referred to as the *distance* prescription, and the power of the reading portion is referred to as the *near* prescription.

8.13. One-Piece Bifocals

Cemented and Ultex-Style Bifocals

The powers of the distance and reading portions of cemented and Ultex-style one-piece bifocals may be analyzed in the following manner. In a sagittal section of a cemented or Ultex-style one-piece bifocal, the lens can be considered as being made of two components: the major lens and the segment. For a cemented bifocal, the *wafer* is the segment. For a one-piece bifocal, both the major lens and the segment are constructed from a solid piece of glass, with the segment usually on the back surface. In such a bifocal, the surface dividing the major lens and the segment is purely *imaginary*, but it can be represented by a continuation of the back surface of the distance portion of the lens (Figure 8–23). The major lens of a cemented or Ultex-style one-piece bifocal encompasses both the distance field and the reading field, but the segment encompasses only the reading field. The glass in the segment has the same index of refraction (1.523) as the glass in the major lens.

For a cemented bifocal, the front side of the segment (which is cemented to the back of the major lens) has a power corresponding to the power of the back surface of the major lens, but it is opposite in sign. The power of the major lens is that of the distance prescription. If F_1 is the front surface power of the distance portion of the lens, the approximate power of the distance portion is given by the formula

$$\text{approximate power of distance portion} = F_1 + F_2. \quad (8.1)$$

If F_3 is the front surface power of the segment and F_4 the back surface power of the segment, the power of the reading addition is equal to the power of the segment and is given by the formula

$$\text{power of reading addition} = F_3 + F_4. \quad (8.2)$$

However, since

$$F_3 = -F_2,$$

the power of the reading addition = $F_4 - F_2$; (8.3)

hence, the power of the reading addition can be determined directly by measuring F_4 and F_2 with a lens measure. This can be done for either a one-piece bifocal or a ce-

mented bifocal (even after the wafer has been cemented to the lens).

For a one-piece bifocal, the segment is ground in such a way that it has a thin edge. The edge represents the intersection of the two spherical surfaces and, consequently, is circular. The *upper* portion of the Ultex A segment therefore has a thin, circular edge, but at the *lower* portion of the lens, the edge of the lens does not extend to the (imaginary) circle represented by the segment, with the result that the lower edge of the segment has a finite thickness (Figure 8–23). However, a one-piece *prism* bifocal has a round prism segment that is thick on one side and thin on the other, and the amount of prism is specified in terms of the prismatic effect at the geometric center of the segment.

The center thickness of a round, feather-edged, one-piece segment can be calculated by use of the following formula, in which h represents one-half the diameter (or one-half the width) of the segment:

$$\text{center thickness} = \frac{h^2 F_{\text{add}}}{2(n' - n)}. \quad (8.4)$$

The Executive Bifocal

This lens can be considered as a single-vision distance lens on which has been placed a reading segment with a power of the required addition, and with a back surface curvature matching the front surface curvature of the single-vision distance lens (Figure 8–24). The segment could be placed toward either the nasal or the temporal side of the lens, which would create a *decentered* segment. In practice, decentration is achieved by grinding the distance center where it is required *after* the back surface of the lens has been finished. In this manner, two different curvatures are ground on the front surface of the blank. The distance portion of the blank is ground with a preselected curvature, and a steeper curve (more plus power) is ground on the lower (reading area) portion of the blank. The difference between the powers of these two surfaces determines the reading addition.

The power of the upper (distance) portion of the lens corresponds to the power of the distance portion in ordi-

FIGURE 8–23.   **An Ultex-style bifocal, showing the imaginary surface dividing the segment and the major lens in the near portion of the lens.**

FIGURE 8–24.   **An Executive-style bifocal considered as a single-vision distance lens with a reading segment.**

nary bifocal terminology, and the power of the lower portion of the lens is the *total power* (distance power plus add) through the reading portion.

The centers of curvature (C_s and C_u) of the two front surface radii (r_s and r_u) fall on the common axis that intersects the lens surface at the point of minimal thickness of the *ledge* (Figure 8–25). The optical center falls on the common axis at the point of minimal ledge thickness. The position of the segment optical center is fixed, as in the case of any semifinished bifocal blank. When the back surface of the reading portion of the lens is finished (surfaced), the position of the optical center of the segment is not changed; it remains as the point of minimum ledge thickness on the front surface. The optical center can, however, be decentered horizontally or vertically, as with any bifocal lens, by specifying its position in relation to the geometric center of the distance portion of the finished lens.

The *base curve* of the lens is the surface power of the distance portion on the segment side of the lens.

8.14. Fused Bifocals

For fused bifocals, three surfaces are considered: (1) the front surface of the major lens, which is continuous with the front surface of the segment and has a radius of curvature r_1; (2) the back surface of the major lens, whose radius of curvature is denoted by r_2; and (3) the back surface of the segment, which contacts and becomes identical with the countersink surface of the major lens, and whose radius of curvature is r_3 (Figure 8–26). If we define the index of refraction of the glass comprising the major lens as n', the index of the glass comprising the segment as n'', the index of air as n, and if we assume that all three surfaces are spherical, the powers of the distance and reading portions of the lens can be represented by the following equations:

power of the distance portion

$$F_D = \frac{n' - n}{r_1} + \frac{n - n'}{r_2}. \tag{8.5}$$

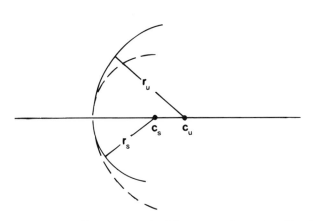

FIGURE 8–25.   **The common axis of the centers of curvature (C_s and C_u) of the two front curves (r_s and r_u) of an Executive-style bifocal.**

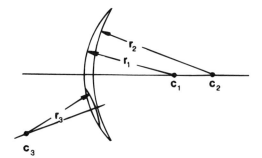

FIGURE 8–26.   **The three radii of curvature in the reading portion of a fused bifocal.**

power of the reading portion

$$F_R = \frac{n'' - n}{r_1} + \frac{n' - n''}{r_3} + \frac{n - n'}{r_2}. \tag{8.6}$$

Fundamentally, the power of the reading addition is equal to the power of the reading portion minus the power of the distance portion, and is given by the following formula:

power of reading addition

$$F_A = \frac{n'' - n}{r_1} + \frac{n' - n''}{r_3} + \frac{n - n'}{r_2} - \frac{n' - n}{r_1} - \frac{n - n'}{r_2}$$

$$= \frac{n'' - n}{r_1} + \frac{n' - n''}{r_3} - \frac{n' - n}{r_1}$$

$$= \frac{n'' - n}{r_1} - \frac{n' - n}{r_1} + \frac{n' - n''}{r_3}$$

$$F_A = \frac{n'' - n'}{r_1} + \frac{n' - n''}{r_3}. \tag{8.7}$$

The term $(n'' - n')/r_1$ is equivalent to the power of the front surface of the segment covered by the material of the major lens, and the term $(n' - n'')/r_3$ is the power of the fused surface between the segment and the major lens.

This condition actually existed for the cemented Kryptok bifocal lens—the segment (instead of being fused into the countersink) was cemented to the front surface of the lens, and the whole front surface was covered with a concentric shell of glass having the same index of refraction as that of the major lens.

Important Note. The power of the segment of a fused bifocal in air is *not* equal to the power of the reading addition, as it is for the wafer of a cemented bifocal or for the imaginary segment of a one-piece bifocal. The reading addition of a fused bifocal lens is obtained by the *gain in power* on the front surface of the segment compared with that of the front surface of the distance portion *plus* the power of the fused surface between the segment and the major lens. Equation 8.7 indicates that the power of the reading addition corresponds to the total power of the segment if the segment is completely embedded in glass having an index equal to n'. Clearly, the gain in power on the front surface of the segment compared with that of the front surface of the distance portion is equal to the front surface power of the segment embedded in the major lens.

If every term of Equation 8.7 is multiplied by the term

$$\frac{n' - n}{n'' - n'},$$

we obtain

$$\frac{n' - n}{n'' - n'} F_A = \left(\frac{n' - n}{n'' - n'} \right) \left(\frac{n'' - n'}{r_1} \right)$$

$$+ \left(\frac{n' - n}{n'' - n'} \right) \left(\frac{n' - n''}{r_3} \right)$$

$$\frac{n' - n}{n'' - n'} F_A = \frac{n' - n}{r_1} + \left(\frac{n' - n}{n'' - n'} \right) (-1) \left(\frac{n'' - n'}{r_3} \right)$$

$$\frac{n' - n}{n'' - n'} F_A = \frac{n' - n}{r_1} - \frac{n' - n}{r_3}.$$

The quantity $(n' - n)/r_1$ represents the power of the front surface as measured by means of a lens measure and may be designated as F_1; the quantity $(n' - n)/r_3$ represents the power of the countersink curve (in air) as measured with a lens measure and is designated as F_C. Therefore,

$$\frac{n' - n}{n'' - n'} F_A = F_1 - F_C. \qquad (8.8)$$

Solving for F_C,

$$F_C = F_1 - \frac{n' - n}{n'' - n'} F_A, \qquad (8.9)$$

and solving for F_1,

$$F_1 = F_C + \frac{n' - n}{n'' - n'} F_A. \qquad (8.10)$$

Equation 8.9 is useful in calculating the countersink curve required to obtain a given reading addition when F_1 has been specified; Equation 8.10 is used to calculate F_1 when the countersink curve and the reading addition are known.

EXAMPLE 1

A 20-mm round bifocal segment is fused into a concave countersink surface having a radius of curvature of 50 cm on the front surface of the lens. The index of refraction of the distance portion of the lens is 1.51, and the index of refraction of the segment is 1.68. To obtain a +2.50-D add, what must the front surface power be?

$$F_1 = F_C + \frac{n' - n}{n'' - n'} F_A$$

$$= F_C + \frac{1.51 - 1.00}{1.68 - 1.57} (2.50)$$

$$F_C = \frac{n' - n}{r_C} = \frac{1.51 - 1.00}{-0.5} = -1.02$$

$$F_1 = -1.02 + \frac{0.51}{0.17} (2.50)$$

$$= -1.02 + 7.50$$

$$= +6.48 \text{ D}.$$

EXAMPLE 2

The refractive index of a fused front surface segment is 1.60, and the refractive index of the distance portion (carrier lens) is 1.50. The power of the front surface is +6.00 D, and the power of the countersink surface (in air) is –1.50 D. What is the power of the add?

$$\frac{n' - n}{n'' - n'} F_A = F_1 - F_C$$

$$\frac{1.50 - 1.00}{1.60 - 1.50} F_A = 6.00 - (-1.50)$$

$$5F_A = +7.50$$

$$F_A = \frac{+7.50}{5}$$

$$= +1.50 \text{ D}.$$

For a *finished lens* received from the laboratory, it is no longer possible to obtain a measurement of the countersink curve with a lens measure. In this case, the power of the add is found by (1) measuring the power of the reading portion by an optical method, (2) measuring the power of the distance portion either with a lens measure or by an optical method, and (3) subtracting the power of the distance portion from the power of the reading portion. In practice, a *lensometer* is used to determine the spherical or sphero-cylindrical formula of the major lens and then the spherical power of the reading portion. The power of the add is found by subtracting the spherical power of the distance portion from the spherical power of the reading portion.

Both the front and back surfaces of the segment are spherical (Figure 8–27); thus, for a *round* fused bifocal,

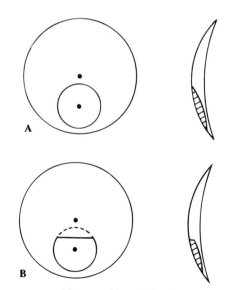

FIGURE 8–27.   **A, With a round fused bifocal, a feathered edge can be obtained; B, with a straight-top fused bifocal, the upper edge of the segment is relatively thick but a feathered edge can be obtained at the bottom of the segment.**

a feather-edged segment can be obtained by letting the two surfaces intersect at the boundary of the segment (A). The optical center lies at the geometric center of the segment, which is also the segment reference point. The upper edge of the segment of a *straight-top* fused bifocal, such as the X-Cel D, is relatively *thick*, but the remainder of the segment boundary is circular and progresses to a feathered edge at the bottom of the segment (Figure 8–27B). The Panoptik style and Vision-Ease C bifocals also have a thick edge at the top and a thin edge around the circular portion of the contour. In each case, the segment optical center lies at the center of the circular portion of the segment, which is also the reference point of the segment.

As stated above, Equations 8.9 and 8.10 indicate that the curvature of the countersink curve is used to obtain the desired amount of add in the finished lens. Because the power of the add is independent of the power of the back surface of the lens, the front surface of a bifocal blank can be finished at the factory; the grinding and polishing of the back surface, to meet the requirements of the patient's prescription, can be left to the laboratory. Semifinished bifocal blanks with adds from +0.50 to +3.00 D or more, in 0.25 D steps, are stocked by prescription laboratories, and a number of manufacturers supply blanks with higher adds by special order.

The term

$$\frac{n' - n}{n'' - n'}$$

is sometimes referred to as the *ratio*. The numerical value of this ratio is determined by the selection of glasses to be used in the two parts of the lens. For ophthalmic crown glass of index 1.523 and flint glass of index 1.69, the ratio is approximately 3/1. This means that the add will be changed by 1 D by changing the value of F_1 by 3 D. Rearranging Equation 8.9,

$$F_A = \frac{F_1 - F_C}{\text{ratio}}. \tag{8.11}$$

If the ratio = 3/1, and if F_1 = +4.50 D, and F_C = −1.50 D, the power of the add is +2.00 D. But if F_1 is increased by 3.00 D to +7.50 D, the power of the add is +3.00 D (increased 1 D in power). Using this relationship, if $n'' < n'$, a minus add is obtained. If enough information is known to calculate the power of the add, the thickness of the segment can easily be found by considering the segment as completely embedded in the distance portion of the lens. The thickness sometimes needs to be known to avoid grinding into the segment while finishing the back surface of the lens. If the segment is considered as completely embedded, as in the cemented Kryptok bifocal, the center thickness can be found by the equation

$$\text{center segment thickness} = \frac{h^2 F_A}{2(n'' - n')}. \tag{8.12}$$

A 22-mm round fused-front-surface bifocal has a distance power of +2.00 D and an add of +3.00 D. The index of refraction of the distance portion of the lens is 1.54 and that of the segment is 1.63. What is the center thickness of the segment?

$$t_C - t_P = \frac{h^2 F_A}{2(n'' - n')}$$

$$t_C - 0 = \frac{(0.011)^2(+3.00)}{2(1.63 - 1.54)}$$

$$t_C = \frac{(0.000121)(3)}{2(0.09)} = \frac{0.00363}{0.18}$$

$$= 0.002 \text{ m} = 2 \text{ mm.}$$

Some segments are available with thick edges all around, which permits the production of *prism segments*. The amount of prism is specified in terms of the prismatic effect at the segment reference point.

As shown in Figure 8–28, the *vertical* position of the segment of a finished lens is specified in terms of the height of the top of the segment above the bottom of the lens or in terms of the distance from the top of the segment to the geometric center of the distance portion of the lens. The *horizontal* position of the segment is specified in terms of the displacement of the segment center to the right or the left of the distance fitting point.

Segments with *toric* countersink surfaces could be produced, but because there is seldom an occasion for using such a lens, bifocals with segments of this type are not maintained as stock items.

For a fused bifocal lens with the segment embedded in the front surface (the usual situation), the front surface of the major lens has a spherical curvature which is identical and continuous with that of the segment; for a fused bifocal with the segment embedded in the back surface, the back surface is spherical and its curvature is continuous with that of the segment. As mentioned earlier, if the prescription for a fused bifocal requires a cylinder, the cylinder is ground on the side of the lens opposite the segment side.

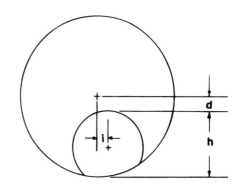

FIGURE 8–28. **Specification of the position of a fused bifocal segment, both vertically and horizontally.**

_____PERFORMANCE CHARACTERISTICS_____

8.15. Vertical Placement of the Optical Center of the Segment

To evaluate the performance of a given bifocal lens, one must know, in addition to the distance and near powers, the positions of the optical centers of the distance portion of the lens and of the segment, and the point in the lens through which the wearer's line of sight will pass during reading or other close work.

As discussed in Chapter 2, Section 2.17, all lenses function at their best when the optic axis of the lens passes through the center of rotation of the eye. Lens designers assume this when they specify the performance in the periphery of a lens. The level of the distance optical center of a bifocal lens, as with a single-vision lens, is determined on the basis of the amount of *pantoscopic tilt* of the lens—the distance optical center is lowered 1 mm from the center of the pupil for every 2 degrees of pantoscopic tilt. Because a pantoscopic tilt of 6 degrees is usually considered cosmetically desirable, the distance optical center is normally located *3 mm below* the point directly in front of the center of the pupil when the eyes are in the primary position (Figure 8–29). The position of the distance optical center of a bifocal lens is usually specified, both laterally and vertically, in relation to the *geometric center* of the lens.

An important respect in which various bifocal styles differ from one another is the distance from the segment pole to the segment top. For fused and one-piece *round* knife-edged segments, the optical center of the segment lies at the geometric center of the segment. For example, the distance from the segment optical center to the segment top in the case of a 22-mm round fused segment is 11 mm; the corresponding distance for a 38 × 19-mm Ultex A-style seg-

ment is 19 mm. These and other segment optical center locations are illustrated in Figure 8–30. For regular or modified *straight-top* fused bifocal segments with thick (rather than knife-edged) segment tops, the segment optical center is located at the center of the circular contour of the segment. For example, for a 22 × 16-mm D-style segment, the distance from the segment optical center to the segment top is 5 mm. For the Executive-style *one-piece* bifocal, the segment optical center is located *at* the segment top. For prism segments with thick edges all around, the contour of the segment is of no assistance in locating the optical center of the segment.

For an individual who does not wear spectacles or who wears single-vision lenses, when the eyes are lowered during reading, the *head* is also lowered. Consequently, for a wearer of single-vision lenses, the lines of sight for the two eyes pass through the lenses at only a slightly lower level for reading than that for distance vision. However, for a bifocal wearer, the head must be kept more or less erect to see through the bifocal segments (some practitioners tell novice bifocal wearers to "point with the chin, rather than with the eyes," when they read). Fry and Ellerbrock[4] found that when a person reads, the foveal line of sight passes through a point in the lens (which they called the *reading center*) approximately 11 mm below the point directly in front of the center of the pupil when the eyes are in the primary position (Figure 8–31). If the lens has a pantoscopic tilt of 6 degrees and the distance optical center is 3 mm below the pupillary level (so that the optic axis of the lens can pass through the center of rotation of the eye), the *reading center* is located approximately 8 mm below the distance optical center. If one assumes that the visible iris diameter in the vertical meridian averages 12 mm, and that

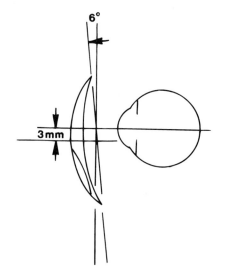

FIGURE 8–29. **A lens with a pantoscopic tilt of 6 degrees, with the distance optical center located 3 mm below the point directly in front of the center of the pupil.**

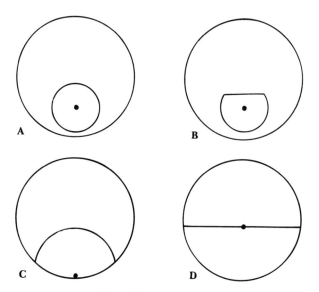

FIGURE 8–30. **Positions of the segment optical center. A, Kryptok segment, 11 mm below segment top; B, straight-top fused, 5 mm below segment top; C, Ultex-style, 19 mm below segment top; D, Executive-style, segment center at segment top.**

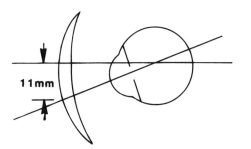

FIGURE 8–31.   **The reading center, located approximately 11 mm below the point directly in front of the pupil.**

the segment top falls at the lower border of the iris (or 6 mm below the center of the pupil), the reading center falls 5 mm below the top of the segment, as shown in Figure 8–32. If it is considered desirable for the wearer to read through the segment at the level of the segment optical center, the segment center should be located *5 mm below* the segment top.

8.16. Lateral Placement of the Optical Center of the Segment

When one determines the specifications for a pair of bifocal lenses, the segment optical centers should be decentered inward from the distance fitting points of the two lenses, so that they coincide with (or fall directly above or below) the reading centers. In reality, the segment optical centers seldom fall exactly at the reading centers; they may be displaced horizontally or vertically.

The inward displacement of the segment optical center from the distance fitting point is referred to as *segment inset.* Segment inset is always *in* unless the segment position is manipulated to provide a horizontal prismatic effect. Segments are inset for two purposes: (1) to ensure that the fields of view through the two segments coincide (or overlap) for the two eyes and (2) to prevent the segment from producing any horizontal prismatic effects at the reading center. When the optical center of the segment is placed

directly above or below the reading center, the segment itself produces no horizontal prismatic effect at the reading center.

The *field of view* is the area of useful vision that can be obtained with the eye held stationary, with the center of the entrance pupil used as the reference point. Field of view may also be thought of as the solid angle of vision for the stationary eye, subtended at the center of the entrance pupil. A distinction must be made between the *field of view* and the *field of fixation,* which is the area of object space within which direct foveal vision can be obtained by moving the eye with the head stationary. The reference point for the field of fixation is the center of rotation of the eye. Field of view and field of fixation are illustrated in Figure 8–33.

The correct amount of segment inset depends on:

1. The distance interpupillary separation (usually referred to as the *distance PD*)
2. The distance from the back pole of the lens to the center of rotation of the eye (usually called the *stop distance*)
3. The fixation distance
4. The power of the distance correction, in the horizontal meridian

Segment inset is normally determined by measuring the distance and near PDs (using the method described in Chapter 9), and then insetting each of the segments one-half the difference between the distance and near PDs. Thus, if the distance PD is 64 mm and the near PD is 60 mm, the segment inset is 2 mm for each lens. A near PD taken without the distance-correcting lenses before the eyes or calculated on the basis of geometric relationships ignores the *prismatic effects* of the distance correction (in the horizontal merid-

FIGURE 8–32.   **A round fused bifocal, showing segment top at lower border of the iris, with reading center located 5 mm below the segment top and 11 mm below the center of the pupil.**

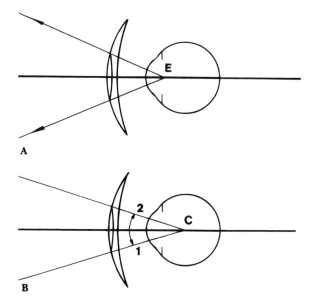

FIGURE 8–33.   **The concepts of field of view of a bifocal segment. A, peripheral field of view, subtended at the center of the entrance pupil, E; B, field of fixation, or macular field of view, subtended at the center of rotation, C.**

ian) on the positions of the segment optical centers. For example, when the eyes of a hyperope wearing plus lenses centered for the distance PD converges on a close object, the visual axes move inward and pass through points in the lenses located nasally from the distance optical centers. At such points, *base-out* prismatic effects are produced, and the eyes must converge *to a greater extent* than is necessary without glasses. On the other hand, for a myope wearing minus lenses centered for the distance PD converging the visual axes produces a *base-in prismatic effect*, with the result that the eyes are required to converge *less* than is necessary without glasses.

Scott Sterling[5] mathematically determined the amount of segment inset required for a 40-cm reading distance to make the reading fields coincide. His calculations depended on the powers of the distance portions of the lenses and were based on the assumptions that the visual axes pass through the segment optical centers and that the distance from the lens to the center of rotation of each eye (the *stop distance*) is 25 mm. The amounts of segment inset for various lens powers and PDs, as determined by Sterling, are shown in Table 8–11. Use of this table is recommended.

Total inset is defined as the lateral displacement of the segment optical center from the geometric center of the lens. When the distance portion of the lens has no power or contains only prismatic power (in the form of a plano prism), total inset may be inward, zero, or outward, depending on the position of the fitting point of the distance lens in relation to the geometric center of the lens. If the fitting point falls *inward, on,* or *not farther than 1.5 mm outward* from the geometric center of the lens, the total inset is *in*. However, if the fitting point falls *2 mm outward* from

the geometric center, the total inset is *zero*. If the fitting point falls *farther than 2 mm* outward from the geometric center, the total inset is *out*. These relationships are illustrated in Figure 8–34.

The following examples will illustrate the concepts of segment inset and total inset.

EXAMPLE 1

Given the distance prescription –2.00 DS with +2.00-D add, both eyes (OU). The frame size is 50 mm with a distance between lenses (DBL) of 18 mm, and the patient's PD is 64 mm for distance vision and 60 mm for near vision. What is the segment inset? the total inset?

Because no prism is prescribed, the optical centers and the fitting points coincide. The *frame PD* is 50 + 18, or 68 mm. Because the patient's distance PD is 64 mm, the optical centers must each be decentered 2 mm inward from the geometric center, or

$$\text{Frame PD} - \text{patient's PD} = 68 \text{ mm} - 64 \text{ mm}$$
$$= 4 \text{ mm}.$$
$$\text{Optical centers} = 2 \text{ mm in, each lens}.$$
$$\text{Segment inset} = (64 - 60)/2$$
$$= 2 \text{ mm in, each lens}$$
$$\text{(from the distance}$$
$$\text{fitting points).}$$
$$\text{Total inset} = (68 - 60)/2$$
$$= 4 \text{ mm in, each lens}$$
$$\text{(from the geometric}$$
$$\text{centers).}$$

TABLE 8–11
Segment Inset Required (for Each Bifocal Segment) to Make the Two Reading Fields Coincide at a 40-cm Reading Distance*

Distance Lens Power, 180° Meridian	Distance PD								
	56	58	60	62	64	66	68	70	72
+14.00 D	2.5	2.5	2.6	2.7	2.8	2.9	3.0	3.1	3.2
+12.00 D	2.3	2.3	2.4	2.5	2.6	2.7	2.8	2.9	3.0
+10.00 D	2.2	2.2	2.3	2.4	2.5	2.5	2.6	2.7	2.8
+8.00 D	2.0	2.1	2.2	2.2	2.3	2.4	2.5	2.5	2.6
+6.00 D	1.9	2.0	2.1	2.1	2.2	2.3	2.3	2.4	2.5
+4.00 D	1.8	1.9	2.0	2.0	2.1	2.1	2.2	2.3	2.3
+2.00 D	1.7	1.8	1.9	1.9	2.0	2.0	2.1	2.1	2.2
0.00 D	1.6	1.7	1.8	1.8	1.9	1.9	2.0	2.1	2.1
–2.00 D	1.6	1.6	1.7	1.7	1.8	1.9	1.9	2.0	2.0
–4.00 D	1.5	1.5	1.6	1.7	1.7	1.8	1.8	1.9	1.9
–6.00 D	1.4	1.5	1.5	1.6	1.6	1.7	1.8	1.8	1.9
–8.00 D	1.4	1.4	1.5	1.5	1.6	1.6	1.7	1.7	1.8
–10.00 D	1.3	1.4	1.4	1.5	1.5	1.6	1.6	1.7	1.7
–20.00 D	1.1	1.2	1.2	1.2	1.3	1.3	1.4	1.4	1.4

*For distances from 30 to 40 cm, add 0.2 mm to the amount of inset for each 5 cm of reading distance nearer than 40 cm.
SOURCE: Adapted from S. Sterling, Modern Bifocal Lenses. *Ophthalmic Lenses: Their History, Theory, and Selection.* Bausch & Lomb Optical Co., Rochester, NY, pp. 53–81, 1935.

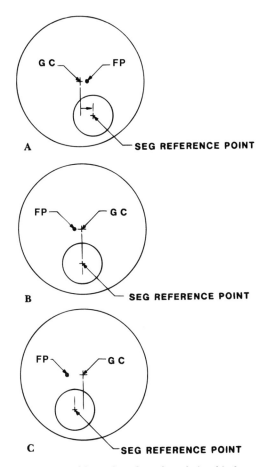

FIGURE 8–34. **Total inset, based on the relationship between the geometric center (GC) and the fitting point (FP) of the lens. A, Total inset is inward (the usual situation); B, total inset is zero; C, total inset is outward.**

EXAMPLE 2

Given the distance prescription +2.00 DS combined with 1 prism diopter base-in, with +2.00-D add, OU. The frame size is 46 mm, with a DBL of 18 mm. The patient's PD is 70/66. What is the segment inset? the total inset?

Because prism is prescribed, the optical centers and the fitting points will not coincide.

$$\text{Frame PD} = 46 \text{ mm} + 18 \text{ mm}$$

$$= 64 \text{ mm}.$$

$$\text{Frame PD} - \text{patient's PD} = 64 \text{ mm} - 70 \text{ mm}$$

$$= -6 \text{ mm}.$$

$$\text{Distance fitting points} = 3 \text{ mm } out, \text{each lens}.$$

$$\text{Segment inset} = (70 - 66)/2$$

$$= 2 \text{ mm in, each lens}$$

$$\text{(from the distance}$$

$$\text{fitting points).}$$

$$\text{Total inset} = (64 - 66)/2$$

$$= 1 \text{ mm } out, \text{each lens}$$

$$\text{(from the geometric}$$

$$\text{centers).}$$

8.17. Differential Displacement (Image Jump)

The optical performance of a bifocal lens can be considered in terms of

1. Differential displacement at the segment top (*image jump*)
2. Differential displacement at the reading level
3. Total displacement at the reading level
4. Chromatic aberration

Fundamentally, any modern bifocal lens can be considered as the equivalent of a cemented bifocal, having a segment wafer cemented to a single-vision lens (Figure 8–35). While reading through the segment, the patient may be considered as looking through two lenses, the distance lens and the added segment wafer. In effect, a bifocal lens may have three centers: (1) the distance optical center; (2) the segment optical center; and (3) the resultant optical center, or the point of zero prism in the segment position. The resultant optical center may actually fall outside the segment area.

As discussed in Chapter 4, prismatic effects exist for a spherical lens at all points on the lens except at the optical center of the lens. Prentice's rule provides an easy formula for the calculation of the magnitudes of these prismatic effects. When the wearer looks through the segment area of a bifocal lens, in addition to the prismatic effect caused by the distance lens there is a prismatic effect caused by the segment itself (unless the patient looks through the optical center of the segment). The prismatic effect at any point in the segment is equal to the sum of the prismatic effects of the distance lens and the segment.

The prismatic power of the segment solely determines the amount of *image jump*, or *differential displacement*. An effective way of demonstrating image jump at various parts of a bifocal segment is to observe a distant horizontal line through a bifocal lens held about 8 inches or more in front of the eye. Differential displacement manifests itself in that the parts of the line seen through the distance portion of the lens and seen through the segment are *not continuous*. Examples of differential displacement are shown in Figure 8–36. By comparing the level of the image seen through

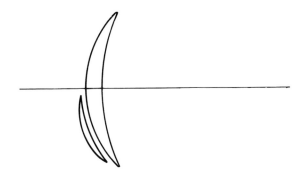

FIGURE 8–35. **A bifocal lens considered as the equivalent of a cement bifocal, made up of a single-vision lens and a segment wafer.**

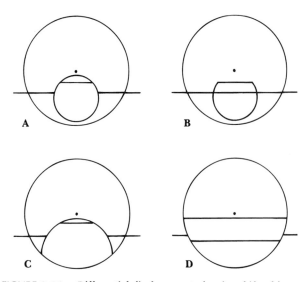

FIGURE 8–36.   **Differential displacement of various bifocal lenses, when viewing a horizontal line through a bifocal lens held about 8 inches in front of the eye. The greater the vertical distance between the line in the distance portion and that in the segment portion, the greater the differential displacement.**

FIGURE 8–37.   **Image jump, or differential displacement at the segment top. Note the base-down prismatic effect, which causes a blind area. The letter *U* is in the blind area, with the result that the word *MAD* is seen.**

the distance portion with that seen outside the field of the lens, it is possible to determine the prismatic effect of the distance portion. In addition, the total prismatic effect at a specified level in the reading area can be determined by comparing the level of the part of the line seen through the segment with the part seen outside the field of view of the lens.

If the prismatic power of the distance portion of the lens at a point on the segment boundary differs from the prismatic effect of the segment, the image "jumps" as the line of sight moves from the distance portion into the segment area. The jump is manifested to the wearer by an apparent alteration in the position of an image of any viewed object as the line of sight passes from the distance portion of the lens to the segment area, or vice versa. Image jump may occur at any point on the boundary of the segment; however, the term *jump* is usually used to describe the phenomenon occurring at the *top* of the segment, where it is particularly bothersome. The amount of jump present at the top of the segment depends entirely on the prismatic effect of the segment at that point. It is simply the differential displacement at the top of the segment. As shown in Figure 8–37, this is a *base-down* prismatic effect, resulting in an apparent *scotomatous* (blind) area.

The amount of jump is independent of the power of the distance portion of the lens but, as indicated by Prentice's rule, it is equal to the distance, *d*, from the segment top to the segment pole times the power of the add, F_A.

Thus,

$$\text{image jump} = dF_A. \qquad (8.13)$$

For a bifocal addition of a given power, image jump depends *solely* on the position of the segment optical center in relation to the segment top.

EXAMPLE

A patient requires the distance prescription +3.00 DS with a +2.00 D add. What is the amount of image jump (1) for a 22-mm round fused bifocal segment; (2) for a 22-mm-wide fused straight-top segment; (3) for a 38-mm round Ultex segment; and (4) for an Executive-style segment?

(1) For the 22-mm round fused bifocal segment (segment optical center 11 mm below the segment top),

$$\text{jump} = 1.1(+2.00)$$
$$= 2.2 \text{ prism diopters, base-down.}$$

(2) For the 22-mm-wide fused straight-top bifocal segment (segment optical center 5 mm below the segment top),

$$\text{jump} = 0.5(+2.00)$$
$$= 1.0 \text{ prism diopter, base-down.}$$

(3) For the Ultex bifocal segment (segment optical center 19 mm below the segment top),

$$\text{jump} = 1.9(+2.00)$$
$$= 3.8 \text{ prism diopters, base-down.}$$

(4) For the Executive-style segment (segment optical center at the top of the segment),

$$\text{jump} = 0(+2.00)$$
$$= 0 \text{ prism diopters.}$$

Size of the Scotoma

For a 40-cm reading distance, the linear height of an apparent scotoma subtending an angle of 1 prism diopter is 40/100 cm, or 0.4 cm. Therefore, the scotomas created for each of the lenses described in the example above have the following heights:

(1) For the 22-mm round segment,

$$2.2(0.4) = 0.88 \text{ cm.}$$

(2) For the straight-top segment,

$$1(0.4) = 0.4 \text{ cm.}$$

(3) For the Ultex segment,

$$3.8(0.4) = 1.52 \text{ cm.}$$

(4) For the Executive segment,

$$0(0.4) = 0 \text{ cm.}$$

As shown in Figure 8–37, jump is expected to cause a blind area at the top of the segment. Whether or not the wearer actually experiences a scotoma depends on the amount of jump and on the *pupil size* and the *vertex distance* of the lenses. For an extremely small pupil, or for a very large vertex distance, seeing any object that fell within the angle between the two beams is *impossible*. However, with a normal pupil, none of the common types of bifocals worn in the usual position before the eyes produce the effect of a blind area.

A bifocal lens with the segment optical center located at or close to the segment top is sometimes referred to by the manufacturer as a *no-jump* bifocal. When these lenses were first developed, some optical dispensers demonstrated the phenomenon of jump with the help of a reading card, such as the one shown in Figure 8–38. The patient was asked to look at the letters on the card while changing fixation from the distance portion to the near portion of the lens. Depending on the position of the line of sight, the patient saw either the word *MAD* or the word *MUD*. With a no-jump bifocal, the word *MAUD* was seen.

A phenomenon that consists of an *overlapping* of the distance and near fields at the top of the segment is also sometimes referred to as a "blind area," but the term *zone of confusion* more aptly describes this phenomenon.

8.18. The Zone of Confusion

When a bifocal wearer attempts to look at an object through the top edge of the segment, the person sees two images because a portion of the bundle of rays entering the pupil passes through the distance lens and a portion passes through the segment. The images formed by these bundles of rays may differ from each other in three ways:

1. In direction (differential displacement)
2. In focus (differences in power)
3. In size (differences in magnification)

The difference in direction depends on the differential prismatic effects at the top of the segment and can be controlled by varying the position of the segment optical center. It is possible to completely eliminate the difference in direction by placing the segment center at the top of the segment. However, this is of questionable value because the differences in image focus and in image size are present.

Zone of confusion may be applied to any portion of the lens where the line of sight traverses the dividing line because the phenomena of change in image vergence and change in image size occur simultaneously. The depth of the zone of confusion depends solely on the *size of the pupil* and the *vertex distance* and occurs relatively independently of the differential displacement at the top of the segment. Consequently, if the goal is to improve the wearer's vision at the top of the segment, there is probably little advantage in attempting to eliminate prismatic effects in that area.

8.19. Differential Displacement at the Reading Level

Figure 8–39 shows that, if the reading level corresponds to the position of the segment center (solid line), the segment causes no prismatic effect; any displacement of the object of regard is the same as that through the distance portion of the lens, and thus there is no differential displacement at the reading level (A). However, if the reading level is *above* the segment center, a *base-down* prismatic effect (caused by the segment) is present (B); if the reading level is *below* the segment center, the segment causes a *base-up* prismatic effect (C).

If the vertical distance between the segment optical center and the reading level is indicated by d_A, and the power of the add by F_A, the differential displacement at the reading level is given by

$$\text{differential displacement} = d_A F_A. \qquad (8.14)$$

If the reading level is above the segment center, the segment contains base-down prism; if the reading level is below the segment center, the segment contains base-up prism.

We can compare differential displacement at the reading level to image jump by using the same prescriptions and the same bifocal segments given in the examples in Section 8.17.

EXAMPLE
Given the distance prescription +3.00 DS with a +2.00 D add, what is the amount of differential displacement at the reading level, if the reading level is 8 mm below the distance optical center of the lens (Figure 8–40) (1) for a 22-mm round fused bifocal segment, whose segment top is 2 mm below the distance center, with a reading

FIGURE 8–38.   **A, Reading card used to demonstrate a no-jump bifocal; B, only the letters *MAD* are seen, unless a no-jump bifocal is used.**

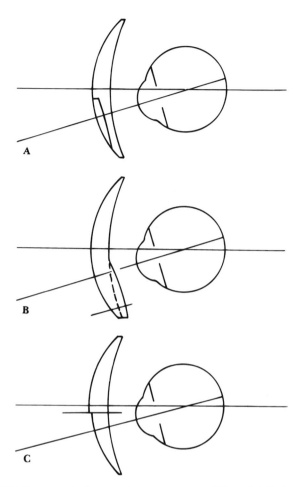

FIGURE 8–39. Influence of segment type on differential displacement at the reading level. A, no displacement; B, base-down prismatic effect; C, base-up prismatic effect.

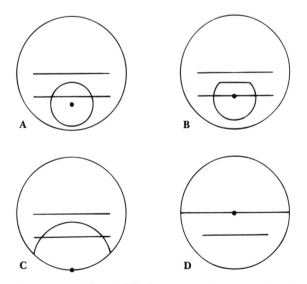

FIGURE 8–40. Differential displacement. A, 22-mm round fused bifocal; B, 22-mm-wide straight-top fused bifocal; C, 38-mm round Ultex A bifocal; D, Executive-style bifocal.

level 6 mm below the segment top (A); (2) for a 22-mm-wide straight-top fused bifocal segment, whose segment top is 3 mm below the distance center, with a reading level 5 mm below the segment top (B); (3) for a 38-mm round Ultex A bifocal, whose segment top is 2 mm below the distance center, with a reading level 6 mm below the segment top (C); and (4) for an Executive-style bifocal, whose distance and near optical centers are both located at the segment top, with a reading level 5 mm below the segment top (D)?

(1) For the 22-mm round fused segment,

differential displacement = 0.5(+2.00)

= 1.00 prism diopter,

base-down.

(2) For the straight-top fused segment,

differential displacement = 0(+2.00)

= 0 prism diopters.

(3) For the Ultex A bifocal,

differential displacement = 1.3(+2.00)

= 2.6 prism diopters,

base-down.

(4) For the Executive-style bifocal,

differential displacement = 0.5(+2.00)

= 1.00 prism diopter

base-up.

Interestingly, the Executive-style bifocal, which induces no image jump at all, is responsible for 1 prism diopter of differential displacement at the reading level, and the Ultex bifocal, which has the largest amount of jump of any of the four bifocal types, has considerably more differential displacement at the reading level than that of the Executive-style bifocal, but opposite in direction.

8.20. Total Displacement at the Reading Level

Image jump and differential displacement at the reading level are independent of the power of the distance portion of the lens, but total displacement at the reading level depends on both the power of the distance lens and the power of the add. Inspection of Figure 8–41 indicates that total displacement is equal to the prismatic effect caused by the distance lens plus that caused by the bifocal add. If we use F_D to indicate the power of the distance portion of the lens, F_A to indicate the power of the add, d_D to indicate the distance from the distance optical center of the lens to the reading level, and d_A to indicate the distance from the segment pole to the reading level,

$$\text{total displacement} = d_D F_D + d_A F_A. \quad (8.15)$$

The displacement caused by the distance portion of the lens, $d_D F_D$, is, in all cases, base-up for a distance lens of plus power, and base-down for a distance lens of minus

FIGURE 8–41. **Total displacement at the reading level, caused by both the power of the distance-vision lens and the power of the segment.**

power. This is shown in Figure 8–42. A comparison of total displacement for a positive and for a negative distance prescription can be made by calculating the total displacement for the four types of segments, each having a +2.00 D add, for (1) a distance prescription of +3.00 DS, as previously used, and (2) a distance prescription of –3.00 DS.

EXAMPLE 1

For the distance prescription of +3.00 DS (with all other values the same as in the example in Section 8.17):

(1) For the 22-mm round fused segment,

$$\text{total displacement} = 0.8(+3.00) + 0.5(+2.00)$$
$$= 2.4 \text{ base-up} + 1.0 \text{ base-down}$$
$$= 1.4 \text{ prism diopters, base-up.}$$

(2) For the straight-top fused segment,

$$\text{total displacement} = 0.8(+3.00) + 0(+2.00)$$
$$= 2.4 \text{ base-up} + 0$$
$$= 2.4 \text{ prism diopters, base-up.}$$

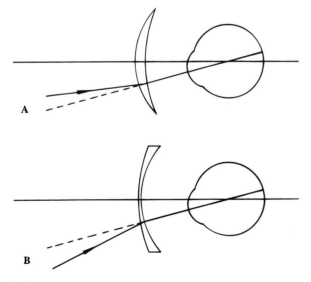

A

B

FIGURE 8–42. **Displacement at the reading level caused by the power in the distance portion of the lens. A, base-up effect for a plus lens; B, base-down effect for a minus lens.**

(3) For the Ultex A segment,

$$\text{total displacement} = 0.8(+3.00) + 1.3(+2.00)$$
$$= 2.4 \text{ base-up} + 2.6 \text{ base-down}$$
$$= 0.2 \text{ prism diopter, base-down.}$$

(4) For the Executive-style segment,

$$\text{total displacement} = 0.5(+3.00) + 0.5(+2.00)$$
$$= 1.5 \text{ base-up} + 1.0 \text{ base-up}$$
$$= 2.5 \text{ prism diopters, base-up.}$$

EXAMPLE 2

For the distance prescription of –3.00 DS (again, with all other values the same as in the previous example):

(1) For the 22-mm round fused segment,

$$\text{total displacement} = 0.8(-3.00) + 0.5(+2.00)$$
$$= 2.4 \text{ base-down} + 1.0 \text{ base-down}$$
$$= 3.4 \text{ prism diopters, base-down.}$$

(2) For the straight-top fused segment,

$$\text{total displacement} = 0.8(-3.00) + 0(+2.00)$$
$$= 2.4 \text{ base-down} + 0$$
$$= 2.4 \text{ prism diopters, base-down.}$$

(3) For the Ultex A segment,

$$\text{total displacement} = 0.8(-3.00) + 1.3(+2.00)$$
$$= 2.4 \text{ base-down} + 2.6 \text{ base-down}$$
$$= 5.0 \text{ prism diopters, base-down.}$$

(4) For the Executive-style segment,

$$\text{total displacement} = 0.5(-3.00) + 0.5(+2.00).$$
$$= 1.5 \text{ base-down} + 1.0 \text{ base-up}$$
$$= 0.5 \text{ prism diopter, base-down.}$$

These examples show that for the +3.00 D lenses the Ultex A provides the smallest amount of total displacement because the base-down effect of the segment opposes the base-up effect of the distance lens. On the other hand, for the –3.00 D distance lens, the Executive style provides the smallest amount of total displacement because the base-up effect of the segment opposes the base-down effect of the distance lens.

Note also that for the straight-top fused bifocal, which has no differential displacement at the reading level because the segment pole is at the reading level, total displacement is caused by the distance lens. Thus, when a wearer of single-vision lenses first begins to wear bifocals, the use of a straight-top bifocal causes the total displacement at the reading level to be no different than it was with single-vision lenses. (However, if we consider that the wearer of bifocal lenses is forced to lower the lines of sight of the eyes more than that of the wearer of single-vision lenses, the total displacement at the reading level is greater than the displacement with single-vision lenses.)

8.21. Transverse Chromatic Aberration

As discussed in Chapter 6, the chromatic aberration of a lens can be considered in terms of either *longitudinal* (axial) or *transverse* chromatic aberration. Because the eye itself has longitudinal chromatic aberration, any longitudinal chromatic aberration caused by a lens only adds to or subtracts from the eye's chromatic aberration. However, for lenses of high power, transverse chromatic aberration can sometimes be a problem. A lens having a large amount of transverse chromatic aberration (*lateral color*) might cause wearer to complain of the presence of "color fringes" when viewing an object through the peripheral portion of the lens.

Transverse chromatic aberration (Figure 8–43) may be expressed in linear form as a difference in image size of the red and blue images (A) or in angular terms as the difference between the refracted red and blue rays (B). As noted in Chapter 6, Section 6.6, transverse chromatic aberration in angular terms is given by Equation 6.6:

$$\text{transverse chromatic aberration} = \frac{dF_d}{V},$$

where d represents the distance from the optical center of the lens to the point in question, F represents the power of the lens, and V represents the Abbe number. When d is expressed in centimeters, the numerator of the equation is the equivalent of Prentice's rule, and the transverse chromatic aberration in angular terms is expressed in prism diopters. Therefore, transverse chromatic aberration depends on the point in a lens through which the foveal line of sight passes.

Transverse chromatic aberration exists for any point in the periphery of a lens and, for a given power, increases as the eye rotates away from the optical center. It does *not* exist at the optical center.

For a *bifocal lens*, the total transverse chromatic aberration for any point within the segment area is found by combining the transverse chromatic aberration caused by the distance lens with that caused by the segment. If the subscript D is used to indicate the distance lens and the subscript A is used to indicate the add, the transverse chromatic aberration at any point within the segment is given by the expression

$$\text{transverse chromatic aberration} = \frac{d_D F_D}{V_D} + \frac{d_A F_A}{V_A}. \quad (8.16)$$

If we are interested in the transverse chromatic aberration at the reading level, the parameters represented by d_D and d_A are those given in Sections 8.15 and 8.17. The transverse chromatic aberration at the reading level is related to the total displacement at the reading level, as described in Section 8.17. For a one-piece bifocal, a comparison of Equations 8.15 and 8.16 indicates that the transverse chromatic aberration at the reading level is caused by the total displacement (expressed in prism diopters) divided by the Abbe number. For example, because the Abbe number of crown glass is 59, the transverse chromatic aberration at the reading level for an Ultex A bifocal having a distance power of +3.00 DS and a +2.00 D add is

$$0.2/59 = 0.003 \text{ prism diopter,}$$

and for an Ultex A having a distance power of –3.00 DS and a +2.00 D add, the transverse chromatic aberration at the reading level is

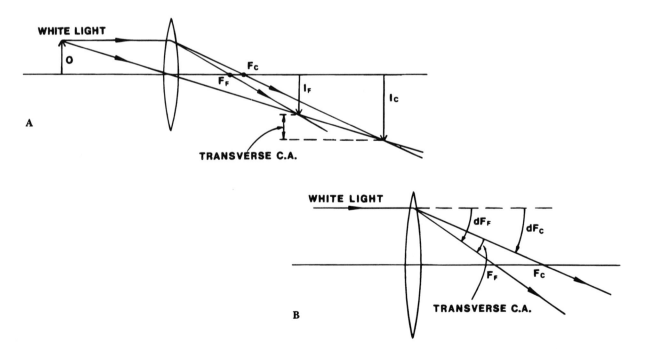

FIGURE 8–43. Transverse chromatic aberration (C.A.). A, expressed in terms of the difference in image sizes for the red and blue rays; B, expressed in angular terms, as the difference in the angles of refraction for the red and blue rays.

5.0/59 = 0.08 prism diopter.

For the Executive bifocal having a distance power of +3.00 DS and a +2.00 D add, the transverse chromatic aberration is

2.5/59 = 0.04 prism diopter,

and for an Executive bifocal having a distance power of –3.00 DS and a +2.00 D add, the transverse chromatic aberration at the reading level is

0.5/59 = 0.008 prism diopter.

For a fused bifocal segment made of flint glass with an Abbe value of only 36, the transverse chromatic aberration caused by the segment itself is approximately twice that caused by the segment of a one-piece bifocal, for a given value of d_A. However, for a straight-top fused bifocal, the segment causes little or no displacement at the reading level, so the lower Abbe value of the flint glass is no problem. Even for the Kryptok bifocal, the value of d_A is sufficiently small that (for the examples used here) the displacement caused by the +2.00-D add, with a distance power of +3.00 D, is only 1.4 prism diopters. This would cause chromatic dispersion at the reading level of only

1.4/36 = 0.04 prism diopter.

Transverse Chromatic Aberration at the Segment Periphery

Although the transverse chromatic aberration caused by a 22-mm flint-segment fused bifocal is negligible at the reading level, it is possible that in a given combination of distance powers and reading additions the transverse chromatic aberration at the *periphery* of the segment could be a problem. We might, for example, consider two extreme cases (Figure 8–44): one in which the wearer of a plus-powered distance lens looks through the lower edge of the segment, and one in which the wearer of a minus-powered distance lens looks through the upper edge of the segment.

If the power of the plus lens is +3.00 DS, the power of the add is +2.00 D, and the segment top is located 3 mm below the distance optical center, the transverse chromatic aberration occurring 1 mm above the lower edge of the segment is

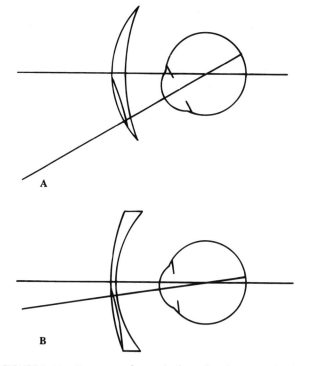

FIGURE 8–44.   **Transverse chromatic aberration. A, wearer of a plus-powered distance lens looking through the lower edge of the segment; B, wearer of a minus-powered distance lens looking through the upper edge of the segment.**

$$\frac{2.4(3)}{59} + \frac{1(2)}{36} = 0.122 \text{ base-up} + 0.056 \text{ base-up}$$

$$= 0.178 \text{ prism diopter, base-up.}$$

For a distance power of –3.00 DS, an addition of +2.00 D, and the segment top located 3 mm below the distance optical center, the chromatic dispersion at a point 1 mm below the segment top is

$$\frac{0.4(3)}{59} + \frac{1(2)}{36} = 0.020 \text{ base-down} + 0.056 \text{ base-down}$$

$$= 0.076 \text{ prism diopter, base-down.}$$

However, even in these extreme cases, the transverse chromatic aberration at the edge of the segment is less than 1 prism diopter. Thus, very few bifocal wearers complain of seeing color fringes.

CLINICAL CONSIDERATIONS

8.22. Theories of Bifocal Selection

The problems of image jump, differential displacement at the reading level, and total displacement at the reading level have led to three theories of bifocal selection:

1. The bifocal segment should be selected so that jump is eliminated. This is done by choosing a bifocal with a segment pole located at the dividing line. Such lenses are called no-jump bifocals. The straight-top one-piece (Executive-style) bifocal satisfies this criterion.

2. The bifocal segment should be selected so that differential displacement at the reading level is eliminated. This is done by choosing a bifocal with a segment pole located at the reading level. The straight-top fused bifocal (with the segment pole 5 mm below the segment top) satisfies this criterion.

3. The bifocal segment should be selected so that the total displacement at the reading level is zero, or as near zero as possible. This can be done by selecting a bifocal with a segment that provides prismatic effect opposite to that provided by the distance lens. Two extreme approaches are available here (Figure 8–45): (1) for a minus distance prescription, the *base-down* prismatic effect at the reading level can be opposed by the *base-up* prismatic effect of an Executive-style segment (A); (2) for a plus distance prescription, the *base-up* prismatic effect of the distance power can be opposed by the *base-down* prismatic effect of an Ultex A segment (B). This was shown quantitatively by examples in Section 8.20.

A number of arguments, pro and con, can be made concerning each of the three theories. Regarding the idea of eliminating *image jump*, because of the finite size of the pupil and the normally used vertex distance, the patient may not be *aware* of the predicted image jump; because of the change in vergence of light and the change in image size when the line of sight crosses the dividing line, there exists a *zone of confusion*, even for a bifocal (such as the Executive) that has no jump. One can make the argument, therefore, that image jump is not a severe problem.

Regarding the theory of attempting to eliminate the *total displacement* at the reading level, wearers of single-vision lenses are accustomed to displacement at the reading level. The only way displacement can be avoided is for the wearer to tip the head forward sufficiently during reading so that the foveal line of sight passes through the optical center of the lens. Wearers of single-vision lenses *are* accustomed to this displacement; therefore, one can argue that there is no point in trying to *eliminate* it when the wearer switches to bifocals. The goal should not be to reduce the prismatic effect at the reading level to zero, but to avoid changing the effect to which the patient has already become adapted.

In a situation in which bifocals are the first pair of glasses to be worn by a patient, he or she is not accustomed to prismatic effects at the reading level. The easiest type of bifocal for this patient to become adjusted to is one that has *no* prismatic effects at the reading level. In such a case the distance correction is not likely to be very strong; to avoid prismatic effects at the reading level, the segment optical center would be placed very close to the reading center.

On the other hand, when a patient requires a strong distance correction, the patient has very likely been wearing glasses; hence, the patient will already be accustomed to the prismatic effect at the reading center caused by the power in the distance portion of the lens. To provide the same prismatic effect that was present in single-vision lenses, the segment optical center must be placed at the reading center.

One may conclude that, of the three problems, the problem of *differential displacement at the reading level* is most likely to be a source of annoyance to the bifocal wearer. Although image jump, along with change in vergence, occurs fleetingly and can, with practice, be ignored (or can be eliminated by *blinking* as the eye crosses the dividing line), differential displacement at the reading level is more difficult to ignore. Fortunately, it can be easily eliminated by prescribing a straight-top fused bifocal with the segment center located approximately 5 mm below the top of the segment.

8.23. Segment Size and Shape

The selection of a bifocal style for a given patient involves a number of considerations in addition to image jump and displacement; one of the most important is the selection of the segment size and shape that most nearly meet the patient's needs.

Segment Width

Just as spectacle lenses have progressively grown larger in recent years, bifocal segments, too, have grown. The fused Kryptok bifocal, invented early in this century, was for many years made in a diameter of 17 mm, but it gradually grew to 19 mm, 20 mm, and finally to 22 mm in diameter. The standard width of the fused straight-top bifocal segment has grown from 19 to 22 mm, with segments as wide as 35 mm available. The epitome of segment width is expressed by the Executive-style bifocal, with a segment width equal to the width of the lens. The early, smaller, bifocal segments were designed to infringe as little as possible on the wearer's dis-

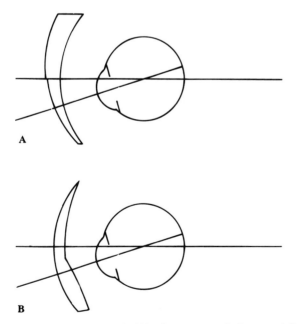

FIGURE 8–45. **Selection of a bifocal segment to eliminate total displacement at the reading level. A, minus distance lens with Executive-style segment; B, plus distance lens with Ultex-style segment.**

tance field of vision (and, incidentally, to make the segment as *invisible* as possible). The large segments now in use were designed mainly for the *desk worker*.

By the use of very simple mathematics it may be shown that, for a 22-mm-wide segment, the width of the macular field of view (field of fixation) for a working distance of 40 cm, neglecting the effect of lens power, is approximately 35 cm (14 inches). Referring to Figure 8–46, for a distance of 2.7 cm from the spectacle plane to the center of rotation of the eye, we find by the use of similar triangles that

$$\text{field width} = \frac{(42.7)(2.2)}{2.7}$$

$$= 34.8 \text{ cm}$$

$$= \text{approx. 14 inches.}$$

The field given here is based on the head remaining in a stationary position. The field can be widened by moving the head. For the Executive-style bifocal with a lens width of 50 mm, the width of the field of view (without moving the head) is

$$\frac{(42.7)(5)}{2.7} = 79 \text{ cm} = \text{approx. 31 inches.}$$

Even though a 22-mm-wide segment is considered wide enough for most everyday near-vision tasks such as reading, writing, or sewing, many patients (whose activities would not seem to require them) request to be fitted with the Executive-style bifocal. One can make the argument that, with a narrower segment, *distance vision* is available on either side of the segment. However, a counterargument to this is that, for a fused, 22- or 25-mm-wide segment, the wearer is aware of the dividing line when the eyes are moved to one side or the other (when looking through the lower part of the lens); a segment that goes across the lens presents no dividing line in the field of view (although the field is blurred for distance vision). Nevertheless, when a patient requests a wide segment, there is usually nothing to be gained by attempting to change the patient's opinion.

FIGURE 8–47. **The ciliary line for the lower lid is normally at the same level as the lower limbus.**

Segment Height

Many patients (and even some eye practitioners and optical dispensers) believe that a bifocal segment should be placed as low as possible in the lens, so as to infringe on the distance field as little as possible. Fitting a bifocal in this manner is almost always a mistake and results in the patient getting a *stiff neck* as a result of throwing the head back to find the bifocal segment. Errors are more often made by fitting bifocal segments *too low* than by fitting them too high.

The reference point most often used in specifying segment height is the *ciliary line* at the top edge of the lower lid. For most people, the ciliary line is on the same level as the lower limbus (corneoscleral junction), as shown in Figure 8–47. However, if a patient's lower lid is very much lower or higher than the lower limbus, the *limbus* should be used as the reference point. Because the vertical extent of the cornea (the visible iris diameter) is usually 11 to 12 mm, the vertical distance from the ciliary line to the center of the pupil is usually very close to 6 mm.

One disadvantage of a *round* bifocal segment is that the widest (and the most useful) part of the segment is a considerable distance below the dividing line. Because of this, the segment top must be fitted higher than that for a straight-top bifocal, whose widest portion is very close to the dividing line (Figure 8–48). As a general rule, a round segment is fitted at about the level of the ciliary line, but a straight-top segment is usually fitted 1 or 2 mm below the ciliary line.

Occupation, head position, and many other factors are important in determining the segment height. In general, the more time the patient spends reading or doing other close work, the higher the segment should be. For an individual whose entire working day involves close work at or near eye level, such as a barber or postal clerk, a reading

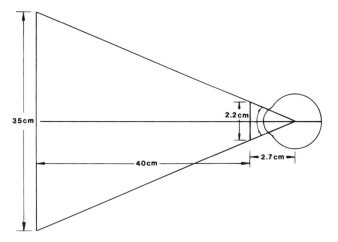

FIGURE 8–46. **Linear width of the field of fixation for a 40-cm reading distance, 27-mm stop distance, and a 22-mm-wide segment.**

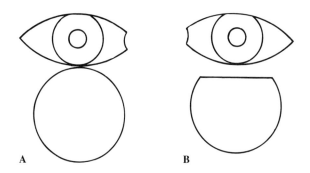

FIGURE 8–48. **A, a round segment is normally fitted at the level of the ciliary line; B, a straight-top segment is fitted 1 or 2 mm below the ciliary line.**

lens with a distance window, such as a very high Executive style or an Ultex AL, should be considered. As for head position, an individual who customarily walks with the head held back may require a somewhat lower segment; one who walks with the head slouched forward requires a somewhat higher segment. It is a good idea to observe a patient's posture, both while walking and reading, before deciding the bifocal segment height.

Segment Shape

Probably the only advantage of a *round* fused segment (with its knifelike edges) is the fact that it is *less visible* than a straight-top fused segment. The least visible segment is a *no-chrome* round segment (made of barium crown glass with an Abbe value very close to that of crown glass) in a tint such as Vision-Ease Pink #1. In years past, a very small, fused round segment, about 12 mm in diameter (called a *spot* or *button* segment), was sometimes recommended for a patient whose occupation required mainly distance vision. Although such segments are no longer manufactured, a small round segment of any size may be obtained by resurfacing the front surface of a 22-mm round fused segment until the desired segment size is reached.

A *ribbon* segment (in particular, a B segment, 9 mm high) should be considered for a worker, such as a construction worker, who may have to climb ladders or other structures, but who must have occasional near vision available. However, for the distance field below the segment to be of any value to this type of patient, the segment must be fitted sufficiently high and with a sufficiently large frame so that the distance portion of the lens below the segment is at least 7 or 8 mm high. The segment height, therefore, should be at least 16 or 17 mm. There is little advantage in fitting the 14-mm-high R segment for such a patient because the segment would have to be fitted *very* high for any distance field to be available below the segment. The most appropriate use of the R segment is for the compensation of differential vertical prismatic effects (see Chapter 10, Section 10.3.)

A final factor that must be considered is the style of bifocal that the patient is *currently wearing*. In most cases, if the patient is completely satisfied with the type of bifocal that he or she has been wearing, the best procedure is *not* to change the bifocal type. For example, a patient having a moderate amount of astigmatism and who has worn Ultex bifocals (which are usually in positive toric form) may not be happy if he or she is switched to an Executive-style or straight-top fused bifocal (in negative toric form), even though the differential displacement at the top of the segment is greatly decreased. An analogous situation arises when a wearer of single-vision lenses made in positive toric form is first fitted with bifocals. The patient may have difficulty adjusting to an Executive-style bifocal made in negative toric form. However, because of the important advantages of negative toric lenses (discussed in Chapter 6) and the increased differential displacement at the segment top often caused by an Ultex bifocal, it is probably best to switch these patients to a negative toric bifocal and to warn them of the possible adaptation problems.

8.24. Horizontal Prismatic Effects

When bifocal lenses are prescribed, unintentional horizontal prismatic effects caused by the *distance* power or the power of the *add* may be induced in the reading portion of the lens. To understand these prismatic effects, the bifocal segment should be thought of as existing *behind* the distance lens, as if it were a cemented bifocal. If the segments have been correctly inset for the wearer's near PD as determined by Sterling's table (presented in Table 8–10), the fields of view for the two eyes will coincide. However, the *distance* power of the lens induces a horizontal prismatic effect at near unless the distance prescription has no power in the horizontal meridian. For example, for a distance correction of +3.00 DS and a PD of 66/62, the prismatic effect at the near PD, caused by the distance power, is

$$0.2(+3.00) = +0.6$$
$$= 0.6 \text{ prism diopter, base-out,}$$

and for a –3.00 DS with the same PD, with the prismatic effect at the near PD caused by the distance power, is

$$0.2(-3.00) = -0.6$$
$$= 0.6 \text{ prism diopter, base-in.}$$

If the wearer's right and left lenses both have the same power (both +3.00 DS or both –3.00 DS), the total prismatic effect is 1.2 prism diopters (base-out for the positive DS and base-in for the negative DS). Note that the prismatic effect, caused by the distance power, is independent of the power of the add. As long as the segments are inset to correspond to the near PD, the addition itself causes no prismatic effect.

Because the addition causes no prismatic effect, when a wearer of single-vision lenses is first fitted with bifocals, the prismatic effect at near is no different than it was for single-vision lenses (assuming that the single-vision lenses had been centered for the distance PD). Therefore, if the patient had no complaints of asthenopia as a result of the prismatic effect induced by the single-vision lenses, one would think the patient would have no complaints as a result of the prismatic effect when the bifocal lenses are worn. However, with the application of the plus addition for reading, the patient becomes more exophoric at near because of the loss of accommodative convergence, and this may precipitate complaints (although Sheedy and Saladin[6] found that many presbyopic patients had no complaints in spite of the exophoria at near). If the patient has been *esophoric* at near before becoming presbyopic, the plus addition reduces the esophoria. However, most presbyopes are exophoric through the reading addition. The *myopic* presbyope obtains some relief from the induced exophoria caused by the plus addition because of the *base-in* effect of the distance correction, but the *hyperopic* presbyope is more likely to be bothered by symptoms of exophoria because of the *base-out* effect of the distance lenses.

If a presbyope has symptoms when doing close work, and the symptoms appear to be caused by exophoria at near, some relief may be obtained by increasing the segment inset to obtain a base-in prismatic effect from the segment. For example, for a +2.50-D addition, if each segment is inset an *additional* 3 mm, the additional inset produces a horizontal prismatic effect of 0.75 prism diopters base-in for each lens, or a total of 1.5 prism diopters base-in.

Care must be taken that the additional segment inset designed to provide a base-in effect through the segment does not create a new problem. Additional inset of small segments should be avoided. The outline of the segment acts as a field stop, which determines the monocular field of fixation; if the segment is small, the temporal limits of the monocular fields of fixation could be significantly reduced. Hence, the overall binocular field of fixation would be appreciably contracted. Large straight-top segments such as the 28- and 35-mm fused segments can undergo additional inset without reducing the binocular field of fixation below that of an average-sized segment. However, these segments have an unusual appearance because of the cutoff appearance on the nasal side of the lens (Figure 8–49). For this reason, when additional segment inset is necessary, the Executive-style bifocal is very suitable because the monocular fields of fixation are maintained with no noticeable change in the appearance of the lenses.

Occasionally, a practitioner may decide to incorporate prismatic power *only in the segment.* This may be done to compensate for a lateral phoria at near or possibly to counteract the prismatic effect induced at near by the distance prescription. Some bifocal manufacturers have available *prism segment* bifocals that can incorporate as much as 2 or 3 prism diopters of base-in or base-out prism. However, prism segment bifocals are always factory orders, and they involve increased cost and a very long delay. Accordingly, their use is recommended only as a last resort.

Another solution to providing horizontal prism only in the segment is the use of Fresnel *Press-on prisms* (discussed in Chapter 4). The Fresnel prism may be cut from a sheet or purchased in precut form. Press-on prisms, however, have the disadvantages of poor appearance and a slight loss of visual acuity. Fortunately, presbyopes usually have no difficulty compensating for a high exophoria at near vision.

8.25. Differential Vertical Prismatic Effects at the Reading Level

If the distance powers of a patient's lenses differ for the two eyes in the vertical meridian, the two eyes experience dif-

ferential prismatic effects at the reading level. For a wearer of single-vision lenses this may not constitute a problem, since the head is normally tilted downward in reading, with the result that the reading level may be very little different than the level used for distance vision. However, a bifocal wearer is forced to read at a level approximately 10 mm below the distance optical centers of the lenses, so differential prismatic effects associated with reading may be troublesome. A number of methods of compensating for differential vertical prismatic effects are available. These are discussed in Chapter 10.

8.26. Ordering and Dispensing Bifocals

A laboratory order for a pair of bifocal lenses must include the following information:

1. The *distance prescription,* as ordinarily specified for single-vision lenses, including for each eye the sphere power, cylinder power and axis, the distance PD, the vertical level of the distance fitting point, and (if prism is prescribed) the amount of prism and the direction of its base.

2. The *power of the add,* specified as a plus sphere addition, for example, +1.50-D add. The total power through the segment area is the sum of the distance prescription and the add.

3. The *bifocal style,* or type. If a trade name (e.g., American Optical Executive, or Vision-Ease FT-22) is specified, the laboratory is obligated to provide the specific trade-name lens. However, if a descriptive term such as "straight-top one-piece bifocal," "straight-top fused bifocal," or even "Executive style" is used, the laboratory is free to fill the order with any manufacturer's lens that fulfills the description.

4. The *segment size.* As with lens sizes in general, the horizontal dimension (measured where the segment is widest) is specified first. The vertical dimension of the segment is the vertical measurement of the *unfinished* lens, before cutting and edging are done. For example, a Kryptok bifocal is specified as 22-mm round and an X-Cel D is specified as 22 × 16 mm, even though the lenses are mounted with the top of the segment only 14 mm high in the frame. It is not necessary to specify the *width* of an Executive-style segment.

5. The *segment height.* The height of the segment is specified as the perpendicular distance from a line tangent to the lowest part of the lens bevel to a line tangent to the highest point on the top of the segment (Figure 8–50). The segment height is specified, for example, as *19 mm high.*

6. The *segment inset.* The segment inset is specified as the distance nasally (inward) from the distance fitting point of the distance portion of the lens to the optical center of the segment (see Figure 8–50). When the horizontal meridian of the distance lens contains no power or has only prismatic power, the *total inset* must be specified from the geometric center.

7. The *frame specifications.* The size of the frame is specified on the basis of the *box system,* such as 50 × 42 mm. The

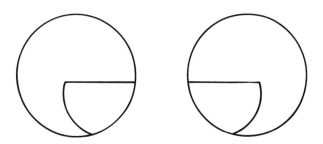

FIGURE 8–49. **Wide fused bifocal segments, inset sufficiently to provide a base-in prismatic effect.**

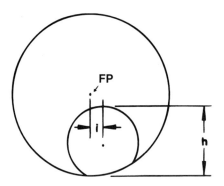

FIGURE 8–50. **Specification of segment height and inset. (FP = fitting point).**

DBL, shape of the frame, color, temple style, and length of the temple must also be specified.

8. The *lens material and tempering process.* Most prescription order forms have a check-off list by which to indicate whether glass or plastic lenses are desired. If *glass* is specified, the method of tempering (heat or chemical) must also be specified. If *plastic* is specified, the order is usually filled with CR-39 plastic with an index of refraction of 1.498. If polycarbonate or another plastic material is desired, it must be specified. The surfaces of polycarbonate lenses are routinely coated with a scratch-resistant coating. If a scratch-resistant coating is desired for CR-39 lenses, it must be specified in the order.

9. *Tint.* As with single-vision lenses, the order must indicate either clear lenses or the specific tint, if a tint is desired.

When the lenses are received from the laboratory, they should be carefully verified (see Section 8.27).

At the *dispensing visit,* the patient should be instructed in the use of the bifocals. This is particularly true for the patient's *first pair* of bifocals. The patient should be told to lower the eyes, rather than the head, when reading, and should be told to try to ignore the dividing line as the line of vision sweeps across it. One way to ignore the dividing line is to *blink* when lowering the eyes.

Some new bifocal wearers tend to worry about whether they are looking through the upper or the lower portions of the lenses. A way to take care of this problem is to suggest that the patient make sure to tilt the head *downward* slightly when looking through the upper part of each lens and tilt the head *upward* slightly when looking through the lower part.

In addition to the mechanical problems of learning how to hold the head and to move the eyes for near vision, some new bifocal wearers have difficulty in adapting to optical factors such as the difference in magnification, difference in reading distance, and differences in the stimuli to accommodation and convergence.

Most new bifocal wearers are pleased to find that "everything looks larger" through their bifocals, although some may have difficulty learning to hold reading material at a sufficiently close distance. It is sometimes disappointing, after prescribing bifocal lenses that definitely improve the patient's near acuity, for the practitioner to receive patient complaints such as "I have to hold my reading too close." Fortunately, most patients adapt to this problem within a few days.

Because bifocal lenses reduce *accommodative demand,* less accommodative convergence is available, which causes the near phoria to change in the *exophoric* direction. Most presbyopes have little difficulty compensating for the exophoria. Sheedy and Saladin[6] hypothesized that presbyopes compensate for exophoria at near vision by *unrestricted use of accommodative convergence.* Because accommodative convergence is not accompanied by the usual amount of accommodation, a presbyope may freely make use of accommodative convergence to compensate for the exophoria.

If the patient perseveres in wearing the bifocals (assuming that they were prescribed and fitted correctly), complete adaptation usually occurs within 2 or 3 weeks. For new bifocal wearers, it is a very good idea to schedule a *progress visit* at the end of 2 or 3 weeks.

8.27. Verification of Bifocals

When the practitioner receives a finished pair of glasses from the laboratory, they must be evaluated in terms of accuracy of workmanship and quality of materials. Procedures for the verification of *single-vision* lenses are discussed in Chapter 9—only the aspects of verification that apply to bifocal lenses are discussed here.

The operations involved in the layout, marking, surfacing, and cutting of bifocal lenses are more complicated than are those for single-vision lenses, and the lenses must be carefully examined to ensure that they have been made according to specifications. In addition to determining the accuracy of the placement of the distance centers, bifocals must be evaluated for segment type, segment width, segment height, segment inset, and power of the add. In verifying segment height, each lens must be measured; for straight-top segments, a straight edge should be used to ensure that both segment tops lie in the horizontal meridian.

As described in Chapter 4, when a lensometer is used to determine the back vertex power of a single-vision lens (or the distance portion of a bifocal lens), the lens is placed in the lensometer with its back pole against the lens stop and the target is moved until the image of the target on the reticle is in sharp focus. Using this procedure, one actually measures the *back focal length* of the lens—the distance from the back pole of the lens to the secondary focal point. Lenses used in refractors or as trial lenses in trial frames are calibrated in terms of back vertex power, and the use of such lenses is appropriate when determining a patient's *distance* lens prescription. The *effectivity,* or effective power, of a lens depends on the distance from the back pole of the lens to the vertex of the cornea; whatever the form or thickness of a lens, lenses with the same back vertex power for parallel light have the same effectivity for axial rays as long as their back poles are placed at the same distance from the corneal vertex.

A different situation exists, however, when a refractor or trial lens is used to determine a patient's *near* prescription. In this situation, the light rays emerging from the test object (a near-point card) are *divergent* rather than parallel, with the result that the concept of back vertex power does not apply. Unless the spectacle lens for the near prescription is made in the same form and thickness as the test lens, it does not have the same near-point effectivity as the test lens—that is, it does not focus the image of a near object at the same position as it did with the test lens. For example, if a +5.00-D lens is needed for distance vision and the total power of the lenses in the refractor or trial frame for a near object is +7.50 D, a single-vision spectacle lens measuring +7.50 D (back vertex power) in a lensometer does not have the same effect as the test lenses unless the spectacle lens and the test lenses have the *same form.* This fact accounts for the discrepancy often found between the clearest working distance obtained with the refractor and that found when the finished spectacle lenses are worn.

The following example illustrates the effects on near-point effectivity when the lenses are made in a different form than that used in the examination.

EXAMPLE

The distance portion of a bifocal lens has a back vertex power of +5.00 D. A +2.50 D add is required for work at 40 cm. The final lens in the refractor head is +7.50 D sphere, in plano-convex form, with a center thickness of 5.0 mm, and with the convex surface facing the eye. For a viewing distance of 40 cm, the vergence leaving the plano front surface (effective F_1) is equal to

$$L' = F_1 + L$$

$$L' = 0.00 + \frac{1}{-0.40} = -2.50 \text{ D.}$$

In the back vertex power formula,

$$F_V = \frac{F_1}{1 - \frac{t}{n}F_1} + F_2,$$

we substitute the value of the vergence leaving the front surface (−2.50 D) for F_1, and solve for F_V, the vergence of light leaving the back surface.

$$F_V = \frac{-2.50}{1 - \frac{0.005}{1.523}(-2.50)} + 7.50$$

$$= \frac{-2.50}{1 - (0.00328)(-2.50)} + 7.50$$

$$= \frac{-2.50}{1 + 0.0082} + 7.50$$

$$= -2.48 + 7.50 = +5.02 \text{ D.}$$

Thus, this lens has a *near-point effectivity* of +5.02 D.

The near prescription of +7.50 D back vertex power is made with a back surface of −5.50 D, a thickness of 6.0 mm, and a diameter of 55 mm. To determine the value of F_1,

$$F_1 = \frac{F_V - F_2}{1 + \frac{t}{n}(F_V - F_2)}$$

$$F_1 = \frac{+7.50 - (-5.50)}{1 + \frac{0.006}{1.523}[7.50 - (-5.50)]}$$

$$F_1 = \frac{13}{1 + 0.00394(13.00)}$$

$$= \frac{13}{1.0512}$$

$$= +12.37 \text{ D.}$$

The vergence of light at the front surface, L_1, for an object at 40 cm (effective F_1) is

$$L_1 = F_1 + L$$

$$= +12.37 + \frac{1}{-0.40}$$

$$= +12.37 - 2.50 = +9.87 \text{ D.}$$

The vergence of light leaving the back surface (near-point effectivity) is

$$F_V = \frac{F_1}{1 - \frac{t}{n}F_1} + F_2$$

$$F_V = \frac{9.87}{1 - \frac{0.006}{1.523}(9.87)} + (-5.50)$$

$$= \frac{9.87}{1 - 0.03889} + (-5.50)$$

$$= \frac{9.87}{0.961} + (-5.50)$$

$$= 10.27 - 5.50 = +4.77 \text{ D}$$

Thus, this lens has a near-point effectivity of +4.77 D.

Comparing the near-point effectivity of the refractor lenses (+5.02 D) to the near-point effectivity of the final lens (+4.77 D), we find that the final lens is *too weak* by the amount of

$$+5.02 - 4.77 \text{ D} = 0.25 \text{ D.}$$

Although it is difficult to duplicate the exact *effectivity* achieved under the test conditions for a near object with either single-vision lenses or bifocal lenses, the difference is usually small, and in most cases it is not necessary to have exact correspondence in effectivity of the test lenses and the patient's lenses. Most patients can make a slight alteration in near working distance without difficulty. It is important, however, that the powers of the lenses fall within the individual patient's tolerance.

Standards published by the American National Standards Institute (ANSI Z80.1-1995)[7] recommend, as do manufacturers of bifocal lenses, that the power of the near portion of a bifocal lens should be measured with the *segment side* of the lens placed against the lensometer stop.

1. For a *back surface segment,* such as an Ultex-style bifocal, the power of both the distance and the near portions

Reading 1

Reading 2

FIGURE 8–51.   **For a back surface bifocal,** *back* **vertex power should be measured. The first lensometer reading is the back vertex power of the distance-vision portion; the second reading is the back vertex power of the near-vision portion. The power of the add is equal to the second reading minus the first reading. A₁ is the position of the front pole or vertex of the distance portion.**

of the lens should be measured by placing the *back* surface of the lens against the lensometer stop to measure the back vertex power (Figure 8–51). The power of the bifocal addition is the back vertex power of the near portion of the lens minus the back vertex power of the distance portion.

2. For a *front surface segment,* such as a fused bifocal, the back vertex power of the distance portion is measured in the usual manner, with the back surface of the lens against the lens stop. To obtain the power of the add, both the distance and near portions of the lens should be measured by placing the lens in the instrument with its *front* surface against the lensometer stop (Figure 8–52) to measure the front vertex power. The power of the bifocal addition is the front vertex power of the near portion of the lens minus the front vertex power of the distance portion.

Confusion exists in the minds of many optometrists concerning the recommended method of measuring the power of the addition of a front surface bifocal segment.[8] With few exceptions, optometrists use refractors with lenses calibrated in terms of back vertex power; logic says that the finished lens should conform to the back vertex power determined by use of the refractor. Furthermore, because the patient looks through the lens from the back, why must the power of the addition be verified by reversing the lens in the lensometer? The answer is that there are limitations in the back vertex power notation.

Whether the lensometer is used to measure back vertex power or front vertex power, for the image of the lensometer target to be seen sharply focused on the reticle, the light between the test lens and the eyepiece must be *parallel* (Figure 8–53).

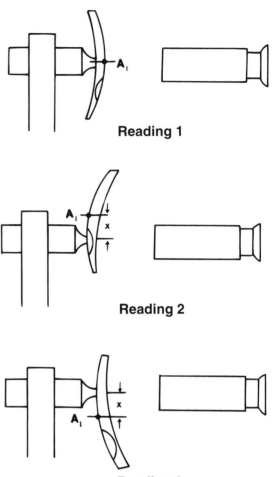

Reading 1

Reading 2

Reading 3

FIGURE 8–52.   **For a front surface bifocal, A₁ denotes the position of the front pole or vertex. The first lensometer reading is the back vertex power of the distance portion, at the distance pole; the second reading is the front vertex power of the reading portion; the third reading is the front vertex power of the distance portion. Note that the distance, x, is the same in the second and third diagrams to balance the effect of thickness. The power of the add is equal to the difference between the second reading and third reading.**

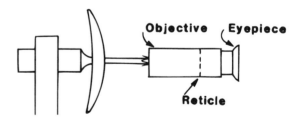

FIGURE 8–53.   **For the image of the lensometer target to be seen sharply focused on the reticle, the light between the test lens and the eyepiece must be parallel.**

A bifocal lens can be considered as a distance lens with a specified back vertex power, having a plus spherical add placed on the front or back surface. The power of the distance lens is correctly verified in terms of back vertex power by placing the back pole of the lens against the lens stop. For a front surface bifocal, it is apparent that the back surface of the lens provides the same change in vergence through both the distance and the near portions of the lens. The difference in vergence of the wavefronts between the distance and near portions is generated solely by the *segment* on the front surface. To measure the difference in effectivity occurring at the front surface of the lens, for a near object, the readings must be made with the front surface of the lens against the lens stop.

Although neither of the two front vertex powers (for the distance and the near-vision portions of the lens) is actually experienced by the wearer, the important consideration is that the *difference* between these two powers determines the power of the add.

The purpose of the bifocal addition is to change the vergence of the light from a near object so that it appears to originate from a greater distance. For an absolute presbyope, the add must render diverging rays from a near object *parallel*, as if they came from infinity. The distance lens then directs the rays toward the far point of the eye, and the optical system of the eye focuses the rays on the retina. This is shown in Figure 8–54.

There is a slight difference in effectivity for near refraction when an add is placed on the front surface instead of the back surface of a lens. Even though the two adds have the same power when each is measured on the segment side of the lens, the effectivity of the back surface segment is slightly less than that of a front surface segment.

For most lenses, the measurement of a front-surface-segment add results in essentially the same power whether the front or the back surface of the lens is placed against the lensometer stop. Any difference is not large enough to be significant. However, for lenses with an *appreciable center thickness* (high plus lenses or industrial safety lenses) the difference in the two methods of measurement often exceed 0.25 D.

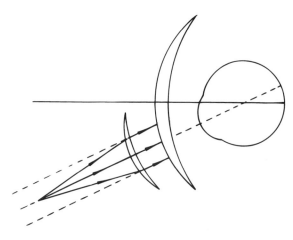

FIGURE 8–54. **For an absolute presbyope, the bifocal add should render diverging rays from a near object parallel, as if they came from the far point of the eye as corrected by the distance-vision lens.**

EXAMPLE
Given the Executive-style bifocal of +8.00 D having a center thickness of 6.0 mm, a back surface power of –6.00 D, and a +2.50 D add, find F_1, for the top and bottom of the lens.

Solving for F_1 for the top of the lens.

$$F_1 = \frac{F_V - F_2}{1 + \frac{t}{n}(F_V - F_2)}$$

$$= \frac{+8.00 - (-6.00)}{1 + \frac{0.006}{1.523}[8.00 - (6.00)]}$$

$$= \frac{14}{1 + 0.00349(14)}$$

$$= \frac{14}{1.055} = +13.27 \text{ D.}$$

Solving for F_1 for the bottom of the lens:

$$F_1 = +13.77 + 2.50 = +15.77 \text{ D.}$$

Solving for F_V for the bottom of the lens:

$$F_V = \frac{F_1}{1 - \frac{t}{n}F_1} + F_2$$

$$= \frac{15.77}{1 - 0.00394(15.77)} + (-6.00)$$

$$= \frac{15.77}{1 - 0.062} + (-6.00)$$

$$= \frac{15.77}{0.938} + (-6.00)$$

$$= +16.81 - 6.00 = +10.81 \text{ D.}$$

The add determined by back vertex power comparison between the top and the bottom is equal to

$$+10.81 - 8.00 = +2.81 \text{ D,}$$

and the measured add determined from the two back surface measurements is +2.81 D.
Since

$$+2.81 - 2.50 = +0.31 \text{ D,}$$

we see that the add is 0.31 D too strong.

The measured add determined from front surface measurements (front vertex power, or neutralizing power) for the top and bottom of the lens can be calculated as follows:

Solving for F_N for the top of the lens:

$$F_N = \frac{F_2}{1 - \frac{t}{n}F_2} + F_1$$

$$= \frac{-6.00}{1 - \frac{0.06}{1.523}(-6.00)} + 13.27$$

$$= \frac{-6.00}{1 + 0.02364} + 13.27$$

$$= \frac{-6.00}{1.02364} + 13.27$$

$$= -5.86 + 13.27 = +7.41 \text{ D}$$

Solving for F_N for the bottom of the lens:

$$F_N = \cfrac{-6.00}{1 - \cfrac{0.06}{1.523}(-6.00)} + 15.77$$

$$= \frac{-6.00}{1 + 0.02364} + 15.77$$

$$= \frac{-6.00}{1.02364} + 15.77$$

$$= -5.86 + 15.77 = +9.91 \text{ D.}$$

$$\text{Add} = F_{N(\text{bottom})} - F_{N(\text{top})}$$

$$= +9.91 - 7.44 = +2.50 \text{ D.}$$

The difference is smaller for strong minus lenses than it is for strong plus lenses for two reasons: (1) Strong minus lenses have smaller center thicknesses than those of strong plus lenses, and (2) strong minus lenses have flatter front surfaces than those of strong plus lenses, which creates smaller vergence changes at the back surface of the lens when it is measured with the back pole of the lens against the lens stop.

In summary, it appears to be almost impossible, for the viewing of a near object, to provide exactly the same effectivity with a spectacle lens (either for a single-vision reading lens or for a bifocal lens) as with the test lenses calibrated in back surface power. The manufacturer places the addition either on the front surface or on the back surface, and if measurements are made through the distance portion and the near portion with the *segment surface* against the lensometer stop, the difference between the two readings equals the addition specified in the prescription. It may appear that the recommended procedure for measuring bifocal additions exists only for the purpose of standardization—that is, to convince all parties to agree with the procedure. This is true, up to a point; however, the recommended procedure *is accurate*.

One other point is important. Most manufacturers make multifocal lenses in *semifinished* form, that is, only the segment side is finished. The add is unalterably fixed before the other parameters (such as distance power, back surface power, and thickness) are known. This procedure applies to all multifocals, whether bifocals, trifocals, or progressive addition lenses, and to segments, whether on the front or back surface.

8.28. Prescribing and Fitting Double-Segment Bifocals

The double-segment bifocal may be the most *underutilized* bifocal style. Experience shows that, when a double-segment bifocal is prescribed (and correctly fitted) for a patient who must make use of near vision above eye level on a routine basis, wearers have little difficulty adjusting to them and usually request them again when the prescription must be changed. A probable reason for underutilization is that many practitioners fail to ask their patients about the need for above-eye-level vision.

The correct method of fitting a double-segment bifocal is illustrated in Figure 8–55. Most double-segment bifocals

FIGURE 8–55. **The correct method of fitting a double-segment bifocal. A, Double Executive and B, double straight-top fused. The top edge of the lower segment is fitted in the usual manner, from 1 to 2 mm below the lower limbus.**

have a separation of *13 mm* between the upper and lower segments. Because the vertical extent of the cornea is about 11 or 12 mm, if the top edge of the lower segment is fitted in the usual manner (at 1 to 2 mm below the lower limbus), the lower edge of the upper segment is approximately at the level of the upper limbus (which is usually slightly *above* the ciliary line of the upper lid).

The double-segment bifocal is *not a trifocal*. For most people, near vision above eye level involves about the same working distance as near vision below eye level. Thus, the power of the add in the upper segment should be the same in most cases as that in the lower segment. As noted in Section 8.4, all double-segment bifocals have the same power in both the upper and lower segments with the exception of the Tillyer Double Executive that has an upper segment with a power approximately two-thirds the power of the lower segment.

8.29. Prescribing and Fitting Trifocals

When a patient requires a +1.75- or +2.00 D add (which usually occurs at about age 50), the practitioner should seriously consider recommending *trifocal* lenses. Like double-segment bifocals, trifocals are generally underutilized. Many practitioners think of trifocals as vocational lenses. However, almost *any* advanced presbyope has difficulty with arm's-length tasks, such as seeing merchandise and prices in a supermarket, through either the upper or lower portion of a bifocal lens.

As a rule, a patient should have to use no more than half the amplitude of accommodation on a sustained basis. For instance, a patient with 2.00 D of accommodation should have to *use* only 1.00 D of accommodation, and therefore should be given (for a 40-cm reading distance) a +1.50 D add. With 2.00 D of accommodation, the near point of accommodation (through the *distance* lenses) is 50 cm; the far point (or the most remote distance that allows clear vision through the *segment*) through a +1.50 D segment is

$$\frac{1}{1.50} = 67 \text{ cm,}$$

and the closest distance of clear vision through the *segment* is

$$\frac{1}{2.00 + 1.50} = \frac{1}{3.50} = 29 \text{ cm.}$$

Figure 8–56 shows that there is an area of *overlap* (A) between the distances at which objects can be seen clearly through the distance and near portions of the lens. Moreover, the depth of field of view of the eye makes this area of overlap even larger.

For a patient who has an amplitude of accommodation of only 1.00 D, only 0.50 D of accommodation should be used on a routine basis; thus, a +2.00-D add is required for a 40-cm working distance. With 1.00 D of accommodation, the near point of accommodation through the *distance* portion of the lens is 1 m, and the range through the near portion of the lens extends outward to

$$\frac{1}{2.00} = 50 \text{ cm}$$

and inward to

$$\frac{1}{+1.00 + 2.00} = \frac{1}{3.00} = 33.3 \text{ cm.}$$

As shown in Figure 8–56B, there is a *gap* from a distance of 1 m to a distance of 50 cm, in which vision is blurred through both the distance and near portions of the lens. Although the depth of field of view adds approximately 0.25 D to the far end of the near range (through the segment) and to the near end of the distance range, there is still a gap extending 80 to 57 cm.

When a practitioner increases a patient's bifocal addition from +1.50 to +2.00 D, the patient believes it is the *practitioner's fault* that the gap exists because the gap did not exist with previous glasses. For this reason, the practitioner must inform the patient that a gap will be present because of the increase in the add to +2.00 D (or even to + 1.75 D). Better yet, the existence of the gap can be *demonstrated* to

the patient, either by the use of the refractor or by the use of trial lenses.

Many presbyopic patients are unaware of the existence of trifocals or do not understand their function, and are therefore unaware of the possibility of improved vision at intermediate distances. A careful analysis of the patient's visual status should consider not only the patient's age and amplitude of accommodation but the patient's occupation, hobbies, and the requirements for clear vision for specific intermediate tasks. As a *routine* matter, the practitioner should demonstrate to any patient requiring a + 1.50 D add (or greater) that clear vision is available at distance, at 40 cm, and at intermediate ranges with appropriate lens powers. Through education and demonstration, the inclusion of this procedure substantially increases the use of trifocals and improves the visual performance of many presbyopes.

Unfortunately, many practitioners are hesitant to suggest trifocals unless the patient specifically complains of blur at an intermediate distance. The hesitancy may occur partially because trifocal lenses are more expensive, but, more important, may be the result of the practitioner's failure to take an adequate case history and to take the time necessary to inform the patient of the problem and to demonstrate the problem (as described above). Practitioners who themselves wear trifocals are in a position to inform their patients in a manner not open to younger practitioners—that of offering personal testimony about the benefits.

Most patients adjust to trifocals at least as easily as they adjust to bifocals, often more easily. When dispensing the glasses, the practitioner should instruct the beginning trifocal wearer in the proper head movements for best vision through the intermediate and near segments.

Trifocals are available in both fused and one-piece styles. For the fused styles, the intermediate segment is made of glass with an index of refraction between that of the distance portion and that of the segment; for the one-piece styles, the intermediate segment has a curvature that is halfway between that of the distance portion of the lens and the bifocal segment. Most trifocals, whether fused or one-piece, are of straight-top construction. The standard power of the intermediate segment is 50% of the power of the lower segment, although some manufacturers of vocational trifocals vary the power of the intermediate segment and use 40% for weaker adds and as much as 70% for higher adds.

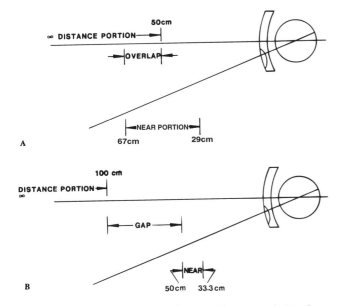

FIGURE 8–56.   **A, For a patient with 2.00 D of accommodation, there is an area of overlap (at distances of 50–67 cm) in which objects may be seen clearly through either the distance portion or the near portion of a bifocal lens; B, for a patient with 1.00 D of accommodation, there is a gap (at distances of 44 cm to 1 m) where vision is blurred in both the distance and the near-vision portions of the lens.**

Field of View

The vertical extent of the field of view through the intermediate-range segment depends on the following parameters:

1. The vertical dimension of the intermediate segment
2. The pupil size
3. The vertex distance
4. The viewing distance
5. The total power through the intermediate segment

As shown in Figure 8-57, the field of view in the vertical meridian is directly proportional to the *vertical dimension* (*depth*) of the intermediate segment (A). The most com-

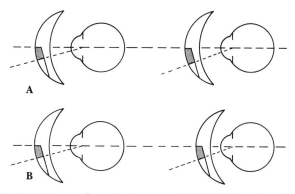

FIGURE 8–57.   **A, The vertical extent of the field of view for an intermediate segment is directly proportional to the vertical dimension (depth) of the intermediate segment; B, the vertical extent of the field of view for an intermediate segment of a given depth depends on the distance of the segment from the eye.**

monly used depth for an intermediate segment is 7 mm, but 6-, 8-, 10-, and even 14-mm segments are available. Although one may imagine that "bigger is better," increasing the vertical extent of the intermediate segment causes an infringement of either the near or the distance portion of the lens. The deeper the intermediate segment, the lower the upper boundary of the *near* portion (or the higher the lower boundary of the *distance* portion).

With a given vertical dimension, the smaller the patient's pupil, the larger the vertical field of view before doubling of the image occurs. If the edge of the intermediate field splits the pupil, two images are seen, varying in position, size, and focus. Fortunately, most presbyopic patients have small pupils.

The vertical extent of the field of view for an intermediate segment of a given depth depends on the distance of the segment from the eye (as shown in Figure 8–57B). The field of view decreases as the *vertex distance* increases. For this reason, the field of view is also influenced by the pantoscopic tilt, the curvature of the segment surface, and whether the segment is placed on the front or the back surface of the lens.

For a constant lens power, the *linear* size of the field of view increases as the *viewing distance* increases, even though the *angular* field of view remains constant. For a pupil size of 3.5 mm, a vertex distance of 12 mm, and a viewing distance of 56 cm (22 inches), Holmes, Jollife, and Gregg[9] showed that the absolute field of view (the field in which there is no diplopia) is:

6.0 cm for a 6-mm intermediate segment
8.3 cm for a 7-mm intermediate segment
10.6 cm for an 8-mm segment

For a viewing distance of 69 cm (27 inches), the absolute field of view is:

7.6 cm for a 6-mm intermediate segment
10.6 cm for a 7-mm intermediate segment
13.5 cm for an 8-mm intermediate segment

The vertical extent of the field of view for the intermediate segment also varies with the *power of the lens* in the in-

termediate portion of the lens. The field decreases with increasing plus lens power and increases with increasing minus lens power.

Segment Height

In the laboratory order, the segment height of a trifocal lens is specified as the distance of the *upper edge* of the intermediate segment from the lower edge of the lens. No other trifocal parameter has been more controversial than that of specification of segment height. Although the purpose of a trifocal lens is to provide the wearer with intermediate-range vision, with few exceptions, the wearer will use the lenses much more often for the normal near-point (reading) range than for the intermediate range. Comfortable near-point vision, therefore, should not be sacrificed for the sake of intermediate-range vision.

The trifocal segment can be considered as sitting on top of the bifocal segment, in the position in which the bifocal segment would be *without* the intermediate segment, as shown in Figure 8–58. For example, if a patient would normally require a 17-mm-high bifocal, the height of the trifocal segment should be specified as 23 mm for a 6-mm segment or as 24 mm for a 7-mm segment. The result of this method of fitting is that the area occupied by the intermediate segment is taken *entirely* from what would otherwise have been the distance portion of the lens. Any substantial departure from this practice, such as placing the top of the intermediate segment at the customary bifocal height, makes the near segment inaccessible for close work. On occasion, the intermediate segment may be placed in a unique position for a specific vocational purpose, but such a situation is rare. For the patient described above, Figure 8–58 shows that if the top of the bifocal segment is 2 mm below the lower limbus, and if the vertical diameter of the cornea is 12 mm with a 3-mm pupil, the top of a 7-mm segment falls slightly above the lower margin of the pupil.

When a trifocal lens is fitted for occupational use (that is, for a person who routinely works at an intermediate distance), the top of the intermediate segment is usually placed at the lower edge of the pupil. Variations in head position and in physical stature, however, must be taken into consideration. For nonoccupational use, the top of

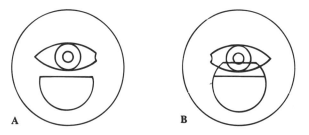

FIGURE 8–58.   **A, Segment height for a bifocal lens; B, trifocal segment height—the top edge of the near segment of the trifocal lens should be in the same position that it would be in without the intermediate segment.**

the intermediate segment is normally placed no more than 1 or 2 mm below the lower margin of the pupil. For a short, stout person or for a chronic "line-noticer," the top of the segment may be placed near the midpoint between the lower limbus and the lower edge of the pupil. However, as with bifocal lenses, many more errors are made in setting segments *too low* than in setting them too high. Fitting a trifocal lens too low makes use of the reading segment very inconvenient—the wearer must tilt the head back excessively, just as the person must do if a bifocal segment is fitted too low.

Several devices are available for measuring segment height for both near and intermediate-range segments. For example, glazed frames may be used for marking trifocal segment height. However, the *most accurate* measurement of segment height is made if the patient wears a fitting sample that corresponds to the frame style, eye size, and DBL of the frame selected by the patient. For a patient's first trifocal prescription it is advisable to use a frame or mounting with *adjustable nose pads* because such a frame allows some latitude in adjusting the segment height after the glasses are dispensed.

INVISIBLE BIFOCALS AND PROGRESSIVE ADDITION LENSES

8.30. Invisible Bifocals

On reaching an age at which a reading addition is required, most ametropic patients readily (although reluctantly) accept the practitioner's advice that bifocal lenses offer the best solution to the problem. Although the use of two pairs of glasses—one for distance vision and one for reading—may be considered as an alternative, most people who try this system eventually find (as Benjamin Franklin did, more than 200 years ago) that switching from one pair to the other becomes very tiresome. However, some people, if given a choice, accept bifocals only on the condition that the bifocal segments be as *invisible* as possible.

An inexpensive method of making bifocal segments *almost* invisible is to use a fused, no-chrome round segment with a light tint. Such a segment has a feathered edge all around, and its invisibility is enhanced because the chromatic dispersion is almost the same for the barium crown glass segment as it is for the ophthalmic crown glass major lens. Although a round-top segment is slightly more difficult for most people to adapt to than is a straight-top segment, the lens, on the whole, provides very good optical performance. One reason for slower adaptation is that the widest portion of the segment is at the center (rather than at or near the top, as with a straight-top segment); as a result, the eyes must be lowered farther into the segment for useful near vision. Another reason is the larger amount of *image jump*, when compared with that for a fused or a one-piece straight-top segment.

An often overlooked advantage of the round segment fused bifocal is its very small amount of *differential displacement at the reading level.* If a 20-mm round segment is fitted with the segment top *2 mm above the ciliary line*, there is only a small amount of differential displacement at the reading level (if we assume a reading level 10 mm below the position of the visual axis in the primary position). Although fitting the segment top at this height may result in a segment that is too high for many patients (depending on lens size and shape, pantoscopic tilt, and anatomical factors) it is, nevertheless, a good idea to fit this bifocal relatively

high—*at least* at the level of the ciliary line to achieve not only a minimum of differential displacement at the reading level but also (and perhaps more important) to eliminate the need for the patient to throw the head back to use the wider portions of the bifocal segment.

No-chrome round fused bifocals, such as the Sola RD and the Vision-Ease CRF, are high-quality, corrected-curve lenses. Although a straight-top segment has obvious advantages over a round segment, when a patient requests an "invisible" bifocal, the practitioner should seriously consider a lightly tinted, fused, no-chrome, round segment bifocal.

Multifocal lenses designed specifically to be *invisible* are available in two categories: (1) blended bifocals and (2) progressive addition lenses. A *blended bifocal* is a one-piece, round segment bifocal in which the transition between the major lens and the bifocal segment has been blended over a relatively small zone to reduce its visibility. A *progressive addition lens* is also a one-piece lens with no visible segment area, but it differs from a blended bifocal in that there is a progressive increase in plus power over a relatively large area between the upper (distance) and lower (near) portions of the lens. The portion of the lens within which the power of the addition varies is known as the *progressive zone*. The power of the addition in this corridor varies, in a continuous manner, from zero in the distance portion of the lens to that of the full add in the near portion. Although progressive addition lenses are advocated to provide a continuity of vision from infinity to the near point, and hence satisfy the needs of the patient who would otherwise wear trifocals, the predominant motivating factor for using this lens (on the part of both practitioners and patients) is often that the segment is *completely invisible.*

8.31. Blended Bifocals

When a blended bifocal lens (Figure 8–59) is made, the procedure by which the one-piece segment is blended results in an annular band, 3 to 5 mm in width, that encircles the segment (A). The width of the annular band varies by manufacturer but also depends on the base curve of the lens and the power of the add. Although the power of a blended bifocal changes gradually (rather than abruptly) from the distance to the near-vision portion of the lens, the blended area is *unusable* to the wearer. There is no usable "progressive zone," as a progressive addition lens has. None of the blended bifocal segments is really completely invisible, especially when viewed obliquely. Each has a *bump* on the front surface; the higher the power of the add, the larger and the more noticeable the bump.

The blended bifocal was first introduced in 1946 by Howard Beach; it was called the Beach Blended bifocal. This lens is no longer available. The Younger Seamless bifocal was introduced in 1954, and is currently available in ophthalmic crown glass, in CR-39 plastic, in photochromic glass, and in High-Lite (high-index) glass. In 1979 Coburn Optical began marketing the Coburn E-Z 2 Vue lens. It is available in CR-39 plastic only. Shortly thereafter many other manufacturers introduced blended bifocal lenses, available only in CR-39 material. American Optical introduced the Ultravue Blended bifocal; Sola Optical followed with the Sola Blend 2000; Silor Optical introduced the Super Blend 25; and Robinson-Houchin designed the Ultimate blended lens.

In the manufacture of a blended bifocal, when the line of intersection between the major lens and the segment is blended, the rate of change of curvature in the radial meridians (the meridians that pass through the segment center in all directions) is substantially more rapid than the rate of change of curvature in the circumferential meridians. The difference between the two curvatures, at any point in the transition zone, represents *cylinder power*, usually referred to by lens designers simply as *astigmatism*. Unwanted astigmatism (Figure 8–59B) is an inevitable con-

sequence of manufacturing a blended bifocal; the astigmatism cannot be avoided. The amount of astigmatism is a function of the rate of change in curvature, which in turn depends on the width of the blended area and the power of the add. The amount of astigmatism decreases as the width of the blend increases; the manufacturer may choose either a wide blended zone, which produces a smaller amount of astigmatism, or a narrow blended zone, which produces a larger amount of astigmatism. And, of course, the narrower the blended area, the narrower the *unusable* portion of the lens.

Knoll[10] found that the magnitude of the cylindrical component in the transition zone of a blended bifocal was roughly equal to the power of the add. For a given distance from the center of the segment, the amount of astigmatism is the same, but the principal meridians of the unwanted cylinder vary with the direction of the patient's gaze because one of the principal meridians is parallel to the direction of the radial meridian and the other principal meridian is parallel to the direction of the corresponding circumferential meridian.

In fitting and dispensing the blended bifocal, the top of the blended zone should normally be placed 1 or 2 mm above the lower ciliary line, which places the astigmatism-free area of the segment in the most favorable position. The manufacturer of a blended bifocal places an ink mark on the lens at the upper end of the blended zone (Figure 8–59A), to assist the practitioner in arriving at the segment height. To provide as large a vertical field of view through the segment as possible, it is important to select a frame with a deep vertical dimension. It is best to use a corneal reflection method of measuring the PD and to fit the segments to the monocular PD to ensure maximum use of the entire segment width. Representative blended bifocals are listed in Table 8–12.

FIGURE 8–59. **A,** A blended bifocal lens has an annular transition area (dashed lines), 3 to 5 mm wide, which is unusable because of unwanted astigmatism. The horizontal line above the transition area is the manufacturer's ink mark, used to gauge segment height. **B,** The annular-shaped zone of unwanted astigmatism in a blended bifocal lens. (Reprinted with permission from American Optical Truvision Progressive Lenses, American Optical Corp., 1984.)

TABLE 8–12
Representative Blended Bifocals

Material	Manufacturer	Name	Size
CR-39	American Optical	Blended bifocal	23–24
	Phillips Lens	Ultimate	25
	Signet Armorlite	Blended 25	25
	Silor	Super Blended 25	25
	Sola	Blended 22	22
		EZ 2 Vue	28
	Vision-Ease	Blended 25	25
	X-Cel	X-Celite Blend 25	25
	Younger	Seamless 22	22
		Seamless 28	28
Crown Glass	Younger	Seamless 22	22

8.32. Progressive Addition Lenses

In progressive addition lenses, there is a continuous downward transition of lens power from a stable distance power in the upper portion of the lens through a *progressive zone* to a stable near-vision portion in the lower area of the lens. The increase in power is caused by an increase in curvature in the progressive zone; that is, there is a progressive decrease in the front surface radius of curvature between the constant radius of the distance portion and that of the near portion. This basic principle is followed in the construction of all progressive addition lenses and is illustrated in Figure 8–60.

A progressive addition lens is a one-piece lens having distance and near portions that are relatively stable in power and free of aberrations; the progressive zone extends across the entire width of the lens and connects the distance and near-vision portions. As shown in Figure 8–61, the central portion, which is the usable area of the progressive zone, is known as the *progressive corridor*. Within the progressive corridor, the power increases continuously from the distance to the near portion of the lens. All powers between the distance and near prescriptions are present in the progressive corridor. There is no visible reading segment and there are no dividing lines; hence there is an absence of image jump.

The advantages of clear vision at all distances and the absence of a visible reading segment are partially offset by areas in which the aberration of *astigmatism* is present. The astigmatism occurs because a progressive addition surface (normally the front surface of the lens) is produced by generating an *aspherical* curvature, a process that produces local and gradual variations in refractive power as well as astigmatism. It is impossible, both mathematically and physically, to design and construct a progressive addition lens that does *not* produce astigmatism in the lateral portion of the progressive zone.

The principal parameters of a progressive addition lens are interrelated, and include (1) the size of the distance and near areas, (2) the types and intensity of the aberrations, and (3) the depth and usable width of the progressive corridor. Differences in lens design reflect differences in the designer's priorities. Compromises must be made between areas of high image performance and the severity of the aberrations.

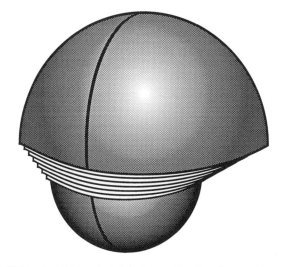

FIGURE 8–60. **Basic principle in the construction of progressive surfaces. There is a constant decrease in the radii of curvature between the radius of the distance portion and that of the near-vision portion. (Reprinted with permission from Carl Zeiss Optical.)**

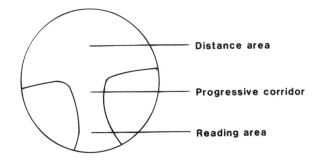

Distance area

Progressive corridor

Reading area

FIGURE 8–61. **Progressive addition lens, showing progressive corridor connecting the distance-vision and near-vision portions.**

When an aspherical surface with a variable radius of curvature is generated, the inherent astigmatism found to the right or left of the line at the center of the progressive corridor (a line known as the *umbilicus*) is proportional to the *rate of change in curvature*. Hence, there are two basic approaches to the design of progressive addition lenses. The approaches are sometimes referred to as *hard* and *soft* designs, referring to the amount and distribution of the astigmatism on the convex lens surface.

1. The *hard* design is created by having a short progressive corridor. Because the amount of surface astigmatism generated is a function of the rate of progression, this design concentrates the intense aberrations into small regions adjacent to the progressive corridor and near add area. Thus, large areas of the lens are free from astigmatism. For the wearer, the advantage of the hard design is the presence of large distance and near-vision zones that are free of astigmatism. Also, the near-vision area is located closer to the distance center and is therefore more accessible with downward rotation of the eyes. The drawback of the hard design is that the areas of high aberrations adjoining the progressive corridor and the near add areas produce strongly blurred vision and spatial distortion.

2. *Soft* designs have a long progressive corridor that extends into the lateral portions of the distance and near areas of the lens. Because there is no heavy concentration of aberrations in any one area, the intensity of the resulting astigmatism and visual disturbances are reduced. However, this design provides smaller areas of high-quality imagery in the distance and near-vision portions of the lens. Also, the soft design imposes a lower location of the near-vision add area, which forces greater eye or head movements to use that area.

Hard designs offer large fields of view for distance and near-vision areas, but they impose more intense peripheral aberrations and spatial distortions adjacent to the progressive corridor and near-vision area. Soft designs offer less noticeable blurring and spatial distortion in the periphery, but provide smaller fields of sharp vision in the distance and near-vision portions of the lens. Figure 8–62 illustrates the differences between hard and soft progressive addition lens designs.

When the visual axes pass through areas of the lenses where astigmatism is present, the wearer's vision not only is blurred but objects in the visual field tend to "rock" or "swim," especially under conditions in which relatively large, and repeated, eye movements are made. These subjective symptoms are directly related to the astigmatism and to changes in magnification that result from the gradual increase in power toward the bottom of the lens; the more severe the symptoms, the longer the adaptation period.

It is possible to calculate the approximate amount of astigmatism adjacent to the progressive corridor.[11] Assume that no astigmatism exists along the center line (umbilicus) of a symmetrical aspherical surface, and that a refractive change of 1 D occurs along the center line over a vertical distance Y (Figure 8–63). Along a vertical line parallel to the center line and at a lateral distance Y from the umbilical line, the astigmatism is approximately 2.00 D.

The Omnifocal Lens

The first commercially successful progressive addition lens introduced in the United States was the Omnifocal, invented by David Volk and Joseph Weinberg in 1961. It was a glass lens, manufactured by Robinson-Houchin, and marketed to the profession in 1965 by Univis Lens Company. The *front* surface of the lens was the aspherical (progressive) surface. On this surface, the radius of curvature in the *vertical* meridian gradually decreased from the top to the bottom of the lens, but the radius of curvature in the *horizontal* meridian did not vary. The power of the cylinder in the horizontal meridian was +0.75 D greater than the power of the desired addition; that is, for a +1.50 D, add, the cylinder on the front surface had a power of +2.25 D. On the front surface of the lens, the spherical power, increasing gradually from top to bottom with a constant amount of astigmatism, created a *plus cylinder, axis 90*; its power was constant in the horizontal meridian. To eliminate the plus cylinder and to produce the correction for the eye's astigmatism, a compensating toric surface had to be ground on the back surface of the lens. This resulted in a *bi-toric* lens, with the axis of the back surface cylinder normally at an oblique angle to the 90° axis of the front surface cylinder. Calculation of the amount and axis of the back surface cylinder for this lens, as well as the manufacturing process, were complicated procedures. These and other problems contributed to the slowness with which this lens was accepted.

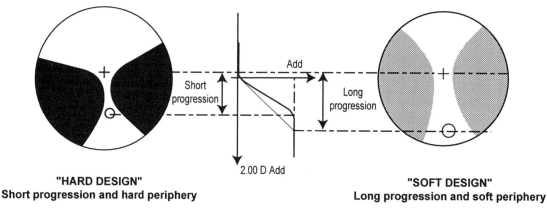

"HARD DESIGN"
Short progression and hard periphery

"SOFT DESIGN"
Long progression and soft periphery

FIGURE 8–62. **Comparison of the power progression path and peripheral aberration between hard and soft progressive addition design. (Reprinted with permission from Essilor International/Varilux Corp.)**

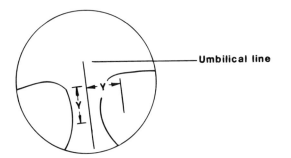

FIGURE 8–63. **The amount of astigmatism at a lateral distance Y from the umbilical line is equal to twice the change in power for the vertical distance Y in this diagram.**

The distance and near-vision centers of the Omnifocal lens are separated by a vertical distance of 25 mm. Because the power in the vertical meridian varies over the entire extent of the lens, the total amount of plus power actually *decreases* from the distance optical center upward, but increases from the distance optical center downward (Figure 8–64).

The increase in plus power, as the line of sight moves downward through the lens, is *nonlinear*, which results in a maximum addition of + 1.75 D for a lowering of the line of sight by 25 mm, but only one-fourth this amount of added plus power is created by lowering the line of sight 12.5 mm. The increase in astigmatism, too, is nonlinear and increases ever more rapidly as the visual axis approaches the bottom of the lens. Because the progression occurred over the entire front surface of the lens (from top to bottom) this lens was the epitome of a soft design. The Omnifocal is no longer available, but many other progressive addition lenses have been introduced.

The Varilux Lens

Developed by Bernard Maitenaz, the original Varilux lens was introduced by Essel Optical of France in 1959. This lens enjoyed considerable success in Europe before it was introduced in the United States by Titmus Optical Company in 1967. The original Varilux lens, now called the Varilux 1, differed from the Omnifocal in that the upper half of the lens had no progression in power. The progression was con-

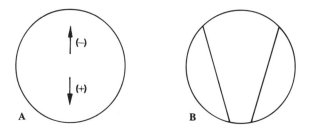

FIGURE 8–64. **The Omnifocal lens. A, The plus power in the distance-vision portion decreases from the distance optical center upward; B, the usable area of the lens is wide at the top and gradually narrows toward the bottom.**

fined to a 12-mm-deep zone in the center of the lens, throughout which the power increased in a linear fashion. Below the progressive corridor was a zone of maximum addition having a constant power and a width of about 22 mm.

The astigmatism-free progressive corridor of the original Varilux lens was approximately 5 mm wide. Outside the hourglass-shaped area containing the distance area were the progressive corridor and the reading area; the amount of unwanted astigmatism increased toward the bottom of the lens. In the areas lateral to the progressive corridor, the axis of the astigmatism varied in such a manner as to cause a sensation of blurring and vertigo. Unfortunately, the usable width of the progressive corridor decreased with increasing power of the add.

The design of the original Varilux lens evolved over a period of 8 years and took place in four principal stages.[12] Although the theoretical problems of surface design were challenging, the design and construction of the surfacing machinery proved to be even more difficult.

As shown in Figure 8–65, the distance portion of this lens has a conventional spherical surface. At the beginning of the progressive zone, without any visible line of demarcation, the radius of curvature begins to shorten and uniformly decreases over a distance of 12 mm until the full power of the addition is reached. At that point, the progressive surface merges into a second portion that is essentially spherical and has the curvature necessary to produce the power for the add. The boundaries of the stabilized near area are invisible. No image jump occurs between the lower portion of the distance area and the beginning of the progressive zone or between the end of the progressive zone and the stabilized near area. Because the progressive surface is confined to a 12-mm-deep zone, rather than extending from top to bottom, the Varilux lens is considered a hard design.

The umbilical line (the line of symmetry at the center of the progressive corridor) has the following property: For small distances around each point on this line, the vertical and horizontal radii of curvature are essentially equal. Hence, for any point along the line of symmetry, quasi-spherical surface properties exist. With the determination of the curvature along the vertical meridian, and with the requirement that the line of symmetry form an umbilical line, the progressive surface and its image properties are largely predetermined.

Varilux lenses are manufactured differentially for the right and left eyes, with the line of symmetry inclined nasally toward the bottom of the lens so that it conforms to the convergence of the visual axes for any point in the progressive zone (Figure 8–66). The inclination provides a segment inset of 2.5 mm from the distance optical center. As a result, equal horizontal eye excursions to the right or the left of the line of symmetry provide uniform power changes (A). Other progressive addition lenses achieve segment inset by rotating the segments nasally; equal horizontal eye movements to the right or left of the line of symmetry do not result in uniform power changes (B). Laboratory finishing to the prescribed distance power, whether spherical or sphero-cylindrical, is accomplished on the *back* surface in the same manner as for any front surface multifocal lens. In the United States, the original Varilux lens was available only in glass.

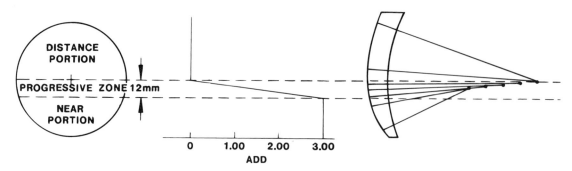

FIGURE 8–65.   The original Varilux lens. The distance portion has no progression of power, but in the progressive zone the radius of curvature decreases over a distance of 12 mm until the full power of the addition is achieved. (Reprinted with permission from *All About Varilux: The Progressive Addition Lens*. Titmus Optical, Petersburg, VA, 1967.)

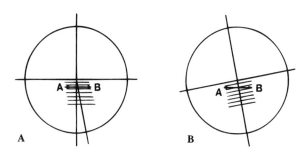

FIGURE 8–66.   A, With the Varilux lens, the line of symmetry is inclined nasally toward the bottom of the lens so that equal horizontal eye movements provide uniform power changes; B, if segment inset is provided by nasalward rotation, equal horizontal eye movements fail to provide uniform power changes. (Reprinted with permission from Essilor Optical.)

In 1972, Essilor Optical patented the Varilux 2 lens, a lens in which the entire front surface, not just the progressive zone, was of aspherical design. As shown in Figure 8–67, the cross-sections of the curves that form the front surface of the Varilux 2 lens are a family of conic sections. Starting in the upper portion of the lens, the conic section is first an oblate ellipse, gradually becomes a circle at the optical center of the lens, below which it gradually changes to increasingly flatter prolate ellipses, then to a parabola, and finally (in the near segment area) becomes increasingly flatter hyperbolas. In any horizontal section of the *upper portion* of the lens, the power (plus spherical power) is at a minimum at the midline and increases toward either side; in the *lower portion* of the lens, the plus power is at a maximum at the midline and decreases toward either side.

This design reduced the intensity of surface astigmatism and distortion in the peripheral areas of the lens, compared with that of the original Varilux. Therefore, the Varilux 2 is a softer design than the original Varilux. At the same time, the distance-vision area and the segment area, where high image resolution is present, are reduced in size. This modification in design not only reduced the amount of unwanted astigmatism in the peripheral portions of the progressive zone, but controlled the axis of the unwanted astigmatism in such a way that the rectangularity of peripherally viewed objects was preserved, which thus reduced the rocking and swaying and the disturbing deformation of the image.

When the original Varilux lens was discontinued, the Varilux 2 lens was called the Varilux lens. It is now called the Varilux Plus, and represents Varilux's general purpose, mono-design, aspheric based, progressive addition lens.

American Optical Progressive Lenses

When the patent on the original Varilux lens expired, other manufacturers quickly began to introduce their own versions of progressive addition lenses. In 1973 American Optical Company introduced the Ultravue lens, a CR-39 plastic lens. This lens had a segment area width of 25 mm, and it was later named the Ultravue 25. It was followed in 1978 by the Ultravue 28 lens, with a segment 28 mm wide. The Ultravue lens differs from the Varilux by having a well-defined distance-vision portion, free of surface astigmatism, and a relatively wide astigmatism-free segment area, but at the expense of a higher rate of progression in the 10- to 12-mm progressive corridor and larger amounts of astigmatism adjacent to the progressive corridor and the segment area. This lens, therefore, is a hard design lens.

The second difference between the Ultravue and Varilux lenses is that the progressive corridor in the Ultravue lens blank lies vertically rather than being angled nasally toward the bottom of the lens. In finishing this lens, the laboratory must rotate the axis of symmetry 10 degrees from the vertical to provide 2.4 mm of segment inset. If a correction for the eye's astigmatism is required, it is incorporated into the back surface of the lens, taking the 10-degree rotation into account.

In 1982, American Optical introduced the Truvision lens, which replaced the Ultravue. This lens was designed by John Winthrop, who also designed the Ultravue lens. Although the Truvision lens is a hard design, it has less astigmatism in the periphery of the progressive corridor than do other lenses in this group because the progressive corridor is lengthened to 15 mm. It has an unaberrated distance area and a fairly wide segment area, but the segment area is positioned lower in the lens blank because of the increased depth of the progressive corridor. The areas and distribution of astigmatism for the Truvision, Varilux 2, and CPS progressive addition lenses are shown in Figure 8–68.

In 1985, Winthrop was issued a patent for a lens that was designed to produce a uniform distribution of the result-

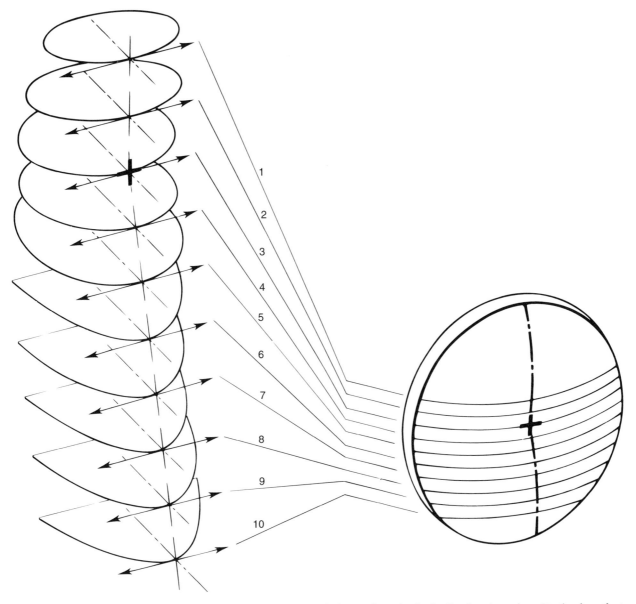

FIGURE 8–67.   **The Varilux lens. The entire front surface is of aspheric design, as shown by the family of conic sections. Starting from the top of the lens as an oblate ellipse (1), it continues as oblate ellipses (2, 3) and gradually becomes a circle (4) in the central area, then varying prolate ellipses (5, 6) and then, successively, parabolas and hyperbolas (7, 8, 9, 10) in the near-vision area. (Reprinted with permission from Essilor Optical.)**

ing peripheral aberrations in a progressive addition lens.[13] The essence of this design is a bipolar configuration and the application of the Dirichlet principle. In thermodynamics, the *Dirichlet principle* is used to determine the distribution of temperature around two points on the surface of a metal sheet, the two points having constant but unequal temperatures. If two points on a thin copper sheet, with dimensions similar to a lens blank, are heated to 0° and 100° C, the resultant isotherms form a regular pattern. In the optical analogue, the distance and near-vision centers of the lens correspond to the points on the metal sheet and their powers correspond to the temperatures. Aligning the power distributions between the distance and near-vision centers similar to the temperature contours in the thermodynamic model is expected to provide a uniform flow

of optical power that minimizes the inherent aberrations. In 1988 American Optical introduced a progressive addition lens, the Truvision Omni, based on the Dirichlet principle. This lens is described by the manufacturers as a soft design with wide intermediate and near-vision zones.

Younger 10/30 and CPS Lenses

Younger Optical introduced the Younger 10/30 lens, a progressive addition CR-39 plastic lens, in 1978. The designation *10/30* is used because the lens has a 10-mm-deep progressive corridor and a 30-mm-wide usable segment area (with no more than 1.00 D of astigmatism). This lens epitomizes the hard progressive addition lens design. Not only is the un-

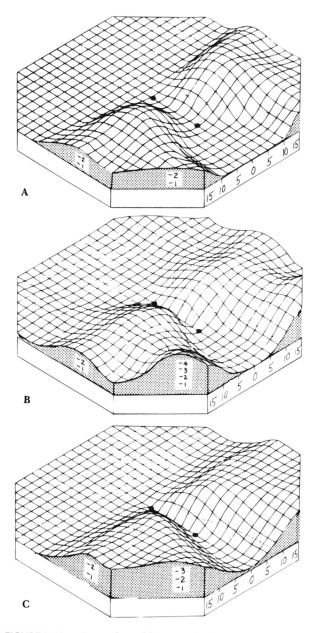

FIGURE 8–68.   **Comparison of the areas of astigmatism. A, Truvision, B, Varilux, and C, Younger CPS progressive addition lenses. The height of each contour represents the amount of astigmatism. (Reprinted with permission from American Optical Truvision Progressive Lenses, American Optical Corp., 1984.)**

aberrated area larger than that of other progressive addition lenses, but image distortion is eliminated both nasally and temporally for a short distance below the mid-horizontal meridian of the lens. The near segment area is spherical, and although designated as 30 mm wide, the usable width depends on the base curve, the power of the add, and the segment height (i.e., the vertical position of the segment area). The effective segment width is usually no greater than about 25 mm.

The Younger 10/30 lens differs from the Varilux and Ultravue lenses in that the progression is *nonlinear*, as with the Omnifocal lens. The first one-third of the power change occurs in the upper 5 mm of the progressive corridor; the remaining two-thirds occurs in the lower 5 mm. This means that the amount of unwanted astigmatism, outside the progressive corridor, increases progressively in the downward direction. Because the lens has unaberrated distance and near areas, the aberrated areas are small (as typified by the hard design). Therefore, the intensity of the aberrations, confined to small areas, is relatively high, and makes these areas unusable.

In early 1982, Younger Optics introduced the Cosmetic Parabolic Sphere (CPS) progressive addition lens. This lens, made of CR-39 plastic, is the counterpart of the Younger 10/30 lens—The Younger 10/30 lens is a hard design; the CPS lens is a soft design. The CPS lens has an unaberrated distance area, a 12.5-mm-deep progressive corridor of reasonable width, and a small reading area. The orientation of vertical and horizontal lines of peripherally viewed images is fairly well controlled.

The Silor Super No-Line Lens

Silor Optical, which had marketed the original Varilux lens since 1969, renamed the Varilux lens the No-Line lens in 1978. In 1980, Silor began marketing the Super No-Line lens, made by Benoit Berthiot of France. This is an improved version of the original No-Line progressive lens, and has a progressive corridor 12 mm deep. It has wide distance-vision and segment areas. The segment area is about 25 mm wide and is therefore a hard design. Although surface astigmatism and distortion are present in the peripheral portions of the progressive corridor, the lens is designed to control the axes of unwanted astigmatism to prevent rotation of vertical and horizontal lines of peripherally viewed objects. The Super No-Line lens is made with the line of symmetry inclined nasally, as is the Varilux lens, with the result that separate blanks are required for right and left lenses.

The Unison Lens

In mid-1980, Univis Lens Company introduced the Unison lens. This lens is a hard design lens. It has a completely spherical distance area, a 12-mm-deep but relatively narrow progressive corridor, and a relatively wide segment area. Astigmatism and distortion are concentrated adjacent to the segment area, with little rotation of vertical or horizontal lines of peripherally viewed objects. In 1983 Univis Lens was sold to Vision-Ease.

Sola VIP and XL

Sola Optical, in 1984, introduced a CR-39 plastic progressive addition lens called the VIP lens. This is a soft design lens, having a large distance-vision area and a relatively large near-vision area, with the unwanted astigmatism distributed in the peripheral portions of the lens. Orientation of vertical and horizontal lines of peripheral objects has been well controlled. Sola Optical has also introduced a lens called the XL, a soft design intended for early presbyopes. Sola recently introduced the VIP Gold and the XL Gold lenses, each made in clear Spectralite plastic and Spectralite Transitions. Spectralite has a refractive index of 1.537 and an Abbe number of 47.0, the highest Abbe number of the high-index plastics.

Other Progressive Addition Lenses

In 1984, Coburn Optical Industries began marketing the Progressiv R, a lens designed by Rodenstock in Germany in 1981. The lens is now being marketed by Rodenstock, rather than Coburn. The lens is a hard design, having a virtually aberration-free distance area, a 12-mm-deep progressive corridor, and a relatively narrow segment area. Although the peripheral portions of the progressive zone contain astigmatism, the orientation of vertical and horizontal lines of peripherally viewed objects is largely retained. The lens must be rotated 8 degrees to obtain 2 mm of segment inset. Rodenstock also manufactures the Progressiv S, a hard design with aspheric surfaces. The most recent Rodenstock lens is the Progressiv Life, described as an integrated design using field-designed aspherics.

In 1986, Seiko Optical Products introduced two progressive addition lenses, the P-2 and the P-3. The P-2, intended for general wear, is a soft design and reduces the magnitude of astigmatism but increases the area containing the astigmatic error. The P-3 is recommended for active patients, and resembles a hard design lens because it has large areas free of astigmatism and more intense levels of astigmatism concentrated in small regions of the lens. Both these lenses have been replaced by the P-6, a plastic lens described by the manufacturer as having linear power progression for the active individual.

PolarLite in 1986 developed a plastic polarized progressive addition lens called the Progressiv M, later called the Polarite Progressive. This lens may be tinted gray or brown. Polarite also produces a nonpolarized progressive addition lens called the High Time Progressive, of refractive index 1.56. This lens is described as having mild progression leading to easy adaptation.

Multi-Design Progressive Addition Lenses

Soft progressive lens designs, with deep progressive corridors and relatively small amounts of astigmatism spread over relatively large areas, tend to be favored by early presbyopes who require an addition of less than +1.50 D; harder designs, with shorter progressive corridors and larger astigmatism-free distance and reading areas, tend to be preferred by presbyopes requiring higher additions. For example, Borish, Hitzeman, and Brookman[14] reported on a double-blind study in which 54 presbyopic patients were fitted with both Varilux 2, a relatively soft design, and Ultravue, a hard design. They found that their younger subjects, requiring low- or medium-power additions, preferred the Varilux 2 by a ratio of approximately 2:1, and the older presbyopes tended to be evenly divided in their preference for the two lenses. To take advantage of the tendency for younger presbyopes to prefer softer designs, *multi-design* progressive lenses were developed.

For most of the time that progressive addition lenses have been available, each manufacturer has tended to use a constant power gradient for the complete range of additions. Such lenses are known as *mono-design* lenses. In these lenses there is a linear relationship between add powers in a lens series. A mono-design lens that starts out in a hard (or soft) design retains its design throughout its entire power range.

Recently, however, lenses with the surface design changed as the add increases have been introduced as a way to provide optimal performance for each addition. These lenses are called *multi-design* lenses. The multi-design lens usually starts out in the soft design made for beginning or early presbyopes; as the add increases, the lenses gradually take on a hard design conformation for mature presbyopes. Thus, a nonlinear relationship exists between add powers. This approach assumes that an early presbyope started on multi-design lenses can maintain an acceptable visual performance as the design evolves with add power increases. However, patient satisfaction is achieved only if the evolving lens design matches the patient's visual requirements.

The first multi-design lens introduced was the Varilux Infinity, in 1988. The lens is designed individually for add power from +0.75 to +3.50 D, with the result that there are 12 individual designs. The lens designs are softest for the low add powers, have gradual progression of power with wide intermediate zones, and spread small amounts of aberration throughout the lens; however, they have the disadvantage of having the near segment located relatively low in the lens. As add power increases, the designs become increasingly harder, with the +3.50-D add having the hardest design. For the higher adds, the hard design has the advantage of a relatively short progressive zone and relatively larger distance and reading areas. Hard, soft, and multi-design lenses are compared in Figure 8–69.

The Varilux Comfort lens was introduced in 1993. This lens is described by the manufacturer as a multi-design lens with a high and wide reading area and a soft, usable, periphery.

American Optical has recently introduced the AO Pro 15 and AO Pro 16 lenses. These lenses are described by the manufacturer as *multi-design* lenses with stabilized distance and reading areas. The lenses adhere to the bipolar design of their predecessor, the Omni lens, based on the Dirichlet principle. They differ from the Omni, however, in using aspheric lens theory, which produces a very flat, thin lens.

Another multi-design lens, the Adaptor No-Line, has been introduced by Silor Optical. This lens has 5 individualized designs, gradually increasing from soft to hard designs as the add power increases. The five lens designs are intended for emerging presbyopes, confirmed presbyopes, mid-range presbyopes, mature presbyopes, and advanced presbyopes.

The *Kodak* progressive lens, manufactured under license by Signet Armorlite, is a custom multi-design with a different design for each add. It follows the soft design model and has an aphericized distance zone.

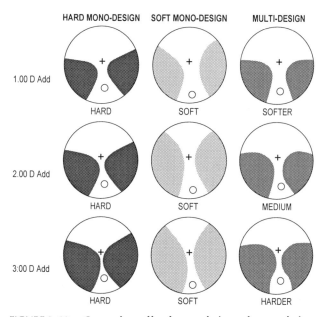

FIGURE 8–69.   **Comparison of hard mono-design, soft mono-design, and multi-design progressive addition lenses as the power of the add changes. (Reprinted with permission from Essilor International/ Varilux Corp.)**

Special Purpose Progressive Addition Lenses

COSMOLIT P

Produced by Rodenstock, the Cosmolit P is designed for patients who have extensive near and intermediate task requirements in recreational and occupational activities. The progressive zone is approximately 30 mm long, and the power change over that zone is approximately 1.50 D; this indicates that the power changes slowly, that is, at about 0.05 D per millimeter. Because the inherent peripheral astigmatism in progressive lens design is a function of how fast the power changes, the peripheral unwanted astigmatism in this design is very low.

The fitting procedure for the Cosmolit P lens is different from that of a conventional progressive addition lens. With the eyes in the primary position of gaze, the *fitting cross* is dropped 0.5 mm downward from the center of the pupil for every 1 degree of pantoscopic tilt. The *reading point* is located 7.0 mm below the fitting cross. With a pantoscopic tilt of 8 degrees, the reading point falls 11 mm below the center of the pupil. The power ordered is the power required for the patient's preferred near-vision distance, and this power is supplied at the reading point. The lens achieves an *addition* of +0.50 D at 10 mm *below* the reading point. At the fitting cross, or 7.0 mm *above* the reading point, the power *decreases* by 0.37 D. At 20.0 mm above the reading point, the power *decreases* (1) by 1.00 D for lenses with a base curve of 5.00 D (signifying a higher add); or (2) by 0.75 D for lenses with a 4.00-D base curve (a low add).

GRADAL RD

The Gradal RD lens was introduced by Zeiss in 1994 and is a progressive addition lens that is solely for intermediate and

near-vision activities. It is available in CR-39 and glass of refractive index 1.604, an Abbe number of 41.7, and a specific gravity of 2.67. The lens has a 30-mm-long progressive corridor, compared with the 15-mm corridor length used in the Zeiss Gradal HS general-purpose progressive addition lens.

The Gradal RD is ordered in the same way as a conventional progressive addition lens, by furnishing the distance prescription and the near-vision add. The laboratory adjusts the powers by adding +0.50 D to the distance prescription and by reducing the near add accordingly to maintain the correct near-vision power. Conventional fitting involves placing the fitting cross level with the center of the pupil, with the eyes in the primary position of gaze. For the patient who spends relatively long periods at near and intermediate-vision tasks, the lens provides fields of view that are uninterrupted, relatively wide, and distortion free.

OVERVIEW

Manufactured by Varilux, the Overview lens is a modified progressive addition lens designed for persons who perform close work above eye level (Figure 8–70). The lower part of the lens is a customary Varilux progressive addition lens, but the upper part carries a 41-mm round bifocal segment. The distance between the central fitting cross and the lower edge of the segment is 9 mm; the addition power is always 0.50 *less* than the engraved progressive addition power.

In fitting the Overview lens, the fitting cross is placed in front of the center of the pupil, with the eyes in the primary position of gaze. A frame that allows sufficient segment height must be chosen to provide the necessary vertical field of view to accomplish the specialized tasks.

READABLES

Readables are progressive addition lenses that extend the range of clear vision for near and intermediate-vision tasks. The lens is manufactured by Varilux. Readables were designed specifically for emmetropic or nearly emmetropic presbyopes.

The power in the Readables changes 1.50 D over a wide corridor in the middle 28 mm of the lens. The prescribed

FIGURE 8–70.   **The Overview lens. (Reprinted with permission from Essilor International/Varilux Corp.)**

near-vision power (the algebraic sum of the distance prescription sphere and the desired add power) is placed at the optical center, which is at the lower lid margin. Above the optical center, the power *decreases* approximately 0.25 D every 4 mm and stabilizes 12 mm above the optical center at 0.75 D less plus (or 0.75 more minus) than the power at the optical center. Below the optical center, the power *increases* approximately 0.25 D every 5 mm until it stabilizes 16 mm below the optical center at 0.75 D more plus (or 0.75 less minus) than the prescribed power at the optical center.

The unwanted astigmatism that necessarily accompanies any progressive lens is more intense at the bottom of the lens than it is at the top.

TECHNICA

The Technica lens is a progressive addition lens introduced by American Optical in 1988. The lens is designed to increase the size of the lens area devoted to intermediate powers. The Technica lens is prescribed in the same manner as a regular progressive addition lens, by prescribing the distance power and the near add suitable for the patient's preferred near-vision distance. The fitting center is placed at the center of the pupil, with the eyes in the primary position.

The distance viewing zone is located 12 mm above the fitting center. At the fitting center, the power is 50% of the near addition power. The intermediate viewing zone is centered 7 mm below the fitting center and the power is 80% of the power of the near-vision addition. There is a large, usable, near-vision area, but the area devoted to the distance prescription is small and located near the top of the lens.

SMARTSEG

Manufactured by Sola, the SmartSeg is a patented 30-mm-wide straight-top bifocal with a progressive zone that is present only in the segment. This lens offers an intermediate range correction with a wide distance and near-vision area. At the top of the segment, the power is suitable for an intermediate distance and then builds gradually to full add power halfway down the segment. The reduced add power at the top of the segment has the following advantages: (1) it extends the intermediate range beyond that of a conventional bifocal, (2) it creates less image jump, and (3) the top of the segment is less noticeable because it is thinner.

The Effect of Pupil Size

For a ray of light passing through any point on the line of symmetry in the progressive corridor, the power is essentially spherical and free from astigmatism. But the situation for the wearer's eye, which has a *pupil of finite size*, when looking through the progressive zone, has rays passing through the pupil's upper margin with different dioptric value than those passing through the lower margin. With a progressive corridor 12 mm deep and a +2.50 D add, the dioptric difference in power for the upper and lower margins of a 6-mm pupil is +1.25 D. In addition, the larger the pupil, the smaller the usable area of the progressive corridor. Fortunately, the pupil tends to become smaller with age, so most candidates for progressive addition lenses have relatively small pupils.

Edge Thickness

Because of the increase in curvature toward the bottom of the lens, which is necessary to obtain the required increase in power, the lower edge of the lens is substantially *thinner* than the upper edge. The difference in thickness creates a *base-up* prismatic effect. The amount of prism created depends on the power of the add and imposes a limitation on the minimal thickness of the finished lens.

To equalize edge thickness, some manufacturers work *base-down* prism over the entire back surface of the lens. The amount of prism required is determined by the difference in edge thickness between the top and bottom of the lens. Because the difference in thickness is the same for both the right and left lenses, the prism is the same for each lens, and no residual vertical imbalance is created. However, both distance optical centers are lowered for plus lenses, and raised for minus lenses. The equalization of the edge thicknesses results in a substantial reduction in overall lens thickness.

Right/Left Lens Designs

Another aspect of lens design is the method of producing right and left lenses. The progressive corridor must be inclined from top to bottom in a nasalwards direction to allow the eyes to follow the middle of the progressvie corridor as the natural convergence of the eyes occurs for near vision.

For optimal conditions of binocular vision at near vision, the wearer should encounter identical sphere, cylinder, and prism power in both lenses when the eyes move right or left. To accomplish this, the lens must have the same surface form on each side of the progressive corridor, which is achieved by designing separate lenses for the right and left eyes, with the inclination of the progressive corridor built into the lens design. Thus, no rotation of the lens is required (asymmetrical design).

The alternate method of achieving the inclination of the progressive corridor is to produce a single lens blank and then rotate the bottom of each lens nasalwards (about 10 degrees) to produce a right and left lens (symmetrical design). In this design, the inclination of the progressive corridor and the natural convergence of the eyes match, but the eyes experience different surface effects when the user looks to the right or the left at near distances.

8.33. Patient Selection

Patient selection is an important consideration in the fitting of progressive addition lenses. Although these lenses have been designed to provide continuous vision for all distances, many practitioners and their patients consider these lenses as "invisible bifocals." If a patient is interested *only* in invisibility, the practitioner should consider the possibility of prescribing either a no-chrome round fused bifocal, which has the advantages of being inexpensive and optically sound (as described in Section 8.30), or a blended one-piece bifocal (as described in Section 8.31). However, a blended bifocal has the disadvantage of a blurred transition area and lacks the advantage of vision for intermediate distances. Progressive addition lenses should therefore be considered for patients who require vision for occasional intermediate distances (who would otherwise require trifocal lenses) *and* for those who request an invisible bifocal.

Patients who resist conventional bifocals or trifocals because of the "lines" are strongly motivated and are excellent candidates for progressive addition lenses. Emerging presbyopes are also good candidates. They understand that they have to adapt to a new optical aid and, therefore, they will be receptive to lenses that provide both cosmetic advantages and functional vision across all distances. The initial add for emerging presbyopes is low in power and the associated aberrations are therefore minimal; adaptation should occur rapidly. Previous bifocal wearers who demonstrate need for a trifocal lens for occasional use may enjoy the flexibility of a progressive addition lens as compared with a conventional trifocal.

Progressive addition lenses should not be recommended indiscriminately for all presbyopic patients, however; discretion should be exercised, especially with the following patients:

1. Patients who are currently wearing bifocals or trifocals (in particular, Executive-style bifocals or trifocals) and who are completely satisfied with their lenses.
2. Patients with large oculomotor imbalances (lateral or vertical) who require prism.
3. Patients who are accustomed to wearing (and are satisfied with) single-vision lenses for near-vision use only.
4. Patients with a significant amount of anisometropia (more than 3.00 D).
5. Patients who need adds of high power and who have large pupils.
6. Patients who are nervous, "tense," impatient, and generally intolerant of health-care devices.

Another important consideration for the wearer to adapt successfully to progressive addition lenses is the wearer's ability to become a "head-mover" rather than an "eye-mover." When the wearer succeeds in learning to move the head to view objects on one side or the other, rather than moving the eyes, complaints of the sensation of blurring or "swimming" no longer occur.

Lewis[15] devised a scoring system designed to rule out patients who are unsuited for progressive addition lens wear. A specified number of points is given for each of three factors: age, refractive error, and various motivational considerations. If a patient has a score less than 20 from a total of 40 possible points, the person is considered not suitable for progressive addition lens wear.

8.34. Matching Design and Patient

Although each progressive addition lens has a different theory of construction, all the lenses share common design problems: (1) producing high-quality image performance for distance and near-vision areas, (2) merging the distance and near-vision zones gradually, and (3) placing the inevitable aberrations and distortions where they least interfere with comfortable vision. As discussed previously in this section, the available lenses vary from one to another in terms of the size of the aberration-free distance area, the power and width of the usable near area, the depth and usable width of the progressive corridor, and the dimensional orientation, intensity, and location of the aberrations and distortions. Because of the differences, the practitioner should become familiar with the characteristics of the available lenses. After determining that the patient is motivated and has the emotional makeup conducive to wearing progressive addition lenses, the practitioner should analyze the patient's visual characteristics and visual requirements for both work and leisure, taking into consideration:

1. The power of the distance correction
2. The power of the add
3. The pupil size
4. Previous experience with multifocals
5. Habitual eye and head movements
6. Height of commonly viewed objects at near vision
7. The frequency of use of near and intermediate-vision ranges

Matching the design to the individual patient increases the potential for patient acceptance. However, appropriate design characteristics can only be selected if the practitioner has sufficient information to make a choice. Most manufacturers of progressive addition lenses provide qualitative descriptions or comparisons of lens design, not *quantitative data*. Unfortunately, quantitative data provided by investigators have not been reported in a standardized format that would permit comparisons of the relevant parameters of lens design.

Plot Diagrams

When a new progressive addition lens is introduced, the manufacturer often supplies some form of physical measurements. For example:

1. *The Grid Plot.* This is produced by taking a photograph through the progressive addition lens (with a plano distance portion) against a black and white grid. The lens can then be judged by the amount of magnification and lack of orthoscopy that occurs as a result of the distortion created by superfluous astigmatism and prismatic effects. This information is difficult to quantify and, more importantly, it does not present a realistic picture of the power variations perceived by the wearer as the line of sight traverses various portions of the lens.

2. *The Eye-Path Profile of Progression.* This plot demonstrates how power varies along the umbilical line of the progressive corridor and may include (1) the rate of power change along the corridor, (2) the length of the corridor, and (3) the stability of the area of near vision (see Figure 8–62).

3. *Three-Dimensional Topographical Plot.* This representation may display the amount and distribution of power changes as well as the amount and location of unwanted astigmatism (see Figure 8–68).

4. *The Contour Plot.* A progressive addition lens (with a plano distance portion) is used to produce a large number of lens power measurements across the entire usable aperture of the lens. A computer program is then used to produce lines of isocylindrical power (sometimes including axis position) and also lines of isospherical equivalent power.

Contour plots may be used to distinguish hard-design lenses from soft-design lenses. A hard design is characterized by contour lines that are concentrated together, make abrupt turns near the progressive zone, and fail to extend into the distance area. A soft design is characterized by contour lines that are more widely separated, curve gently, and spread throughout large portions of the lens, including the distance area (Figure 8–71).

Contour plots can also be used to distinguish mono-design from multi-design formats. For a mono-design, the *mean power* contour lines for different add powers in a lens series coincide when superimposed. For example, if adds of +1.00, +2.00, and +3.00 D are selected from the same lens series, and the contour plot lines for adds of +0.50, +1.00, and +1.50

D are superimposed, the plots coincide in a mono-design format. However, for a multi-design format, the mean power contour lines do not coincide for different add powers.

Examination of contour plots by an experienced eye can also determine whether the lens is manufactured with symmetrical design (rotation of the progressive corridor nasalward), or asymmetrical design (right and left lenses manufactured separately).

Contour plots are helpful in comparing lenses from different manufacturers, but only if the method used to determine the plot is understood. Contour plots of aberrational astigmatism must be used cautiously in selecting a progressive addition lens. The plots are only one indication of lens performance. Contour plots cannot show, with any degree of certainty, whether a particular lens is suitable for an individual. The optical and physical characteristics are important in progressive addition lenses, but they have probably been overemphasized in relation to other factors. For instance, the success rate in fitting progressive addition lenses is strongly influenced by the attitude, knowledge, and fitting skills of the practitioner.

Any valid assessment of lens performance can be achieved only by controlled clinical studies involving a large number of subjects with a variety of visual requirements and a range of prescriptions. Clinical studies are expensive and time consuming. In view of the continued rapid development of progressive addition lenses, the results of such studies would probably become available only after the lenses in question had been superseded by newly introduced lenses.

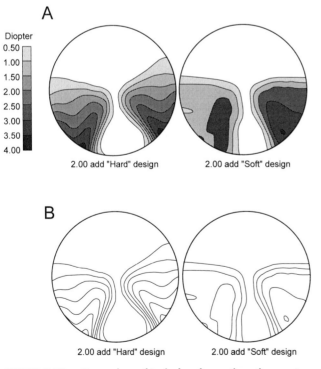

FIGURE 8–71. **Comparison of typical surface astigmatism contour plots for +2.00-D add hard and soft designs of progressive addition lenses. A, with shading and legend; B, without shading. (Reprinted with permission from Sola Optical USA, Inc.)**

8.35. Dispensing Considerations

In general, the fitting of progressive addition lenses is more demanding than the fitting of conventional multifocals. The success rate strongly depends on the fitting and dispensing ability of the practitioner.

Essential Fitting Measurements

The measurements necessary for fitting progressive addition lenses differ from those for the fitting of conventional segment multifocal lenses in two respects:

1. Interpupillary distance is measured *monocularly*, as opposed to a single measurement taken with a millimeter ruler.
2. The reference point in the vertical meridian (analogous to segment height for a conventional multifocal lens) is the *center of the pupil* rather than the ciliary line.

Because of the relatively narrow width of the progressive corridor, the fitting of progressive addition lenses must be done very precisely. Monocular distance PD measurement is *essential* to ensure that the line of sight of each eye remains in the progressive corridor as the eyes turn downward. Measurement may be done by means of a corneal reflection pupillometer or by the use of a special device made available by the manufacturer of the lens.

When the monocular distance PD measurement has been made, it is necessary to measure the vertical distance (Figure 8–72) from the center of the pupil to a horizontal line tangent to the lowest point on the bottom edge of the lens (while the patient's head is held erect and the visual axes are in a horizontal plane) (A). The manufacturer places a temporary marking called a *fitting cross* on the finished lens at a point on the lens corresponding to the center of the pupil.

The vertical distance measurement should be made on the exact frame (in the correct eye size and bridge size) in which the patient's lenses will be mounted. One method of making this measurement, for an unglazed frame, consists of placing a strip of clear tape on the frame with the adhesive side toward the fitter, with the tape approximately centered across the pupil. The fitter holds a penlight in a position level with the patient's eye, instructs the patient to look at the penlight, and observes the patient's corneal reflex. Using a felt pen, a dot is placed on the tape directly in front of the corneal reflex (Figure 8–72B). Other methods of making the measurement include the use of segment measuring devices and special templates supplied by lens manufacturers.

Two systems designed especially for progressive addition measurements are the Grolman Fitting System, supplied by American Optical, and the Magna/Mark System. The Grolman Fitting System attaches directly to the patient's frame and has movable horizontal and vertical scales to determine the necessary measurements. The Magna/Mark System employs magnetically held translucent target spots that move over a plastic lens mounted into the eyewire of the frame. When the target spots are centered before each pupil, the frame is removed and the target spot location is transferred to the plastic lens by a finepoint pen.

For most lenses, the progressive corridor begins about 2 mm *below* the fitting cross. Although the manufacturer's recommendations should be kept in mind, there are times when this fitting technique should be modified. For many patients, the technique causes the reading area to be *too low in the lens* to be useful. For a wearer who would like to make considerable use of vision at intermediate distances, the fitting cross needs to be placed 1 or 2 mm *above* the center of the pupil. Factors such as head posture, location of near-vision tasks (in relation to the vertical level of the lenses), and pupil size are important considerations.

As stated in Section 8.33, patients who have large oculomotor imbalances requiring prism are not good candidates for progressive addition lenses. Brooks and Riley[16] suggested

that these patients may encounter difficulty with progressive addition lenses because of the position of the fitting cross. They recommended that, when prism is prescribed in progressive addition lenses, the position of the fitting cross be modified from its traditional position in front of the center of the pupil. Measurements of the pupillary position are normally made under conditions of binocular fusion with the chosen frame in place but without lenses.

If *lateral* prism is worn, the eye rotates toward the apex of the prism, by the amount of the prism, but the fitting cross on the lens does not move. In effect, the center of the pupil and the fitting cross are no longer aligned, with the result that the eye does not track the center of the progressive corridor, which causes difficulty in viewing objects at intermediate distances. If *vertical* prism is worn, the center of the pupil of one eye is higher than that of the other, and the eyes are not be aligned vertically with the fitting crosses. This causes one eye to move down the corridor ahead of the other; the result is that the add power increases unequally for the two eyes. To rectify these problems, the fitting cross should be adjusted *0.3 mm per prism diopter*, in the following manner:

1. *For horizontal prism.* Monocular PDs should be modified 0.3 mm per prism diopter by increasing the PD for base-in prism and decreasing the PD for base-out prism.
2. *For vertical prism.* The fitting cross heights should be modified the same 0.3 mm per prism diopter by raising the fitting cross height for base-down prism and lowering the fitting cross height for base-up prism.

Frame Selection

The frame selected should provide a minimum vertical distance of *22 mm* from the center of the pupil to a horizontal line tangent to the lowest point on the bottom edge of the lens. For a lens with a 12-mm progressive zone beginning 2 mm below the pupil, the reading area (which has the full power of the addition) would then be 8 mm deep. As shown in Figure 8–73, this generally means that the B (vertical) measurement must be a minimum of 38 mm. If the distance below the pupil is less than 22 mm, the effective depth of the full-power reading area is so small that the lower rim of the frame intrudes into the patient's visual field during reading (particularly for a patient who has large pupils).

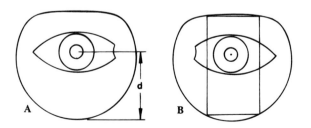

FIGURE 8–72. **Necessary measurements for fitting progressive addition lenses. A, vertical distance measurement; B, tape-and-dot vertical distance measurement (see text for explanation).**

FIGURE 8–73. **The vertical box measurement of a frame for a progressive addition lens should be a minimum of 38 mm.**

Lens shapes with cutaway nasal portions, such as goggle shapes that rapidly slope away from the nose, should be avoided, particularly if a large amount of inward decentration is necessary. To provide a wide lateral field of view through the progressive corridor and the stabilized near-vision area, the patient's frame should be fitted at as close a vertex distance as possible (no greater than 12–13 mm) and should have a pantoscopic tilt of 12 to 15 degrees with a slight amount of face forming. As with other multifocals, adjustable nose pads allow flexibility in positioning the frame, both at the time of dispensing and later.

Verification of Progressive Addition Lenses

Most progressive addition lenses have two sets of markings, a temporary set and a permanent set, to assist in verification of power and in fitting the lenses to the patient's face (Figure 8–74). The temporary markings usually consist of a fitting cross, which should fall at the center of the pupil, and a distance reference center and a near-reference center to use in checking the powers of the distance and near segment areas (Figure 8–74A). The PD and the vertical height of the fitting cross are confirmed by placing the lens on the manufacturer's centering or verification chart. The temporary markings should be left on the lens until the position of the fitting cross can be verified on the patient's face.

The permanent markings are semi-invisible, and consist of two engraved circles that establish the horizontal line at the beginning of the progressive corridor (Figure 8–74B). Some manufacturers also place their own identification mark and the power of the add near the engraved circle on the temporal side of the lens. In the event that the tempo-rary markings are removed, they can be reconstructed by locating, marking, and placing the engraved circles over the manufacturer's centration chart. If the lens is placed against a dark background and viewed with an intense light, the circles can be seen more easily.

Patient Communication

Patient instruction, demonstration, and follow-up are important aspects of progressive addition lens fitting. The patient must be told exactly how to use the lenses and should be scheduled for at least one return visit after the lenses have been dispensed, to evaluate progress in adapting to the lenses. The patient should understand the importance of maintaining the lenses in correct adjustment. Return visits for readjustment need to be scheduled more frequently than those for wearers of conventional multifocal lenses.

Patient Acceptance of Progressive Addition Lenses

Numerous reports[17–21] indicate that success rates for progressive addition lenses (calculated on the basis of patient acceptance) are as high as 90% or even higher. The report by Jan[21] indicates a success rate of more than 90% for Varilux 1, Varilux 2, Ultravue, and Younger 10/30 lenses. Given the differences in the design philosophies of these lenses, Jan's results suggest that lens design is not a critical factor in patient acceptance, but that other factors (such as patient selection, meticulous fitting, fabrication, verification, and dispensing procedures) together with patient instruction may be very important.

Young and Borish[22] have stated that 75% marks the acceptance rate for an adept prescriber of progressive addition lenses. A major conclusion of their study was the *extreme importance* of fitting skills. More than 15% of the practitioners in the study fell below the 75% minimum, with most failures isolated to relatively few practices—some practices had acceptance levels of less than 40%.

Despite reports of high success rates, and despite aggressive marketing campaigns by some manufacturers to the eye-care professions and to the public, progressive addition lenses have failed to penetrate the multifocal market in the United States to the extent that they have in Europe.

However, the use of progressive addition lenses seems to be gaining momentum as "Baby Boomers" move into presbyopia and second-generation wearers of progressive addition lenses need stronger additions or move on to improved designs. Progressive addition lenses now account for about one-third of the multifocal market in the United States.[23]

Although the reasons for their lack of use in the United States are hard to determine, the perceived advantages of progressive addition lenses are apparently not yet great enough to override the accepted benefits of conventional multifocal lenses. However, the market for progressive addition lenses will undoubtedly expand as a result of consumer awareness; an increase in the knowledge, skill, and confidence of many practitioners; the positive recommendations of practitioners currently wearing the lenses; referrals by suc-

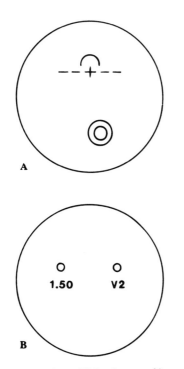

FIGURE 8–74. **Progressive addition lens markings. A, temporary markings; B, permanent semi-invisible markings.**

cessful progressive addition lens wearers; improvement in lens design; and an expansion in available lens options.

Design Evolution and Future Developments

Since the introduction of the original Varilux lens in the United States in 1967, progressive addition lenses have undergone a gradual evolution:

1. *Expanded Availability of Materials.* Early lenses were available in crown glass and CR-39 plastic. Currently, lenses are available in high-index glass, high-index plastic, glass and plastic photochromic materials, and polycarbonate. The materials available for representative progressive addition lenses are listed in Table 8–13.

2. *Extended Prescription Range.* The prescription range has been extended for spheres, cylinders, adds, and base curves.

TABLE 8–13
Materials Available for Representative Progressive Addition Lenses*

Manufacturer	Name	Materials	
		Glass	Plastic
American Optical	Pro 15	1.523, PGX, PBX	CR-39, TR
	Pro 16	1.60, PGX, PBX	1.58 HR, PC
	TruVision Omni	1.523, PGX, PBX	CR-39, PC
	TruVision	1.523, PGX	CR-39
	Prima		CR-39
Gentex	Profile Progressive		PC
Hoya	Hoyalux EP		CR-39
	Hoyalux EX		1.60 HR
Optima	Hyperview 166		1.66 PU
Orcolite	LineFree		CR-39, PC
Pentax	Progressive		CR-39
	Lite 1.60 Zoom		1.60 PU
Polarite	High Five Progressive		1.56 HR
	PolarLite Progressive		CR-39 POL, GR, BR
Rodenstock	Progressiv S	1.60, PBX	CR-39; 1.60 HR, TR
	Progressiv R	1.523, PGX	CR-39
	Progressiv Life	1.523	CR-39
Seiko	P-6		CR-39
	P-6 Thin		1.55 HR
Signet Armorlite	Progressive Elegance		CR-39, PC; 1.56 HR
	Kodak Vision		CR-39 PC; 1.56/1.60 HR, TR
	PE II		CR-39
Silor	Super No-Line	1.523, PGX	CR-39
	Adaptor No-Line	1.523, PGX	CR-39, 1.60 HR, TR, PC
	Essilor Natural	1.60, PGX	CR-39
Sola	VIP	1.523, PGX	CR-39, TR, PC
	XL	1.523, PGX	CR-39, TR, PC
	VIP Gold		SP, SP–TR
	XL Gold		SP, SP–TR
Varilux	Infinity	1.60, PGX	CR-39; 1.60 HR, TR
	Plus	1.523, PGX, PBX	CR-39 PC
	Comfort	1.60, PGX	CR-39, 1.60 HR, PC, TR
Vision-Ease	Delta	1.523, PGX, PBX	CR-39 PC
	Varivue		1.56 HR, PC
	Varivue Sungrays		PC, GR
X-Cel	Freedom	1.523, PGX, PBX	CR-39, POL, GR
Younger	10/30		CR-39
	CPS		CR-39
Zeiss	Gradal HS	1.60, 1.80	CR-39, 1.60 HR
	Gradal	1.70	

* BR = Brown; GR = Gray; HR = Hard Resin; PBX = Photobrown Extra; PC = Polycarbonate; PGX = Photogray Extra; POL = Polarized; PU = Polyurethane; SP = Spectralite; TR = Transitions.

3. *Control of Aberrations.* Progressive addition lenses are necessarily aspheric in the vertical section; but lenses with aspheric horizontal sections, to control aberrations, have been introduced.

4. *Longer Progressive Corridors.* Lengthening the progressive corridor reduces the rate of change in the progressive zone, and hence reduces the amount of aberrational astigmatism. Large-aperture frames permit longer progressive corridors. The disadvantage is that a larger degree of downward ocular rotation is required to use the near add portion.

5. *Special Purpose Lenses.* There has been a slow but steady proliferation of special purpose progressive lenses of nonconventional design. These lenses emphasize near or intermediate-vision ranges.

6. *Multi-Design.* These designs are optimized so that all prescriptions in the range achieve reasonable performance compared with the performance of early lenses in which the design was optimized around a 6.00 D base curve and a 2.00 D addition.

7. *Asymmetrical Design.* An increasing number of manufacturers are adopting the design of separate right and left lenses with asymmetical progressive corridors, rather than having a single design that requires rotation of each lens to achieve progressive corridor inclination.

New, general-purpose progressive addition lenses with minor modifications to existing designs are likely to be introduced. Current lens designs will continue to expand with use of materials already available and with materials yet to be developed. There will be an increasing number of nonconventional designs for special uses. However, given the limited degrees of freedom accessible to the lens designer, basic improvement over present designs will be possible only in very small steps. Perhaps the next breakthrough in presbyopic correction will originate from a totally different concept and use new technology such as liquid crystal lenses, gradient-index lens materials, diffractive optics, and deformable lenses.

References

1. Sheedy, J. E., Parsons, S. D. The Video Display Terminal Eye Clinic: Clinical Report. *Optom. Vis. Sci.*, Vol. 67, pp. 622–626, 1990.
2. Collins M. J., Goode, A., and Atchison, D. A., The Effectiveness of Computer Screen Filters. *Clin. Exp. Optom.*, Vol. 76, pp. 91–100, 1993.
3. Barresi, B. T., and Rosenthal, J. *New York Occupational Vision Benefit Plan Study: An Evaluation of a Vision Plan for VDT Users and Office Workers.* New York: State University of New York, State College of Optometry, 1986.
4. Fry, G. A., and Ellerbrock, V. J. Placement of Optical Centers in Bifocal Lenses. *Optom. Weekly*, Vol. 37, No. 35, pp. 989–996, 1941.
5. Sterling, S. Modern Bifocal Lenses. *Ophthalmic Lenses: Their History, Theory, and Selection*, Bausch & Lomb Optical Co., Rochester, NY, pp. 53–81, 1935.
6. Sheedy, J. E., and Saladin, J. J. Exophoria at Near in Presbyopia. *Am. J. Optom. Physiol. Opt.*, Vol. 52, pp. 474–481, 1975.
7. American National Standard Recommendation for Prescription Ophthalmic Lenses, Z80.1-1995. American National Standards Institute, Inc., New York, 1995.
8. Field, K. The "Correct" Method of Checking Bifocals. *Opt. J. Rev. Optom.*, Vol. 103, pp. 19–20, 1966.
9. Holmes, C., Jollife, E., and Gregg, J. *Guide to Occupational and Other Visual Needs*, Vol. 1. Silverlake Lithographers, Los Angeles, 1958.
10. Knoll, H. The Optical Characteristics of Beach Blended Bifocals. *Am. J. Optom. Arch. Am. Acad. Optom.*, Vol. 29, pp. 150–154, 1952.
11. Davis, J. K. Aspheric Lenses: What's Possible and What Isn't. *Rev. Optom.*, Vol. 115, No. 5, pp. 68–74, 1978.
12. Maitenaz, B. Four Steps That Led to Varilux. *Am. J. Optom. Arch. Am. Acad. Optom.*, Vol. 43, pp. 441–450, 1966.
13. Sullivan, C. M., and Fowler, C. W. Progressive Addition and Variable Focus Lenses: A Review. *Ophthalmol. Physiol. Opt.*, Vol. 8, pp. 401–414, 1988.
14. Borish, I. M., Hitzeman, S. A., and Brookman, K. E. Double-Masked Study of Progressive Addition Lenses. *J. Am. Optom. Assoc.*, Vol. 51, pp. 933–943, 1980.
15. Lewis, R. *Conquest of Presbyopia.* R & M Lewis, Sydney, Australia, pp. 42–45, 1983.
16. Brooks, C. W., and Riley, H. R. Effect of Prescribed Prism on Monocular Interpupillary Distance and Fitting Heights for Progressive Addition Lenses. *Optom. Vis. Sci.*, Vol. 71, pp. 401–407, 1994.
17. Wittenberg, S. Field Study of New Progressive Addition Lens. *J. Am. Optom. Assoc.*, Vol. 49, pp. 1013–1021, 1978.
18. Chapman, D. T. One Clinic's Experience with Varilux 2—The First 400 Patients. *Optom. Monthly*, Vol. 69, pp. 946–949, 1978.
19. Betouray, A. A Study of 250 Varilux 2 Prescriptions. *Optom. Monthly*, Vol. 70, pp. 885–888, 1979.
20. Augsburger, A., Cook, S., Dietrich, R., Shackleton-Hardenstein, S., and Wheeler, R. Patient Satisfaction with Progressive Addition Lenses in a Teaching Clinic. *Optom. Monthly*, Vol. 75, pp. 67–72, 1984.
21. Jan, D. The Results of Fitting Progressive Addition Lenses. *Opt. Index*, Vol. 55, pp. 77–78, 1980.
22. Young, J. M., Borish I. M. Adaptability of Broad Spectrum of Randomly Selected Patients to a Variable Design Progressive Lens: Report of a Nationwide Clinical Trial. *J. Am. Optom. Assoc.*, Vol. 65, pp. 445–450, 1994.
23. Bennett, I. The Optical Industry in the United States 1995. *Optical World*, Vol. 23, No. 176, pp. 14–16, 1995.

Questions

1. A bifocal lens is to be made to the following specifications:

OD +2.00 DS
Add +3.00 D (22-mm round fused seg, 16 mm high)
Lens size 46 × 40 mm

Assume that the bifocal inset is zero and that the distance optical center is located at the geometric center of the lens. What is the jump at the top of the segment?

2. A bifocal lens is to be made to the following specifications:

OD +2.00 DS
Add +2.00 D (22-mm round fused seg, 16 mm high)
Lens size 44 × 40 mm

The patient reads through a point 9 mm below the distance optical center. Assume that the bifocal inset is zero and that the distance-optical center is located at the geometric center of the lens. If the reading distance is 50 cm, what is the jump at the top of the segment *expressed in centimeters?*

3. A bifocal lens is to be made to the following specifications:

    OD +4.25 DS –1.75 DC x 180
    Add +2.00 D (22-mm round fused seg, 16 mm high)
    Lens size 44 × 40 mm

    The patient reads through a point 9 mm below the distance optical center. Assume that the bifocal inset is zero and that the distance optical center is located at the geometric center of the lens. What is the differential displacement at the reading level?

4. A bifocal lens is to be made to the following specifications:

    OD +3.25 DS +1.75 DC x 180
    Add +2.00 D (22-mm round fused seg, 16 mm high)
    Lens size 44 × 40 mm

    The patient reads through a point 10 mm below the distance optical center. Assume that the bifocal inset is zero and that the distance optical center is located at the geometric center of the lens. What is the total vertical displacement at the reading level?

5. If a prescription is –2.00 DS, add +2.00 D, Ultex A bifocal, lens size 46 × 40 mm, segment 17.0 mm high, distance optical center at geometric center of lens, what is the vertical prismatic effect everywhere in the segment?

6. The prescription is OD +1.50 DS, OS +1.50 DS; +2.00 D add. The top of the segment is 6 mm below the distance optical center. The reading level is 6 mm below the top of the segment. What size round bifocal gives *zero vertical prismatic effects* at the reading level?

7. A bifocal lens is to be made to the following specifications:

    OD +2.00 DS
    Add +1.50 D (Ultex A, 17 mm high)
    Lens size 42 × 38 mm

    Assume that the bifocal inset is zero and that the distance optical center is located at the geometric center of the lens. Where is the combined optical center or point of zero vertical prismatic effect of the segment located?

8. In a front surface fused bifocal, the power of the distance portion is –6.00 D and the power through the near portion is –4.00 D. The power of the fused surface formed by the rear surface of the segment and the countersink surface is +2.00 D. What is the power of the back surface of the distance portion?

9. What is the dioptric value of the countersink surface in air of a front surface fused bifocal whose specifications are –4.00 DS, +2.00 D add, +10.00 D base curve, index of refraction of glass for distance lens = 1.50, index of refraction of segment glass = 1.60?

10. A 20-mm round Kryptok bifocal is made with a +10.00 D curve on the front side of the distance portion. The power of the segment in air is +18.00 D. The index of the glass of the major lens is 1.5, and the index of the segment is 1.6. What is the power of the add?

11. A fused front surface bifocal has a carrier portion (for distance) made with an index of refraction of 1.50 and a segment made with an index of refraction of 1.60. The power of the add is +2.50 D. What is the power of the segment in air?

12. A fused trifocal is made with a +6.00 D front surface on the distance portion with a countersink surface of –2.00 D. The index of refraction of the distance portion is 1.48 and the near add is +2.00 D. If the intermediate add is to be half that of the near add, what are the indices of refraction of near and intermediate segments?

13. The index of refraction of the segment flint glass is 1.69; the index of refraction of the carrier crown glass is 1.53. If the reading add is +2.00 D, and the segment is 22 mm, round, what is the center thickness of the segment?

14. A 20-mm round fused bifocal has a distance prescription of –4.00 D and a +3.00 D add. The surface power on the distance front side is +6.00 D, index of refraction of carrier is 1.52, and index of refraction of segment button is 1.65. After the segment of this lens has been fused to the carrier lens, what powers must be ground on the front and back surfaces of the distance portion to obtain a +7.00-D add and a distance prescription of –9.00 D?

15. A 20-mm round front surface fused bifocal has a distance power of –4.00 D and a +4.00 D add, +6.00 D base curve, index of refraction of the carrier = 1.52; index of refraction of the segment = 1.65. The lens size is 52 × 42 mm and the bifocal height is 19 mm. If the center of the back of the segment is covered by 0.6 mm of the distance portion, what is the center thickness of the distance-vision lens?

16. A golfer requires a low-segment fused 20-mm round bifocal. The round bifocal lens blank is 56 mm in size. The lower edge of the segment is 6 mm above the lower edge of the blank, and the finished lens size is 48 × 40 mm. What is the minimal segment height obtainable?

17. A lens measure on the front surface of an Ultex B lens reads: +6.00 D along the 180° meridian and +7.50 D along the 90° meridian. The back surface spherical curve is –6.50 D and the segment surface power is –4.25 D. What is the approximate prescription of this lens?

18. An Executive bifocal prescription, +2.00 DS –1.50 DC x 180, add +2.00 D, is made on +6.50 D base curve. What are the surface powers on the back surface in the principal meridians?

19. The pupil of a patient wearing progressive addition lenses with an add of +2.75 D is 6 mm in diameter. It is assumed that the progressive zone is 14 mm deep and that the power increases linearly in the zone. When the entire pupil is in the progressive zone, what is the approximate difference in power of a ray passing near the upper edge of the pupil and near the lower edge of the pupil?

20. A 20-mm round fused front surface bifocal is made with a +8.50 D front surface of the distance portion. The distance power is +4.50 D and the add is +2.00 D. The

index of refraction of the major lens is 1.55, Abbe number = 60. The index of refraction of the glass of the segment is 1.66, Abbe number = 40. What is the total longitudinal chromatic aberration through the reading portion of the lens?

21. A fused bifocal is made with a tinted carrier glass with an index of refraction of 1.54 and a white (clear) segment with an index of refraction of 1.63. The distance portion has a power of +3.00 D with 2.7 prism diopters base-up; the add is +3.00 D. The front surface power of the distance portion is +9.00 D. The round segment is 22 mm in diameter. At the geometric center, the lens is 4 mm thick. The top of the segment is located 1 mm below the geometric center. If the transmission is 10.0% through the geometric center, what is the *difference* in transmission through the geometric center and through the optical center of the segment?

22. A trial lens (n = 1.523) has a back vertex power of +10.00 and a plano front surface. The center thickness is 7.0 mm, and the lens properly corrects the eye for 40 cm. The finished spectacle lens (n = 1.523) has a back vertex power of +10.00 D, a back surface power of −3.00 D and a thickness of 7.0 mm. What is the effectivity of the finished spectacle lens compared with that of the trial lens assuming both lenses are worn at the same vertex distances?

CHAPTER NINE

Eyewear Design and Dispensing

No matter how careful the practitioner has been in his or her examination, and no matter how expertly a pair of ophthalmic lenses have been prescribed, they will be of little value to the intended wearer unless they are mounted in a well-fitting and cosmetically pleasing frame or mounting. Attention to the design of eyewear—including the frame or mounting as well as the lenses—is an important aspect of the vision care practitioner's daily work.

Although optometrists have historically performed the functions of eyewear design and dispensing themselves, in recent decades this task has largely been delegated to assistants. However, this work is sufficiently important so that the practitioner should be fully conversant with it. The practitioner should be able to evaluate (and to criticize, if necessary) the work of the assistant and—because relatively few optometric assistants have had previous training—be able to train newly hired assistants.

Whether eyewear design and dispensing are done by the optometrist or by an assistant, extreme care must be taken in all phases of the work, from the physical measurements such as interpupillary distance (PD) and segment height to frame selection, verification of the finished eyewear, and adjustment of the eyewear to the patient's face.

This chapter describes various types of spectacle frames and mountings and then presents the principles involved in measurement of PD, frame selection, ordering materials, and verification and dispensing of eyewear.

SPECTACLE FRAMES AND MOUNTINGS

9.1. Historical Background

Although an optical device intended for use by only one eye is known as an *eyeglass* or a *spectacle*, such a device intended for use by both eyes may be referred to as a pair of *eyeglasses*, a pair of *spectacles*, or simply as a pair of *glasses*. As discussed in Chapter 1, the art of glassmaking and the use of glass for a variety of purposes occurred hundreds of years before the invention of spectacles. Evidence suggests that the first visual aid was a simple magnifying glass, or *eyeglass*, mounted in a rim of wood, metal, bone, horn, or leather, and was held in front of the eye by means of a short handle. Eventually, two such devices were hinged in such a way that an eyeglass could be placed before each eye (Figure 9–1); the device constituted a rudimentary pair of eyeglasses or spectacles.

The inventor of spectacles is not known, but the honor has been attributed to several individuals: Roger Bacon, a monk at Oxford who died in 1294; Alexandria de Spina, a monk at Pisa who died in 1313; and Salvino d'Armati of Florence who died in 1317. Bacon, in his *Opus Magnus*, written in 1267, described the magnification of letters or small objects brought about by a strong plano-convex lens held on a page of manuscript. He concluded that such an instrument could be useful for persons having weak eyes. No evidence exists that Bacon moved the lens to the eye or mounted lenses in any frame-like structure. The reference to the invention of glasses by de Spina can be found in a manuscript belonging to St. Catherine's monastery in Pisa. The claim of d'Armati is made on an epitaph in the church of Santa Maria Maggiore in Florence. The inscription (translated from the Italian) reads:

HERE LIES
SALVINO D'ARMATI OF THE ARMATI
OF FLORENCE
INVENTOR OF SPECTACLES
MAY GOD FORGIVE HIM HIS SINS
IN THE YEAR OF OUR LORD 1317

Because of a lexigraphic error on the epitaph and a discrepancy between the age of the bust on his tomb and the

FIGURE 9–1.   **An early spectacle frame.**

date of the epitaph, investigators believe that d'Armati's claim is spurious. The earliest written evidence of the invention of spectacles was given in a sermon by the monk Giordano da Rivalto, who stated in 1305 that it had not been quite 20 years since the art of making eyeglasses had been found.[1] This statement places the invention of spectacles at about 1285. The sermon was recorded and is still in existence in the Medicio-Laurenziana Library in Florence.

From their inception, early spectacles, because of their weight and construction, were difficult to mount securely before the eyes. Initially, hinged or riveted spectacles, clamped to the nose, were uncomfortable and often interfered with breathing. Later, various devices in the form of headbands were used. Late in the sixteenth century, Spanish spectacle makers used loops of silk or cord attached to the outer edge of the frames, and the loops extended securely over the ears. Around 1730 Edward Scarlett, an English optician, is credited with perfecting rigid sidepieces (temples), which became the precursors of the temples of modern spectacles.

9.2. Modern Frames and Mountings

The various types of devices used for supporting spectacle lenses before the eyes can be classified in two categories: *frames* and *mountings*. Although these terms are often used interchangeably, the terms have different meanings.

A *frame* has three parts: a *front*, which encircles the lenses, a *bridge*, and a pair of *temples*. The frame may be made of either metal or plastic (Figure 9–2). A *combination frame* combines both metal and plastic—the upper part is made of plastic and the lower part (and in some cases the entire eyewire) is made of metal. Typically, a metal frame or a combination frame is provided with adjustable *pads*, designed to fit against the sides of the nose; a plastic frame has stationary pads or none at all.

A *mounting* is a device that holds the two lenses in front of the eyes but does not completely encircle the lenses. Mountings are typically made of gold-filled materials and are classified as either rimless or semi-rimless.

A *rimless mounting* (Figure 9–3) has five parts: a *center*, or bridge, that holds the two lenses together nasally; two *endpieces*; and two *temples*. Two holes must be drilled in each lens, one nasally (to attach to the center) and one temporally (to attach to the endpiece). The center, or bridge, is provided with two adjustable pads, fitting against the sides of the nose and carrying the weight of the mounting and the lenses. Each pad has an extension, called the *pad arm*, holding it to the center. The *strap* is a device that butts up against the lens at both the endpiece and the center.

A *semi-rimless mounting* has three parts: a *front* that includes the bridge and two arms, and two *temples*. There are two versions of the semi-rimless mounting. The first version developed, the American Optical Numont (Figure 9–4), attaches only to the nasal side of the lens and requires only

FIGURE 9–2.   **Modern spectacle frames: A, metal; B, plastic; C, combination.**

one hole per lens. This is a very lightweight mounting that uses a *tri-flex spring* located where the lens attaches to the mounting. Although the Numont mounting looks fragile, the spring tends to keep the lenses from breaking in the presence of bumps and shocks.

Later versions of the semi-rimless mounting are the American Optical Rimway (Figure 9–5) and the Shuron Shurset. The mounting attaches to both the nasal and the temporal sides of each lens and requires two holes per lens. Although appearing to be less fragile than the Numont mounting, this mounting has the problem that the temporal corner of the lens may break if the glasses are bumped; thus, it may be more fragile than the Numont.

In addition to conventional frames or mountings (which have bridges and temples), other devices are available for holding a pair of lenses in front of the eyes (or a single lens in front of one eye). The term *pince-nez*, as well as the term *eyeglasses*, is used for a pair of lenses that is attached to the head by pinching the nose (there are no temples). The term *lorgnette* indicates either a pair of lenses or a single lens held in front of the eyes by means of a handle. The term *monocle* is used to designate a single lens (which looks very much like a trial case lens) usually used only for occasional wear and which is held in front of the eye by means of pressure exerted by the facial and brow muscles.

Frames and mountings can be made of almost any material, but most are made from metals, plastics, or metal and plastic combinations. Each material has numerous advantages and disadvantages, and thus offers options that help to determine the material most appropriate for each patient.

FIGURE 9–3.   **A rimless mounting.**

FIGURE 9–4.   **A Numont semi-rimless mounting.**

FIGURE 9–5.   **A Rimway semi-rimless mounting.**

9.3. Metal Frame and Mounting Materials

Commonly used metal frame and mounting materials are gold, aluminum, nickel silver, titanium, stainless steel, cobalt, monel, and beryllium. Gold has many desirable attributes for a frame material: It is easily worked, corrosion resistant, acid resistant, does not tarnish readily, and can be alloyed with many other metals to change its color and strength.

Pure gold frames (24 karat) are too soft for frame making and are heavy and very expensive. Solid gold alloy frames, usually 18, 14, or 12 karat, are now rarely seen because they are expensive, but they are made by a small group of frame manufacturers. The frames usually carry designer names and are meant to confer status in both prestige eyeglasses and sunglasses. If there is no marking (engraving) on a metal frame, the frame can be made of *any* material, but it is illegal to represent the frame as "gold" unless the gold content is specified. A spectacle frame or mounting that is said to contain gold must meet specific government standards.

The chemically pure, unalloyed metal is known as *fine gold*. Because a spectacle frame or mounting made of fine gold is too soft to be useful, other metals are added to improve the gold's hardness and durability. According to the *karat* system of designation, *fine gold* is 24-karat gold. In any gold alloy, the proportion (by weight) of fine gold to the weight of other metals is expressed in terms of karats, that is, as a multiple of 1/24 times the total weight. Thus, "10-karat gold" means 10 parts of gold combined with 14 parts of other materials.

According to the Federal Trade Commission, the word *gold* used alone (without a karat designation) indicates fine gold of 24-karat quantity. The term *solid*, when used with respect to fine gold or gold alloy, refers not to the fineness or the karat quality of the gold but to the fact that the article is "solid" rather than "hollow" (or rather than containing a core of a base metal, such as a wire-core temple). The term *solid gold* (or solid 10-karat gold) is properly used only as a descriptive term for an article that is made entirely of fine gold (or of 10-karat gold) and that is solid rather than hollow or having a core made of a base metal. The term solid, used with respect to a gold alloy article, must immediately *precede* the karat marking, that is, solid 12-karat gold. If an alloy having a fineness of *less than 10 karat* is used, it cannot be represented as "karat gold."

Most metal frames and rimless or semi-rimless mountings with any appreciable gold content are categorized as *gold-filled*. The soaring cost of gold has made gold-filled stock materials a costly and risky investment, and fewer frame manufacturers hold stocks of this expensive product. Gold-filled material consists of a base metal (usually a special steel or copper alloy) to which a layer of gold has been bonded by the use of heat and pressure. The term *gold-filled* actually has two meanings: the *process* by means of which the material is made and as a *mark of quality*.

In an article that is marked gold-filled, the weight of the gold must be at least 1/20 of the total weight of the item, and the fineness must be at least 10 karat. Gold-filled may be spelled out or may be abbreviated *GF*. The fraction does not have to be included in the marking as long as the gold material is at least 1/20 of the total weight. For a marking "10 K GF," 1/20 is implied. If an article is made by the gold-filled process and the weight of the gold is *less than* 1/20 of the total weight, the term gold can be used with the correct descriptive term, such as *gold plate*, *gold overlay*, or *rolled gold plate*. However, the fraction (karats) must be specified. For example, the abbreviation "1/30 10 K GP" means 1/30 10-karat gold plate.

Gold may also be applied to the base metal by means of an *electroplating* process. The layer of gold must be at least 7-millionths of an inch thick, but *heavy gold electroplating* is 100-millionths of an inch thick. Abbreviations cannot be used for gold applied by electroplating; the words must be spelled out to avoid any misunderstanding.

If the word gold is used alone, it implies *pure* gold; the use of terms such as "embodying gold," "dura-gold," "mira-gold," "gold-craft," and "gold-effect" are misleading if not illegal.

The responsibility for the correct marking of gold can be placed at any point in the distribution of a spectacle frame or mounting—with the manufacturer, the importer (if a foreign frame), the distributor, or the dispenser. Mislabeling or misrepresentation is a misdemeanor punishable by a fine of not more than $5,000 or imprisonment of not more than 1 year, or both, for *each article* improperly represented. The criminal provisions of the National Stamping Act are enforced by the U.S. Department of Justice. In addition, competitors injured by mislabeling practices in the jewelry trade associations may bring civil action.

A very high proportion of gold-like spectacle frames are now produced by electrolytically plating a base metal with just enough gold alloy (1–2 microns) to impart gold color to the frame. To protect the thin gold layer from a relatively harsh environment, a thin polymer coating is deposited on the gold layer. The polymer coating is usually an epoxy resin or polymethyl methacrylate (PMMA). Practitioners should be wary of describing these frames as "gold."

Aluminum is stain and tarnish resistant, durable, and lightweight. It can be anodized to alter the surface to the oxide form, which is more resistant to corrosion. It can be painted or colored in many attractive colors. Aluminum is strong and very rigid and although the frames are durable in wear, their rigidity causes problems in fitting lenses to the frame (glazing) and adjusting. Aluminum conducts heat readily and becomes especially cold in the winter.

Nickel silver has a misleading name because the alloy contains no silver. It is composed of approximately 60% copper, 20% nickel, plus zinc and other materials. The material is rigid and lustrous, but not very malleable. It is the metal of choice for the base metal in gold-filled frames.

Titanium is a metallic element that is lightweight, flexible (easy to adjust), corrosion resistant, abrasion resistant, and has excellent memory retention. It is expensive and the colors are limited.

Stainless steel is a steel alloy containing 74% iron, 18% chromium, and 8% nickel. It is durable, flexible, strong, nonmagnetic, and extremely resistant to oxidation and corrosion. Stainless steel allows numerous matte or shiny finishes and an endless color range secured with an enameling process.

Cobalt with an alloy is the primary ingredient used for frames. The material is ductile and makes durable, flexible, lightweight, and resilient frames. The material is noncorrosive and takes many colors with a lustrous finish. It is relatively expensive.

Monel is an alloy of 68% nickel, 30% copper, and 2% iron. It is corrosion resistant and can be coated with many colors. It is used mostly for temples and bridges because the eyewires are difficult to shape. It takes strong solder joints and has a durable finish.

Beryllium is a hard, light, metallic element used in an alloy with copper, nickel, and cobalt for frames. The frames are very light, strong, and resilent.

9.4. Plastic Frame Materials

Plastic materials possess the following properties for producing frames that are relatively inexpensive, easy to adjust, and attractive:

1. Dimensional stability
2. Dermal compatibility
3. Colorfastness
4. Mechanical durability
5. Low specific gravity
6. Good strength-weight ratio
7. Good thermal-electrical insulation
8. High resistance to chemicals
9. Ease of production

As discussed in Chapter 1, there are two types of plastic materials, thermosetting and thermoplastic. A *thermosetting* material begins as a liquid and becomes solid during the manufacturing process because of the application of heat and pressure. Once the product has been manufactured, it never again softens to any significant extent, even at elevated temperatures or with the application of pressure—under these circumstances it decomposes. Examples of thermosetting plastics are *melanines* (used, e.g., to make dishes known by the trade name Melmac); *phenolics* (Bakelite); *polyesters* (used for clothing and other materials); and *allyls*. The plastic lens material CR-39 is *allyl diglycol carbonate*.

A *thermoplastic* material has the property of softening when heated and hardening when cooled. No matter how often the process is repeated, the basic structure of the material remains unchanged. Examples of thermoplastic materials are *acrylics* (known by trade names Plexiglas, Perspex, and Lucite), including *polymethyl methacrylate*, used to make hard contact lenses; *polycarbonate*, the toughest spectacle lens material available; two materials used for the manufacture of spectacle frames, *cellulose nitrate* and *cellulose acetate*, and *vinyl* (used for seat covers and upholstering).

Although cellulose nitrate and cellulose acetate are similar in appearance, when used for spectacle frames, they have very different properties. Cellulose nitrate, also called *zylonite* (called *celluloid* by the film industry), is superior to cellulose acetate in the following respects:

1. Cellulose nitrate is tougher than cellulose acetate, and because of its inherent toughness, frames can be made thinner with it than with cellulose acetate.
2. The surface of cellulose nitrate is harder, which allows it to take a better and more easily maintained polish.
3. Cellulose nitrate is somewhat easier to work because it can be stretched when heated and shrunk when cooled without measurable deterioration.
4. The softening point of cellulose nitrate is higher than that of cellulose acetate and its water absorption is lower; thus, it has better dimensional stability in warm and humid climates.

On the other hand, cellulose acetate is superior to cellulose nitrate in three respects:

1. Cellulose acetate can be produced faster than cellulose nitrate.
2. Cellulose acetate frames are more *colorfast* than frames made of cellulose nitrate.
3. More important, cellulose acetate frames are far *less combustible* than frames made of cellulose nitrate.

Although cellulose acetate frames can burn, the propagation of flames is slow; frames made of cellulose nitrate are highly inflammable—they ignite very easily, with almost an explosive force, and the flames propagate rapidly. Because of its flammability, cellulose nitrate has been banned for the manufacture of spectacle frames in the United States since 1950, although some foreign manufacturers still use it.

On casual inspection, it is difficult to differentiate a frame made of cellulose acetate from one made of cellulose nitrate. However, *camphor* is commonly used as a plasticizer in the manufacture of cellulose nitrate (but not for cellulose acetate); if the frame is rubbed briskly with a cloth, an odor of camphor is produced. Both these materials are soluble in ketones such as *acetone*, but neither is very soluble in alcohol. Acetone is frequently used to repolish or repair frames made from both materials.

Acrylic is the common name for the family of thermoplastic materials that includes polymethyl methacrylate. In addition to its use for hard contact lenses, the material has been used, on occasion, for the manufacture of spectacle frames. It has many desirable characteristics for this purpose, including dimensional stability, clarity, colorfastness, surface hardness, good wear resistance, lightness in weight, and flame resistance; if heated properly, frames made of this material can be easily adjusted. However, its hardness is offset by brittleness and low impact resistance, both of which have been found to be major handicaps. This material is therefore not often used for spectacle frames.

Nylon is a generic name given to a class of thermoplastic polymers known as *polymides*. The nylon material is too expensive if produced in sheet form, so an injection-molding technique is used. Nylon is tough and hard, but its usefulness is limited by its inherent handicaps of brittleness, lack of transparency, poor color selection, and high rate of water absorption. Nylon frames are currently available but are not often used.

Optyl, a modified thermosetting material, is an epoxy resin introduced in 1968 by an Austrian frame maker, Wilhelm Anger. An Optyl frame is made by casting a liquid at high temperature followed by a curing process. It is colorless when molded, and is dyed or sprayed (either partially or successively) with various colors on different parts and at various angles. The advantages of Optyl include hardness, high luster, nonflammability, dimensional stability, and lightness in weight.

Unlike traditional thermosetting materials, Optyl becomes soft and pliable when heated above 87°C, and can be bent or shaped with the fingers to any desired form. When cool, it retains the adjustment indefinitely. It has a *locked-in* chemical memory; that is, when reheated, the frame returns to its original shape. Because the frame is cast in the final form, the plastic eyewires do not stretch or shrink to any extent, as do those made of cellulose nitrate and cellulose acetate; thus, lenses must be edged to the *exact* size to fit the frame. Optyl has the disadvantage that it must be heated to a higher temperature than that required by a cellulose acetate frame, and the frame will break if an attempt is made to adjust it while it is cold.

In recent years, another ester of the cellulose family, *cellulose propionate*, has entered the plastic frame market. It has many attributes similar to Optyl, including manufacture by a molding process. Frames made of this material are strong, lightweight, and can be made with strong elements of styling, such as sculptured effects.

Polymide(Co-Polymide) is a nylon blend that features durability, reduced weight, and flexibility. It is considered to be hypoallergenic. It is produced by injection molding; the color and design possibilities are almost infinite.

Carbon fiber and carbon are added to plastic frames to give them the strength of metal frames, but keep them lightweight. These frames offer durability and shape retention. Finished frame colors are opaque, but frame colors can be bright and vibrant with high-sheen enamel finish. However, flexibility and adjustments are difficult.

In summary, although a great many materials have been used for the manufacture of plastic frames, most plastic frames are currently made of the thermoplastic material *cellulose acetate*.

9.5. Bridge and Temple Styles for Plastic Frames

Bridges

A metal frame or a rimless or semi-rimless mounting makes no contact with the nose (contact is made by means of adjustable pads), but a plastic frame is designed so that the bridge itself makes contact with the sides of the nose. Bridges of plastic frames can be classified as saddle bridges, keyhole bridges, or as modifications of either form.

FIGURE 9–6.   **Plastic frame with a saddle bridge.**

A *saddle bridge* (see Figure 9–6) rests directly on the crest of the nose and has no pads to contact the sides of the nose. For a saddle bridge to fit correctly, the shape of the saddle must fit the contour of the nose. There are also *modified* saddle bridges, designed to shorten the apparent length of the nose. A very few *metal* frames (mainly older styles that are now considered antiques) have saddle bridges.

A *keyhole bridge* (Figure 9–7) makes contact only on the sides of the nose. The contact is made by means of fixed, nonadjustable pads made of the same material as that of the frame. Although usually fitting the wearer's nose more precisely than a saddle bridge, a keyhole bridge sometimes has the cosmetic disadvantage of accentuating the length of the nose. Some plastic frames have bridges that are, in effect, compromises between saddle and keyhole bridges.

Bridge width is specified, for rimless and semi-rimless mountings and for plastic and metal frames, as the shortest distance between the two lenses (DBL) and is specified in millimeters (Figure 9–8).

Temples

The major types of temples available are the skull temple, the library temple, the riding bow temple, and the comfort cable temple (Figure 9–9).

FIGURE 9–7.   **Plastic frame with a keyhole bridge.**

FIGURE 9–8.   **Specification of bridge width. Distance between lenses (DBL).**

FIGURE 9–9. **Types of temples. A, skull; B, library; C, riding bow; D, comfort cable.**

The *skull* temple is the most commonly used type for plastic frames. It is bent downward behind the ear and conforms to the contours of the skull. There are many modifications of the skull temple; they vary from the "standard" skull temple mainly in terms of *width*. Most skull temples (in particular, the thinner styles) have a *wire core* to provide added strength.

The *library* (Hollywood, spatula) temple extends straight back over the ear and has no bend. This type of temple is difficult to fit because the glasses must stay on the head by pressure exerted by the temples on the sides of the skull. However, this type of temple is convenient for a person who wears glasses only occasionally and for brief periods of time.

The *riding bow* temple encircles the back and lower part of the wearer's ear. It is a plastic temple with a metal core and is used for children's frames and safety frames.

The *comfort cable* temple also encircles the back and lower part of the ear, but differs from the riding bow temple in that all or part of the temple (particularly the part encircling the ear) is made of a coiled metal cable rather than plastic. The terms *riding bow* and *comfort cable* are to some extent used synonymously; a comfort cable is considered as a type of riding bow temple. Metal frames and mountings usually have comfort cable (riding bow) temples.

A relatively new addition to temple styles is the *spring hinge* temple. A number of different spring mechanisms are in use, and they can be found on both plastic and metal frames. Spring hinges are designed to remove the stress placed on a temple when the glasses are repeatedly removed by the wearer with only one hand. The spring is not designed to act as a holding device. Spring hinge frames require normal temple spread and mastoid bone bends to be effective.

Temple length was formerly specified in terms of "length to bend" or "overall length." However, temples are currently specified only in terms of overall length. Although other frame measurements (lens size and DBL) have always been specified in millimeters, temple length was formerly specified in inches. At the present time, almost all manufacturers specify overall temple length in millimeters.

SELECTING FRAMES AND ORDERING MATERIALS

9.6. Measuring Interpupillary Distance

The first step in the design and ordering of eyewear for a patient is the measurement of the patient's PD. Both distance PD and near PD are measured.

The desired measurements for distance and near vision, respectively, are the separation between the two visual axes where they intercept the spectacle plane. For distance vision, the lines of sight are parallel, and their separation is the same whether measured at the centers of rotation, the plane of the cornea, or the spectacle plane. However, when the eyes converge for near work, they rotate about their centers of rotation with the result that the separation of the lines of sight decreases from the centers of rotation to the corneal plane and decreases further at the spectacle plane (Figure 9–10).

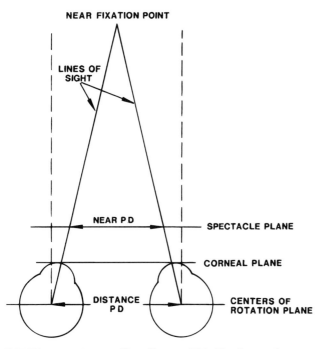

NEAR FIXATION POINT

LINES OF SIGHT

NEAR PD ——— SPECTACLE PLANE

——— CORNEAL PLANE

DISTANCE PD   CENTERS OF ROTATION PLANE

FIGURE 9–10.   **Interpupillary distance (PD). The distance between the visual axes of the two eyes where they intersect the spectacle plane.**

To measure the *distance PD*, the examiner faces the patient at a distance of approximately 40 cm and holds a millimeter ruler in the patient's spectacle plane (Figure 9–11). The patient is instructed to look at the examiner's left eye, and the examiner aligns the temporal edge of the patient's right pupil with the *zero* on the scale of the millimeter ruler. He then instructs the patient to look at his right eye, and notes the millimeter reading which is

aligned with the nasal edge of the patient's left pupil (Figure 9–11A). For patients having dark irides, it is usually necessary to align the scale reading on the millimeter ruler with the temporal limbus (corneoscleral junction) of the right eye and the nasal limbus of the left eye.

In measuring the *near* PD, the examiner again faces the patient at a distance of approximately 40 cm and instructs the patient to fixate either his right or left eye (which is positioned on the patient's midline). The examiner aligns the temporal edge of the patient's right pupil with the zero on the scale, and notes the scale reading corresponding to the nasal edge of the left pupil (Figure 9–11B). For a 40-cm distance, the near PD is usually about 4 mm less than that of the distance PD.

Instead of measuring the near PD, it is probably more accurate to carefully measure the distance PD and then determine the near PD by calculation or by reference to a table. A simple formula for calculating the near PD may be derived with the aid of Figure 9–12. For *each eye*, the difference between the distance and near PD, *x*, is given by the equation

$$\frac{x}{27} = \frac{\frac{1}{2}\, \text{distance PD}}{427},$$

$$x = \frac{27\left(\frac{1}{2}\, \text{distance PD}\right)}{427}.$$

EXAMPLE 1

For a distance PD of 60 mm,

$$x = \frac{27(30)}{427} = 1.9,$$

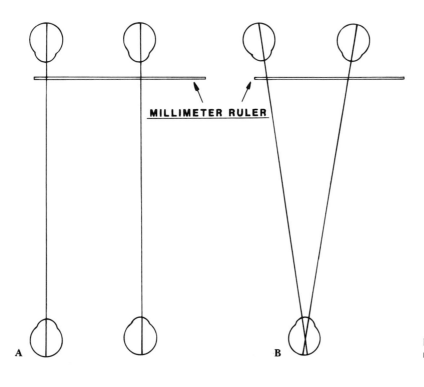

MILLIMETER RULER

A   B

FIGURE 9–11.   **Measurement of PD. A, distance; B, near.**

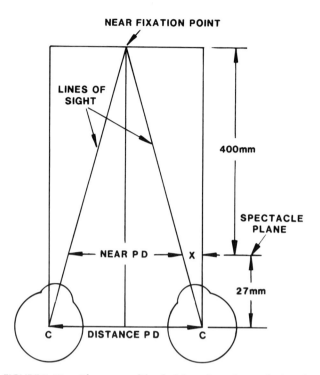

NEAR FIXATION POINT

LINES OF SIGHT

400mm

SPECTACLE PLANE

NEAR P D — X

27mm

C   DISTANCE P D   C

FIGURE 9–12.   **Diagram used for deriving a formula to calculate the near PD.**

and

$$\text{near PD} = 60 - 2(1.9) = 56.2 \text{ mm}.$$

EXAMPLE 2
For a distance PD of 70 mm,

$$x = \frac{27(35)}{427} = 2.2,$$

and

$$\text{near PD} = 70 - 2(2.2) = 65.6 \text{ mm}.$$

A compilation of near PD values, as a function of the distance PD, is given in Table 9–1.

The Use of a Pupillometer

Many practitioners and dispensers prefer to use an instrument known as a *pupillometer*, rather than a millimeter ruler, to measure PD. Use of such an instrument has the advan-

tage that the *monocular PD* can be measured. As discussed in Chapter 8, monocular PD measurement is necessary in the fitting of progressive addition lenses.

9.7. Frame Selection

The primary purpose of a spectacle frame is to hold the prescribed lenses in such a way as to provide the optimal visual efficiency. In addition, the frame should be physically comfortable, attractive in appearance, and meet the expectations of the patient.

A skilled dispenser may make sure that the requirements for optical performance and comfort are fulfilled by (1) specifying lens parameters meticulously for refractive power, lens centration, base curve specification, lens material, multifocal type, and tint; (2) selecting a bridge design that is stable, provides the proper weight distribution, and helps maintain the glasses in the desired position in front of the face; (3) fitting the lenses as close to the face as possible; (4) providing the appropriate pantoscopic tilt and the corresponding vertical centration; (5) selecting the appropriate temple style and length, adjusted to conform to the contour of the ear and the shape of the mastoid process. If these requirements are not met, the visual performance may not be as the prescriber intended, and the patient may become uncomfortable from a sore nose, sore ears, or both.

Before frame selection is begun, circumstances that may influence frame selection should be assessed. For example, the powers of the lenses along with the probable size of the lenses affects thickness and weight of the lenses; and multifocal or progressive addition lenses may require a particular minimum vertical frame dimension. The patient's PD as related to the frame PD indicates whether the eyes will look approximately centered laterally in the frame, and whether the lenses can be cut from standard uncut blanks. The purpose or purposes for which the glasses are to be worn must also be considered to avoid unsuitable frame types.

Fitting the Bridge

Although the percentage of weight of the spectacles carried by the nose varies with both the style of the frame and the patient's head position, most weight is normally borne by the nose when the head is held in an erect position. To prevent irritation of the nose, the bridge of the frame should distribute the weight of the spectacles over as large an area as possible. Because the fitting of the bridge is so impor-

TABLE 9–1
Calculated Near PD Values, as a Function of Distance PD, for a Near Working Distance of 40 cm

Distance PD	58	60	62	64	66	68	70	72
Near PD	54.5	56	58	60	62	63.5	65.5	67.5

tant, the bony angular configuration of the nose should be determined by palpating the bridge of the nose with the thumb and forefingers. The pads of the frame should closely match both the frontal angle and the transverse, or splay, angle of the nose (Figure 9–13). The *frontal angle* is the angle through which each side of the nose departs from a vertical line through the midline of the nose, as shown in Figure 9–13A, whereas the *transverse angle* (splay angle) is the angle formed by the side of the nose with the median sagittal plane (the anterior–posterior plane through the midline of the nose), as shown in Figure 9–13B.

Fitting the Temples

As the head is tilted forward, the weight of the spectacles shifts from the nose to the ears. This can create a problem if library or skull temples are worn because they can hold the glasses in place only by pressure of the sides of the temples against the head in the region behind the ears. Riding bow temples, on the other hand, encircle the ears and secure the frame by making contact at the lower arc of the crotch of the ear.

The important features in the fitting of temples are (1) the shape of the *crotch* or angle of the external ear in relation to the side of the head, in terms of both the top of the ear and the back of the ear, and (2) the shape of the mastoid process. It is therefore necessary for the dispenser to get an unimpeded view of the back of the ear and the mastoid process before deciding on the type of temple to be fitted.

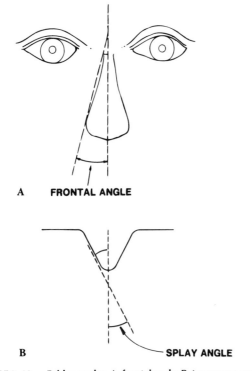

A   FRONTAL ANGLE

B   SPLAY ANGLE

FIGURE 9–13.   **Bridge angles. A, frontal angle; B, transverse, or splay, angle.**

Fashion in Eyewear Design

Once the optical and comfort criteria have been met, the features that satisfy the esthetic and cosmetic components are a matter of choice, taste, and fashion. Fashion is not new in eyeglasses. One needs only to glance through *Fashions in Eyeglasses*[2] to appreciate the variety of eyewear styles that have been introduced since the invention of glasses. Until the 1930s, developments in eyewear styles arose from the nature of the materials available and the skill of the optical artisans. In the 1940s, designers of spectacle frames began to study fashion trends and based their designs on these trends. Since that time, eyewear has become an increasingly important component of the fashion picture, a component that is not likely to go away. Not surprisingly, the public is convinced that attractiveness in eyeglasses, as judged in relation to current fashion norms, is not an option but a necessity.

Emphasis on fashion has served a useful purpose by making it easier for many patients to accept their practitioner's advice that corrective lenses are needed. Although optometrists understandably feel competent concerning the visual performance and comfort the patient may expect with the lenses being prescribed and fitted, lack of formal training in the fields of fashion and cosmesis may lead to a less secure feeling concerning the more esthetic and personal aspects of frame selection. However, most practitioners eventually come to realize that the patient's desire for attractive eyewear can be used as a justifiable means toward a desirable end.

Having undergone several years of professional training, some newly licensed optometrists resent the fact that a spectacle frame, which they believe should be considered only as a "clinical appliance," is instead considered an item of style and fashion. The emphasis on fashion does, after all, focus attention on products rather than on the services the optometrist has been trained to provide. In recent years, emphasis on fashion has progressed to the point that manufacturers consider fashion to be of greater importance than fitting requirements—as witnessed by the increasingly large number of designer frames that are available only in one size!

Since fashion in eyewear is here to stay, the practitioner who does not wish to deal with this aspect of optometric practice is well advised to delegate the task of frame selection to a well-trained assistant. Eyewear styling is a complex matter of color, texture, shape, size, and bridge and temple design. To a great extent it is an individualist undertaking, with the patient often having strong ideas concerning frame styling rather than seeking the advice of the optometrist or the dispenser. In matters of esthetic suitability the patient must have the final say, but patients are receptive to the guidance of a dispenser if he or she demonstrates a strong grasp of cosmetic principles and a keen eye for facial structures. The patient can be assisted in making a choice if the dispenser is able to demonstrate how a particular facial shape is modified by eyewear that creates balance and emphasizes positive facial features while minimizing ones that may be considered negative.

Multiple Pairs

For many years, eyewear manufacturers and distributors have carried out promotional campaigns intended to convince the public of the necessity of owning more than one pair of glasses. Using slogans such as "The right eyewear at the right time" and "A second pair for outdoor wear," these campaigns have been only moderately successful. Most members of the ametropic public have not been convinced that different occasions require different frame styles, but many have become aware of the value of a second pair of glasses in the form of absorptive lenses for outdoor wear. However, during the past decade, with the availability of photochromic lenses, many patients are electing (often at the suggestion of the optometrist or the dispenser) to order only one pair of glasses, with the result that "second pair" campaigns tend to lose momentum.

When the patient decides to obtain only one pair of glasses, compromises must often be made among factors of color, comfort, weight, durability, and other factors. For example, the wearer of high minus lenses, normally a candidate for plastic lenses, may decide on a single pair of photochromic glasses—which are not widely available in plastic—and thus avoid the expense of a second pair of spectacles but have to put up with the extra weight of glass lenses. Detailed descriptions of frame selection are given by Sasieni,[3] Brooks and Borish,[4] and Stimson.[5]

9.8. Fitting Principles

Assuming that a spectacle frame or mounting has been properly *aligned* by the manufacturer or the laboratory, the correct fitting (to the patient's face) may be discussed in terms of the fitting triangle, the pantoscopic tilt, and the temple angle.

The Fitting Triangle

A frame or mounting can be considered as fitting like a *triangle*, as shown in Figure 9–14, with points of contact at the crest of the nose and the tops of the ears. When the head is held erect, approximately two-thirds of the weight of the spectacles should be borne by the nose, and one-third by the ears. When the head is tilted downward, the weight of the frame is shifted to the ears. A common problem occurring with library temples is a tendency for the frame to slip down on the nose when the head is tilted downward. Solving this problem requires a significant increase in the pressure of the temples against the sides of the head.

Because most of the weight of a pair of spectacles is borne by the nose, it is often necessary to *cushion* the load on the nose. For frames with adjustable pads, it is important to make sure that the *entire surface* of the pad makes contact with the nose. For patients who have sensitive noses, the area of contact of the pad may be increased by the use of *jumbo* pads. Most plastic frames lack adjustable pads; thus,

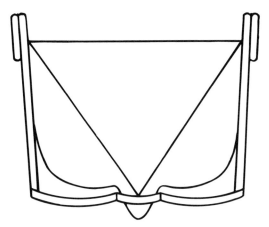

FIGURE 9–14. **The fitting triangle.**

the frame selected must be one that provides as large an area of contact with the nose as possible. A saddle bridge must fit mainly on the *crest* of the nose; this frame style is appropriate for a patient who has a relatively wide, protruding bridge, or has a high bridge. For patients with very narrow bridges or flat, recessed bridges (often the case with blacks or Asians), a keyhole bridge or an adjustable pad bridge may be required.

Pantoscopic Tilt

The *pantoscopic tilt* of a frame is defined as the amount of inward tilt of the front, away from the vertical (Figure 9–15). The provision of a pantoscopic tilt makes it possible to bring the lower edges of the lenses closer to the wearer's cheeks. Not only does this increase the field of view and afford greater protection from flying objects, but it also improves the appearance of the glasses. The optical principles relative to pantoscopic tilt were presented in Chapter 2, Section 2.20.

To adjust a pair of glasses, if one lens is higher than the other on the patient's face, the two lenses may be made level by increasing the pantoscopic angle for the lens that is low (or by decreasing the pantoscopic angle for the lens that is high). Tilting a lens so that the lower part of the lens tilts *away* from the face is called a *retroscopic* tilt. This tilt should be used only if absolutely necessary to achieve a satisfactory fit on the wearer's face.

Temple Angle

The *temple angle* is defined as the angle (in the horizontal plane) that the front makes with the temple, as shown in Figure 9–16. Although the temple angle depends on several factors, including the width of the front and the width of the patient's head, in most cases the temples are bent *outward* a few degrees. However, with the popularity of large-size frames, it is sometimes necessary to bend the temples *inward* slightly.

FIGURE 9–15.   **Pantoscopic tilt.**

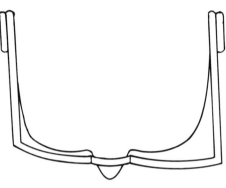

FIGURE 9–16.   **Temple angle.**

FIGURE 9–17.   **Unequal temple angles.**

Whether the two lenses are equally distant from the patient's brow (as determined by having the patient bend his head downward) depends on the temple angles for the two lenses. If the temple angle on one side is *too small*, an excessive amount of pressure occurs on the side of the head, as shown in Figure 9–17 and causes the lens to extend outward in comparison to the other lens. This problem can be solved by increasing the temple angle on the protruding side (and, in some cases, also decreasing the temple angle on the other side).

9.9. Frame Alignment

The fitting principles described in the foregoing section apply when one selects a frame or mounting for a patient before ordering the spectacles from the laboratory and when one adjusts the completed spectacles to the patient's face. Although one might assume that the frame has been placed in standard alignment ("trued") by the manufacturer or the laboratory, this is not always the case, so the task of alignment is often left to the dispenser. To make sure that a frame or a pair of spectacles is properly aligned, the first procedure is to verify the alignment of the front itself; the remaining procedure is to verify the alignment of the temples as they relate to the front.

Alignment of the Front

Alignment of the front involves two steps, each of which requires the use of a straightedge (usually a millimeter ruler). The straightedge is first used to verify the *horizontal* alignment of the front. As shown in Figure 9–18, the straightedge is placed against the back of the frame, below the endpieces (usually at the level of the tops of the pads), while the frame is held horizontally. When this is done, the left and right endpieces should be at equal distances above the straightedge. If not, the bridge must be adjusted to raise (or lower) one endpiece with respect to the other.

The straightedge is then used to verify the *vertical* alignment of the front, as shown in Figure 9–19. The frame is held vertically, with the temples extending upward, and the straightedge is placed along the back of the frame underneath (or possibly above) the pads or pad arms. Normally, a "four-point touch" is expected—the straightedge should touch the eyewire above each lens (or the back surfaces of each lens, for a rimless mounting) at the nasal and temporal edges. However, some spectacle frames are designed with the front bowed *outward* slightly (known as *face-form*, as shown in Figure 9–20); the nasal edges of the front will fail to make contact with the straightedge. This is particularly true of aviation-type goggles or sunglasses. If a four-point touch (or the desired amount of face-form) is not present, it can be corrected by appropriate adjustment of the bridge.

Occasionally, on verifying the vertical alignment of the front, the two lenses are not in the same vertical plane—

FIGURE 9–18.   **Checking horizontal alignment of the front.**

FIGURE 9–19.   **Checking vertical alignment of the front.**

FIGURE 9–20.   **Face-form.**

one lens is tilted inward (or outward) with respect to the other. This condition, shown in Figure 9–21, is known as *X-ing*, and is corrected with an adjustment of the bridge.

Alignment of the Temples

Temple alignment involves two adjustments described in the previous section: for pantoscopic tilt and for temple angle. Normally, a properly aligned frame has a small amount of pantoscopic tilt (usually no more than about 10 degrees) and the angle of each temple should be somewhat greater than a right angle (about 95 degrees). To make sure that both sides of the frame have the same amount of pantoscopic tilt, the frame is placed on a tabletop with the temples downward, as shown in Figure 9–22. If one temple fails to make contact with the table, the endpiece on that side has a greater amount of pantoscopic tilt than the one on the other side. Both sides should have the same temple angle, which is easily verified by inspection. Specific procedures for adjusting spectacle frames or mountings to remedy various maladjustments are given in Table 9–2.

9.10. Frame and Mounting Specifications

When ordering a frame or mounting for a patient, the following parameters must be specified:

Name. Each frame or mounting has a name or a number (usually a name). This label must be specified, along with the name of the manufacturer.

Color. Metal frames or mountings are usually available in yellow or white gold. However, some newer metal frames are available in darker colors, such as bronze, brown, gray, or black. Plastic frames are typically available in an assortment of colors. Frame colors (as well as the other specifications listed below) are available in manufacturers' catalogs and in references such as the *Frame Fax* catalog.

Size. Eye size is usually specified in terms of the *boxing system* (described in Chapter 4); thus the horizontal box measurement is normally specified. Bridge size is normally specified in terms of DBL. Temple length is normally specified in terms of overall length. All specifications are given in millimeters.

Temple Style. Temple style should be specified if, as sometimes occurs, the frame is available with more than one style of temple.

Lens Shape. Sometimes lens shape must be specified because a frame or mounting may be available with more than one lens shape. This is particularly true of rimless and semi-rimless mountings.

9.11. Lateral Placement of Optical Centers

The correct specification of the optical center of each lens is of importance (1) to manage prismatic effects and (2) to control the placement of the optic axis of each lens relative to the center of rotation of the eye. The management of pris-

SIDE VIEW

A

B   **TOP VIEW**

FIGURE 9–21.   **X-ing of a frame. A, side view; B, front view. (Modified from C. W. Brooks and I. M. Borish,** *System of Ophthalmic Dispensing,* **Professional Press, Chicago, 1979.)**

FIGURE 9–22.   **Unequal pantoscopic angles.**

matic effects involves both the lateral and vertical placement of the lens centers; controlling the placement of the optic axis relative to the center of rotation of the eye depends not only on the lateral and vertical placement of the centers but also on the amount of pantoscopic tilt of the lenses.

In Chapter 3, the *prism reference point* was defined as the point on a lens, as specified by the manufacturer, at which the prism value of the finished lens is to be measured. If no prismatic effect is specified, the prism reference point coincides with the optical center, or pole, of the lens. If a prismatic effect is specified, the prism reference point for each lens is the point intersected by the line of sight of the eye

when the eyes are in the primary position, with reference to both the vertical and horizontal meridians. The optical center (if no prism is to be incorporated) or the prism reference point for each lens is usually specified for *distance vision*; when the correction is intended primarily for near visual tasks, specification for *near vision* may be considered (see Section 9.13). In any event, the position of the prism reference point must be considered in terms of both its lateral and vertical placement.

Lateral placement of the optical centers, if no prismatic effects are called for in the prescription, depends simply on the relationship between the patient's PD and the frame PD. As discussed in Chapter 4 (and illustrated in Figure 9–23) the frame PD is equal to the horizontal box measurement plus DBL. With today's large lens sizes, the optical center of the lens usually must be decentered *nasalward* to make the separation of the optical centers of the lenses equal to the patient's PD. For example, if a patient having a distance PD of 64 mm is fitted with a 50/20 frame, and if the glasses are to be centered for distance vision, the optical center of each lens must be decentered inward 3 mm.

TABLE 9–2
Spectacle Adjustments: Common Maladjustments and Their Remedies

Condition	Possible Causes	Remedy
Pads dig into nose evenly	Pads too tight	Widen distance between pads
	Temple tension too great	Reduce temple tension
	Pads too small for weight of glasses	Use large pads
	Tender skin	Toughen skin with alcohol or other means
Pads dig into nose unevenly	Pads do not fit flatly against nose	Correct pads to fit flatly against nose
	Temple angle greater on one side	Correct temple angles
Spectacles slide down on nose	Distance between pads too great	Bring pads closer together
	Temple tension too weak or temples too long	Increase tension or replace with shorter temples
Lashes touch lenses	Distance between pads too great	Bring pads closer together or use deeply curved lenses
	Temple tension too great	Reduce tension
	Temples too short	Replace with longer temples
	Pad arms too short	Lengthen pad arms
Eyewires touch cheeks	Too great a distance between pads	Bring pads closer together
	Too great a pantoscopic tilt	Reduce pantoscopic tilt
	Lenses too large in vertical dimension	Refit with smaller eye size
Lenses touch brow	Lenses inset too far	Lengthen pad arms
	Resting point on nose too high	Lower spectacles by raising pad arms or pads
	Too much retroscopic tilt	Reduce retroscopic tilt
One lens higher than the other	Temples not adjusted to different ear heights	Correct pantoscopic tilt for one or both lenses
	One pad arm and pad lower than the other	Adjust to balance
	Deformed nose	Compensate for difference with pad arm and pad
One lens farther out than the other	Temple angle uneven	Correct temples in reference to angle
	One side of face larger than the other	Widen temple angle on larger side of face
Temples hurt behind ears	Tension too great	Loosen temple tension or fit larger temples
	Uneven pressure	Bend temples to conform to shape of ears
	Area of contact between temple and ear too small	Use temple tubing to increase temple surface
	Temples too short	Fit longer temples
	Temples ride too far out on top of ear	Bend tip of temple to correct
	Temple tip rides too far out at base of ear	Bend tip of temple in
Lenses too far from eyes	Pads improperly fitted	Spread pads
	Pad arms too long	Shorten pad arms
Bifocal segments cause blurred area	Segments too high	Raise pad arms or use more pantoscopic tilt
	Segments too high	Lower pad arms or use less pantoscopic tilt

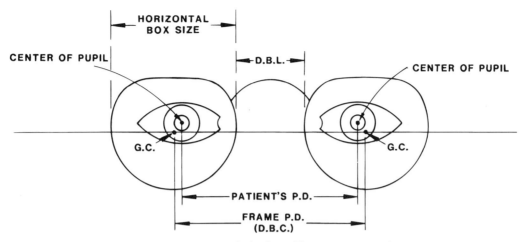

FIGURE 9–23.   **Frame PD. The horizontal box measurement plus DBL.**

Lateral placement of the optical centers may be altered to help relieve a particular patient's binocular vision problem. For example, if a myope has exophoria at near vision, centering the lenses for the distance PD induces *base-in* prismatic effect at near, which reduces the amount of exophoria. Likewise, if a hyperopic patient is esophoric at near, centering the lenses for distance induces a *base-out* prismatic effect at near, which reduces the esophoria. Samples of such cases were given in Chapter 4.

If, for the patients described above, a patient also has a *distance* phoria, and if the phoria is in the same direction at both distance and near vision, decentering the lenses with respect to the patient's distance PD should be considered. For the exophoric myope, decentering the lenses *outward* provides base-in prism at both distance and near vision; for the esophoric hyperope, decentering the lenses *outward* provides base-out prism for both distance and near vision (in both cases the amount of prismatic effect is greater at near than at distance vision). The same principle may be applied for the esophoric myope (whose lenses may be decentered *inward* to provide more base-out prism at distance than at near vision), and for the exophoric hyperope (whose lenses may be decentered *inward* to provide more base-in prism at distance than at near vision).

Thus, for a decision concerning lateral placement of the optical centers of the lenses, each case should be considered in terms of its own particular merits. However, if the frame selection is done by a dispenser or a technician (rather than by the practitioner who examined the patient) he or she normally centers the lenses for either distance or near vision, as stated in the prescription. The lenses will not be decentered inward or outward to reduce a phoria unless the prescription calls for such decentration.

9.12. Vertical Placement of Optical Centers

Although the horizontal position of the optical center receives close scrutiny, the vertical position is largely neglected. Various authors have recommended optimal vertical positions for optical centers. Waters[6] stated that the lenses should be "so positioned that the optical center of the area used is as close as possible to the normal level of the eyes"; Maxwell[7] claimed that the lenses should be mounted "so that the visual axes, when directed straight ahead, will pass through the lenses 3 mm above their centers." Laurance[8] suggested that the heights of the optical centers should be determined on the basis of the use that is made of the glasses and listed three possible positions depending on whether the glasses would be used for distance vision only, for constant wear (for both distance and near vision), or for near vision only.

For glasses to be worn for distance vision only, Laurance suggested that the optical centers be positioned so that they are pierced by the lines of sight when the eyes are directed toward a point on the ground at a distance of 12 m, or halfway to the ground at a distance of 6 m. For a person whose eye level is 5 feet, 6 inches from the ground, and for a stop distance of 25 mm, those points would fall 3.5 mm below the centers of the pupils (Figure 9–24). For constant wear, the optical centers would be lowered about 1.5 mm or would be placed 5 mm below the centers of the pupils. For close work only, the optical centers would be placed in line with the lower borders of the irides, or about 6 mm below the centers of the pupils.

In general, it is desirable to vertically position the optical centers at the *most used* portions of the lenses for two reasons:

1. Prismatic effects are absent at the optical centers of the lenses. Therefore, when one looks through the optical centers, objects are not subject to apparent displacement.
2. Chromatic aberration is absent at the optical centers; thus, objects are not affected by color dispersion.

For a lens of a given design to perform at its maximal potential, it must be worn as its designer intended. As discussed in Chapter 6, physiological approaches to lens design vary from one lens designer to another and serve to differentiate one particular lens or lens series from another.

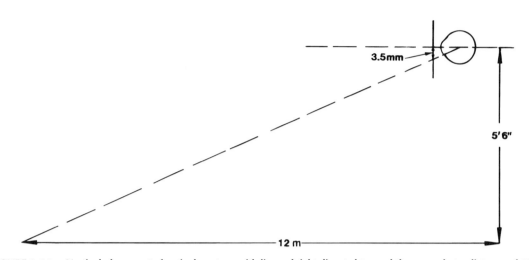

FIGURE 9-24.   **Vertical placement of optical centers, with lines of sight directed toward the ground at a distance of 12 m.**

However, in every lens design there is agreement on one basic assumption: The optic axis of the lens should pass through the center of rotation of the eye.

When the optic axis of the lens passes through the center of rotation of the eye, the optic axis and the visual axis coincide when the wearer looks through the optical center of the lens; that is, the visual axis is perpendicular to both lens surfaces. For any other viewing angle, a lens designer is able to anticipate the specific location in the lens through which the visual axis will pass. Therefore, by appropriate design, the designer can predict and can control image quality.

When the optic axis of the lens fails to pass through the center of rotation of the eye, the chief ray of the image-forming bundle, which essentially coincides with the visual axis, intersects the lens surfaces at locations and at angles of incidence not anticipated by the designer. The mismatch between the designer's intention and the actual use of the lens creates differences in the angles of incidence in the tangential and sagittal planes and, therefore, differences in the tangential and sagittal foci, which causes the aberration of *oblique astigmatism*. Differences in the angles of incidence in the tangential and sagittal planes occur even at the optical center; hence, the refracted bundle of rays entering the eye is astigmatic, even though the lens is a spherical lens.

When one looks through the optical center of a lens when the optic axis of the lens fails to pass through the center of rotation of the eye, the region of the optical center of the lens suffers both an increase in spherical power and a cylindrical power effect. A plus cylinder effect is created for a plus spherical lens, and a minus cylindrical effect is created for a minus spherical lens. Formulas for calculating these effects were given in Chapter 2, Section 2.19. The axis of the induced cylinder is always *parallel* to the axis of rotation of the lens tilt. For example, the axis is 180° for a pantoscopic tilt, and 90° for a face-form tilt.

The formulas for calculating these effects, which occur when the optic axis of the lens fails to coincide with the visual axis, apply *only* to the area of the optical center of the lens. However, the lens also fails to perform as intended in the peripheral portions.

A Note of Caution. The student may conclude that, when any lens is tilted, power changes occur at the optical center. This is incorrect. A lens *can be tilted* without bringing about power changes at the optical center *as long as the optic axis of the lens passes through the center of rotation of the eye* (see Figure 9–15). However, oblique astigmatism occurs in the peripheral portions of the lens, and the amount of oblique astigmatism depends on the particular lens design (i.e., on the amount of bend).

If we adhere to the principle that the optic axis of the lens should pass through the center of rotation of the eye, the required level of the optical center depends on the pantoscopic tilt necessary to bring the lens into the proper relationship with the wearer's eyebrows and cheeks. In a given case, it is best to provide the pantoscopic tilt that gives the *best appearance* and to lower the optical centers of the lenses from the pupillary level (when the eyes are in the primary position) *1 mm for each 2 degrees of pantoscopic tilt*, as explained in Chapter 2, Section 2.20. One can estimate the pantoscopic tilt, or use a protractor to approximate the tilt, of the front relative to the vertical plane when the head is held in the primary position.

It is a common laboratory procedure, unless the dispenser specifies otherwise, to place the optical center at the level of the *geometric center* of the lens. Because the level of the geometric center is usually about 3 to 5 mm below the wearer's eye level, the placement of the optical center is consistent with the typical "cosmetic" pantoscopic angle of 6° to 10°; thus, the lens functions as the designer intended. An exception may occur, however, with *very large lens sizes*, for which the level of the geometric center of the lens may be as far as 8 to 10 mm below the wearer's eye level. For large lenses, the dispenser should specify the position of the optical center of the lens, on the basis of the amount of pantoscopic tilt, so that it can fall somewhat *above* the geometric center. Fortunately, the average levels of the lines of sight for various visual tasks tend to be consistent with the level usually selected for the optical center on the basis of the amount of pantoscopic tilt required to conform to the structure of the wearer's face.

Except in cases of large amounts of anisometropia, it is not desirable to place the optical centers of the lenses higher than usual when glasses are to be worn for *distance only,* or to place the optical centers lower than usual when the glasses will be worn for *near vision only.* To change placement would require that the glasses be tilted at an unattractive angle to make the optical axes of the lenses pass through the centers of rotation of the eyes.

9.13. Centering Problems and Solutions

Centering Lenses for Near Work Only

An interesting question arises in regard to the centration of lenses made solely for close work: Should the lenses be centered for the distance PD or for the near PD? The answer depends on whether it is considered more important (1) to avoid inducing horizontal prismatic effects or (2) to ensure that the optical axes of the lenses pass through the centers of rotation of the eyes. Placing the optical centers of the lenses so that they coincide with the *near* PD produces zero prismatic effects for close work, but the optic axes do not pass through the centers of rotation. On the other hand, positioning the optical centers so that they coincide with the *distance* PD results in the optic axes passing through the centers of rotation of the eyes, and therefore controlling oblique astigmatism, but with the prism induced as the eyes converge for close work.

Although most practitioners would normally position the optical centers of the lenses for the near PD, both approaches should be considered, and the decision made on the basis of the alternative that will best serve the patient.

Face-Forming

Face-forming refers to the process of curving a frame in such a way as to conform to the wearer's face. As shown in Figure 9–20, the procedure involves both an outward bowing of the bridge and a widening of the temple angles. Although face-forming improves the appearance of a large frame, it is responsible for two problems:

1. If the optical centers are placed so that they coincide with the patient's distance PD, face-forming causes the optic axes to pass *nasalward* to the centers of rotation of the eyes (Figure 9–25), which changes the effective performance of the lenses. This can be corrected by decentering both lenses outward (with the result that the optic axes of the lenses pass through the centers of rotation of the eyes); unfortunately, this procedure induces unwanted horizontal prism.

2. The laboratory normally places the distance fitting points so that the sum of their respective distances from the nasal edges plus the DBL is equal to the specified PD. If the frame has face-form, the shortest distance between the distance fitting points is *smaller* than the PD. In prac-

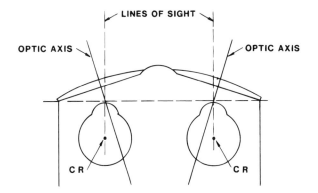

FIGURE 9–25. **Face-forming, with optical centers coinciding with the wearer's distance PD, which causes the optic axes of the lenses to pass nasalward to the centers of rotation of the eyes.**

tice, the shortest distance between the distance fitting reference points should correspond to the distance PD, but unless allowance is made for face-forming, the PD of the finished spectacles will not match the patient's PD.

Although the effect of pantoscopic tilt on the direction of the optic axis can be corrected by lowering the optical centers of the lenses 1 mm for each 2 degrees of tilt, the problems created by face-forming have no satisfactory solution. Therefore, face-forming a frame, especially one with lenses of high power, results in inferior optical performance of the lenses for foveal vision.

Hyper-Eye

Hyper-eye is defined as the condition in which one eye is positioned higher in the head than the other (like the little man on the cover of *MAD* magazine). Hyper-eye is not the same as *hyperphoria,* in which the visual axis of one eye is aimed higher than that of the other eye when dissociated. When writing an order for a pair of glasses for a patient with hyper-eye, the dispenser must decide where to specify the vertical positions of the optical centers of the two lenses. In making this decision, the dispenser must consider the relationship between the patient's eyes and eyebrows—specifically (as shown in Figure 9–26), the relationship between the imaginary line between the two eyebrows and that between the centers of the two pupils.

From an esthetic point of view, the appearance of a pair of glasses on a patient's face (Figure 9–27) is usually more pleasing if the frame is roughly parallel to the *eyebrow level* (A) rather than to the *eye level* (B). However, in many cases a compromise is the best solution. Once the most acceptable solution has been decided, the dispenser should determine the relative vertical positions of the centers of the patient's pupils when the frame (the same style and size as the frame in which the finished lenses will be mounted) is worn in the desired position on the patient's face. This may be done by measuring the vertical distance from the bottom rim of the frame to the center of the pupil, for each eye. Using the familiar rule that the optical center of each lens should be placed 1 mm below the center of

FIGURE 9–26.   **Hyper-eye. The center of the pupil of the right eye is approximately 4 mm higher than that of the left eye.**

the pupil for each 2 degrees of pantoscopic tilt, the dispenser should specify the vertical position of the optical center for each lens.

If the power of the prescription in the vertical meridian is plano or is very low (e.g., +1.00 DS –0.75 DC axis 180), it is not necessary to specify differential vertical positions for the optical centers. However, if *multifocal lenses* are being ordered, failure to specify differential positions of the centers means that one segment top will be farther below the eye than the other. For a hyper-eye patient who has already worn bifocals, the optometrist or dispenser should check the segment heights of those bifocals. Some patients have no complaints of asthenopia despite the fact that one segment is 2 or 3 mm lower (with respect to the center of the

FIGURE 9–27.   **Hyper-eye. A, with frame parallel to the eyebrow level; B, with frame parallel to the eye level.**

pupil) than the other. If the patient is well adapted to this situation, differential vertical placement of the segments in new glasses will cause complaints of asthenopia.

9.14. Bifocal Segment Inset

As stated briefly in Chapter 8, Section 8.16, there are two reasons for specifying *segment inset* in an order for a pair of bifocal lenses: to ensure that the segments do not induce unwanted prismatic effects, and to ensure that the reading fields of the two segments coincide.

The first step in deciding the amount of segment inset is the patient's *near PD*. The near PD may be measured, along with the distance PD, or it can be determined by reference to a table (see Table 9–1). Even when the bifocal segments are inset for the exact near PD, so that the segments themselves induce no prismatic effects, the *distance prescription* (unless it has zero power in the horizontal meridian) will induce a prismatic effect at near vision.

As discussed in Chapter 8, Section 8.24, the distance lens may be considered as existing *behind* the segment (which actually is the case for a one-piece bifocal) and will induce horizontal prismatic effects at near vision because of the distance prescription. Because a bifocal add always has *plus* power, insetting the segments closer than required by the near PD induces *base-in* prism. Therefore, for a hyperopic patient, whose distance lenses induce a *base-out* prismatic effect at near, the effect can be counteracted to some extent by increasing the segment inset; for a myopic patient, whose distance lenses induce a *base-in* prismatic effect at near, decreasing the segment inset helps to counteract this effect.

Because most presbyopes are exophoric at near, the *hyperopic* patient is of most concern to the practitioner. For this patient, an additional 2 mm of segment inset, for a +2.00-D add, induces a total base-in prismatic effect of 0.8 prism diopter (for the two lenses). However, an excessive amount of segment inset tends to cause the reading fields for the two eyes to fail to coincide completely; therefore, additional segment inset should be accompanied by use of a reasonably wide segment (instead of the usual 22-mm-wide fused segment). A 28- or 35-mm-wide segment could be used, or an Executive-style segment. Fortunately, the reading fields coincide reasonably well, even with excessive amounts of bifocal inset, unless the patient requires relatively high-powered lenses, which may be a problem in aphakia, particularly. The relationship between distance lens power and segment inset on the coincidence of the reading fields is illustrated by the data in Chapter 8, Table 8–11.

9.15. Prescription Order Forms

Prescription laboratories normally supply their clients with their own prescription order forms. A typical laboratory order form is shown in Figure 9–28. Although one form differs from another in minor details, they all have provision for the lens and frame information necessary to order a pair

687859

	SPHERE	CYLINDER	AXIS	DECENTER DISTANCE	PRISM	BASE	LENS COLOR

PATIENT _____ DATE

ADDRESS _____ ☐ MAIL TO PATIENT

| DIST. {R L} | | | | | | | GRAY 1-2-3 |
| | | | | | | | PINK 1-2 |

	SEG. HGT.	SEG. WIDTH	INSET	TOTAL INSET			GREEN 1-2-3
ADD {R L}					☐ 3.0 M.M. INDUSTRIAL SAFETY		PHOTOGRAY
				OTHER:	☐ PLASTIC		OTHER COLORS

BIFOCAL ▶

KRYPTOK	FLAT-TOP	CURVE-TOP (F.V.)	OTHER:	☐ LENSES UNCUT	
TILLYER D	EXECUTIVE	ULTEX A-AL B			COATED LENS

TRIFOCAL ▶

FLAT-TOP	OTHER:	DUAL SEG.	☐ AR	☐ HARDCOTE®
EXECUTIVE		TYPE	☐ COLOR ___	

LENS SHAPE | SIZE | P.D. | SPECIAL Rx DETAIL

| | FRAME | BRIDGE | DIST. | NEAR |

FRAME NAME & COLOR

TEMPLE TYPE, COLOR, & LENGTH

CERTIFICATE: This certifies that the prescribing physician or optometrist has specified that these lenses are NOT to be hardened.	FRAME
X _____ (SIGNATURE)	☐ SUPPLY ☐ ENCLOSED
NOTICE: Glasses are hardened for impact resistance as required by the F.D.A. unless otherwise exempted by law as certified above.	☐ NOT ENCLOSED

LENSES	
COLOR/COAT	
HARD-COTE®	
EDGING	
TEMP. D.B.	
FRAME	
MISC.	
TOTAL	

↑ DO NOT WRITE BELOW THIS LINE

INVOICE NO. 687859

TRAY

DATE

FIGURE 9–28.   **A typical prescription order form.**

of finished glasses. However, most prescription order forms *do not* have spaces for information concerning base curve, cylinder location (front or back surface), or thickness (center or edge).

A prescription laboratory usually deals with one or two lens suppliers. If, for example, the laboratory routinely supplies Gentex polycarbonate lenses, the optometrist or dispenser can expect base curves of the Gentex series; if the laboratory supplies lenses from almost any other manufacturer, the polycarbonate lenses will have whatever base curves are used in the particular series. Most laboratories are pleased to supply customers with information about available series of lenses and charts showing the base curve ranges on the basis of lens powers.

The optometrist or dispenser may wish to specify the trade name of the lens (e.g., Younger Seamless, American Optical Executive, Photogray Extra). When this is done, the manufacturer is obligated to supply the exact product ordered (although, if the laboratory does not deal with the manufacturer of the specified lens, a substitute will probably be offered). However, many *bifocal* lenses made by different manufacturers are sufficiently similar so that the practitioner may wish

to specify an "Executive-style" bifocal, a "blended" bifocal, and the like. When this is done, the laboratory is *not* required to supply an American Optical Executive or a Younger blended bifocal, but may supply a lens that looks and performs like the trade-name lens. In many cases, "look-alike" lenses are available because the original patents have expired. The custom of substitution does *not* apply to *progressive addition* lenses. Lens design in this field has not yet reached the point where one manufacturer's lens performs much the same as that of another manufacturer.

If the optometrist or dispenser plans to order both lenses and frame from the same laboratory and plans to have the laboratory assemble the glasses, he or she needs to know which frame manufacturers the laboratory deals with, and, more important, which frame styles (and sizes and colors in each style) the laboratory carries *in stock*. Specifying a frame that the laboratory must order from the factory is sure to result in unnecessary delay. The laboratory manager should be asked to supply this information. As already noted, there are a number of catalogs and indexes, such as *Frame Fax*, that list complete (and current) information on all available frames and mountings.

VERIFICATION AND DISPENSING

9.16. Verification

After the completed glasses arrive from the laboratory, they should be examined for accuracy of the prescription and for quality of the workmanship. To ensure that no phase of inspection is overlooked, a routine method of evaluation should be established. Furthermore, the accuracy and quality of workmanship must be judged against a preexisting list of tolerances, usually referred to as a *standard*.

Ophthalmic Lens Standards

The American National Standards Institute (ANSI) is a nationally recognized, nongovernmental body whose job is to act as a coordinator of voluntary standards development and as a clearinghouse for information on national and international standards. ANSI approval procedures for standards strive for a consensus among those within its scope and affected by its provisions. Ophthalmic lens standards were first developed in 1964, revised in 1972, 1979, 1987, and again in 1995. The Z80.1-1995 Standard refractive tolerances for the power in each principal meridian and the value of the cylinder for single-vision and standard multifocal lenses are displayed in Table 9–3; the refractive tolerances for progressive addition and aspheric lenses are shown in Table 9–4. Tolerances for cylinder axis position are listed in Table 9–5.

The most significant change in the standard is the tolerance for refractive power. Tables 9–3 and 9–4 give the tolerances for the two principal meridians and the power of

the cylinder (the difference between the two principal meridians). Different tolerances exist for single-vision and standard multifocal lenses (Table 9–3) and for progressive addition and aspheric lenses (Table 9–4). The different tolerances recognize that it is more difficult to tightly control progressive addition and aspheric lens powers than it is for single-vision and standard multifocals.

The second significant change in the standard is that of the power error between a *pair* of lenses. A footnote to Tables 9–3 and 9–4 states that "The distance refractive power error between a pair of lenses in each meridian cannot exceed 2/3 the sum of the tolerances for each lens for that meridian." The footnote addresses the condition in which one lens is on the strong side of the tolerance and the other lens is on the weak side of the tolerance. This tolerance is imposed on the two principal meridians, but *not* on the cylinder power.

The Z80.1-1995 Standard applies to all ophthalmic prescription lenses, whether edged lenses or lenses mounted in a frame. It also applies to uncut lenses supplied by an optical laboratory in filling a specific prescription. However, all relevant optical specifications and tolerances included in the standard are considered as *recommendations*, not as specific requirements. The standard serves as a guide for tolerances, but is not restrictive. A lens may meet or exceed all specifications of the standard and be judged by the dispenser as unacceptable, or a lens not in conformance with the standard may be considered acceptable by the dispenser.

The optometrist should come to an agreement with the laboratory as to what his or her acceptable tolerances are.

TABLE 9–3
Refractive Tolerances for Single-Vision and Multifocal Lenses

Meridian of Highest Absolute Power	Tolerance on Each Principal Meridian*	Tolerance on Nominal Value of the Cylinder			
		0.00–0.75	>0.75–4.00	>4.00–6.00	>6.00
0.00–3.00	±0.12	±0.09	±0.12	±0.18	±0.25
>3.00–6.00	±0.12	±0.12	±0.12	±0.18	±0.25
>6.00–9.00	±0.12	±0.12	±0.18	±0.18	±0.25
>9.00–12.00	±0.18	±0.12	±0.18	±0.25	±0.25
>12.00–20.00	±0.25	±0.18	±0.25	±0.25	±0.25
>20.00	±0.37	±0.25	±0.25	±0.37	±0.37

*The distance refractive power error between a *pair* of lenses in each meridian cannot exceed 2/3 the sum of the tolerances for each lens for that meridian.
SOURCE: Adapted from the American National Standards Institute, Inc.

If the optometrist wishes to impose stricter tolerances than those specified in Z80.1-1995, this may be done, as long as the optical laboratory agrees. A copy of the adopted standards should be posted, for reference, in the verification area of the optometric office.

The optical laboratory includes with the completed glasses a copy of the prescription order form (this is usually a carbon copy of the form submitted by the optometrist, unless the glasses were ordered by telephone, in which case a laboratory employee will have completed the form). Because orders may contain clerical errors, the laboratory copy should be checked against both the optometrist's order form and the original examination record to make sure that all agree. In this way, any transcription errors will be found before the patient is notified that the glasses are ready for dispensing.

Verification of the completed eyewear should include the following procedures, performed in any sequence that seems appropriate.

Lens Verification

1. The lens material (ophthalmic crown glass, high-index glass, CR-39 plastic, high-index plastic, or polycarbonate) should be verified. High-index glass and high-index plastic can be identified by the lower *approximate power* as determined by the lens gauge (the lens gauge is calibrated for the index of refraction of ophthalmic crown glass). CR-39 and polycarbonate plastic can be identified on the basis of weight (they are approximately half the weight of crown glass). One can differentiate polycarbon-

TABLE 9–4
Refractive Tolerances for Progressive Addition and Aspheric Lenses

Meridian of Highest Absolute Power	Tolerance on each Principal Meridian*	Tolerance on Nominal Value of the Cylinder			
		0.00–0.75	>0.75–4.00	>4.00–6.00	>6.00
0.00–3.00	±0.12	±0.12	±0.18	±0.18	±0.25
>3.00–6.00	±0.12	±0.12	±0.18	±0.18	±0.25
>6.00–9.00	±0.18	±0.18	±0.25	±0.25	±0.25
>9.00–12.00	±0.18	±0.18	±0.25	±0.25	±0.25
>12.00–20.00	±0.25	±0.18	±0.25	±0.25	±0.25
>20.00	±0.37	±0.25	±0.25	±0.37	±0.37

*The distance refractive power error between a *pair* of lenses in each meridian cannot exceed 2/3 the sum of the tolerances for each lens for that meridian.
SOURCE: Adapted from the American National Standards Institute, Inc.

TABLE 9–5
Tolerances in Degrees on the Direction of the Cylinder Axis

Nominal value of the cylinder power	0–0.37	>0.37–0.75	>0.75–1.50	>1.50
Tolerance of the axis (°)	±7	±5	±3	±2

SOURCE: Adapted from the American National Standards Institute, Inc.

ate from CR-39 plastic by the surface power found with use of the lens gauge because CR-39 has a lower index of refraction (1.498) than that of crown glass and polycarbonate has a higher index (1.586) than that of crown glass.

2. The lens should have the specified tint and coating.

3. If the lens has been toughened by *air-tempering*, it should exhibit a typical strain pattern when placed between the crossed polarizing filters of a polariscope. Two modified versions of the polariscope are available (the Tempr-a-Scope by Kirk and the Chem-Check by American Optical) to identify a lens that has been *chemically tempered*. These instruments are designed on the basis of the following principle: If the edge of a chemically tempered lens is immersed in a cell containing glycerin (between crossed polarizing filters), the edge of the lens shows a characteristic ring of light.

4. The lens media should be free of defects such as stress, veins, bubbles, and foreign particles.

5. The lens surface should be free of defects that would impair its function, such as grayness, scratches, pits, abrasions, waves, cloth marks, and water marks.

6. The accuracy of the prescription specifications (spherical power, cylinder power and axis, prism power and base direction, and centration) should be verified, by using a lensometer. The optical center (or the prism reference point if prism is prescribed) should be marked and measured, in terms of its position both horizontally and vertically from the geometric center.

7. For multifocal lenses, the segment type, width, height, and inset should be verified.

8. The base curve (if specified in the order) should be verified, as well as the side (front or back) on which the cylinder is ground.

9. Center thickness (minus lens) or edge thickness (plus lens) should be verified with a caliper. If thickness was not specified in the order, the lens should be no thicker than the amount required to provide mechanical stability and impact resistance.

Frame Verification

1. The frame should be verified as the correct type (indicated by the manufacturer's trade name or number), color, eye size (usually the box measurement), bridge size (DBL), and temple style and length. The frame should be inspected to ensure that it is in good condition with no scratches, plier marks, or other damage.

2. The quality of workmanship in mounting or glazing should be verified. The lenses should not wobble or feel loose in the frame. No air spaces should be present between the lens and the frame. The bevel should be examined for evenness and for the absence of chips. Screws used on hinges, on rimless mountings, or to attach trims on plastic frames should be checked to ensure that excess length has been properly cut off, filed smoothly, and peened over to prevent the screws from backing out.

3. For rimless mountings or metal frames, the lenses should be checked between crossed polarizers of a polariscope for visible evidence of strain at the mounting points

and around the metal rim. Excessive strain may cause the lenses to fracture or chip.

4. Alignment of the frame should be checked, to make sure that the frame was in standard alignment when it left the laboratory. Temples should open easily, and adjustable pads should swivel freely.

In the interest of time, errors detected on inspection should be corrected in the office, if possible. If errors of workmanship not correctable in the office are present, or if the lens parameters do not meet the specified tolerances, the glasses should be returned to the laboratory for correction. Errors should be described precisely, so there will be no doubt of the validity of the cause for rejection. Although the patient will be disappointed by the delay, most patients will be pleased to know that their doctor requires accuracy on the part of the laboratory. Furthermore, the laboratory manager quickly learns whether a given practitioner demands accuracy and good workmanship or is one who accepts substandard merchandise.

Augsburger[9] described a method of ophthalmic material verification that results in both better service by the laboratory and a lowered rejection rate. He attributes success to the fact that, when glasses must be returned, the laboratory is supplied with thorough documentation of the evaluation process. Much time can be saved and aggravation avoided by selecting a laboratory that has high standards of accuracy and workmanship and that is capable of handling any prescription, no matter how complicated, and entrusting most (if not all) the prescription work to this laboratory.

9.17. Dispensing and Adjusting

The most convenient method of dispensing and adjusting the finished glasses is for the practitioner or dispenser to face the patient, seated on the opposite side of a small table. Relatively little adjusting should be required if the frame fitting was done accurately and if the glasses were received from the laboratory in standard alignment. In the standard alignment procedure, laboratory personnel normally provide a temple angle slightly greater than 90° (although this should *not* be done with very large frames), a small amount of pantoscopic tilt, and (depending on the type of frame) possibly a small amount of face-forming. (The procedures for determining whether the glasses are in standard alignment are described in Section 9.9.) If the glasses, when received from the laboratory, are *not* in standard alignment, they should be aligned before they are dispensed to the patient. Procedures for alignment are also described in Section 9.9.)

Alignment with Facial Features

One of the first things to be checked, when the glasses have been placed on the patient's face, is whether they are level with the patient's eyebrows and other facial features. A significant number of people have one ear higher than the other or one eyebrow slightly higher than the other, with the result that the glasses look crooked in relation to the face. The solution to this problem is to increase the pantoscopic angle of the temple on the low side or to decrease the pantoscopic angle on the high side. As a part of this process, the pantoscopic angle for each lens may have to be increased or decreased to maximize both the cosmetic effect and the optical performance. For example, the pantoscopic angle must be *increased* if the distance between the lower edges of the lenses and the cheekbones is too great (more than the thickness of a finger) or if the upper edges of the lenses are too close to the eyebrows. The angle must be *decreased* if the bottoms of the lenses are too close to the cheekbones or the tops are too far from the eyebrows. If the frame fitting and lens ordering were done correctly, the resulting pantoscopic tilt (in degrees) should be approximately twice the distance (in millimeters) between the optical center of each lens and the center of the patient's pupil.

Often, adjusting the glasses so that the front appears to be properly aligned with the patient's face is a matter of compromise. This is particularly true for patients with *hyper-eye*, or for patients who have two eyes on the same level but one eyebrow higher than the other. (For a discussion of hyper-eye, see Section 9.13.)

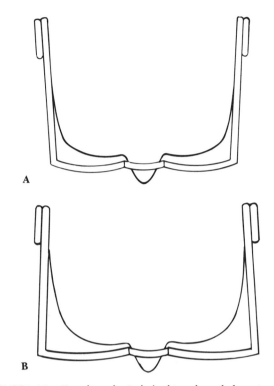

FIGURE 9–29.   **Temple angle. A, desired temple angle for a standard-sized frame; B, temple angle for an extra-large frame.**

Temple Adjustments

In addition to angling the endpieces to make the glasses level on the patient's face and to provide the correct amount of pantoscopic tilt, it may be necessary to adjust the temple angles and to adjust the temples where they wrap around the patient's ears.

If the temple angles are correct, the temples should contact the sides of the head lightly but not great enough to make grooves in the skin (Figure 9–29). The temples of a standard-sized frame (i.e., less than 50 mm wide) usually contact the sides of the head from just behind the temporal angle of the orbit (A); temples of an extra-large frame may contact the head only for an inch or so in front of the ear (B). Such a frame may require temple angles of *less than 90°*. Whatever the frame size, if the temple makes no contact with the side of the head, the temple angle must be decreased, and if there is forceful contact, the temple angle must be increased. As a part of the temple angle adjustment, the patient should be asked to bend the head downward, and the dispenser should make sure that the top of the frame is equally close to both upper orbital ridges (in the region of the eyebrows). If this is not the case, the temple angles are unequal (as shown in Figure 9–17), and the temple angle should be *increased* on the side that is too far from the brow region.

The position of each temple where it bends over and behind the patient's ear should be carefully noted and, if necessary, the temple should be adjusted by bending it so that it will gently contact the skin in the area of the temple crotch (at the top of the ear) and in the region of the mastoid bone, without putting pressure on the outer ear. If the bend is in front or behind the crotch of the ear, it should be corrected. For most temples (particularly plastic temples) the best way to make the adjustment is to straighten the temple (almost completely removing the bend), and then to place the bend where it is needed.

Occasionally, the "length to bend" of both temples is either too long or too short. In such a case, an error was made at the time of frame selection and ordering, and the temples should be replaced with ones of the correct length. Unfortunately, for some currently available fashion frames, only one or two temple lengths are available, so it is occasionally necessary to "make do" with temples that are really too short or too long for an optimal fit by judicious positioning of the bend and adjustment behind the ears.

Bridge Adjustments

If the glasses being dispensed incorporate a plastic frame with no adjustable pads, little can be done to improve the fitting of the bridge. However, if a bridge frame with pads is used, the pads can easily be adjusted to move the glasses up or down on the patient's face or to move them closer or farther away from the eyes. Adjusting the pads downward moves the glasses upward on the patient's face; moving them upward allows the glasses to fit lower on the face; spreading the pads apart makes the glasses fit closer to the eyes, and moving the pads closer together moves the glasses away from the eyes. However, in any pad adjustment, care must be taken to ensure that the pressure of the pads is spread evenly over each side of the nose—a pad that digs in at the bottom or top edge, or at the back or front edge, is sure to cause discomfort. If a patient has a tender nose (particularly if heavy lenses, a heavy frame, or both, are being dispensed), it is a very good idea to replace the pads that come with the frame with *jumbo* pads.

Verifying Visual Acuity

At the dispensing visit, the patient should be given an opportunity to read the letters on the distance Snellen chart with the new glasses; if the glasses are intended mainly for near vision (or if they are multifocals) the patient should be asked to read the letters on a reduced Snellen chart or a reading card. The optometrist may be very sure that the patient has 20/20 vision or better with the new glasses, but many patients are disappointed if they are not given the opportunity to try out new glasses by reading the eye chart. For this reason, some optometrists routinely do all dispensing in the refracting room, with the patient seated in the refracting chair (even though frame selection and other aspects of dispensing are done by a dispenser or technician with the patient seated at a fitting table). Not only can the glasses be conveniently adjusted in the refracting chair, but the patient does not have to be moved to another room for the visual acuity check.

Checking Centration of Finished Spectacles

If the practitioner is concerned about the centration of the patient's lenses, this may be checked by the use of a retinoscope or ophthalmoscope in a semidarkened room. With the spectacles in place, the patient is asked to fixate the instrument light while the examiner observes the patient's eye through the instrument's peephole. The examiner sees two images of the light reflected from the front and back surfaces of the spectacle lens; by moving about, the two images can be made to coincide (students will recognize this procedure as reminiscent of that of lining up the reflected images from the cornea of a schematic eye when they practice retinoscopy).

At this point, the examiner's line of sight coincides with the optical axis of the lens. A third image, the corneal reflex, is also seen. Because the corneal reflex lies near the patient's visual axis (which passes through the center of rotation of the eye) the separation of the two superimposed images and the corneal reflex indicates the discrepancy between the optical axis of the lens and the visual axis. By altering the pantoscopic tilt or by raising or lowering the spectacles, the two lens reflections may be aligned with the corneal reflex. The optical axis of the lens then passes through the center of rotation, so the fitting criteria match the designer's assumption for optimal performance.

Care and Maintenance of Glasses

Once the adjustment of the glasses has been completed, the dispenser should instruct the patient about their care and maintenance, particularly if the glasses are the patient's

first pair. The patient should be cautioned not to spread the temples apart when putting the glasses on (it is surprising how many people do this) but to put the glasses on by tilting the temples over the ears. The patient should also be told that the glasses should be taken off evenly with a hand on each temple. They should be put in a case, placed upside down on a table or other surface with the temples wide open, or folded and placed in such a way that they rest on the folded temples. They should *not* be placed with the front surfaces of the lenses in contact with the table (again, it is surprising how many patients do this, if not warned against it). The patient should understand that if the lenses are *plastic lenses*, extra care should be taken to avoid scratching them. Lenses (whether glass or plastic) should never be cleaned with a dry cloth; they should be cleaned by rubbing the lenses between the fingertips moistened by a liquid detergent and held under running tap water. A soft cloth or tissue should be used to dry the lenses. Glass lenses may be wiped dry, but plastic lenses should be *patted* dry.

Advice About Use of Glasses

After the glasses have been properly adjusted, the patient should be instructed (even if this has been done during the examination) about what to expect from the new glasses. If a substantial change has been made in the prescription, the patient should be informed of the likely perceptual changes that may be encountered and advised that the changes should disappear with time.

For a patient who is wearing his or her first bifocals, trifocals, or progressive addition lenses, adequate instruction should be given for their use during walking (particularly in going up and down steps or curbs) and for the positions of the head, eyes, and arms that result in comfortable reading posture.

Subsequent Adjustments

When the glasses are dispensed, the patient should be told that the glasses may need further adjustment after they have been worn for several days and should be encouraged to return for readjustment. Many optometrists routinely schedule each patient to return in approximately 2 weeks for a progress check, to make sure the glasses are performing as intended. At this time, clinical findings, such as visual acuity, may be verified, but, more important, the *adjustment* of the glasses should be verified. More patients are lost to other practitioners by *poor dispensing or adjusting* than by poor refracting or prescribing! The reader's attention is again called to the common maladjustments and remedies listed in Table 9–2.

References

1. Gasson, W. The Florentine Legend. *Ophthalmic Optician*, Vol. 9, No. 17, pp. 924–928, 1969.
2. Corson, R. *Fashion in Eyeglasses*. Peter Owen Ltd., London, 1970.

3. Sasieni, L. S. *Principles and Practice of Optical Dispensing and Fitting*, 3rd edition. Butterworths, London, 1975.
4. Brooks, C. W., and Borish, I. M. *System for Optical Dispensing*. Professional Press, Chicago, 1979.
5. Stimson, R. L. *Ophthalmic Dispensing*, 3rd edition. Charles C Thomas, Springfield, IL, 1979.
6. Waters, E. H. *Ophthalmic Mechanics*, Vol. 1, Edward Brothers, Ann Arbor, p. 262, 1964.
7. Maxwell, J. T. *Outline of Refraction*, Medical Publishing Co., Omaha, p. 380, 1937.
8. Laurance, L. *Visual Optics and Sight Testing*, School of Optics, London, p. 399, 1920.
9. Augsburger, A. Evaluation of Ophthalmic Materials. *Am. J. Optom. Physiol. Opt.*, Vol. 55, pp. 700–705, 1978.

Questions

1. What is the pure gold content of a center stamped 1/10 12 K GF?

2. A patient has a distance PD of 70 mm. Assume the distance from the spectacle plane to the centers of rotation is 2.7 cm. What is the calculated near PD for a viewing distance of 25 cm from the spectacle plane?

3. Assume that the distance from the spectacle plane to the center of rotation is 27 mm. If the near PD is 56 mm for a point 25 cm from the spectacle plane, what is the calculated distance PD?

4. Given the prescription
   OD +4.00 DS 1 prism diopter, base-in
   OS –2.00 DS 1 prism diopter, base-in
   Add = +2.00 D
   and the prism is obtained by decentration,
   PD 62/58 mm
   DBL = 20 mm
   Horizontal box size = 46 mm
   What is the bifocal segment inset (amount and direction) of the right and left lenses, respectively?

5. Given the prescription
   OD +4.00 DS 1 prism diopter, base-in
   OS –2.00 DS 1 prism diopter, base-in
   Add = +2.00 D
   and the prism is obtained by decentration,
   PD = 62/58 mm
   DBL = 20 mm
   Horizontal box size = 46 mm
   What is the total inset (amount and direction) of the right and left lenses, respectively?

6. The distance PD is 64 mm and the near PD is 60 mm. The prescription is
   OD +1.50 D
   OS +1.50 D
   +2.00-D add
   If we wish to have *zero horizontal prismatic effects* at the reading level, what must be the bifocal segment inset for each lens?

7. A frame is 52 × 44 mm in size and will be worn with a pantoscopic tilt of 10°. The center of the pupil falls at a point 24 mm from the bottom of the frame. Assuming we use corrected-curve lenses and wish them to function as such, where is the vertical location of the optical center in this frame?

8. An emmetropic presbyope requires an add of +2.50 D OU (both eyes) for normal close work and reading at 40.0 cm. The person stands 25 cm from a plane mirror while shaving and experiences difficulty seeing well enough to get a close shave. What prescription in single-vision lenses would be most satisfactory in solving his shaving problem?

9. The outside surface of a Kryptok bifocal is resurfaced with the original surfacing tool to remove scratches. The segment was reduced in size, with the optical center of the segment remaining in the same position. The segment originally measured 18 mm high, 22 mm wide. If the segment height is reduced to 16.0 mm, what is the segment width?

10. Discuss the characteristics of cellulose acetate and cellulose nitrate as frame materials.

11. Give the variables that determine the near PD.

12. Discuss the importance of the fitting triangle as a foundation for spectacle adjustments.

13. Discuss the merits of centering for the distance PD or the near PD in single-vision lenses for near use only.

14. Describe the adjustment procedure when the left lens is farther from the face than is the right lens.

15. Describe the adjustment procedure when the right lens is higher on the face than it is for the left lens.

16. Outline the procedures for evaluating an order for spectacles received from a laboratory.

CHAPTER TEN

Anisometropia and Aniseikonia

For most wearers of glasses or contact lenses, the refractive error differs little for the two eyes. However, for a small number of wearers, the refraction differs by a significant amount, which causes the condition known as *anisometropia*. Anisometropia—both in the uncorrected and corrected states—is responsible for several problems. For example, an individual with uncorrected anisometropia is not able to have sharply focused images on the retinas of both eyes simultaneously. This, in extreme cases, may lead to suppression and even to amblyopia. When anisometropia is corrected, it is responsible for base-in and base-out prismatic effects whenever the eyes are rotated horizontally—the visual axes fail to correspond to the optic axes of the lens and produce differential vertical prismatic effects when the visual axes are lowered for reading.

One of the most bothersome problems caused by corrected anisometropia, however, is induced *aniseikonia*—a condition in which the retinal images for the two eyes differ in size or in shape. Whether or not aniseikonia is induced, for a given patient, depends on the nature of the patient's ametropia (whether caused mainly by the axial or refractive properties of the eyes) and on the magnification characteristics of the correcting lenses.

ANISOMETROPIA

10.1. Problems Caused by Anisometropia

Anisometropia is considered to exist when the spherical equivalent refraction of the two eyes differs by 1.00 D or more. Anisometropia of this amount or greater, whether uncorrected or corrected, can be responsible for a number of problems.

Uncorrected Anisometropia

As pointed out in Chapter 5, Section 5.8, Hering's law of equal innervation tells us that the two eyes respond with equal amounts of accommodation. Therefore, when uncorrected anisometropia exists, the eyes may accommodate, in any given situation, so that the retinal image of one eye or of the other is in focus, or so that the two retinal images are more or less equally out of focus. For a child under the age of 5 or 6 years, uncorrected anisometropia may lead to the development of functional amblyopia or other binocular vision problems. If the child is emmetropic in one eye and has uncorrected *hyperopia* in the other, the more hyperopic eye never has a sharply focused retinal image because it is easier for the child to use the emmetropic eye for vision at *any* distance; as a result, functional amblyopia may develop in the more hyperopic eye. On the other hand, if the child is emmetropic in one eye and has uncorrected *myopia* in the other eye, the child is likely to use the emmetropic eye for distance vision and the myopic eye for near vision, and amblyopia is not likely to develop. However, poor stereopsis or other binocular vision problems may result. If an older child or an adult has uncorrected anisometropia, normal binocular vision seldom exists, but in many cases it can be restored by prescribing appropriate lenses.

Corrected Anisometropia

Problems that may arise when lenses are worn for the correction of anisometropia may involve (1) the accommodative system; (2) the vergence system; and (3) the relationship between the retinal image sizes for the two eyes. Problems involving the accommodative system (discussed in Chapter 5, Section 5.8) occur because the lens *effectivity* differs for different fixation distances. Lenses that are equally effective for the two eyes of an anisometrope for distance vision are not equally effective for near vision. Problems involving the vergence system occur as a result of differential prismatic effects that are present when the visual axes pass through points in the lenses other than the optical centers. These effects can be considered in terms of either the horizontal or the vertical meridian, although they are present also for oblique meridians. (Problems involving retinal image size differences for the two eyes are discussed later in the chapter.)

10.2. Horizontal Prismatic Effects

When lenses of unequal powers are worn to correct anisometropia, any amount of movement of the visual axes away from the optical centers of the lenses brings about a prismatic imbalance. The amount and direction of the imbalance can easily be calculated with the aid of Prentice's rule.

EXAMPLE
If a patient wears the prescription OD +3.00 D sphere and OS +1.00 D sphere, centered for the distance PD, we can easily calculate the prismatic effects resulting, during distance fixation, when the two visual axes pass through points in the lenses (1) 20 mm to the *left* of the optical centers and (2) 20 mm to the *right* of the optical centers.

(1) As shown in Figure 10–1, when the visual axes are turned toward the left, the right eye is subject to a *base-out* prismatic effect, and the left eye is subject to a *base-in* prismatic effect; the base-out prismatic effect is the greater of the two.
    OD $P = dF = 2(+3.00) = 6$ prism diopters, base-out.
    OS $P = dF = 2(+1.00) = 2$ prism diopters, base-in.
    Resultant prismatic effect = 4 prism diopters, base-out.

(2) As shown in Figure 10–2, when the visual axes are turned toward the right, the right eye is subject to a *base-in* prismatic effect and the left eye is subject to a *base-out* prismatic effect, the base-in effect being the greater.
    OD $P = dF = 2(+3.00) = 6$ prism diopters, base-in.
    OS $P = dF = 2(+1.00) = 2$ prism diopters, base-out.
    Resultant prismatic effect = 4 prism diopters, base-in.

These results indicate that when horizontal conjugate (versional) movements are made, the visual system must somehow compensate for an ever-increasing base-out prismatic

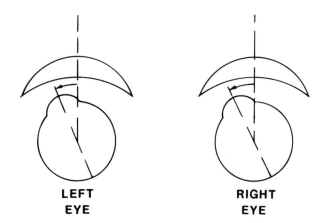

LEFT EYE   **RIGHT EYE**

FIGURE 10–1. **Prismatic effects induced when the visual axes are turned toward the left while wearing the prescription OD +3.00 DS and OS +1.00 DS.**

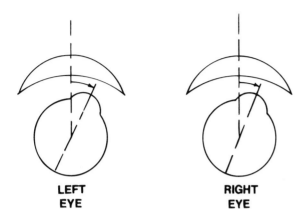

FIGURE 10–2. **Prismatic effects induced when the visual axes are turned toward the right while wearing the prescription OD +3.00 DS and OS +1.00 DS.**

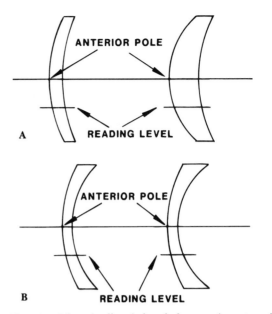

FIGURE 10–3. **Prismatic effects induced when an anisometrope lowers the visual axes for reading. A, for an anisometropic hyperope; B, for an anisometropic myope.**

effect when looking toward the left, and an ever-increasing base-in prismatic effect when looking toward the right. Although our calculations show that the resultant prismatic effect is caused by the excess prismatic power of the *right* lens, in any direction of gaze, the prismatic effect is considered to be shared equally by the two eyes.

Compensating for these horizontal prismatic effects seldom causes a problem for the anisometrope because the visual system is capable of horizontal fusional vergence movements of reasonably large amplitude (*positive* fusional vergence movements to overcome base-out prism, and *negative* fusional vergence movements to overcome base-in prism).

10.3. Differential Vertical Prismatic Effects at the Reading Level

Because the eyes are capable of vertical fusional movements of only a small amplitude, vertical prismatic effects that differ for the two eyes are likely to cause symptoms of eyestrain. Such effects can occur when a corrected anisometrope either elevates or lowers the visual axes to look through points in the lenses considerably above or considerably below the optical centers of the lenses. These effects are most likely to become a problem when the visual axes are lowered for reading. If the lenses are centered in front of the wearer's pupils for distance vision, lowering the visual axes for reading induces a *base-up* prismatic effect for the more hyperopic eye of an anisometropic hyperope or a *base-down* prismatic effect for the more myopic eye of an anisometropic myope (Figure 10–3).

For a wearer of single-vision lenses, the differential prismatic effects at the reading level may not be a problem because the head is normally tilted downward in reading, with the result that the reading level may be very little different than the level used for distance vision. However, a bifocal wearer must read through a level that is approximately 10 mm below the distance optical centers, with the result that differential vertical prismatic effects at near vision can become a problem. For moderate amounts of anisometropia,

the vertical imbalance at the reading level can be overcome by means of vertical fusional movements, but because the amplitude of vertical fusional movements is usually very small, a patient with a significant anisometropia may have to use virtually all his or her vertical fusional vergence amplitude just to achieve single vision. For anisometropic patients who do a great deal of close work, the possibility of a vertical imbalance at the reading level should be considered. Any asthenopia or other symptomatology accompanying near work should suggest an evaluation of an induced vertical imbalance.

EXAMPLE
If a bifocal wearer is given the distance prescription
     OD +1.50 DS –1.00 DC x 180
     OS +2.50 DS
the powers in the vertical meridian are +0.50 D for the right lens and +2.50 D for the left lens. If the patient reads at a level 10 mm below the distance optical centers, the vertical prismatic effects (see Figure 10–3) are
     OD $dF = 1(+0.50) = 0.50$ prism diopters, base-up
     OS $dF = 1(+2.50) = 2.5$ prism diopters, base-up,
     and the differential prismatic effect is
     2.0 prism diopters, base-up, left eye.

Note that the power of the *add* does not enter into the situation as long as it is the same for both eyes. In fact, it is not necessary to specify the power of the add.

As shown in this example, when a patient's lenses are spherical or when the cylinder axes are horizontal or vertical, determination of the vertical imbalance at the reading level is easily done by the application of Prentice's rule. However, for cylinders of oblique axes, calculation of the vertical imbalance must be done by the method described in Chapter 4. On occasion, casual inspection of the patient's prescription may suggest that induced vertical imbalance at the reading level is a potential problem, but for prescriptions with strong oblique cylinders, it may not be readily apparent that vertical imbalance is a potential problem. Fischer[1] developed aids to assist in making a rapid determination of the induced vertical imbalance.

Individual tolerance for induced vertical imbalance varies considerably from one patient to another. Ellerbrock and Fry[2] found that some anisometropic patients developed the capacity to compensate for prismatic inequalities at the reading level. Compensation was defined as the difference between a measured vertical phoria and the calculated vertical imbalance. Cusick and Hawn[3] pointed out that it was not uncommon to find a patient who was wearing a 5.00-D difference in the corrections for the two eyes and who had no measurable hyperphoria with a Maddox rod during downward gaze through the lenses. As already indicated, an additional problem that may occur in anisometropia is asthenopia caused by the image size differences between the two eyes (i.e., induced aniseikonia). However, Ellerbrock[4] recommended that prismatic corrections be provided for anisometropic patients who are uncomfortable at the reading position before any consideration is given to aniseikonia and its correction.

Duke-Elder[5] suggested that, as a general rule, a differential vertical prismatic effect at the reading level is not apt to cause symptoms of asthenopia unless it amounts to 1 prism diopter or more. The practitioner should keep in mind the possibility of a differential prismatic effect at the reading level for any patient having *1 diopter or more* of anisometropia in the vertical meridian because for a reading level of 10 mm below the distance optical centers, each diopter of anisometropia causes 1 prism diopter of differential vertical prismatic effect. Comparison of the *spherical powers* of the two lenses is not sufficient as it was in the above example because a cylindrical correction for only one eye (or a stronger cylinder for one eye than for the other) can greatly increase the difference in the powers of the two lenses in the vertical meridian.

Any one of eight procedures may be used to compensate for differential vertical prismatic effects at the reading level:

1. Lowering the distance optical centers
2. Prescribing single-vision lenses for reading only
3. Prescribing dissimilar bifocal segments for the two eyes
4. Prescribing compensated bifocal segments
5. Prescribing prism segments
6. Prescribing a slab-off lens
7. Prescribing a Fresnel Press-on prism
8. Prescribing contact lenses

1. *Lowering the Distance Optical Centers.* For the patient who is not yet presbyopic, a possible method of alleviating a vertical imbalance at the reading level is to lower the optical centers of the lenses. For example, if the optical centers are dropped 3 mm relative to their normal positions, the amount of vertical imbalance is reduced by a factor of 0.3 multiplied by the amount of anisometropia in the vertical meridian. The amount of vertical imbalance not present at the reading level is present at the positions of the

original optical centers (but opposite in direction). For this reason, this method is apt to prove unsatisfactory and should be used cautiously, if at all.

2. *Prescribing Single-Vision Lenses for Reading Only.* Some pre-presbyopic patients may be willing to accept the idea of wearing two pairs of glasses, one for distance vision and one for reading. The distance lenses are centered in the usual manner, with the optical centers positioned in front of the pupils for distance vision. For the near-vision lenses, the optical centers are positioned lower in the lenses, usually from 5 to 10 mm lower than their placement for distance vision. The patient should be observed while reading, and the points where the lines of sight cross the lenses marked with a grease pencil or a felt pen. The most effective way to do this is to sit at a table opposite the patient and use a small mirror held next to the reading material. For *presbyopic* patients, two pairs of glasses can be prescribed, a pair of bifocals for general wear and a pair of single-vision glasses with the optical centers lowered for reading. The bifocals are worn for distance vision and for short periods of near work, but the single-vision glasses are worn for prolonged periods of close work.

3. *Prescribing Dissimilar Bifocal Segments.* Segments of different size or construction, with their centers at different levels, may be used to compensate for an induced vertical imbalance at the reading level. The amount of compensation is equal to the vertical separation of the segment centers multiplied by the power of the add. As an extreme example, assume that an Ultex A segment (having its center 19 mm below the segment top) is worn on one eye and an Executive segment (having its center at the top of the segment) is worn on the other, with the segment tops at the same level for both eyes (Figure 10–4). If the power of the bifocal addition is +2.00 D, the arrangement compensates for an induced vertical prismatic effect of

$$1.9(+2.00) = 3.8 \text{ prism diopters.}$$

If a 22-mm round fused bifocal (having its segment center located 11 mm below the segment top) is worn on one eye and a straight-top fused bifocal (having its segment center 5 mm below the segment top) on the other (Figure 10–5), for a +2.00-D add, the amount of compensation is

$$0.6(+2.00) = 1.2 \text{ prism diopters.}$$

To minimize the difference in the appearance of the segments, it is desirable for the two segments to be as nearly similar in shape as possible. For example, one may use two round fused bifocals with different diameters, or an Ultex

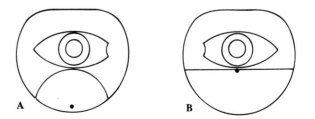

FIGURE 10–4. **Prescribing dissimilar bifocal segments. An Ultex A bifocal is worn on one eye and an Executive bifocal on the other eye.**

FIGURE 10–5. **Prescribing dissimilar bifocal segments. A round fused bifocal is worn on one eye and a straight-top fused bifocal is worn on the other eye.**

A and an Ultex B bifocal. Judicious selection of the two segments allows compensation of a wide range of vertical imbalances. Table 10–1, listing conventional bifocal lenses according to the distance from the segment top to the segment center, is useful for this purpose. The segment with its center at the *greatest* distance from the segment top is always prescribed for the eye requiring the *most plus or least minus power* in the vertical meridian. Although the use of dissimilar segments is a straightforward, inexpensive, and readily available method of solving the problem, it is likely that many patients will resist the idea of wearing differently shaped segments for the two eyes.

4. *Prescribing Compensated Bifocal Segments.* A more cosmetically acceptable method of compensating for differential prismatic effects is to use compensated ribbon segments. The 14-mm-deep R-compensated segment has been designed for this purpose. Although the normal position of the optical center of the R segment is at the center of the segment (7 mm below the segment top), it can

be specified anywhere from 4 to 10 mm below the segment top. With the segment centers in the extreme positions of 4 and 10 mm below the segment tops, one segment is upside down with respect to the other, as shown in Figure 10–6. For a +2.00-D add, the resulting prismatic compensation is

$$0.6(+2.00) = 1.2 \text{ prism diopters.}$$

An R-compensated segment is produced by regrinding the front surface of a regular R-segment lens blank. The resurfacing process moves the segment center from its original position to a higher or lower position. To move the segment center to a lower position, more of the upper edge of the segment is ground away than it is at the lower edge. To move the center higher, more of the lower segment edge is removed than of the upper edge.

As a result of this resurfacing process, it is obvious that the two segments are *not* identical in shape; however, not enough difference exists to be cosmetically unacceptable.

FIGURE 10–6. **R-compensated bifocal segments. The segment optical center is 4 mm below the segment top for one eye and 10 mm below the segment top for the other eye.**

TABLE 10–1
Conventional Bifocal Lenses Listed According to the Distance from the Segment Top to the Segment Center

	Bifocal	*Segment Size (mm)*	*Segment Top to Segment Center (mm)*
Glass	Executive-style one-piece		0.0
	Vision-Ease B-9	22 × 9, 26 × 9	4.5
	X-Cel Ribbon Seg	22 × 9	4.5
	Straight-top fused	22 × 16, 25 × 17.5	5.0
		28 × 19, 35 × 22.5	5.0
	Curved-top fused	22 × 16	5.0
		25 × 17.5, 28 × 19	5.0
	Vision-Ease R-14	22 × 14, 26 × 14	7.0
	X-Cel Ribbon Seg	22 × 14	7.0
	Round fused	22 round	11.0
	Round one-piece B	22 round	11.0
	Round fused	25 round	12.5
	Hemispheric one-piece	38 × 19, 38 × 30	19.0
		40 × 19, 40 × 20, 40 × 35	20.0
Plastic	Executive-style one-piece		0.0
	Straight-top one-piece	22, 25, 28, 35, 45 wide	5.0
	Curved-top one-piece	25, 28, 40 wide	5.0
	Round one-piece	15 round	7.5
		22 round	11.0
		24 round	12.0
		25 round	12.5
		26 round	13.0
		28 round	14.0
	Hemispheric one-piece	40	20.0

The use of R-compensated segments therefore constitutes a subtle application of the concept of dissimilar segments. This method is more expensive than other methods of using dissimilar segments, and is limited to an amount of prism equal to 0.6 multiplied by the power of the add, but the extra cost is often justified by the improved appearance.

As stated above, the segment with its center at the *greatest* distance from the segment top is always prescribed for the eye requiring the *most plus or least minus power* in the vertical meridian.

5. *Prescribing Prism Segments.* A few bifocal manufacturers make available segments incorporating vertical prism power. These lenses are expensive, excessively thick, and are factory orders, involving a delay of several months. Their use is not recommended because other methods (particularly the use of R-compensated segments and the provision of a slab-off lens, discussed below) are effective, less expensive, and do not require a factory order.

6. *Prescribing a Slab-Off Lens.* A *slab-off* lens is made by a procedure known as *bi-centric grinding* (Figure 10–7). The front surface is finished in the usual manner (A), after which a dummy lens is cemented onto the front surface (B). The front surface is then reground, using the same tool originally used for that surface, but ground in such a way that the dummy is ground away in the upper portion of the lens but remains attached to the lower portion. The back surface is then finished with the remaining dummy considered as an integral part of the blank (C). The thickness of the blank is then equal at the top and bottom unless the prescription calls for prism in the distance portion. When the lens is finished, the remaining dummy on the lower portion is then removed (D). The dummy is a base-down prism;

therefore, this procedure results in the removal of base-down prism in the lower portion of the lens, or in the addition of *base-up* prism in the lower portion of the lens.

The center of curvature of the front surface of the lens, in the lower portion, is displaced upward, with the result that the front surface has *two* centers of curvature, one for the upper portion and one for the lower portion, even though the upper and lower portions have the same curvature. This process results in a unique optical axis for each of the two portions of the lens.

Thus, bi-centric grinding results in the removal of base-down prism (whether used on a minus lens or a plus lens), without changing the refractive power below the slab-off line. It is therefore used for the lens that induces the lesser amount of base-up (or the greater amount of base-down) prism, which is always the lens having the *less plus or more minus power* in the vertical meridian. For example, for the prescription

OD –1.00 DS
OS –4.00 DS

bi-centric grinding would be used for the *left* lens.

Bi-centric grinding results in a horizontal line across the width of the lens (Figure 10–8) and provides a very acceptable cosmetic result when the line coincides with the segment top of a straight-top bifocal. It may be done on either the front or the back surface of the lens. *Front surface* bi-centric grinding is used for single-vision glass lenses, straight-top fused bifocals, and one-piece glass bifocals (such as the Ultex) having the bifocal on the back surface. *Back surface* bi-centric grinding is used for one-piece straight-top glass Executive-style bifocals and trifocals and for plastic single-vision lenses, bifocals, and trifocals.

Recently, Younger Optics and Aire-o-Lite have introduced plastic single-vision and bifocal lenses with a slab-off lens molded or cast with *base-down* prism in the segment area, rather than individually generating a base-up prismatic effect by bi-centric grinding. These lenses are known as *reverse slab-off* lenses. Because the compensating prism is base-down rather than base-up, the slab-off lens is prescribed for the eye requiring the *more plus or less minus* power in the vertical meridian. These lenses can be maintained in the laboratory's inventory as semifinished lenses, which makes possible much faster delivery than that for individually produced slab-off lenses.

Slab-off lenses are not usually produced for less than 1.25 prism diopters of compensation because in such cases a

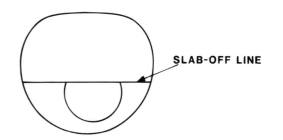

FIGURE 10–7. **Bi-centric grinding, producing a slab-off lens. This procedure produces a horizontal line across the lens.**

FIGURE 10–8. **A straight-top fused bifocal with slab-off prism, resulting in a horizontal line across the lens.**

sharp, horizontal, straight line is difficult to produce. When more than 1.25 prism diopters of compensation is required, the use of a slab-off lens is the method of choice. The slab-off line is relatively inconspicuous and, in straight-top fused bifocals, the slabbed-off area extends beyond the segment to the distance portion of the lens.

Although bi-centric grinding is more expensive than the use of R-compensated segments, it has the advantage that a larger amount of prism can be provided. The amount of prism possible is limited only by the thickness of the lens, but for the R-compensated bifocal, the amount of prism possible (as already noted) is limited to 0.6 times the power of the add. Bi-centric grinding can be done by any prescription laboratory and thus does not require a factory order.

In the case of a finished lens, the amount of slab-off may be verified, using a lensometer, by comparing the vertical prismatic effects of the two lenses at the reading level. The amount of the slab-off is the difference between the calculated amount of vertical imbalance and the amount found by the lensometer at the reading level.

Peters[6] suggested a much simpler method of determining the amount of slab-off. His method, illustrated in Figure 10–9, employs a standard lens gauge with separations of the

fixed legs of 20.8 mm. The lens gauge is first used to measure the front surface power *above* the slab-off line (Figure 10–9A). The second reading is taken with the three points of the lens gauge arranged vertically and with the middle pin directly on the slab-off line (Figure 10–9B). The difference between the initial reading and the second reading (in diopters of refracting power) is the amount of slab-off, in prism diopters.

7. *Prescribing a Fresnel Prism.* A Fresnel prism, as described in Chapter 5, is a plastic "press-on" prism, based on the Fresnel principle, that can be placed on an ordinary spectacle lens. A Fresnel prism can be placed on the back of the segment area of a bifocal lens, as a temporary measure before ordering a more expensive correction with compensated segments or bi-centric grinding. Disadvantages of Fresnel prisms are that they give the lens a striated appearance and lower the wearer's visual acuity by about one line of letters on the Snellen chart.

8. *Prescribing Contact Lenses.* For an anisometrope who is motivated to wear them, prescribing contact lenses can be an effective method of avoiding differential vertical prismatic effects at the reading level. Contact lenses may be considered as the treatment method of choice for some pre-presbyopic patients because well-fitted, single-vision contact lenses remain centered with respect to the pupils when the eyes move downward for reading.

Although bifocal contact lenses have achieved only limited acceptance by both practitioners and wearers, it is likely that the reading level for a wearer of these lenses is considerably higher than that for a wearer of bifocal spectacle lenses. There should be a much smaller differential prismatic effect than that induced by the wearing of bifocal spectacles. The very popular *monovision* method of fitting presbyopes with contact lenses (fitting a distance lens for one eye and a reading lens for the other) is also effective in eliminating differential prismatic effects at the reading level. Differential prismatic effects also can be avoided for a presbyope if the person is willing to wear contact lenses for general wear, supplemented by spherical spectacle lenses for reading. If the contact lenses are removed, the presbyope may use a separate pair of glasses (centered for the reading level) for reading.

Should the Prismatic Effect Be Fully Compensated?

For an assumed reading level at a given distance below the distance optical centers, the vertical imbalance may be precisely calculated. The amount of calculated imbalance, the amount of close work, and the degree of compensation as determined by dissociated and associated phorias can assist in determining whether any correction for vertical imbalance should be prescribed. If a *full correction* is applied for a given reading level, the correction, being a constant, is an *undercorrection* for any level lower than the assumed reading level or an *overcorrection* for any level higher than the assumed reading level. Because the assumed reading level is an estimate, it is usually best to provide an *undercorrection*, no matter which method of compensation is used.

FIGURE 10–9. **Using a standard lens gauge to determine the amount of slab-off prism.**

ANISEIKONIA

10.4. Historical Background

It has been known for many years that the correction of anisometropia by spectacles can introduce unequal image sizes for the two eyes, with consequent disturbances in binocular vision. Donders[7] was one of the early writers who was aware of the dimensional changes in the retinal images introduced by the correction of anisometropia.

The researches initiated by Ames, and implemented by his associates at the Dartmouth Eye Institute,[8] established the basic principles underlying the measurement of image size differences and their equalization in clinical practice. Lancaster,[9] in 1938, coined the term *aniseikonia*, deriving it from Greek word roots, literally meaning "not equal images."

Aniseikonia is defined as the relative differences in the sizes and/or shapes of the *ocular* images of the two eyes. The term ocular image includes not only the *retinal* image formed by the dioptrics of the eye (with any correcting lens) but also the modification of the retinal image by the distribution of the nerve endings in the retina and their representation in the visual cortex. Because the absolute sizes of the ocular images, as just defined, are incapable of measurement, we measure the relative difference in their sizes, and state this difference in terms of the *percentage magnification* of afocal magnifying lenses (or "size" lenses) required to equalize the two images.

10.5. Etiology of Aniseikonia

As a result of the lateral separation of the two eyes of 60 to 70 mm, differences in the sizes and shapes of the retinal images are routinely experienced in everyday life. Separation of the eyes, which provides two different views of all surfaces and contours, forms the basis for normal binocular stereopsis and space perception. The resulting differences in retinal image size and shape are more pronounced when a person views a nearby object that is displaced to one side because the view requires asymmetrical convergence of the eyes (Figure 10–10). As a result of the asymmetrical convergence, the retinal image of the nearer eye is *larger* than that of the farther eye. The image differences are compensated psychologically and cause no symptoms, but they provide clues that assist in spatial localization of objects.

The term *anomalous aniseikonia* is used to include all forms of aniseikonia other than the standard aniseikonia just described. The etiology of anomalous aniseikonia can be classified as either *anatomical* or *optical*. Anatomical causes for aniseikonia include such factors as the degree of separation (density) of the retinal receptors and the functional organization of the terminal neural visual pathways in the cortex. For example, one could argue that if the neural elements were more widely separated in the retina of one eye than in that of the other, the perceived image would be smaller because fewer retinal elements

IMAGE   **IMAGE**

LEFT EYE   **RIGHT EYE**

FIGURE 10–10. **When a person views a nearby object that is displaced to one side, the retinal image of the nearer eye is larger than that of the farther eye.**

would be stimulated. Ogle[10] reported that in about one-third of the cases of aniseikonia studied, the measured image differences were seemingly unrelated to the dioptric characteristics of the anisometropia present, which indicated that the aniseikonia could have been anatomical in origin.

Optical aniseikonia has two origins: *inherent* and *induced.* *Inherent aniseikonia* depends solely on the dioptric system of the eye itself; induced aniseikonia is caused by the magnification properties of the lenses worn for the correction of a refractive error, more specifically for the correction of either anisometropia or astigmatism.

The types of image size differences occurring in aniseikonia are classified as follows.

Symmetrical Differences

1. *Overall,* in which the ocular image of one eye is increased or decreased in size (equally in all meridians) as compared with that of the other eye (Figure 10–11).
2. *Meridional,* in which the ocular image of one eye is increased or decreased symmetrically in one meridian, compared with that of the other eye (Figure 10–12). The meridian of magnification may be vertical (A), horizontal (B), or oblique (Figure 10–13).

Asymmetrical Differences

1. A progressive increase or decrease in the image size in one meridian, as would be produced by an ordinary flat prism (Figure 10–14).
2. A progressive increase or decrease in image size in all directions from the visual axis, as illustrated by barrel or pincushion distortion (Figure 10–15). Although barrel (A) and pincushion (B) distortion are not usually thought of as manifestations of aniseikonia, they nevertheless are embraced by its definition.

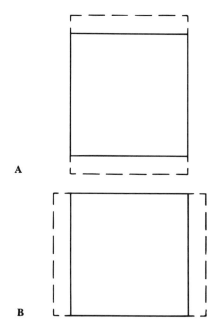

FIGURE 10–12.   **Meridional aniseikonia. The ocular image of one eye is increased or decreased symmetrically in one meridian. A, in the vertical meridian; B, in the horizontal meridian.**

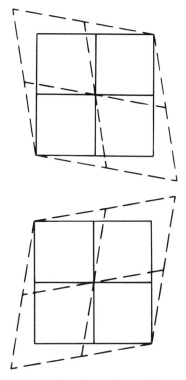

FIGURE 10–13.   **Meridional aniseikonia. The ocular image of one eye is increased or decreased symmetrically in an oblique meridian.**

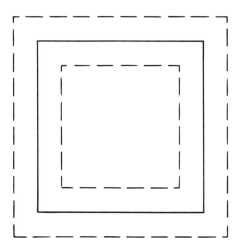

FIGURE 10–11.   **Overall aniseikonia. The ocular image of one eye is increased or decreased in size (equally in all meridians).**

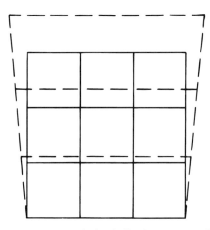

FIGURE 10–14.   **Asymmetrical aniseikonia. A progressive increase or decrease in image size in one meridian, as would be produced by a flat prism.**

10.6. Significance of Aniseikonia

The correction of ametropia and oculomotor imbalance provides optimal visual acuity and comfort for most patients. However, some patients fail to obtain relief, even though they see clearly and even though ocular or systemic abnormalities have been ruled out by a routine visual examination. After careful correction of the ametropia and alleviation of oculomotor imbalance by appropriate lenses, prisms, or training, the occurrence of any unexplained visual symptoms should suggest the possibility of aniseikonia.

Aniseikonia has its primary effects on fusion and spatial organization. To produce a single mental image from a single object, the images formed by the two retinas must undergo sensory fusion, or unification. The greater the degree of similarity between the two images, the easier the process of fusion. A significant difference in the sizes or shapes of the two images impedes the fusional process and compromises the binocular status.

The perception of space is served by two mechanisms. The first of these, binocular in nature, is an innately determined mechanism derived from the slight disparity of the retinal images as a result of the lateral separation of the two eyes, and causes normal binocular stereoscopic perception. The second mechanism, uniocular in nature, consists mostly of learned clues such as geometric perspective, motion parallax, overlay, light and shadow, and the expected sizes and distances of known objects. Our orientation in space is a result of the constant interrelation and summation of the uniocular and binocular factors.

Normal stereoscopic vision is based on the normal disparity of the retinal images. When significant amounts of disparity are present, the result is anomalous spatial perception with apparent changes in one's environment.

Aniseikonia, with an abnormal size or shape relationship between the two ocular images, causes anomalous binocular spatial localization with rotation and distortion of binocular stereoscopic perception. The effects that image size differences evoke are so predictable and so characteristic that they are used to measure aniseikonia by means of an instrument called a *space eikonometer.*

The distortion of stereoscopic space perception affects the integration and efficiency of the space orientation process. The symptoms encountered by patients with aniseikonia most likely result from efforts to retain former patterns of perception or to adapt to the new visual condition.

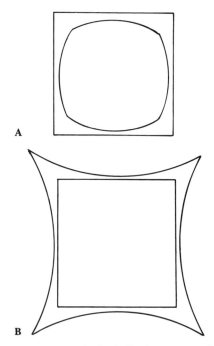

FIGURE 10–15.   **Asymmetrical aniseikonia. A progressive increase or decrease in image size in all directions from the visual axis, as illustrated in A, by barrel distortion and B, by pincushion distortion.**

Symptoms of Aniseikonia

The symptoms of aniseikonia mimic those reported by patients having uncorrected errors of refraction, oculomotor imbalance, or both. The symptoms of aniseikonia are different, however, in that the symptoms persist (or have their onset) when lenses have been prescribed to correct the ametropia or oculomotor imbalance. Patients complain not so much about distortion of space but about how their eyes "feel." Ocular symptoms include asthenopia in and around the eyes, usually associated with concentrated use of the eyes. Other symptoms are headaches, photophobia, giddiness, and nervousness.

An important diagnostic test for aniseikonia as the cause of asthenopia is monocular occlusion. If the symptoms disappear under monocular occlusion, aniseikonia should be strongly suspected as the underlying cause.

10.7. The Spectacle Magnification Formula

The size of the retinal image, formed by the optical system of the eye, can be discussed in terms of *spectacle magnification* or *relative spectacle magnification.* Spectacle magnification concerns the change in the retinal image size of a single eye brought about by a correcting lens (either a spectacle lens or a contact lens); relative spectacle magnification concerns the size of the retinal image in corrected ametropia as compared with that of the emmetropic eye.

The ratio of the retinal image size with the correcting lens compared to that without the lens, or spectacle magnification, may be expressed mathematically as

$$SM = \frac{\text{retinal image size in the corrected eye}}{\text{retinal image size in the uncorrected eye}}. \quad (10.1)$$

Spectacle magnification provides the factor by which the initial size of the retinal image is magnified or minified. *Percentage* spectacle magnification may be expressed as

$$\%SM = (SM - 1)(100), \quad (10.2)$$

where SM refers to the spectacle magnification expressed as a ratio, as in the previous equation. Hence, spectacle magnifications of 1.05 and 0.94, respectively, indicate a magnification of 5% and a minification of 6%.

Spectacle magnification is a type of angular magnification that is always present in ophthalmic correcting devices. The simplest way to approach the spectacle magnification of a lens is to imagine the lens separated into two components. A lens intended for distance vision can be imagined as composed of an *afocal* (telescopic) component and a *power* component, as shown in Figure 10–16. The afocal component has the same thickness as the composite (real) lens, and the power component has zero thickness.

The front surface of the afocal component is the same as that of the composite lens, but because the afocal component has zero back vertex power, its back surface can be computed in the following manner, using the classic back vertex power formula:

$$F_V = \frac{F_{1A}}{1 - \frac{t}{n}F_1} + F_{2A},$$

where F_v = the back vertex power of the afocal component, F_{1A} = the front surface power of the afocal component, and

F_{2A} = the back surface power of the afocal component. Since the unit is afocal, $F_v = 0$, and therefore

$$F_{2A} = -\frac{F_{1A}}{1 - \frac{t}{n}F_{1A}}. \quad (10.3)$$

Considering now the power component, the front surface curvature of this component matches the curvature of the back surface of the afocal component, and hence its power is numerically equal to the power of the back surface of the afocal component, but *opposite in sign*. If we let F_{1P} equal the front surface power of the power component,

$$F_{1P} = +\frac{F_{1A}}{1 - \frac{t}{n}F_{1A}}. \quad (10.4)$$

The back surface of the power component is also the back surface of the composite lens. Because the power component is infinitely thin, its power is equal to the sum of its two surface powers. If we let F_P equal the back vertex power of the power component, and if we let F_{1P} and F_{2P} equal, respectively, the front and back surface powers of the power component,

$$F_P = F_{1P} + F_{2P}$$

or

$$F_P = \frac{F_{1A}}{1 - \frac{t}{n}F_{1A}} + F_{2P}. \quad (10.5)$$

This is identical with the back vertex power of the composite lens, and can be measured by means of a lensometer.

It should be understood that the afocal component, taken by itself, has no effect on the clarity of vision when a distant object is seen through the lens because it does not change the vergence of the incident rays, but it does bring about a change in the apparent size of the object and is therefore said to have *magnifying power*, which can be expressed by computing its angular magnification. In Figure 10–17, an incident ray of light, MP, is directed toward the center of curvature, C_1, of the front surface. This ray is not refracted at the front surface because it is normal to it, but is refracted at the second surface, deviated in the direction PQ. If E is located in the focal plane of the front surface, a ray of light from E through C_2 passes through the back surface unrefracted but is refracted at the front surface in the direction OS, parallel to MP. If E also lies in the primary focal plane of the back surface, the ray PQ must be parallel to OE and, hence, the parallel incident rays (SO and MP) emerge from the lens as a parallel bundle. This accords with the principle that the afocal component has zero back vertex power.

The angular magnification is defined as the ratio of the slope of the emerging rays to the slope of the incident rays with respect to the optic axis of the lens, and can be expressed as follows:

$$AM_A = \frac{\alpha}{\beta} = \frac{\dfrac{RE}{C_2R}}{\dfrac{RE}{C_1R}} = \frac{C_1R}{C_2R} = \frac{l_1' - r_1}{l_2 - r_2},$$

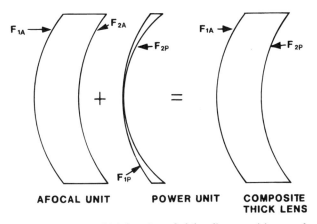

AFOCAL UNIT   POWER UNIT   COMPOSITE THICK LENS

FIGURE 10–16. **A thick lens intended for distance vision can be thought of as being composed of an afocal (telescopic) component and a power component of zero thickness.**

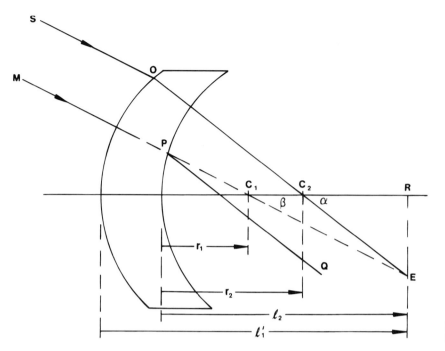

FIGURE 10–17.   **Diagram for determining the angular magnification of the afocal component.**

but since

$$l_1' = \frac{n}{F_1}, \quad \text{and} \quad r_1 = \frac{n-1}{F_1},$$

$$l_1' - r_1 = \frac{n - n + 1}{F_1} = \frac{1}{F_1}.$$

And since

$$l_2 = -\frac{n}{F_2}$$

then

$$l_2 = \frac{\dfrac{n}{F_1}}{1 - \dfrac{t}{n} F_1},$$

$$r_2 = \frac{1-n}{F_2}$$

and

$$r_2 = \frac{\dfrac{1-n}{F_1}}{- 1 - \dfrac{t}{n} F_1},$$

$$r_2 = \frac{\dfrac{n-1}{F_1}}{1 - \dfrac{t}{n} F_1},$$

$$l_2 - r_2 = \frac{\dfrac{n-n+1}{F_1}}{1 - \dfrac{t}{n} F_1} = \frac{1 - \dfrac{t}{n} F_1}{F_1}$$

$$AM_A = \frac{l_1' - r_1}{l_2 - r_2} = \frac{\dfrac{1}{F_1}}{\dfrac{1 - \dfrac{t}{n} F_1}{F_1}}$$

$$AM_A = \left(\frac{1}{1 - \dfrac{t}{n} F_1} \right). \tag{10.6}$$

The principles involved in computing the angular magnification of the power unit are illustrated in Figure 10–18. The ray TC from an object Q at infinity passes through the optical center, C, of the lens. The ray SP from Q, parallel to TC, is refracted at P and passes through the center of the entrance pupil, E, and crosses the ray TC at the point Q', which lies in the secondary focal plane of the lens. Without the lens, Q is seen in the direction OR; with the lens it is seen in the direction OP. The angular magnification of the power unit is derived as follows:

$$AM_P = \frac{\alpha}{\beta} = \frac{f'}{f' - h} = \frac{1}{1 - \dfrac{h}{f'}},$$

but since

$$\frac{1}{f'} = F_P,$$

$$AM_P = \left(\frac{1}{1 - hF_P} \right). \tag{10.7}$$

The angular magnification (spectacle magnification) of the composite lens is equal to the product of the angular magnifications of the afocal unit (also called the *shape*

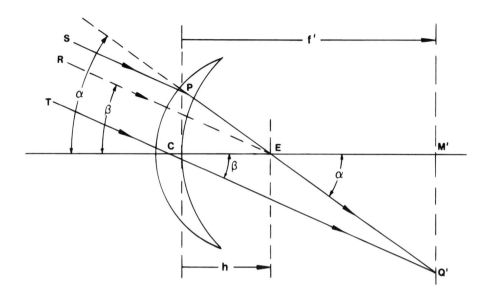

FIGURE 10–18. **Diagram for determining the angular magnification of the power component.**

factor M_S) and the power unit (also called the *power factor, M_P*).

$$AM = SM = (M_S)(M_P)$$

$$SM = \left(\frac{1}{1 - \frac{t}{n}F_1}\right)\left(\frac{1}{1 - hF_V}\right) \quad (10.8)$$

where F_1 = the power (F_{1A}) of the front surface of the lens, F_V = the back vertex power (F_P) of the composite lens, t = the lens thickness, n = the index of refraction of the lens material, and h = the distance from the back vertex of the lens to the entrance pupil of the eye. (The distance from the front surface of the cornea to the entrance pupil of the eye is normally assumed to be 3 mm.)

Inspection of the shape factor shows that spectacle magnification increases with an increase in front surface power or with an increase in lens thickness and decreases with an increase in the index of refraction of the lens material. Inspection of the power factor indicates that spectacle magnification varies directly with back vertex power, with the retinal image size increasing with increasing plus lens power and decreasing with increasing minus lens power. Any spectacle lens, by virtue of its power, changes retinal image size—as a plus lens is moved closer to the eye, decreasing the value of h, there is a *decrease* in retinal image size; whereas when a minus lens is moved closer to the eye there is an *increase* in image size.

The spectacle magnification formula shows that it is possible to construct a series of lenses having the same back vertex power but with various spectacle magnification values, depending on the thickness, the power of the front surface, and the position of the lens relative to the entrance pupil of the eye. However, if the lens should have *zero power*, only the afocal unit is used, and its distance from the entrance pupil of the eye does not affect its spectacle magnification. If one or both surfaces are *toric* rather than

spherical, the spectacle magnification must be computed separately for each principal meridian.

10.8. Clinical Application of the Spectacle Magnification Formula

The use of the spectacle magnification formula is illustrated by the following examples.

EXAMPLE 1
A patient who has previously worn no correction is found to require –2.00-D spheres for both eyes. What is the spectacle magnification if the front surface power is +6.00 D, the center thickness is 2.2 mm, the index of refraction is 1.523, and the vertex distance is 12 mm? If we assume that the distance from the front surface of the cornea to the entrance pupil is 3 mm, the value of h (for a vertex distance of 12 mm) is 15 mm. Therefore,

$$SM = \left(\frac{1}{1 - \frac{0.0022(6)}{1.523}}\right)\left(\frac{1}{1 - 0.015(-2)}\right)$$

$$= (1.009)(0.971) = 0.980.$$

$$\%SM = (SM - 1)(100)$$

$$= (0.980 - 1)(100)$$

$$= -2.0\%.$$

The above example shows why even a small amount of minus power can cause a patient to notice that "everything looks smaller" with the new correction.

EXAMPLE 2
A patient who has previously worn no correction is found to require +2.00 D spheres for both eyes. What is the spectacle magnification if the front surface power is +8.00 D, the center thickness is 2.5 mm, the index of refraction is 1.523, and the vertex distance is 12 mm?

$$SM = \left(\cfrac{1}{1 - \cfrac{0.0025(8)}{1.523}} \right) \left(\cfrac{1}{1 - 0.015(+2)} \right)$$

$$= (1.013)(1.031) = 1.044.$$

$$\%SM = (SM - 1)(100)$$

$$= (1.044 - 1)(100)$$

$$= +4.4\%.$$

Important Note. It is clear from the above examples and from examination of Equation 10.8 that spectacle magnification is always greater than unity for a plus lens, and always less than unity for a minus lens. This is true not only for a spectacle lens but also for a contact lens. Although the *amount* of magnification is different for a contact lens than that for a spectacle lens because of the much shorter distance between the lens and the entrance pupil of the eye, the *direction* of the magnification change is identical for corrections of equal sign; that is, spectacle magnification is greater than unity for either a spectacle lens or a contact lens of plus power, and is less than unity for either a spectacle lens or a contact lens of minus power.

If a correcting lens were to be infinitely thin and placed at the entrance pupil of the eye, the shape factor and the power factor would each be 1.0, with the result that spectacle magnification would be *unity*, whatever the refractive error. This condition is most nearly approximated by either a contact lens or an intraocular lens.

The computation of spectacle magnification is useful in predicting the effect on the image size (for a single eye) in any of the following circumstances:

1. A change in a patient's prescription, for any reason
2. A change in the vertex distance of a spectacle lens
3. The change from spectacles to contact lenses or vice versa
4. A change in the thickness of a lens
5. A change in the bend, or form, of a lens

In addition, an understanding of the principles of spectacle magnification makes it possible to manipulate the variables in such a way as to equalize the sizes of the retinal images of the two eyes, and thus minimize induced aniseikonia (see Section 10.21).

10.9. Spectacle Magnification and Vertex Distance

An eye's ametropia is corrected when the secondary focal point of the correcting lens coincides with the far point of the eye. If the vertex distance is altered, the secondary focal length must be changed to ensure that the secondary focal point still falls on the far point of the eye. With the correcting lens in place, the image of the eye's far point is conjugate to the retina. If we assume the correcting lens is infinitely thin and the object at infinity, the retinal image size is proportional to the size of the image formed at the far point plane of the eye—this is true for either a spectacle lens or a contact lens.

In Figure 10–19, a plus correction lens is located in position 1 (A and B); in (C) and (D) the correction lens is moved farther from the eye, to position 2. In each position, the object subtends the angle, α, at the optical center of the lens. When the positive correction lens is moved from position 1 to position 2, which increases the secondary focal length, the image formed (h_2' in Figure 10–19C and D) is *larger* than the image formed when the lens was in position 1 (h_1' in Figure 10–19A and B). In position 2, the angular size of the retinal image as subtended from the eye's nodal point (α_2' in Figure 10–19D) is larger than the angular size of the retinal image in position 1 (α_1 in Figure 10–19B). Hence, as the vertex distance of a plus correction lens increases, the spectacle magnification also *increases*, and vice versa.

In Figure 10–20, a minus correction lens is moved from position 1 to a farther distance from the eye at position 2. In each position, the object subtends the angle, α, at the optical center of the lens. Again, when a minus correction lens is moved farther from the eye to position 2 (shortening the secondary focal length) the image formed (h_2' in Figure 10–20C and D) is *smaller* than the image formed when the lens was in position 1 (h_1' in Figure 10–20A and B). In position 2, the angular size of the retinal image as subtended from the eye's nodal point (α_2' in Figure 10—20D) is smaller than the angular size of the retinal image in position 1 (α_1' in Figure 10–20B). Hence, as the vertex distance of a minus correction lens increases, the spectacle magnification *decreases* (minification), and vice versa.

From Figures 10–19 and 10–20, it is apparent that the retinal image size is directly proportional to the secondary focal length or inversely proportional to the refracting power of the correction lens. The greatest change in vertex distance occurs when the patient changes from spectacle lenses to contact lenses, or vice versa. Therefore, in going from spectacle lenses to contact lenses,

$$\frac{\text{retinal image size with a contact lens}}{\text{retinal image size with a spectacle lens}} = \frac{f_C'}{f_S'} = \frac{1/F_C}{1/F_S} = \frac{F_S}{F_C}$$

or in going from contact lenses to spectacle lenses,

$$\frac{\text{retinal image size with a spectacle lens}}{\text{retinal image size with a contact lens}} = \frac{f_S'}{f_C'} = \frac{1/F_S}{1/F_C} = \frac{F_C}{F_S}.$$

EXAMPLE 1
A patient wears + 14.00-D spectacles at a vertex distance of 12 mm. If the patient is fitted with contact lenses of appropriate refracting power, fitted *on K* (i.e., so that the radius of curvature of the back surface of each lens is equal to the apical radius of the corresponding cornea in the flattest meridian), what is (1) the required contact lens power and (2) the percentage change in "spectacle magnification" when the contact lenses are worn rather than glasses?

(1) The required contact lens power is

$$\cfrac{1}{\cfrac{1}{14} - 0.012} = \frac{1}{0.0714 - 0.012} = +16.83 \text{ D.}$$

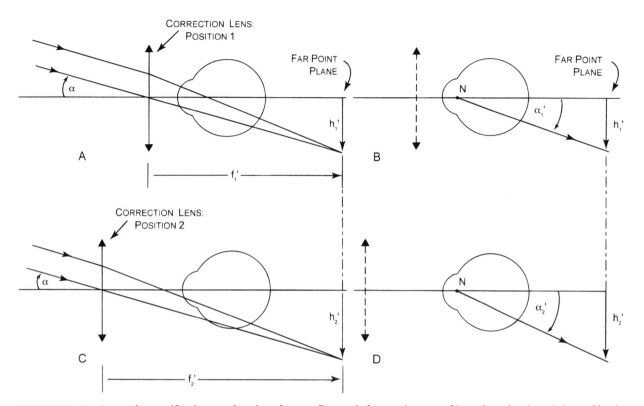

FIGURE 10–19.   Spectacle magnification as a function of vertex distance in hyperopia. A, an object of angular size α is imaged by the correction lens (position 1) at the far point plane as h_1'; B, the angular size of h_1', as subtended at the eye's nodal point, is α_1'; C, if the correction lens is moved farther from the eye (to position 2) it forms an image, h_2', that is larger than h_1'; D, the retinal angular size, α_2', at the eye's nodal point, is larger than α_1'. (Modifed from Katz, M. The Human Eye as an Optical System. In A. Safir, Ed., *Refraction and Clinical Optics*, Harper and Row, Hagerstown, 1980.)

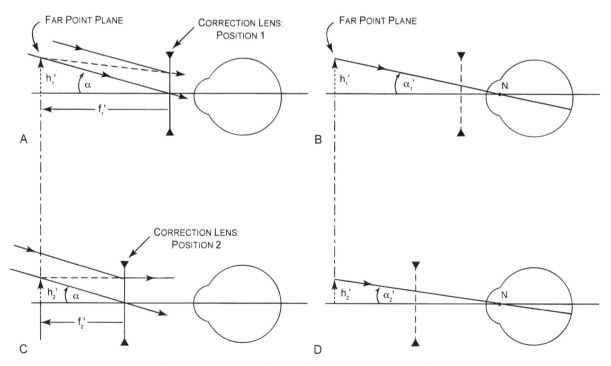

FIGURE 10–20.   Spectacle magnification as a function of vertex distance in myopia. A, an object of angular size α is imaged by the correction lens (position 1) at the far point plane as h_1'; B, the angular size of h_1', as subtended at the eye's nodal point, is α_1'; C, if the correction lens is moved farther from the eye (to position 2) it forms an image, h_2', that is smaller than h_1'; D, the retinal angular size, α_2', at the eye's nodal point, is smaller than α_1'. (Modifed from Katz, M. The Human Eye as an Optical System. In A. Safir, Ed., *Refraction and Clinical Optics*, Harper and Row, Hagerstown, 1980.)

(2) The change in spectacle magnification is

$$\frac{F_S}{F_C} = \frac{+14.00}{+16.83} = .832.$$

The percentage spectacle magnification change is

%SM change = $(0.832 - 1)100 = -16.8\%.$

EXAMPLE 2

A patient wears a +16.83-D contact lens, fitted on K. If the patient is fitted with appropriate spectacle lenses worn at a vertex distance of 12 mm, what is (1) the required power of the spectacle lens and (2) the percentage change in spectacle magnification?

On casual inspection it may seem that the answer is a +16.8% increase in spectacle magnification. However, this is incorrect:

(1) The required spectacle lens power is

$$\frac{1}{\dfrac{1}{16.83} + 0.012} = \frac{1}{0.5941 + 0.012} = +14.00 \text{ D.}$$

(2) The change in spectacle magnification is

$$\frac{F_c}{F_g} = \frac{+16.83}{+14.00} = 1.202.$$

The percentage spectacle magnification change is

%SM change = $(1.202 - 1)100 = +20.2\%.$

EXAMPLE 3

A patient wears −10.00-D contact lenses fitted on K. If the patient is fitted with appropriate spectacle lenses worn at a vertex distance of 12 mm, what is (1) the required power of the spectacle lenses and (2) the percentage change in spectacle magnification?

(1) The required spectacle lens power is

$$\frac{1}{\dfrac{1}{10} - 0.012} = \frac{1}{0.10 - 0.012} = -11.36 \text{ D.}$$

(2) The change in spectacle magnification is

$$\frac{F_C}{F_S} = \frac{-10.00}{-11.36} = 0.88.$$

The percentage spectacle magnification change is

%SM change = $(0.88 - 1)100 = -12.00\%.$

Therefore, when going from contact lenses to glasses for this myopic patient, the retinal image size decreased by 12%.

EXAMPLE 4

A patient wears spectacle lenses having a power of −11.36 D at a vertex distance of 12 mm. If this patient is fitted with appropriate contact lenses fitted on K, what is (1) the required power of the contact lenses and (2) the percentage increase in spectacle magnification?

(1) The required spectacle lens power is

$$\frac{1}{\dfrac{1}{-11.36} - 0.012} = \frac{1}{-0.0880 - 0.012} = -10.00 \text{ D.}$$

(2) The change in spectacle magnification is

$$\frac{F_S}{F_C} = \frac{-11.36}{-10.00} = 1.136.$$

The percentage spectacle magnification change is

%SM change = $(1.136 - 1)100 = +13.6\%.$

Therefore, in going from spectacle lenses to contact lenses, the retinal image size increased 13.6% for this patient.

Important Note. In none of the four examples was the actual spectacle magnification calculated for spectacles or contact lenses. What was calculated was the *percentage change* in spectacle magnification when going from one form of correction to the other.

10.10. Spectacle Magnification in Astigmatism

When a lens incorporates a correction for astigmatism, the spectacle magnification differs in the two principal meridians. If the lenses compensate for the patient's refractive error, the retinal image is distorted; it is larger in one principal meridian than in the other. The retinal image is larger in the direction of the *axis of the minus cylinder* that corrects the astigmatism. If we assume that the vertex distance for a spectacle lens is 12 mm and the distance from the anterior corneal surface to the entrance pupil of the eye is 3 mm, calculation of the power factor,

$$\frac{1}{1 - hF_V},$$

for each of the principal meridians indicates that the percentage difference between the two meridians is about 1.5% per diopter of astigmatism for a spectacle lens but only about 0.3% per diopter of astigmatism for contact lenses. Although the value of the shape factor may alter the amounts slightly, the differences in spectacle magnification can be substantial. The difference could be a source of perceptual difficulties that some patients experience when changing from spectacles to contact lenses, or vice versa.

Although contact lenses tend to be more difficult to fit on highly astigmatic corneas than on eyes having mainly spherical corneas, if a patient with highly astigmatic corneas does not object to being fitted with contact lenses, their use should be seriously considered because the difference in image size for the two principal meridians is decreased by a factor of 5. In addition, in many cases of astigmatism, use of contact lenses markedly reduces the amount of induced aniseikonia as compared with that induced by spectacle lenses (see Section 10.14).

10.11. Relative Spectacle Magnification

To compare the retinal image size of one eye with that of another eye, *relative spectacle magnification* may be used. *Relative spectacle magnification* is defined as the ratio of the retinal image size (for an object at infinity) of the corrected ametropic eye in question to that of the standard emmetropic eye. It can be expressed by the formula

$$\text{RSM} = \frac{\text{image size for a corrected ametropic eye}}{\text{image size for a standard emmetropic eye}}. \quad (10.9)$$

When a patient's anisometropia is corrected by spectacles or by contact lenses, the concept of relative spectacle magnification may be used to compare the sizes of the clear retinal images of each of the two eyes to the size of the retinal image of the standard emmetropic eye. The ratio of the actual retinal image sizes for the two eyes can then be expressed as the ratio of the relative spectacle magnification of one eye to that of the other:

$$\text{magnification ratio} = \frac{\text{RSM}_R}{\text{RSM}_L}. \quad (10.10)$$

For such a comparison to be made, it must be known whether the patient's anisometropia is caused by primarily *refractive* or *axial* differences in the two eyes. Clinical indications of the presence of refractive ametropia include (1) significant differences in the keratometric readings for the two eyes; (2) the development of cataracts, more advanced in one eye than in the other; and (3) aphakia. In the absence of A-scan ultrasonographic equipment for measuring the axial length of the eye, the main indication for axial ametropia is the presence of structural changes at the posterior pole of the eye (as viewed with the ophthalmoscope) caused by axial elongation.

As pointed out in the discussion in Chapter 5, Sorsby et al.[11] found that, for small amounts of ametropia, the axial length of the eye is usually within the range for the emmetropic eye, but for eyes having ametropia of ±4.00 D or more, the axial length is almost always outside the range for the emmetropic eye.

If the source of the ametropia of each eye is known, a relationship can be developed. The size of the retinal image of a corrected ametropic eye is directly proportional to the equivalent focal length of the system or inversely proportional to the equivalent power of the system. Therefore,

$$\text{RSM} = \frac{f'_E}{f'_{ST}}, \quad (10.11)$$

where f'_E is the secondary equivalent focal length of the lens/eye system and f'_{ST} is the secondary equivalent focal length of a standard emmetropic eye. Consequently,

$$\text{RSM} = \frac{F_{ST}}{F_E}, \quad (10.12)$$

where F_{ST} is the equivalent power of the standard emmetropic eye and F_E is the equivalent power of the system composed of the correcting spectacle lens, F_{SP}, and the refracting power of the ametropic eye, F_A. Therefore, if the distance from the secondary principal point of the spectacle lens to the primary principal point of the eye is denoted by d, it follows that the equivalent power of the lens/eye system is

$$F_E = F_{SP} + F_A - dF_{SP}F_A \quad (10.13)$$

and, substituting for F_E in Equation (10.12),

$$\text{RSM} = \frac{F_{ST}}{F_{SP} + F_A - dF_{SP}F_A}. \quad (10.14)$$

10.12. Relative Spectacle Magnification in Axial Ametropia

If the source of the ametropia is purely axial, the power of the ametropic eye, F_A, is equal to the power of the standard emmetropic eye, F_{ST}, or $F_A = F_{ST}$. Substituting F_{ST} for F_A in Equation 10.14,

$$\text{RSM}_{(\text{axial ametropia})} = \frac{F_{ST}}{F_{SP} + F_{ST} - dF_{SP}F_{ST}}. \quad (10.15)$$

If the spectacles are placed at the anterior focal point of the eye,

$$d = \frac{1}{F_{ST}},$$

and

$$\text{RSM}_{\text{axial ametropia}} = \frac{F_{ST}}{F_{SP} + F_{ST} - \dfrac{1}{F_{ST}}F_{SP}F_{ST}}$$

$$= \frac{F_{ST}}{F_{ST}} = 1.00. \quad (10.16)$$

This equation mathematically illustrates *Knapp's law*, which states that for an axially ametropic eye, if the correcting lens is placed so that its secondary principal point coincides with the anterior focal point of the eye, the size of the retinal image is the same as if it were the standard emmetropic eye.

If it is assumed that the refracting power of the standard emmetropic eye is +58.50 D, the distance from the first primary principal point of the eye to the anterior focal point of the eye is 17.1 mm. If the distance from the cornea to the first principal plane (or, with negligible error, the center of the entrance pupil) of the eye is considered to be 3 mm, the anterior focal point of the axially ametropic eye can be considered as 14 mm from the cornea.

For the purely axially ametropic eye, the optical system of the eye is of *normal* focal length (i.e., that of the standard emmetropic eye), with the result that the primary focal length is the same for the axially ametropic eye as for the emmetropic eye. Reference to Figure 10–21 illustrates Knapp's law diagrammatically, showing that, if the correcting lens is placed so that its secondary principal point coincides with the primary focal point of the eye, the resulting retinal image size is the same as that of the standard emmetropic schematic eye.

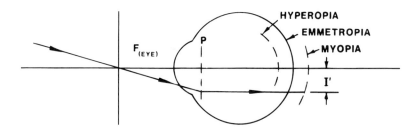

FIGURE 10–21.   **Diagram illustrating Knapp's law. If the correcting lens for an axially ametropic eye is placed in the primary focal plane of the eye, the resulting image size is the same as that for the emmetropic schematic eye.**

Four conditions are necessary for Knapp's law to apply:

1. The ametropia must be *purely axial.*
2. The correcting lens must be located so that its secondary principal point coincides with the primary focal point of the eye. The position of the principal planes moves as the bend of a lens is increased—the move is toward the surface with the greatest curvature. The secondary principal point of a plus meniscus lens is located a short distance anterior to the front surface of the lens, and the secondary principal point of a minus meniscus lens is located a short distance behind the back surface. Therefore, the back vertex of a plus meniscus lens must be located somewhat *closer* than 14 mm from the cornea and a minus meniscus lens must be placed *farther* than 14 mm from the cornea.
3. The refracting power of the eye must be equal to that of the standard emmetropic eye.
4. The shape factor of the correcting lens must be unity (in reality, the shape factor for both plus and minus lenses is *greater than* 1 if the front surface is convex).

An additional factor to be considered is that Knapp's law applies only to *induced* aniseikonia. As stated earlier, ametropic eyes may suffer *anatomical* aniseikonia, which results from the differences in receptor densities for the two eyes. This is particularly expected in axial ametropia because the density of the receptors is being spread out in a large axially myopic eye and is more closely packed in a small, hyperopic eye. This condition, in addition to the four conditions listed above, makes the clinical application of Knapp's law a somewhat inexact procedure.

In the case of axial ametropia corrected by a *contact lens,* the power of a contact lens, fitted on K, can be considered as equal to the ocular refraction, F_O. Consequently, substituting F_O for F_{SP} in Equation 10.15, we obtain

$$\text{RSM} = \frac{F_{ST}}{F_O + F_{ST} - dF_O F_{ST}}, \qquad (10.17)$$

but since d may be considered as negligible for a contact lens,

$$\text{RSM} = \frac{F_{ST}}{F_O + F_{ST}} \qquad (10.18)$$

when a contact lens is used for the correction of axial ametropia.

If contact lenses are to correct an anisometropic patient whose anisometropia is axial in origin, the relative spectacle magnification is *not* unity, and differences in retinal image sizes for the two eyes result.

10.13. Relative Spectacle Magnification in Refractive Ametropia

If the source of the ametropia is assumed to be refractive, the power of the ametropic eye, F_A, is *not* equal to the power of the standard emmetropic eye, F_{ST}, but the *axial length* of the eye is equal to that of the standard emmetropic eye. If the spectacle correction, F_{SP}, is known, the effective power of the spectacle correction at the primary principal point of the eye (the ocular refraction, F_O) added to the power of the ametropic eye, F_A, must be equal to the power of the standard emmetropic eye, F_{ST}. Therefore,

$$F_{ST} = \frac{F_{SP}}{1 - dF_{SP}} + F_A,$$

or

$$F_{ST} = \frac{F_{SP} + F_A - dF_{SP}\,F_A}{1 - dF_{SP}}.$$

Since the general Equation 10.14 is

$$\text{RSM} = \frac{F_{ST}}{F_{SP} + F_A - dF_{SP}F_A},$$

and substituting for F_{ST},

$$\text{RSM} = \frac{\dfrac{F_{SP} + F_A - dF_{SP}\,F_A}{1 - dF_{SP}}}{F_{SP} + F_A - dF_{SP}\,F_A},$$

or

$$\text{RSM} = \frac{1}{1 - dF_{SP}} \qquad (10.19)$$

for refractive ametropia.

Important Note. It is obvious that the relative spectacle magnification for ametropia that is *refractive* in origin is essentially equal to the *spectacle magnification*, if the lens is considered to be a thin lens. That is, in refractive ametropia,

$$\text{SM} = \text{RSM}.$$

Therefore, if spectacle lenses are to be used to correct an eye whose ametropia is refractive in origin, the relative spectacle magnification is *not* unity—the correcting lens is likely to bring about a marked change in image size as compared with the situation for axial ametropia in which a normal retinal image size may result. More specifically, a plus lens creates a magnification greater than unity, and a minus lens creates a magnification less than unity.

Inspection of Equation 10.19 indicates that, for refractive ametropia, relative spectacle magnification increases with increasing values of d, and is at a minimum when d is at a minimum.

Therefore, if a *contact lens* rather than a spectacle lens is fitted, the vertex distance is zero and the value of d is at a minimum. If the distance d is considered to be negligible (i.e., if it is considered that the distance from the corneal surface to the principal plane of the eye is equal to zero), the relative spectacle magnification approaches unity. Therefore, in a situation in which the practitioner wishes to minimize the amount of relative spectacle magnification for an eye that is known to have *refractive* ametropia, the practitioner should consider prescribing a contact lens.

10.14. Relative Spectacle Magnification in Astigmatism

When a patient has a significant amount of astigmatism, the *cornea* is almost always the source of the astigmatism; the lens is responsible only on rare occasions. However, in either case, astigmatism is obviously a form of *refractive* ametropia. It follows, then, that the magnification difference between the two principal meridians of an astigmatic eye is maximal if glasses are worn but minimal if contact lenses are worn. As pointed out in Section 10.10, when astigmatism is corrected by a minus cylinder in the form of a spectacle lens, the retinal image size is greatest in the axis meridian of the correcting minus cylinder and least in the power meridian.

For a single eye, the fact that the shape of the retinal image with a correcting lens is not a true representation of the shape of the object may not be a problem for the wearer. Our concern here, however, is whether or not the retinal image shapes *differ for the two eyes* (Figure 10–22). For example, if a patient has 2.00 D of with-the-rule astigmatism in each eye, corrected with plus cylinders, axis 90°, each lens has its greatest magnification in the horizontal meridian but the shape and orientation of the retinal images is the same for both eyes (Figure 10–22A).

However, if the patient has 2.00 D of oblique astigmatism with symmetrically placed plus cylinder axes (e.g., 45° and 135° for the right and left eyes, respectively), the shapes of the two retinal images are the same, but the orientation is decidedly different (Figure 10–22B). The greatest magnification in this situation is 135° for the right eye and 45° for the left. As a result of the meridional magnification differences, a significant amount of aniseikonia is induced. As noted in Section 10.10, the magnification difference for the two principal meridians is approximately 1.5% per diopter of astigmatism for a spectacle lens, but only about 0.3% per diopter for a contact lens. Therefore, when a significant amount of astigmatism is present (particularly oblique astigmatism with symmetrically placed axes, or in with-the-rule astigmatism in one eye and against-the-rule in the other), a much smaller amount of meridional aniseikonia is induced if contact lenses are worn rather than glasses.

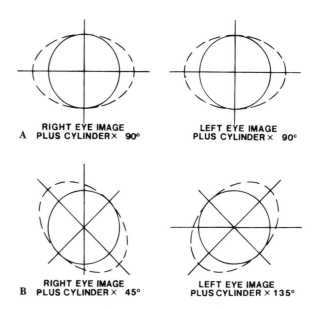

FIGURE 10–22.   A, With 2.00 D of astigmatism in each eye corrected with plus cylinders with their axes at 90°, the shape and orientation of the retinal images are the same for both eyes; B, with 2.00 D of symmetrical astigmatism corrected with plus cylinders with axes at 45° and 135°, the shapes of the retinal images are the same for the two eyes but the orientation differs.

Many highly astigmatic patients who have worn spectacles for a number of years have no complaints traceable to induced meridional aniseikonia. These patients have adapted to the situation very well. If such a patient is switched to contact lenses, he or she may initially have difficulty adapting to the lenses because of the decrease in the accustomed amount of induced aniseikonia. This, however, is not sufficient reason *not* to switch the patient to contact lenses, but he or she should be warned of the possible adaptation problems.

On the other hand, if a spectacle-wearing person with high astigmatism has difficulty adapting to spectacles, he or she should be advised that the adaptation problem may be minimized if contact lenses rather than spectacles are worn. In any case, because contact lenses are considered by most people as mainly a *cosmetic* form of visual correction—something one can wear to avoid wearing glasses—an astigmatic patient (like any other patient) should not be urged to wear contact lenses unless some degree of motivation for their wear is present.

10.15. The Dilemma of Relative Spectacle Magnification

Although relative spectacle magnification is a rigorous mathematical concept, making use of this concept in routine optometric care often presents the practitioner with an insolvable dilemma. Relative spectacle magnification can be determined accurately only if both the equivalent power and the axial length of the eye are known. Unfortunately, the equivalent power of the eye is difficult to determine; and A-scan ultrasonography, although a highly developed and accurate technology for measurement of the axial length of the eye, is not available in most practitioners' offices. Nevertheless, relative spectacle magnification is a useful concept in the presence of anisometropia.

THE QUESTION: Is the anisometropia axial or refractive?
THE ANSWER: Examine the keratometer findings!

If the keratometer findings are essentially equal for the two eyes, it is a fair assumption that the equivalent power (because of the corneal power, anterior chamber depth, and lens power) is the same for the two eyes and therefore the anisometropia is *axial* in origin. On the other hand, if the keratometer findings manifest the same dioptric difference as the magnitude of the anisometropia, it is likely that the axial lengths are equal and that the anisometropia is *refractive* in origin.

Use of the keratometer findings in determining whether anisometropia is axial or refractive is illustrated by the following examples.

EXAMPLE 1
Given the following clinical findings, is the patient's anisometropia due to axial or refractive ametropia?
Keratometer: OD 44.50 D
     OS 44.50 D
Refraction: OD −2.50 DS
     OS plano

Because the keratometer findings are the same for both eyes, the fact that the right eye is myopic but the left eye is emmetropic is explained on the basis of the right eye being longer than the left eye. The ametropia is therefore axial in origin, and the relative spectacle magnification will approach unity when spectacle lenses are worn (and differ significantly from unity if contact lenses are worn).

EXAMPLE 2
Given the following clinical findings, is the patient's anisometropia caused by axial or refractive ametropia?
Keratometer: OD 44.50 D
     OS 42.00 D
Refraction: OD −2.50 DS
     OS plano

Because the patient's anisometropia can be accounted for entirely by the difference in the keratometer findings, the anisometropia is the result of the right eye having *refractive* myopia. In this situation, the relative spectacle magnification will approach unity when contact lenses are worn but differ significantly from unity if spectacles are worn.

With use of A-scan ultrasonography at the University of Houston, the keratometer findings and axial lengths of both eyes of a number of anisometropic subjects were measured and, for amounts of anisometropia as low as 1.50 to 2.00 D, the anisometropia was almost always accounted for by a difference in the *axial lengths* of the eyes. Following is a typical example:

Keratometer: OD 42.50 D
     OS 42.75 D
Refraction: OD +2.75 D
     OS +4.25 D
Axial length: OD 23.6 mm
     OS 23.1 mm

In the absence of a significant difference in the keratometer findings, the anisometropia can be assumed to occur because the more hyperopic eye is 0.5 mm *shorter* than the less hyperopic eye. (The accuracy of the ultrasonic measurements is about 0.2 mm when five readings are taken, but the 0.5-mm difference far exceeds the error of measurement.)

10.16. Clinical Considerations in Anisometropia and Astigmatism

The clinical management of anisometropia and astigmatism concerning induced aniseikonia is summarized in the following sections.

Axial Ametropia

In uncorrected anisometropia caused by axial ametropia, the equivalent powers (corneal power and lens power) are the same for the two eyes but the retinal image sizes are different because of the axial length difference. If spectacle lenses are worn, the retinal image size difference is offset by the spectacle magnification produced by the correcting lenses, which causes (as stated by Knapp's law) the relative spectacle magnification for each eye to be essentially unity and induces little or no aniseikonia. If, on the other hand, axial ametropia is corrected by contact lenses, the spectacle magnification is much less than that for spectacle lenses, with the result that the relative spectacle magnification for each eye differs significantly from unity and a significant amount of aniseikonia is induced. Thus, if ametropia is axial in origin, the prescribing of spectacle lenses is the treatment of choice to minimize induced aniseikonia.

Refractive Ametropia

In uncorrected anisometropia caused by refractive ametropia, the axial lengths of the two eyes are considered to be equal, with the result that the retinal image size for each eye is essentially equal to that of the standard emmetropic eye. If spectacle lenses are worn, the spectacle magnification produced by the lenses causes an inequality in the sizes of the two retinal images, with the result that relative spectacle magnification for each eye differs from unity, and a significant amount of aniseikonia is induced. Contact lenses cause very little spectacle magnification, with the result that relative spectacle magnification differs little from unity, and a minimum amount of aniseikonia is induced. Thus, if the ametropia is refractive in origin, the prescribing of contact lenses is the treatment of choice to minimize induced aniseikonia. A comparison of image sizes in ametropia with those in emmetropia is given in Table 10–2; the indication of the presence or absence of aniseikonia in uncorrected and corrected anisometropia is given in Table 10–3.

Astigmatism

Because astigmatism is a form of *refractive* ametropia, wearing of contact lenses rather than glasses results in a minimum of induced meridional aniseikonia for any patient who has high astigmatism with the axes positioned symmetrically for the two eyes.

TABLE 10–2
Retinal Image Sizes in Ametropia Compared with Those in Emmetropia

Ametropia	Uncorrected	Spectacle Correction	Contact Lens Correction
Axial myopia	Larger than emmetropia	Equal to emmetropia	Larger than emmetropia
Axial hyperopia	Smaller than emmetropia	Equal to emmetropia	Smaller than emmetropia
Refractive myopia	Equal to emmetropia	Smaller than emmetropia	Equal to emmetropia
Refractive hyperopia	Equal to emmetropia	Larger than emmetropia	Equal to emmetropia

TABLE 10–3
Presence or Absence of Aniseikonia in Uncorrected and Corrected Anisometropia

Ametropia	Uncorrected	Spectacle Correction	Contact Lens Correction
Axial anisometropia	Present	Absent	Present
Refractive anisometropia	Absent	Present	Absent

PRESCRIBING TO ELIMINATE OR MINIMIZE INDUCED ANISEIKONIA

When prescribing to eliminate or minimize induced aniseikonia, one must consider not only the optical principles of aniseikonia (described earlier in this chapter) but also the clinical indications of the presence of aniseikonia, methods of measuring and estimating image size differences, methods of avoiding induced aniseikonia with ordinary spectacle lenses, and the design of *eikonic* lenses—lenses that produce magnification in such a way as to avoid or minimize induced aniseikonia. (Although this textbook concentrates on the optical principles and practical applications of lenses used for the correction of visual anomalies, with a minimum of attention given to patient care procedures, it is difficult in the management of aniseikonia to separate the strictly *optical* aspects of management from the *patient care* aspects. This chapter, therefore, includes discussion of all aspects of the management of aniseikonia.)

10.17. Indications of the Presence of Aniseikonia

The most important clues to the presence of aniseikonia are

1. The presence of a significant amount of anisometropia or astigmatism.

2. The presence of an impaired binocular vision status with reduced fusional amplitudes, reduced quality of fusion, or both.

3. Complaints of symptoms, usually asthenopia and headache, after use of the eyes, which occurs *after* proper correction of any refractive error, oculomotor imbalance, or both.

4. The report of more comfortable and satisfactory vision when using only one eye, especially for prolonged visual tasks. Because aniseikonia is a binocular anomaly, *monocular occlusion* is a useful diagnostic procedure—if occlusion brings relief of symptoms, the symptoms may possibly arise from aniseikonia. On the other hand, monocular vision is more disturbing to some people than stressful binocular vision, so if monocular occlusion fails to bring relief, aniseikonia cannot absolutely be eliminated as a source of the problem.

5. The presence of symptoms having their onset coincident with the replacement of a broken lens or with the prescription of new glasses. In such a case, the symptoms may be the result of a change in base curve or thickness or a change from a negative to a positive toric form

(or vice versa) or, in the case of new glasses, from a change in lens powers or vertex distance. The use of a lens gauge and thickness calipers is essential for monitoring lens design.

6. A report of space distortion such as slanting floors, tilted walls, or the ground appearing to be too close or too far away.

Many patients experience symptoms of distortion and discomfort when they first wear glasses or when a significant change is made in the prescription. Most patients get used to the symptoms within about 2 weeks. However, adaptation does not mean that the aniseikonia is no longer present, only that the individual has undergone a conditioning process whereby he or she responds to the familiar empirical clues for space localization and learns to ignore the stereoscopic clues. One would not expect physiologic compensation for the aniseikonia to occur, because neither the innate retinal correspondence nor the disparity of the ocular images has changed.[12] This conclusion is reinforced by the fact that when a patient who has adapted to such space distortions is asked to view a *leaf room* (a visual environment devoid of empirical clues for the perception of space, as shown in Figure 10–23) the space distortions instantly reappear.[13]

The important consideration is whether or not the patient can adapt without undue discomfort and without compromising visual efficiency. Many patients adapt without consequence, although others adapt only with severe asthenopia or loss of visual efficiency. The patient's response, unfortunately, cannot be reliably predicted. (One of us has made a longstanding promise to students to deliver a "tolerance level indicating device" which, when connected to the patient, will separate those who can adapt to new lenses from those who cannot. The list of orders is lengthy!)

FIGURE 10–23.   **A leaf room. The visual environment is devoid of empirical clues for the perception of space. (Reprinted with permission from R. E. Bannon, *Clinical Manual on Aniseikonia*, American Optical Corp., Buffalo, NY, 1954, Figure 28.)**

10.18. Measurement of Image Size Differences

A clinical instrument designed to measure the differences in the magnification of the retinal images of the two eyes is known as an *eikonometer*. In 1951, American Optical introduced the Office Model of the Space Eikonometer (Figure 10–24). The design of this instrument was based on that of Ogle's space eikonometer, a research instrument large enough to fill a small room. The space eikonometer makes it possible to measure image size differences on the basis of their effects on binocular space perception. For many years American Optical made available to practitioners a "translation" service, which interpreted Space Eikonometer findings, designed a pair of lenses that corrected the aniseikonia, and provided the appropriate refractive correction. These lenses were known as *iseikonic* lenses; the shortened version, *eikonic*, seems now to be preferred. A few years ago, American Optical discontinued the manufacture of the Space Eikonometer and no longer provides the translation service.

The Keystone View Company developed a set of stereoscopic cards that are reproductions of the Space Eikonometer target and are used to estimate the amount of aniseikonia present. The cards are designed to be used with the Keystone Orthoscope, a stereoscope with "minimum-distortion" lenses. Although the American Optical Space Eikonometer uses adjustable afocal magnification units, by means of which the magnification can be changed optically to correct the manifested aniseikonia, the Keystone series of cards offers a number of graded stereoscopic targets with built-in aniseikonic errors. The stereogram that appears normal to the patient (that is, demonstrates no distortion of binocularly perceived space) indicates the approximate amount of aniseikonic error.

The nature of the test of aniseikonia with both the Space Eikonometer and the Orthoscope requires that the patient have single binocular vision, normal retinal correspondence, and at least 20/60 visual acuity in each eye. A patient without these visual characteristics cannot be measured for aniseikonia with either instrument. Bannon[14] stated that the patient's intelligence level should be equivalent to that of a normal 6-year-old to understand the questions, make the necessary observations, and give unequivocal responses.

Screening Devices

Because of these limitations and because of the interest in simplification and reduced cost, many clinicians have been interested in designing "screening" devices for detecting and prescribing for the approximate correction of aniseikonia. However, an instrument designed for screening is of no value unless it is as sensitive and as accurate as an instrument designed for the measurement of aniseikonia.

Elvin[15] used the Turville Infinity Balance Test and size lenses to measure the aniseikonia in the vertical meridian of

FIGURE 10–24.   **The American Optical Space Eikonometer target. (Reprinted with permission from R. E. Bannon,** *Clinical Manual on Aniseikonia,* **American Optical Corp., Buffalo, NY, 1954, Figure 31.)**

an anisometrope (Figure 10–25) and arrived at a finding of 2.4% overall aniseikonia, the correction of which provided clear, comfortable vision. Brecher[16] used a Maddox rod placed in front of one eye and two separated light sources, arranged in the meridian of investigation. The patient saw two spots of light and two streaks. The difference between the spot and streak separation constituted the amount of aniseikonia; afocal size lenses were used in front of the eye without the Maddox rod to measure the size difference. Brecher, Winters, and Townsend[17] proposed the measurement of aniseikonia by alternating between the images of the two eyes slowly enough to prevent binocular fusion but fast enough for a subjective comparison of image size.

Baldwin[18] described an instrument called the Zeiss Polatest, designed for binocular refraction, which made use of a target (Figure 10–26) intended to measure the amount of aniseikonia in the vertical meridian by estimating the vernier displacement in terms of target line thickness. Grolman,[19] in 1971, patented a series of Vectographic Nearpoint Cards designed to facilitate binocular refraction at the near point. One of the cards, No. 4 (Figure 10–27), is intended for use in screening the differences in overall and meridional image size. A determination of the magnitude of an indicated meridional or overall aniseikonia could be made by eliciting from the patient an estimate of the vernier displacement in terms of target line thickness.

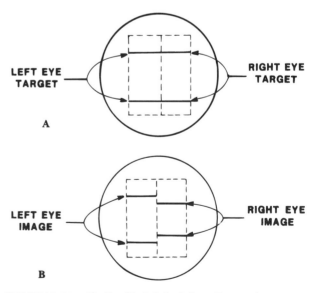

FIGURE 10–25.   **The Turville Infinity Balance Test used to measure aniseikonia in the vertical meridian. A, no aniseikonia is present; B, aniseikonia is present in the vertical meridian. (Reprinted with permission from F. T. Elvin,** *Am. J. Optom. Arch. Am. Acad. Optom.,* **Vol. 26, pp. 78–82, 1949.)**

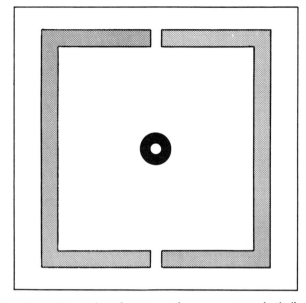

FIGURE 10–26.   **Zeiss Polatest target for measurement of aniseikonia. (Reprinted with permission from *Illustrations for The Polatest*, 1966, Carl Zeiss, Inc., Thornwood, NY.)**

Most screening devices lack reliability and can detect only gross differences in image size. If an individual has normal binocular vision, image size differences greater than 5% are rarely encountered.[20] Image size differences exceeding that amount result in loss of binocularity and are not apt to create asthenopia or other problems. Most patients struggling with aniseikonia have *small* differences in image size, and these small differences would be missed by gross screening methods. For example, Bannon[21] reported that most image size differences in clinical cases were between 1.0 and 2.0%—differences too small to be

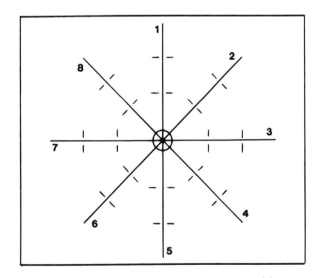

FIGURE 10–27.   **Grolman Vectographic Nearpoint Card for screening differences in overall image size. For each radial line, the vernier line on one side is seen by the right eye and that on the other side is seen by the left eye. (Reprinted with permission from *Introduction for Vectograph Nearpoint Cards*, Reichert Ophthalmic Instruments, Buffalo, NY.)**

detected with most screening instruments (the scale on the Space Eikonometer extends only to an image size difference of ±4%).

A correction for aniseikonia based on accurate measurement by the Space Eikonometer can be made with the greatest of confidence, but a close approximation of the amount of aniseikonia can be obtained with the stereograms designed for the Keystone Orthoscope. Although the Space Eikonometer is no longer manufactured, it may be available for use by referral to another practitioner or to an optometric educational institution.

10.19.   Estimating the Amount of Aniseikonia

If neither the Space Eikonometer nor the Keystone instrumentation is available, the practitioner may reasonably estimate the amount of aniseikonia present and make use of some method of determining the necessary correction. Linksz and Bannon[22] expressed belief that when it is not possible to make eikonometer measurements for a patient who has worn an anisometropic correction but is uncomfortable, a correction for *estimated* aniseikonia is better than no correction, and that there is a place for intelligent guessing about aniseikonia. The same authors stated that even a general familiarity with aniseikonia and its effects enables the practitioner to avoid or minimize the effects of aniseikonia when prescribing and designing a patient's glasses.

Anisometropia and aniseikonia are often concomitant, although not highly correlated.[23] The problem, as stated earlier, is that of differentiating axial from refractive anisometropia. If the determination can be made, it follows that, if anisometropia is axial, ordinary spectacle lenses constitute the most suitable form of refractive correction, but if the anisometropia is refractive, contact lenses are indicated for maximal visual efficiency and comfort.

As stated in Section 10.15, a comparison of the keratometric and refractive findings may provide some insight into the origin of the anisometropia. Although spherical anisometropia may be refractive, axial, or both, it may be incorrect to assume that, in a given case, anisometropia is *entirely* axial or refractive. However, clinically significant levels (more than 2.00 D) of anisometropia are typically axial in nature.[24] In addition, an easy clinical test can assist the practitioner in deciding whether a patient's anisometropia is axial or refractive in origin: While the patient is wearing spherical correction (without the minus cylinder correction, if required), the eyes are dissociated by a vertical prism and a simple direct comparison of the size of the two ocular images is made. If the images are perceived to be equal in size, axial anisometropia is assumed; if the images appear to be of unequal size, refractive anisometropia is assumed.

All astigmatism, as stated earlier, is considered to be *refractive* in origin, and routine refractive changes occurring in adults are also usually refractive in origin. After years of refractive stability, the factors most likely to change are the dioptric elements of the eye rather than the length. For example, the increase in manifest hyperopia in early presbyopia is a common phenomenon, and although this usually occurs binocularly, it occasionally occurs mainly in one eye. Also, it is a rather common experience that sudden changes in refraction can occur from changes in the index of refraction of the crystalline lens as a result of progressive nuclear sclerosis. Frequently, the change occurs more rapidly in one eye than the other, and the correction of such refractive changes may induce aniseikonia.

In the case of the refractive type of ametropia, Ogle[25] estimated that the percentage change in magnification of the retinal image in the corrected eye compared with that in the normal eye is 1.5% per diopter of correction in the case of corneal astigmatism and 2% for a refractive error arising from the crystalline lens.

Linksz and Bannon,[22] on the other hand, suggested that if the image size difference is associated with anisometropia of refractive origin, we can expect it to be about 1.5% per diopter of anisometropia, but because ametropia may be partly axial, an estimate of 1.0% per diopter is more realistic. The eye with the least hyperopia or the more myopia is expected to have the smaller retinal image, and therefore is the one to require magnification. If the patient has astigmatism, the estimate must be made separately for each principal meridian.

In the same article, Linksz and Bannon noted that there are patients for whom a spherical anisometropia of several diopters has been fully corrected by ordinary lenses, and eikonometer measurements have shown no significant aniseikonia. These are cases of *axial* ametropia, and those findings are consistent with the findings of Sorsby et al.,[11] that ametropia of ±4.00 D is usually caused by an abnormally long or short axial length. Linksz and Bannon commented that most patients were myopes, and that clinical experience shows that there are many cases of spherical anisometropia in which this result is *not* obtained, which indicates that ametropia may not always be caused by axial factors.

Ryan[26] published tables of relative spectacle magnification based on *power* magnification only (ignoring the shape factor in the spectacle magnification formula), which show that, for a 12-mm vertex distance, relative spectacle magnification changes at the rate of 1.4% per diopter for purely refractive ametropia but only 0.25% per diopter for purely axial ametropia. Ryan pointed out that if the lens is worn closer to the eye than the primary focal plane (closer than a vertex distance of 12 mm) the relative spectacle magnifications of the axial and refractive components vary *in opposite directions* and therefore tend to compensate for one another if present in the right proportions.

10.20. Avoiding or Minimizing Induced Aniseikonia

A number of procedures have been recommended for prescribing to avoid or to minimize induced aniseikonia for patients who have anisometropia or astigmatism.

Anisometropia

In anisometropia, a partial refractive correction for the more ametropic eye has long been advocated. Donders[7] recommended the prescribing of reading lenses of equal power for presbyopic patients having anisometropia if they have not previously worn a full correction for the anisometropia and have not experienced discomfort. Such a procedure has the advantage of not inducing aniseikonia and its associated asthenopic symptoms but it fails to provide optimal visual acuity for each eye and fails to provide normal binocular vision.

For younger patients, the best thing may be to prescribe a correction that provides maximal visual acuity in each eye and the best possible binocular vision. A partial correction that reduces vision and impairs binocularity may cause failure of the vision requirements set forth by schools, industry, military services, civil services, and driver's licensing bureaus. However, full correction may produce aniseikonia with annoying symptomatology (although children tend to adapt to distortions more readily than do adults). Again, large amounts of ametropia tend to be at least partially *axial* in origin, and in such cases a full correction in spectacle lenses may induce little or no aniseikonia.

Astigmatism

Rayner[27] stated that the spectacle-wearing patient with intact binocular vision most likely to have aniseikonia is one with cylindrical anisometropia of 1.00 to 1.50 D, with a difference in the axes. Because the powers (and possibly the base curves) vary in the principal meridians of a cylindrical or toric lens for an astigmatic eye, unequal magnification effects occur in the various meridians of the eye. This meridional magnification produces monocular distortion and rotation (tilting) of all lines toward the meridian of greatest magnification (except those meridians parallel to the principal meridians). The amount of tilting of vertical lines is known as the *declination error*. Maximal tilting of vertical lines occurs when the principal meridians of a correcting lens are 45° and 135°.

Monocular distortion and tilting are not, by themselves, a problem because their effects are small. Ogle and Madigan[28] showed that when the axes are at 45° and 135°, which gives maximal amount of distortion, the resulting tilt of vertical lines is only 0.43 degree per diopter of astigmatism. When binocular vision is present, a significant clinical problem occurs. Declination errors, when they exist between the images of the two eyes, are important sources of induced aniseikonia because they produce a unique type of false spatial localization for objects seen stereoscopically. A startling effect is generated, in that objects appear to be *inclined*, with the top either away from or toward the observer (Figure 10–28). For example, if a +1.00 D cylinder axis 135 is worn for the right eye and a +1.00 D cylinder axis 45 is worn for the left eye, for a vertical pole 3 m away, the declination error is only 0.43 degree for each eye, seen monocularly—an amount hardly detectable. However, in *binocular* vision, the vertical pole appears to be tilted toward the subject *more than 30 degrees.*[28]

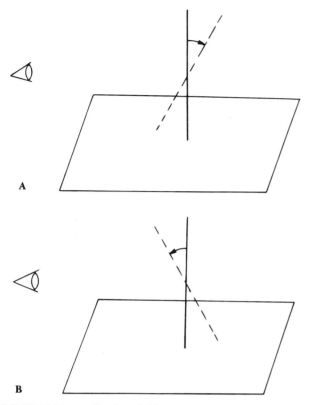

FIGURE 10–28.   **Inclination of objects away from and toward an observer caused by declination error (tilt of vertical lines) arising from correcting cylinders with oblique axes.**

As mentioned in Section 10.17, most patients adapt to anomalous spatial localization by learning to supress stereoscopic clues and depend instead on empirical clues acquired through experience, such as perspective, known size and shape, knowledge of location, and perpendicularity. Some patients make this adaptation easily, but others adapt with difficulty or not at all and are extremely sensitive to anomalous spatial localization.

In order to reduce anomalous spatial orientation, one can minimize the monocular distortion that produces it. Two things can be done for spectacle lenses to reduce monocular distortion with no sacrifice in visual acuity.

1. Specify in the prescription *negative toric* lens construction. With a spherical front surface, the shape factor of the spectacle magnification formula is constant for the two principal meridians and, hence, does not contribute to the meridional size difference.

2. Use as short a vertex distance as possible. Because astigmatism is *refractive* in origin, meridional size differences caused by the power factor are reduced as the vertex distance is made shorter. Of course, if the vertex distance is reduced to zero, with contact lenses, the monocular distortion arising from astigmatism is essentially eliminated.

Monocular distortion can be further reduced by manipulation of the correction, although this results in a failure to fully correct the refractive error and, therefore,

reduces the sharpness of the retinal image. Such manipulations include the following:

1. Reduction of the power of the cylinder, but at the correct axis. Because the amount of meridional magnification is a function of the power of the cylinder, reduction of the power decreases meridional magnification. This leaves some astigmatism uncorrected and causes some blur. Tentatively, when this is done, the spherical power should be altered accordingly, to maintain the same spherical equivalent, but the final sphere power should be one that subjectively provides the best visual acuity.

2. If the cylinder axes are oblique, the axes can be rotated toward the 180° or 90° position, depending on which is closer. The rationale underlying this manipulation is that distortion is usually better tolerated when the axis is either horizontal or vertical. The direction of the meridional magnification is determined primarily by the axis position of the correcting cylinder, regardless of whether it is the correct axis.

If the axis of a cylinder is rotated to make the direction of meridional magnification more tolerable, the cylinder should be reduced in power to minimize the amount of residual astigmatism. The Jackson cross-cylinder, used at the new axis location for the refinement of cylinder power, automatically gives the optimum cylinder power to result in a minimum of residual astigmatism for a unique axis error.[29] The optimal power for the new axis position may also be determined by rotating any two-meridian astigmatic chart (such as the "rotating T") in alignment with the principal meridians for the new axis setting and by balancing the sharpness of the two lines by manipulating cylinder power.

Patients who wear glasses only intermittently for distance vision may not adapt to space distortions during short periods of wear. In such cases, the astigmatic correction may be altered as previously discussed or may be eliminated entirely.

Some presbyopic patients with slight or moderate amounts of astigmatism refuse to wear glasses for distance vision but need assistance for close work. Again, it is probably best to alter the astigmatic correction or eliminate the correction, because adaptation to space distortions may not readily occur.

10.21. Prescribing and Lens Design

When the practitioner concludes that a patient's symptomatology is caused by the presence of induced aniseikonia, the following factors, suggested by Bannon,[30] may be considered to decide whether to prescribe an aniseikonic correction:

1. The age of the patient
2. The nature of the previous correction
3. The patient's occupation and hobbies
4. The patient's temperament

5. The patient's interest in the appearance of the glasses
6. The cost of the correction
7. The nature of the patient's complaint, and the practitioner's assessment of the likelihood of partial or total relief

As shown by Equation 10.8, developed in Section 10.7, spectacle magnification depends on the combination of the shape factor (M_S) and the power factor (M_P):

$$SM = (M_S)(M_P)$$
$$= \left(\frac{1}{1 - \frac{t}{n}F_1}\right)\left(\frac{1}{1 - hF_V}\right),$$

with the shape factor, M_S, caused by the front surface curvature, F_1, and the thickness, t, of the lens; and the power factor, M_P, caused by the power, F_V, of the lens and the distance, h, from the lens to the center of the entrance pupil of the eye.

Although the refractive power of the lens, F_V, participates in the power factor, the powers of the patient's lenses cannot be changed if the ametropia is to be properly corrected. Therefore, the following factors are the *only* ones that can be altered without significantly affecting the refractive power of the lenses:

1. The front surface power of the lens
2. The center thickness of the lens
3. The distance of the lens from the center of the entrance pupil

The spectacle magnification formula is an *exact* formula, and a rather awkward one, but by using approximations, the formula can be simplified with no significant degree of error. Thus, if t/n is small, as it usually is, the spectacle magnification formula can be expanded to

$$M \cong 1 + \frac{t}{n}F_1 + hF_V.$$

Since

$$\%M = 100(M - 1),$$
$$\%M \cong 100\frac{t}{n}F_1 + 100hF_V,$$

with t and h expressed in meters.

If $n = 1.50$ and t and h are expressed in millimeters,

$$\%M = \frac{tF_1}{15} + \frac{hF_V}{10}. \tag{10.20}$$

This formula gives a first approximation of the effect of changes in the front surface power, thickness, and vertex distance on spectacle magnification. An examination of the formula indicates the approximate magnification effects of varying each parameter, which may be stated by the following "rules of thumb":

1. If all other factors are held constant, for every diopter increase in front surface power, the percentage magnifica-

tion is increased (for both plus and minus lenses) by *1/15* of the center thickness. The percentage change in shape magnification per diopter of change in front surface power is given by

$$\Delta\%M_S = \frac{\Delta F_1(t)}{15}. \tag{10.21}$$

2. If all other factors are held constant, for every millimeter increase in center thickness, the percentage magnification is increased (for both plus and minus lenses) by *1/15* of the front surface power. The percentage change in shape magnification per millimeter of change in thickness is given by

$$\Delta\%M_S = \frac{\Delta t(F_1)}{15}. \tag{10.22}$$

3. If all other factors are held constant, for every millimeter the vertex distance is changed, the percentage magnification is changed by *1/10* of the refractive power. Magnification *increases* as a plus lens is moved away from the eye and a minus lens is moved toward the eye; and magnification *decreases* as a plus lens moves toward the eye and a minus lens moves away from the eye. The percentage change in the power magnification, per millimeter of vertex distance change, is given by the relationship

$$\Delta\%M_P = \frac{\Delta h(F_V)}{10}.$$

These rules do not work independently of each other. For example, if the front surface curvature is steepened and the back vertex power remains constant, the back surface curvature must be steepened essentially the same amount to maintain the specified back vertex power, with the result that the back vertex of the lens is *farther* from the eye. For plus lenses, the change causes an additional increase in magnification. Increasing the front surface curvature for a minus lens also produces an increase in magnification, but this is combined with a decrease in magnification as a result of a consequent increase in the vertex distance.

Linksz and Bannon[22] pointed out that the decrease in magnification brought about by increased vertex distance of a minus lens begins to cancel out the magnification caused by the increased curvature as the power of the lens approaches −2.00 D. They suggest that because strong minus lenses have thick edges, it is possible to change the position of the bevel and thus bring the lens closer to the eye, and, hence, preserve the magnification achieved by the increase in front surface power. Linksz and Bannon have developed tables (Tables 10–4 and 10–5) that illustrate the approximate magnification changes associated with changes in front surface curvature and vertex distance (eyewire distance) for lenses of various powers.

Table 10–4 may be used in the following manner. Suppose that the practitioner determines (by measurement or by estimation) that a patient's right lens, having a back vertex power of +2.00 D and a center thickness of 2.7 mm, requires an increase in magnification of 1%. The table shows that, for this lens, an increase in magnification of 1.1% results if the front surface power is increased by 4.00 D. This

TABLE 10–4
Approximate Magnification Changes (%) Associated with Changes in Front Base Curves for Various Lens Powers

Vertex Power of Lens (D)	Average Center Thickness (mm)	Change in Front Base Curve					
		−4.00 D	−2.00 D	+2.00 D	+4.00 D	+6.00 D	+8.00 D
+8.00	7.0	−3.5	−1.7	+1.7	+3.5	+5.2	+6.9
+7.00	6.2	−3.0	−1.5	+1.5	+3.0	+4.5	+6.0
+6.00	5.4	−2.6	−1.3	+1.3	+2.6	+3.9	+5.2
+5.00	4.6	−2.2	−1.1	+1.1	+2.2	+3.3	+4.4
+4.00	3.9	−1.8	−0.9	+0.9	+1.8	+2.8	+3.7
+3.00	3.2	−1.5	−0.7	+0.7	+1.5	+2.2	+2.9
+2.00	2.7	−1.1	−0.6	+0.6	+1.1	+1.7	+2.2
+1.00	2.2	−0.8	−0.4	+0.4	+0.8	+1.2	+1.6
0.00	1.8	−0.5	−0.2	+0.2	+0.5	+0.7	+1.0
−1.00	1.4	−0.2	−0.1	+0.1	+0.2	+0.3	+0.3
−2.00	1.0	+0.1	+0.1	−0.1	−0.1	−0.2	−0.3
−3.00	0.9	+0.4	+0.2	−0.2	−0.4	−0.5	−0.7
−4.00	0.9	+0.6	+0.3	−0.3	−0.6	−0.8	−1.1
−5.00	0.9	+0.8	+0.4	−0.4	−0.8	−1.1	−1.5
−6.00	0.9	+1.0	+0.5	−0.5	−1.0	−1.4	−1.9
−7.00	0.9	+1.2	+0.6	−0.6	−1.2	−1.7	−2.3
−8.00	0.9	+1.4	+0.7	−0.7	−1.4	−2.0	−2.7

SOURCE: Adapted from A. Linksz and R.E. Bannon, *International Ophthalmologic Clinics*, Vol. 5, No. 2. Little, Brown, Boston, pp. 515–534, 1965.

table takes into consideration the change in *vertex distance* that occurs when the front surface power is changed. For example, the table shows that, for a −3.00 D lens, an increase in front surface power of 2.00 D actually causes a *minification* of 0.2%, because of the increase in vertex distance that accompanies the steepening of the front surface.

Magnification changes associated with changes in vertex distance are shown in Table 10–5. In this table, a positive sign indicates an increase in vertex distance, and a negative sign indicates a decrease in vertex distance. As mentioned previously, an increase in the vertex distance results in an increase in magnification for a plus lens and a decrease in magnification for a minus lens. On the other hand, a decrease in the vertex distance produces a decrease in magnification for a plus lens and an increase in magnification for a minus lens.

For a minus lens, the practitioner may decide not to alter the front surface power but to bring about the desired magnification by changing *only* the vertex distance. For example, if one wishes to bring about a 1.2% increase in the magnification of a −6.00-D lens, the table shows that this may be accomplished by moving the lens toward the eye (by moving the bevel forward) 2 mm. It is obvious from Table 10–5 that much greater magnification changes can be obtained with plus lenses than with minus lenses. For this reason, the design of eikonic lenses should always begin with the lens that has the *most plus or least minus power*; the shape magnification of this lens is reduced to a minimum.

Although magnification can be increased by increasing lens thickness, any increase in thickness must be modest to keep from making the lenses unattractive or excessively heavy. However, when one attempts to increase magnification of a minus lens, if thickness is increased while a constant front bevel (such as a hide-a-bevel), is maintained, a sub-

TABLE 10–5
Approximate Magnification Changes (%) Associated with Changes in Eyewire Distance for Various Lens Powers

Vertex Power of Lens (D)	Change in Eyewire Distance			
	Lens Moved toward the Eye			
	−1 mm	−2 mm	−3 mm	−4 mm
+10	−1.0	−2.0	−3.0	−4.0
+ 8	−0.8	−1.6	−2.4	−3.2
+ 6	−0.6	−1.2	−1.8	−2.4
+ 4	−0.4	−0.8	−1.2	−1.6
+ 2	−0.2	−0.4	−0.6	−0.8
− 2	+0.2	+0.4	+0.6	+0.8
− 4	+0.4	+0.8	+1.2	+1.6
− 6	+0.6	+1.2	+1.8	+2.4
− 8	+0.8	+1.6	+2.4	+3.2
− 10	+1.0	+2.0	+3.0	+4.0
	Lens Moved away from the Eye			
	+1 mm	+2 mm	+3 mm	+4 mm
+10	+1.0	+2.0	+3.0	+4.0
+ 8	+0.8	+1.6	+2.4	+3.2
+ 6	+0.6	+1.2	+1.8	+2.4
+ 4	+0.4	+0.8	+1.2	+1.6
+ 2	+0.2	+0.4	+0.6	+0.8
− 2	−0.2	−0.4	−0.6	−0.8
− 4	−0.4	−0.8	−1.2	−1.6
− 6	−0.6	−1.2	−1.8	−2.4
− 8	−0.8	−1.6	−2.4	−3.2
−10	−1.0	−2.0	−3.0	−4.0

SOURCE: Adapted from A. Linksz and R.E. Bannon, *International Ophthalmologic Clinics*, Vol. 5, No. 2. Little, Brown, Boston, pp. 515–534, 1965.

stantial increase in magnification can be obtained. Assuming a constant front bevel, the following formula expresses the change in magnification by a change in thickness:[31]

$$\Delta\%M = \Delta t\left(\frac{F_1}{15} - \frac{F_V}{10}\right). \qquad (10.23)$$

In cases in which there is a correction for astigmatism, the power in each of the two principal meridians must be considered separately.

Berens and Bannon[32] recommend that induced aniseikonia be only *partially* corrected. They compared this correction to the partial correction of heterophoria by prisms. An approximate correction provides not only therapeutic value but also diagnostic information. If an approximate correction provides partial relief from the symptoms, it may be worthwhile to have a thorough eikonometric examination to determine a more exact correction.

10.22. The Use of Eikonic Lenses in Fit-Over Form

Before making up the correction in final form, some practitioners have found it useful to conduct a confirmation test using a *fit-over afocal magnifying lens* with the patient's glasses. The fit-over lens is placed before the lens with the smaller predicted image size. If relief is reported after wearing the fit-over lens for a few days, one may feel confident in prescribing the correction. Some practitioners find it helpful to *reverse* the afocal fit-over lens, and put the lens before the opposite eye, to increase rather than correct the image size difference. Intensification of symptoms by the reversal, tends to confirm the diagnosis.

Because afocal telescopic lenses change the magnification of the retinal image without changing the power of the refractive correction, they are frequently called *size lenses*. Because the back vertex power is zero, the magnification of an afocal lens is given by the shape factor alone,

$$M_S = \frac{1}{1 - \frac{t}{n}F_1}. \qquad (10.24)$$

Since

$$F_V = \frac{F_1}{1 - \frac{t}{n}F_1} + F_2,$$

$$F_1 = \frac{F_V - F_2}{1 + \frac{t}{n}(F_V - F_2)},$$

and, substituting for F_1, in Equation 10.24,

$$M_S = \frac{1}{1 - \frac{t}{n}\left(\dfrac{F_V - F_2}{1 + \frac{t}{n}(F_V - F_2)}\right)}$$

$$= \frac{1}{\dfrac{1 + \frac{t}{n}(F_V - F_2) - \frac{t}{n}(F_V - F_2)}{1 + \frac{t}{n}(F_V - F_2)}}$$

$$= \frac{1 + \frac{t}{n}(F_V - F_2)}{1 + \frac{t}{n}(F_V - F_2) - \frac{t}{n}(F_V - F_2)}$$

$$= 1 + \frac{t}{n}(F_V - F_2),$$

and since for an afocal lens, $F_V = 0$,

$$M_S = 1 - \frac{t}{n}F_2. \qquad (10.25)$$

One may easily design a set of afocal lenses to serve as a trial eikonic lens ("size lens") set. Once the thickness has been selected, either Equation 10.24 or Equation 10.25 may be used to design the lenses. For overall magnifiers, spherical curves should be used. Meridional magnifying lenses, having maximum magnification in one meridian and no magnification in the opposite meridian, are bitoric lenses, made by grinding toric surfaces both on the front and on the back of the lens, with the axes precisely aligned.

Rayner[27] provided the lens specifications for afocal lenses with various magnifications. Tables 10–6 and 10–7 may be used to select the front surface power, thickness, and back surface power needed to provide the desired magnification. The most useful areas of each table fall between the heavy lines that exclude very thin lenses and very thick lenses (more than 8 mm thick). For example, a 3.00% afocal magnifier could be manufactured with a front surface power of +6.00 D, a center thickness of 7.49 mm, and a back surface power of –6.18 D, or with a front surface power of +12.00 D, a center thickness of 3.75 mm, and a back surface power of –12.36 D.

10.23. Frame Selection for Eikonic Lenses

The correct fitting and adjustment of the frame are critical for an eikonic correction. Because these lenses are thicker and therefore heavier than most other lenses, the eye size should be kept small, both to reduce weight and to allow fitting the lens at as short a vertex distance as possible. A plastic frame conceals the thick edge better than a metal frame or a rimless mounting. An eikonic lens tends to have highly curved surfaces and a correspondingly curved bevel and therefore may be difficult to mount without warping the frame. A *symmetrical* lens shape is therefore recommended, that is, a shape having a small difference between the "A" and "B" measurements.

The patient should be seen often during the first few weeks after the correction is dispensed to check adjustment and to provide reassurance and additional instruction if needed.

TABLE 10–6
Plano-Powered Lenses with Desired Percentage Magnification: Required Center Thickness (t) in Millimeters and Inside 1.53 Curve (D_2) for a Selected 1.53 Front Curve (D_1)

% Mag.	1.53 D_t	2.00	2.50	3.00	3.50	4.00	4.50	5.00	5.50	6.00	6.50	7.00	7.50	8.00	8.50
0.50	t	3.84	3.07	3.56	2.19	1.92	1.71	1.54	1.40	1.28	1.18	1.10	1.02	0.96	0.90
	D_2	2.01	2.51	3.02	3.52	4.02	4.52	5.03	5.53	6.03	6.53	7.04	7.54	8.04	8.54
0.75	t	5.74	4.60	3.83	3.28	2.87	2.55	2.30	2.09	1.91	1.77	1.64	1.53	1.44	1.35
	D_2	2.02	2.52	3.02	3.53	4.03	4.53	5.04	5.54	6.05	6.55	7.05	7.56	8.06	8.56
1.00	t	7.64	6.11	5.09	4.37	3.82	3.33	3.06	2.78	2.55	2.35	2.18	2.04	1.91	1.80
	D_2	2.02	2.53	3.03	3.54	4.04	4.55	5.05	5.56	6.06	6.57	7.07	7.58	8.08	8.59
1.25	t	9.52	7.62	6.35	5.44	4.76	4.23	3.81	3.46	3.17	2.93	2.72	2.54	2.38	2.24
	D_2	2.03	2.53	3.04	3.54	4.05	4.56	5.06	5.57	6.08	6.58	7.09	7.59	8.10	8.61
1.50	t	11.4	9.12	7.60	6.52	5.70	5.07	4.56	4.15	3.80	3.51	3.26	3.04	2.85	2.68
	D_2	2.03	2.54	3.05	3.55	4.06	4.57	5.08	5.58	6.09	6.60	7.11	7.61	8.12	8.63
1.75	t	13.3	10.6	8.85	7.58	6.63	5.90	5.31	4.83	4.42	4.08	3.79	3.54	3.32	3.12
	D_2	2.04	2.54	3.05	3.56	4.07	4.58	5.09	5.60	6.11	6.61	7.12	7.63	8.14	8.65
2.00	t	15.1	12.1	10.1	8.64	7.56	6.72	6.05	5.50	5.04	4.65	4.32	4.03	3.78	3.56
	D_2	2.04	2.55	3.06	3.57	4.08	4.59	5.10	5.61	6.12	6.63	7.14	7.65	8.16	8.67
2.25	t	17.0	13.6	11.3	9.70	8.49	7.55	6.79	6.17	5.66	5.22	4.85	4.53	4.24	3.99
	D_2	2.05	2.56	3.07	3.58	4.09	4.60	5.11	5.62	6.14	6.65	7.16	7.67	8.18	8.69
2.50	t	18.8	15.1	12.5	10.8	9.41	8.36	7.53	6.84	6.27	5.79	5.38	5.02	4.70	4.43
	D_2	2.05	2.56	3.08	3.59	4.10	4.61	5.13	5.64	6.15	6.66	7.18	7.69	8.20	8.71
2.75	t	20.7	16.5	13.8	11.8	10.3	9.18	8.26	7.51	6.88	6.35	5.90	5.51	5.16	4.86
	D_2	2.06	2.57	3.08	3.60	4.11	4.62	5.14	5.65	6.17	6.68	7.19	7.71	8.22	8.73
3.00	t	22.5	18.0	15.0	12.8	11.2	9.99	8.99	8.17	7.49	6.91	6.42	5.99	5.62	5.29
	D_2	2.06	2.58	3.09	3.61	4.12	4.64	5.15	5.67	6.18	6.70	7.21	7.73	8.24	8.76
3.25	t	24.3	19.4	16.2	13.9	12.1	10.8	9.71	8.83	8.09	7.47	6.94	6.48	6.07	5.71
	D_2	2.07	2.58	3.10	3.61	4.13	4.65	5.16	5.68	6.20	6.71	7.23	7.74	8.26	8.78
3.50	t	26.1	20.9	17.4	14.9	13.1	11.6	10.4	9.49	8.70	8.03	7.45	6.96	6.52	6.14
	D_2	2.07	2.59	3.11	3.62	4.14	4.66	5.18	5.69	6.21	6.73	7.25	7.76	8.28	8.80
3.75	t	27.9	22.3	18.6	15.9	13.9	12.4	11.2	10.1	9.30	8.58	7.97	7.44	6.97	6.56
	D_2	2.08	2.59	3.11	3.63	4.15	4.67	5.19	5.71	6.23	6.74	7.26	7.78	8.30	8.82
4.00	t	29.7	23.7	20.8	17.0	14.8	13.2	11.9	10.8	9.89	9.13	8.48	7.91	7.42	6.98
	D_2	2.08	2.60	3.12	3.64	4.16	4.68	5.20	5.72	6.24	6.76	7.28	7.80	8.32	8.84
4.25	t	31.5	25.2	21.0	18.0	15.7	14.0	12.6	11.4	10.5	9.68	8.99	8.39	7.86	7.40
	D_2	2.09	2.61	3.13	3.65	4.17	4.69	5.21	5.73	6.29	6.78	7.30	7.82	8.34	8.86
4.50	t	33.2	26.6	22.2	19.0	16.6	14.8	13.3	12.1	11.1	10.2	9.49	8.86	8.31	7.82
	D_2	2.09	2.61	3.14	3.66	4.18	4.70	5.23	5.75	6.27	6.79	7.32	7.84	8.36	8.88
4.75	t	35.0	28.0	23.3	20.0	17.7	15.6	14.0	12.7	11.7	10.8	10.0	9.33	8.75	8.23
	D_2	2.10	2.62	3.14	3.67	4.19	4.71	5.24	5.76	6.29	6.81	7.33	7.86	8.38	8.90
5.00	t	36.7	29.4	24.5	21.0	18.4	16.6	14.7	13.4	12.3	11.3	10.5	9.80	9.18	8.64
	D_2	2.10	2.63	3.15	3.68	4.20	4.73	5.25	5.78	6.30	6.83	7.35	7.88	8.40	8.93

SOURCE: Adapted from A. Rayner, *Am. J. Optom. Arch. Am. Acad. Optom.*, Vol. 43, pp. 617–632, 1966.

10.24. Aniseikonia: Clinical Considerations in Anisometropia and Astigmatism

In summary, in cases of significant anisometropia or astigmatism:

1. The practitioner can predict the amount of image size difference that results for the two eyes by using one of the rules above and by remembering that, although high refractive errors are most likely axial, moderate or low refractive errors are more likely caused by axial-refractive combinations.

2. Once the prediction has been made, tables such as those prepared by Linksz and Bannon and by Rayner may be used to determine the lens parameters necessary to minimize the induced aniseikonia.

3. It is normally preferable to design lenses that only *partially* correct for the induced aniseikonia.

TABLE 10–7
Plano-Powered Lenses with Desired Percentage Magnification: Required Center Thickness (t) in Millimeters and Inside 1.53 Curve (D_2) for a Selected 1.53 Front Curve (D_1)

% Mag.	1.53 D_1	9.00	9.50	10.00	10.50	11.00	11.50	12.00	12.50	13.00	13.50	14.00	14.50
0.50	t	0.85	0.81	0.77	0.73	0.70	0.67	0.64	0.61	0.59	0.57	0.55	0.53
	D_2	9.05	9.55	10.05	10.55	11.06	11.56	12.06	12.56	13.07	13.57	14.07	14.57
0.75	t	1.28	1.21	1.15	1.09	1.04	1.00	0.96	0.92	0.88	0.85	0.82	0.79
	D_2	9.07	9.57	10.08	10.58	11.08	11.59	12.09	12.59	13.10	13.60	14.11	14.61
1.00	t	1.70	1.61	1.53	1.45	1.39	1.33	1.27	1.22	1.18	1.13	1.09	1.05
	D_2	9.09	9.60	10.10	10.61	11.11	11.62	12.12	12.63	13.13	13.64	14.14	14.65
1.25	t	2.12	2.01	1.90	1.81	1.73	1.66	1.59	1.52	1.47	1.41	1.36	1.31
	D_2	9.11	9.62	10.13	10.63	11.14	11.64	12.15	12.66	13.16	13.67	14.18	14.68
1.50	t	2.53	2.40	2.28	2.17	2.07	1.98	1.90	1.82	1.75	1.69	1.63	1.57
	D_2	9.14	9.64	10.15	10.66	11.17	11.67	12.18	12.69	13.20	13.70	14.21	14.72
1.75	t	2.95	2.79	2.65	2.53	2.41	2.31	2.21	2.12	2.04	1.97	1.90	1.83
	D_2	9.16	9.67	10.18	10.68	11.19	11.70	12.21	12.72	13.23	13.74	14.25	14.75
2.00	t	3.36	3.18	3.03	2.88	2.75	2.63	2.52	2.42	2.33	2.24	2.16	2.09
	D_2	9.18	9.69	10.20	10.71	11.22	11.73	12.24	12.75	13.26	13.77	14.28	14.97
2.25	t	3.77	3.57	3.40	3.23	3.09	2.95	2.83	2.72	2.61	2.52	2.43	2.34
	D_2	9.20	9.71	10.23	10.74	11.25	11.76	12.27	12.78	13.29	13.80	14.32	14.83
2.50	t	4.18	3.96	3.76	3.58	3.42	3.27	3.14	3.01	2.89	2.79	2.69	2.60
	D_2	9.23	9.74	10.25	10.76	11.28	11.79	12.30	12.81	13.33	13.84	14.35	14.86
2.75	t	4.59	4.35	4.13	3.93	3.75	3.59	3.44	3.30	3.18	3.06	2.95	2.85
	D_2	9.25	9.76	10.28	10.79	11.30	11.82	12.33	12.84	13.36	13.87	14.39	14.90
3.00	t	4.99	4.73	4.49	4.28	4.09	3.91	3.75	3.60	3.46	3.33	3.21	3.10
	D_2	9.27	9.79	10.30	10.82	11.33	11.85	12.36	12.88	13.39	13.91	14.42	14.94
3.25	t	5.40	5.11	4.96	4.63	4.42	4.22	4.05	3.89	3.74	3.60	3.47	3.35
	D_2	9.29	9.81	10.33	10.84	11.36	11.87	12.39	12.91	13.42	13.94	14.46	14.97
3.50	t	5.80	5.49	5.22	4.97	4.74	4.54	4.35	4.17	4.01	3.87	3.73	3.60
	D_2	9.32	9.83	10.35	10.87	11.39	11.90	12.42	12.94	13.46	13.97	14.49	15.01
3.75	t	6.20	5.87	5.58	5.31	5.07	4.85	4.65	4.46	4.29	4.13	3.98	3.85
	D_2	9.34	9.86	10.38	10.89	11.41	11.93	12.45	12.97	13.49	14.01	14.53	15.04
4.00	t	6.59	6.25	5.93	5.65	5.40	5.16	4.95	4.75	4.57	4.40	4.24	4.09
	D_2	9.36	9.88	10.40	10.92	11.44	11.96	12.48	13.00	13.52	14.04	14.56	15.08
4.25	t	6.99	6.62	6.29	5.99	5.72	5.47	5.24	5.03	4.84	4.66	4.49	4.34
	D_2	9.38	9.90	10.43	10.95	11.47	11.99	12.51	13.03	13.55	14.07	14.60	15.12
4.50	t	7.38	6.99	6.64	6.33	6.04	5.78	5.54	5.32	5.11	4.92	4.75	4.58
	D_2	9.41	9.93	10.45	10.97	11.50	12.02	12.54	13.06	13.59	14.11	14.63	15.15
4.75	t	7.77	7.37	7.00	6.66	6.36	6.08	5.83	5.60	5.38	5.18	5.00	4.83
	D_2	9.43	9.95	10.48	11.00	11.52	12.05	12.57	13.09	13.62	14.14	14.67	15.19
5.00	t	8.16	7.73	7.35	7.00	6.68	6.39	6.12	5.88	5.65	5.44	5.25	5.07
	D_2	9.45	9.98	10.50	11.03	11.55	12.08	12.60	13.13	13.65	14.18	14.70	15.23

SOURCE: Adapted from A. Rayner, *Am. J. Optom. Arch. Am. Acad. Optom.*, Vol. 43, pp. 617–632, 1966.

References

1. Fischer, L. G. Analytical Aids for Determining Induced Vertical Prism Imbalance in Anisometropia. *Am. J. Optom. Physiol. Opt.*, Vol. 53, pp. 249–258, 1976.
2. Ellerbrock, V. J., and Fry, G. A. Effects Induced by Anisometropia Corrections. *Am. J. Optom. Arch. Am. Acad. Optom.*, Vol. 19, pp. 444–459, 1942.
3. Cusick, P., and Hawn, H. Prism Compensation in Cases of Anisometropia. *Arch. Ophthalmol.*, Vol. 25, pp. 651–654, 1941.
4. Ellerbrock, V. J. A Clinical Evaluation of Compensation for Vertical Prismatic Imbalances. *Am. J. Optom. Arch. Am. Acad. Optom.*, Vol. 25, pp. 309–325, 1948.
5. Duke-Elder, S. *Ophthalmic Optics and Refraction*, Vol. 5. Henry Kimpton, London, 1970.
6. Peters, H. B. Measurement of a "Slab-Off" Ophthalmic Lens with a Lens Gauge. *Am. J. Optom. Arch. Am. Acad. Optom.*, Vol. 26, pp. 16–18, 1949.
7. Donders, F. C. *On the Anomalies of Accommodation and Refraction of the Eye.* New Sydenham Society, London, 1864. (Reproduced by Hatton Press, London, 1952.)

8. Burian, H. M. History of Dartmouth Eye Institute. *Arch. Ophthalmol.*, Vol. 40, pp. 163–175, 1948.
9. Lancaster, W. Aniseikonia. *Arch. Ophthalmol.*, Vol. 20, pp. 907–912, 1938.
10. Ogle, K. N. Some Aspects of the Eye as an Image Forming Mechanism. *J. Opt. Soc. Am.*, Vol. 33, pp. 506–512, 1943.
11. Sorsby, A., Benjamin, D., Davey, J. B., Sheridan, M., and Tanner, J. M. *Emmetropia and Its Aberrations.* Her Majesty's Stationery Office, London, 1957.
12. Bannon, R. E. *Clinical Manual on Aniseikonia*, American Optical Corp., Buffalo, NY, p. 95, 1954.
13. Ogle, K. N. *Researches in Binocular Vision*, W. B. Saunders, Philadelphia, p. 282, 1950.
14. Bannon, R. E. Space Eikonometry in Aniseikonia. *Am. J. Optom. Arch. Am. Acad. Optom.*, Vol. 30, pp. 86–93, 1953.
15. Elvin, F. T. Aniseikonia—A Simplified Method of Measurement and a Case Report. *Am. J. Optom. Arch. Am. Acad. Optom.*, Vol. 26, pp. 78–82, 1949.
16. Brecher, G. A. A New Method of Measuring Aniseikonia. *Am. J. Ophthalmol.*, Vol. 34, pp. 1016–1021, 1951.
17. Brecher, G. A., Winters, D. M., and Townsend, C. A. Image Alternation for Aniseikonia Determination. *Am. J. Ophthal.*, Vol. 45, pp. 253–258, 1958.
18. Baldwin, W. R. Binocular Testing and Distance Correction with the Berlin Polatest. *J. Am. Optom. Assoc.*, Vol. 34, pp. 115–125, 1962.
19. Grolman, B. Vectographic Near Point Cards (Instructions). American Optical Corp., Buffalo, NY, 1971.
20. Ogle, K. N. *Researches in Binocular Vision*, W. B. Saunders, Philadelphia, p. 300, 1950.
21. Bannon, R. E. Aniseikonia and Binocular Vision. *Am. J. Optom. Arch. Am. Acad. Optom.*, Vol. 26, pp. 240–250, 1949.
22. Linksz, A., and Bannon, R. E. Aniseikonia and Refractive Problems. *International Ophthalmologic Clinics*, Vol. 5, No. 2, Little, Brown, Boston, pp. 515–534, 1965.
23. Carleton, E. H., and Madigan, L. F. Relationships between Aniseikonia and Ametropia. *Arch. Ophthalmol.*, Vol. 18, pp. 237–247, 1937.
24. Sorsby, A., Leary, G. A., and Richards, M. J. The Optical Components in Anisometropia. *Vision Res.*, Vol. 2, p. 4351, 1962.
25. Ogle, K. N. *Researches in Binocular Vision*, W. B. Saunders, Philadelphia, p. 264, 1950.
26. Ryan, V. I. Predicting Aniseikonia in Anisometropia. *Am. J. Optom. Physiol. Opt.*, Vol. 52, pp. 96–105, 1975.
27. Rayner, A. W. Aniseikonia and Magnification in Ophthalmic Lenses. *Am. J. Optom. Arch. Am. Acad. Optom.*, Vol. 43, pp. 617–632, 1966.
28. Ogle, K. N., and Madigan, L. F. Astigmatism at Oblique Axes and Binocular Stereopsis Spatial Localization. *Arch. Ophthalmol.*, Vol. 33, pp. 116–127, 1945.
29. Guyton, D. L. Prescribing Cylinders: The Problem of Distortion. *Survey Ophthalmol.*, Vol. 22, pp. 117–188, 1977.
30. Bannon, R. E. *Clinical Manual on Aniseikonia*, American Optical Corp., Buffalo, NY, p. 27, 1954.
31. Brown, R. H., and Enoch, J. M. Combined Rules of Thumb in Aniseikonia Prescriptions. *Am. J. Ophthalmol.*, Vol. 69, pp. 118–126, 1970.
32. Berens, C., and Bannon, R. E. Aniseikonia: A Present Appraisal and Some Practical Considerations. *Arch. Ophthalmol.*, Vol. 70, pp. 181–188, 1963.

Questions

1. Given:

   OD −4.00 DS −2.00 DC x 180

   OS −3.00 DS −0.50 DC x 180

   +2.00 D add; D-25 bifocal

   The reading center is 10 mm below the distance center. What is the slab-off prism required to eliminate the vertical imbalance at the reading center?

2. A +5.00 DS, add +2.00 D, 22-mm-wide, 16-mm-high straight-top bifocal is made with the optical center of the distance lens and the top of the segment at the geometric center of the finished lens. If the lens is made with a 3-prism diopter slab-off, what is the total prismatic power 10 mm below the geometric center?

3. Given:

   OD −1.00 DS −0.75 DC x 180

   OS +1.00 DS −0.75 DC x 180

   +2.50 D add

   Segs 18 mm high

   Distance optical center located at geometric center (GC)

   Reading level 10 mm below distance centers

   Lens size 46 × 40 mm

   If you decide to reduce the vertical imbalance at the reading level by using R-compensated segs, what are the R segments that come closest to leaving the patient with a residual vertical imbalance of 1 prism diopter?

4. A patient required the following lens correction:

   OD −0.75 DS −2.00 DC x 180

   OS +0.75 DS −1.00 DC x 180

   +2.00-D add

   Segs 20 mm high

   Distance optical center located at GC

   Reading level 10 mm below distance centers

   Lens size 50 × 44 mm

   You decide to prescribe different segment types for the eyes to reduce the vertical imbalance at the reading level. Which of the following pairs of segment types comes closest to eliminating the vertical imbalance *without overcorrection* at the reading level?

   (a) OD: Kryptok; OS: Ultex A

   (b) OD: Ultex A; OS: Executive

   (c) OD: 16 × 22-mm-wide flat top; OS: Ultex A

   (d) OD: Kryptok; OS: Executive

   (e) OD: Executive; OS: Kryptok

5. Given:

   OD −1.25 DS −1.75 DC x 180

   OS +1.50 DS −0.75 DC x 180

   Refractive index = 1.50

   Distance optical center located at GC

   Reading level 8 mm below distance centers

   Lens size 46 × 40 mm

A slab-off prescription is used to totally correct the vertical imbalance at the reading level. If the slab-off line is 18 mm high, what is the difference in thickness of the upper and lower edges of the slabbed-off lens?

6. A lens clock is used to measure the amount of slab-off prism on a flat-top 22-mm bifocal lens with a correction of +0.50 DS –1.00 DC x 180, +2.00 D add, and 5 prism diopters of slab-off. The base curve of the lens is +6.50 D. When the legs of the lens clock properly straddle the line perpendicularly, what is the clock dial reading?

7. Given:

OD –1.00 DS

OS –4.00 DS

The distance center is located at the GC. The reading level is 10 mm below the distance centers; the lens size is 46 × 40; the slab-off line is 16 mm high. If the left lens is slabbed off 3 prism diopters, where is the optical center of the slabbed-off portion located?

8. Given the following prescription:

OD +2.00 DS –0.75 DC x 180

OS –0.50 DS –0.75 DC x 180

Reading level 10 mm below distance optical centers

The patient views a near object through these lenses. You measure a vertical phoria of 1.5 prism diopters right hyperphoria in this position. If you remove the lenses and repeat the measurement, what vertical phoria would you expect to find?

9. Given the following prescription:

OD –0.50 DS –0.75 DC x 180

PD +2.00 DS –0.75 DC x 180

Reading level 10 mm below distance optical centers

The patient views a near object through these lenses. You measure a vertical imbalance of 2.5 prism diopters left hyperphoria in this position. If you remove the lenses and repeat the measurement, what is the expected vertical phoria?

10. A +3.00 DS +1.00 DC x 45 lens of ophthalmic crown glass with an index of refraction of 1.52 is made with minus cylinder construction, a center thickness of 3.0 mm, and a base curve of +8.00 D. What is the difference in magnification in the two principal meridians if the lens is fitted 18.0 mm from the entrance pupil?

11. A –4.00-D lens with an index of refraction of 1.50 is worn 15 mm from the entrance pupil. If the thickness is 6 mm, what must be the back surface power to produce a total spectacle magnification of 4%?

12. A +8.00-D lens with a front surface power of +12.00 D has an axial thickness of 4.5 mm. The lens is made of glass with a refractive index of 1.50 and the lens rests 15 mm from the entrance pupil. The total spectacle magnification of this lens should increase to 20% (1.20) with a change in lens thickness. If the back surface power is held constant, what must be the thickness of the lens?

13. To produce a pair of plano lenses, $n = 1.50$, for a case of aniseikonia, the right lens is made on a base curve of +6.00 D (3.0 mm in thickness). If the left lens (3.00 mm in thickness) is to have a 1% greater overall magnification than the right lens, what should be the base curve of the left lens?

14. An aphakic patient who has been wearing contact lenses of the appropriate power decides to switch to spectacle lenses. A spectacle refraction done at a vertex distance of 12 mm is found to be +14.00 D. In switching from contact lenses to spectacles, what is the *percentage change* in image size?

15. A patient who has been wearing contact lenses of –10.00 D decides to switch to spectacle lenses worn at a vertex distance of 12 mm. If we assume both lenses to be thin, what is the *percentage change* in retinal image size in switching to spectacle lenses from contact lenses?

16. If a lens with a back vertex power of –10.00 D is fit 3.00 mm closer to the face, how much does the magnification approximately change?

17. If a lens with a thickness of 3 mm is made with an increase in front surface curvature of 5.00 D, what is the approximate change in magnification?

18. If a lens with a front surface power of +10.00 D is made 3.00 mm thicker, how much is the magnification changed approximately?

19. A lens with a back vertex power of +12.50 D is 6 mm thick and rests 15 mm from the entrance pupil. The refractive index is 1.50 and the secondary principal plane falls inside the lens 2.0 mm from the back surface. What is the spectacle magnification of the lens?

20. A lens of refractive index 1.50 has a back vertex power of +10.00 D and an equivalent power of +8.00 D. The lens is 8 mm thick and rests 15 mm from the entrance pupil. What is the spectacle magnification of this lens?

21. An afocal size lens is to give a magnification of 5%. The lens is made of glass with a refractive index of 1.50 and an axial thickness of 8 mm. The back pole of the lens rests 20 mm from the entrance pupil. What is the back surface power of the lens?

22. A patient wears a +5.00 D lens, index 1.50, 6.0 mm thick, and a front surface power of +10.00 DS. In addition, the patient requires an eikonic correction, which is temporarily provided by an afocal 5% magnifier mounted in front of the spectacle lens. We wish to design a single lens of +5.00 D, which provides the same magnification effects as the original spectacle lens and the afocal 5% magnifier. The lens rests 15 mm from the entrance pupil. If the back surface of the final correction is –6.00 D, what is the lens thickness?

23. An afocal size lens placed 20 mm from the entrance pupil has a magnification of 5%. If the refractive index is 1.5 and the back surface is –6.00 D,

  (a) What is the thickness?
  (b) What is the front surface power?

CHAPTER ELEVEN

Lenses for High Refractive Errors

Patients who have high refractive errors must contend with a number of problems that do not exist for most spectacle wearers. The most obvious of the problems are the greater thickness and weight of the lenses. Perhaps less obvious is that lenses of high refractive power are subject to aberrations, magnification properties, and visual field limitations that can be extremely annoying to the wearer.

Lens weight tends to be a problem for wearers of high plus lenses, and lens thickness tends to be a problem for wearers of high minus lenses because of the thick edges of these lenses. Magnification and visual field problems exist for wearers of high plus lenses because of the increased magnification and the decreased extent of the visual field of these lenses.

Of patients who have refractive errors in excess of ±10.00 D, the largest group consists of *aphakics*—individuals who have had one or both crystalline lenses removed because of cataracts; these patients require very strong plus lenses. High hyperopia (apart from aphakia) is relatively uncommon; very few people require lenses stronger than +4.00 or +5.00 D. Although very few myopes need lenses in the range of 10.00 D or greater, a considerable number of myopes require lenses stronger than –4.00 or –5.00 D. Fortunately, the practitioner has many methods of reducing lens weight and thickness and of controlling aberrations and magnification.

LENSES FOR APHAKIA AND HIGH HYPEROPIA

Aphakia ("without lens"), a term proposed by Donders,[1] is used to indicate the absence of the crystalline lens from the dioptric system of the eye. The lens is usually removed by surgery, but in some cases aphakia results from trauma that causes the lens to be lost as a result of perforation of the globe or displacement from the pupil (subluxation). Rarely, the lens may be congenitally subluxated or even congentially absent.

11.1. The Cataract Patient

As life expectancy has increased in recent years, the proportion of geriatric patients seen in optometric offices has correspondingly increased. One of the most common causes of acquired visual loss in older patients is cataract; if an individual lives long enough, some form of cataract invariably develops. Not surprisingly, when even a small amount of visual loss has been experienced, a patient may become apprehensive about the possibility of going blind.

Some types of cataracts (particularly nuclear and posterior subcapsular cataracts) can cause a severe visual handicap for distance vision, particularly on a sunny day, even though the patient achieves reasonably good acuity in the practitioner's refracting room. There are two reasons for this: (1) scattering of light by the opacities in the lens is a greater problem outdoors, in bright light, than it is indoors, and (2) as shown in Figure 11–1, the reduced pupil size in bright light tends to limit the bundle of rays available to the retina to the opaque portion of the lens (particularly in the case of a posterior subcapsular cataract, which is located very close to the nodal point of the eye).

In bilateral cataract, surgery is normally done first on the eye with the more advanced cataract to prevent both eyes from being susceptible to complications at the same time; surgery on the second eye is done at a later date.

When the cataract is *unilateral*, the decision whether to recommend surgery is more difficult. If good binocular vision is essential to the patient's normal activities, a unilateral cataract may be operated on at any stage, but the patient will be able to achieve binocular vision only by the use of a contact lens or an intraocular lens. On the other hand, if a unilateral cataract is operated on, and spectacles, rather than a contact lens or an intraocular lens, are used, binocular vision will be impossible. Thus, the operated eye is usually not corrected. This allows suppression of vision for the operated eye.

The rapidly increasing popularity of intraocular lenses has been fostered, to some extent, by the belief of many that aphakic spectacle lenses are thick, heavy, and difficult to adapt to because of the resulting aberrations and high magnifications. Although adaptation to aphakic lenses remains a problem (as indicated in the following sections), improvements in the design of aphakic lenses have occurred at a rapid pace during the past several years—during the same period of time in which both intraocular lenses and extended-wear contact lenses have become increasingly popular.

Unless an intraocular lens has been implanted, the patient is given a pair of single-vision spectacles for temporary wear immediately after surgery. The power of the temporary lenses is usually about +11.00 D. After a period of about 6 weeks, the eyes normally have healed and the corneal curvature has stabilized sufficiently so that permanent aphakic spectacle lenses can be ordered.

11.2. Optical Consequences of Cataract Surgery

There are many optical consequences of cataract surgery, even when no postoperative complications occur, which can affect the patient's visual performance. The cornea may be distorted, which induces against-the-rule or oblique astigmatism. The size, shape, and mobility of the pupil may be affected, which induces aberrations and alters the amount and distribution of light reaching the retina as well as the depth of focus of the eye.

The absence of the lens in the dioptric system of the eye is responsible for some significant changes in visual function. Because the lens is responsible for accommodation, all accommodation is abolished, and the patient is essentially an absolute presbyope (however, apparent accommodation has been claimed to take place in an aphakic patient[2]).

The removal of the crystalline lens also deprives the eye of about one-fourth its refractive power, which usually results in very high hypermetropia. Gullstrand's exact schematic eye has a refracting power of +58.64 D and an anterior focal length of 17.05 mm, but Gullstrand's schematic aphakic eye has a refracting power of +43.05 D (caused by the cornea only) and an anterior focal length of 23.22 mm. The optical system of the aphakic eye is greatly

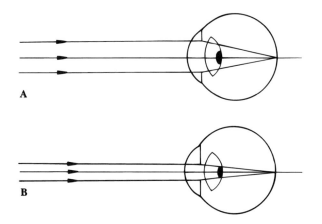

FIGURE 11–1.   **When the pupil is reduced in size because of bright light, the bundle of rays available to the retina may be limited to the opaque portion of the lens, particularly in posterior subcapsular cataract. A, large pupil; B, small pupil, in bright light.**

simplified; essentially it is reduced to a single spherical refracting surface (the cornea) separating air from the aqueous and vitreous humors, which may be regarded as a single medium with a uniform index of refraction. Additional optical problems exist when aphakia is corrected with spectacle lenses. These are discussed in Section 11.4.

11.3. Predicting the Power of an Aphakic Lens

Formulas have been proposed to predict the power of the spectacle lens required postoperatively in aphakia. Laurance[3] estimated that the power of the crystalline lens in the spectacle plane averages about +11.00 D and suggested that the power of a spectacle lens required to correct an aphakic eye could be calculated by the use of the formula

$$F_{aphakic} = +11.00 \text{ D} + \tfrac{1}{2}F_{pre\text{-}aphakic}. \qquad (11.1)$$

Thus, for an eye having 2.00 D of hyperopia before surgery, the required aphakic lens is approximately +12.00 D; for a pre-aphakic eye having 4.00 D of myopia, the required aphakic lens is approximately +9.00 D. Emmetropia is achieved after surgery if the patient is myopic by 22.00 D. Sanders, Retzlaff, and Kraff[4] described a formula for predicting aphakic refraction based on linear regression analysis. Their formula is

$$F_{aphakic} = 80.4 - 1.65 \; L - 0.7 \; K, \qquad (11.2)$$

where L is the axial length of the eye, in millimeters, determined by ultrasonography, and K is the preoperative keratometer finding, in diopters.

This formula correctly predicted, for the patients studied, postoperative spectacle correction to within 1.0 D in 82% of patients (98 of 120 eyes) and to within 2.0 D for 99% of patients (119 of 120 eyes).

11.4. Problems with Aphakic Spectacles

Of the three types of optical devices currently available for the correction of aphakia, spectacle lenses produce the most disturbing visual problems for the wearer. Unlike a contact lens or an intraocular lens, a spectacle lens must be mounted at an appreciable distance from the eye, and it does not move when the eye rotates. Fortunately, most problems caused by aphakic spectacles can be minimized, if not completely solved, by the careful selection of aphakic lenses and frames. Inherent optical defects of convex lenses, which go unnoticed in lenses of low power, become so noticeable in high plus lenses that they cause a number of problems for the wearer. These problems include the following:

1. Increased retinal image size
2. Decreased field of view
3. Presence of a ring scotoma
4. Increased ocular rotations
5. Increased lens aberrations
6. Motion of objects in the field of view
7. Appearance of the wearer
8. Demands on convergence

Each of these problems and their solutions (to the extent that solutions are available) is discussed below.

Increased Retinal Image Size

As discussed in Section 11.2, Gullstrand's schematic emmetropic eye has a refracting power of +58.64 D and an anterior focal length of 17.05 mm, but the aphakic schematic eye has a refracting power of +43.05 D and an anterior focal length of 23.23 mm. If a correcting lens is placed at the anterior focal point of the eye, the size of the retinal image is directly proportional to the anterior focal length and inversely proportional to the refracting power of the eye. That is,

$$\frac{\text{retinal image size in aphakia}}{\text{retinal image size in emmetropia}} = \frac{23.23}{17.05} = \frac{58.64}{43.05}$$
$$= 1.36,$$

or an increase in retinal image size of 36%.

In practice, the lens is placed much closer to the eye than 23.23 mm, and the closer distance decreases the size of the retinal image, but even then the retinal image size is appreciably larger than it would be in the emmetropic phakic eye.

To find the power of the correcting lens required at the anterior focal point of an aphakic eye, the far point of the eye must be located. The length of Gullstrand's schematic eye is 24.38 mm. Therefore, with a refractive power of 43.05 D, the point conjugate to the retina, or the far point of the eye, may be found as follows (Figure 11–2):

$$F = \frac{n'}{l'} - \frac{n}{l},$$

where F = the refracting power of the eye, n' = the index of refraction of the aphakic eye (1.336), l' = the axial length of the eye (24.38 mm), n = the index of refraction of air

FIGURE 11–2. **Diagram for determining the power of the correcting lens for an aphakic eye, based on Gullstrand's schematic eye.**

(1.0), and l = the distance from the far point to the corneal vertex. Hence,

$$43.05 = \frac{1.336}{0.02438} - \frac{1}{l},$$

$$43.05 = 54.80 - \frac{1}{l},$$

and

$$l = \frac{1}{11.75} = 0.085 \text{ m} = 85.0 \text{ mm}.$$

Therefore, the point conjugate to the retina is a virtual object point located 85.0 mm behind the cornea. The distance from this point to the anterior focal point of the eye is

$$85.0 + 23.23 = 108.23 \text{ mm}.$$

The lens needed at the anterior focal point, to correct this aphakic eye, has a power of

$$\frac{1}{0.10823} = +9.24 \text{ D}.$$

If the correcting lens is placed at a vertex distance of 12 mm rather than at the anterior focal point of the eye, the required power is

$$\frac{1}{0.085 - 0.012} = \frac{1}{0.097} = +10.31 \text{ D}.$$

The equivalent power of a thin lens having a power of +10.31 D and a +43.05-D cornea separated by a distance of 12 mm is equal to

$$F_e = F_1 + F_2 - \frac{t}{n} F_1 F_2$$

$$= +10.31 + 43.05 - 0.012(10.31)(43.05)$$

$$= +48.03 \text{ D}.$$

The retinal image size for this aphakic eye is, therefore, equal to

$$\frac{58.64}{48.03} = 1.22,$$

or 1.22 times larger than the retinal image of the schematic emmetropic eye, an increase of 22%.

Thus far, the correcting spectacle lens was considered to be infinitely thin. It is obvious that a lens of approximately +10.00 D, having a diameter of 44 mm or more, is not a thin lens, and, even when the back surface power of the lens is relatively low (about −3.00 D), the front surface power is rather high in a lens of this power. Since the formula for the shape factor is

$$\frac{1}{1 - \frac{t}{n} F_1},$$

it is apparent that both the large thickness value and the steeply curved front surface tend to increase the magnification. For a lens that is 6 mm thick, with a front surface power of +12.00 D, the shape factor is approximately

$$\frac{1}{1 - \frac{0.006}{1.5}(+12)} = \frac{1}{1 - 0.048} = 1.05.$$

The magnitude of the shape factor for high plus lenses cannot be ignored. The total spectacle magnification of the +10.31-D lens with a front surface power of +12.00 D and a center thickness of 6.0 mm, placed at a vertex distance of 12 mm, is therefore equal to

$$SM_T = (1.22)(1.05) = 1.28, \text{ or } 28\%.$$

In bilateral aphakia, if both eyes somewhat resemble Gullstrand's emmetropic eye, the retinal image sizes for the two eyes may be essentially the same, but each is magnified about 28% as compared with the retinal image of the emmetropic eye. The greatly increased magnification means that the aphakic patient must adapt to new size–distance relationships in his or her daily environment—familiar objects not only appear to be much larger, they also appear to be much closer. A unilateral aphakic patient has a more serious problem because the magnification differences between the two eyes make binocular vision impossible with spectacle lenses (discussed further in Section 11.8). Ironically, the same magnification that causes so many problems when aphakia is corrected by a spectacle lens sometimes enables the aphakic patient to achieve central visual acuity that exceeds the best visual acuity obtained before surgery. This single positive outcome of the greatly increased magnification may permit the prescribing of a weaker reading addition than that for the phakic presbyope of the same age and, therefore, extend the range of vision through the bifocal segment and reduce the convergence demand.

Ogle[5] has offered a unique explanation of the magnification effects in an aphakic eye (Figure 11–3). In this figure, (A) represents a normal emmetropic eye in which the crystalline lens has not been removed. The optical result of the removal can be represented as though an infinitely thin minus lens had been inserted at the center of the crystalline lens (B). The resulting hyperopia is then corrected by a convex spectacle lens placed before the eye at a specified distance from the hypothetical minus lens (C). The combination of the convex spectacle lens and the hypothetical concave lens forms an afocal Galilean telescopic system for an otherwise normal eye. The angular magnification of a Galilean telescope, as developed in Chapter 12, Section 12.2, is

$$M = -\frac{f_1}{f_2} = -\frac{F_2}{F_1}, \tag{11.3}$$

where F_1 is the power of the objective lens (the correcting lens, in this case) and F_2 is the power of the eyepiece (the hypothetical minus lens).

of the correcting lens is +10.50 D, then

$$M = \frac{1}{1 - 0.0175(10.50)}$$
$$= \frac{1}{1 - 0.184} = \frac{1}{0.816}$$
$$= 1.23,$$

which is essentially the same magnification as that obtained by using the spectacle magnification formula.

Decreased Field of View

The base-to-the-center prismatic effect of a high plus lens (Figure 11–4) reduces the size of the field of view through the lens, just as the base-to-the-edge prismatic effect increases the size of the field of view through a minus lens.

In discussing the field of view of a spectacle lens, we can think in terms of (1) the peripheral field of view or (2) the macular field of view, or field of fixation. The *peripheral field of view* is the field of view for the steadily fixating eye, subtended at the entrance pupil (Figure 11–5), and is given by

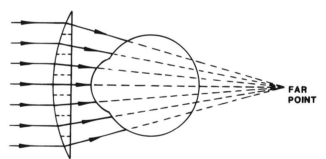

FIGURE 11–4. **A high-powered plus lens acts as a prism, base toward the center, whose power gradually increases toward the periphery.**

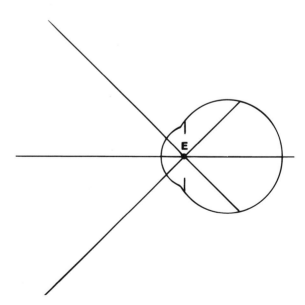

FIGURE 11–5. **The peripheral field of view for a steadily fixating eye, subtended at the center of the entrance pupil.**

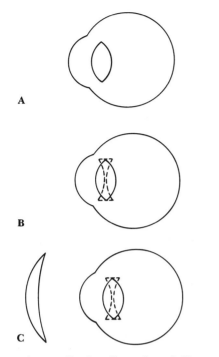

FIGURE 11–3. **The magnification effects of an aphakic eye. A, a normal emmetropic eye before removal of the crystalline lens; B, the optical result of the removal of the lens, represented as an infinitely thin minus lens inserted at the center of the crystalline lens; C, the combination of a convex spectacle lens and the hypothetical concave lens forms a Galilean telescopic system for an otherwise normal eye. (Adapted from K. N. Ogle, *Researches in Binocular Vision*, W. B. Saunders, 1950, p. 258, by permission of Mayo Foundation.)**

For an afocal Galilean telescope, the equivalent power is

$$F_e = F_1 + F_2 - \frac{t}{n} F_1 F_2 = 0,$$

or

$$-F_1 = F_2 - \frac{t}{n} F_1 F_2$$
$$-F_1 = F_2 \left(1 - \frac{t}{n} F_1\right).$$

Substituting for F_1 in Equation 11.3,

$$M = \frac{F_2}{F_2 \left(1 - \frac{t}{n} F_1\right)} = \frac{1}{\left(1 - \frac{t}{n} F_1\right)}.$$

But since $n = 1$,

$$M = \frac{1}{1 - tF_1},$$

where t is the distance between the correcting lens and the hypothetical thin minus lens at the center of the crystalline lens.

If the average distance from the correcting lens to the center of the crystalline lens is 17.5 mm, and if the power the equation

$$\tan\phi = y(E - F),\qquad(11.4)$$

where ϕ = one-half of the angular field of view, y = one-half the lens aperture, in meters, E = the vergence of light at the entrance pupil of the eye, and F = the power of the correcting lens.

On the other hand, *macular field of view* is the field of view for the moving eye, subtended at the center of rotation of the eye (Figure 11–6), and is given by the equation

$$\tan\theta = y(S - F)\qquad(11.5)$$

where θ = one-half of the angular field of view, y = one-half the lens aperture, in meters, S = the vergence of light at the center of rotation of the eye, and F = the power of the correcting lens.

The relationship between the field of view and the field of fixation can be demonstrated by the use of an example.

EXAMPLE

Consider an aphakic patient who requires a +12.50-D spectacle lens with a horizontal width of 50 mm, fitted at a distance of 13 mm from the entrance pupil of the eye and 25 mm from the center of rotation of the eye. What are the peripheral and macular fields of view?
Peripheral field of view:

$$\tan\phi = 0.025(76.92 - 12.50) = 1.6106$$
$$\phi = 58.165°$$
$$2\phi = 116.33°.$$

Macular field of view:

$$\tan\theta = 0.025(40.00 - 12.50) = 0.6875$$
$$\theta = 34.51°$$
$$2\theta = 69.02°.$$

These fields of view may be compared with those for the same eye in the pre-aphakic condition by assuming that the refractive error before surgery was +2.00 D. By substituting +2.00 for +12.50 D in each of

the above equations, the results for the pre-aphakic condition are:
Peripheral field of view:

$$\tan\phi = 0.025(76.92 - 2.00) = 1.873$$
$$\phi = 61.90°$$
$$2\phi = 123.80°.$$

Macular field of view:

$$\tan\theta = 0.025(40.00 - 2.00) = 0.950$$
$$\theta = 43.53°$$
$$2\theta = 87.06°.$$

A comparison of these results with those for the +12.50 D lens shows that the aphakic patient suffers more from loss of macular field of view than from loss of peripheral field of view. The loss of peripheral field is only about 7 degrees, but the loss of macular field is 17 degrees. The loss of both peripheral and macular field of view when a person wears a high plus lens is responsible for the *ring scotoma* (discussed below).

Inspection of Equation 11.5 shows that the macular field of view can be made larger by increasing the size of the lens (increasing the value of y) or by fitting the lens closer to the eye (decreasing the stop distance and therefore the value of S).

Presence of a Ring Scotoma

The presence of a ring scotoma, seen by a wearer of an aphakic lens, may be understood with the help of Figure 11–7. As described previously, the base-toward-the-center prismatic effect of a strong plus lens causes an angular gap in object space completely around the lens; the patient sees nothing either through the lens or beyond the lens unless

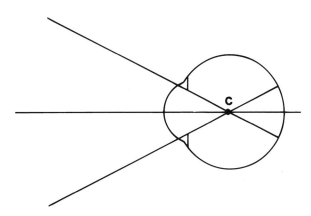

FIGURE 11–6. **The macular field of view for a moving eye, subtended at the center of rotation of the eye.**

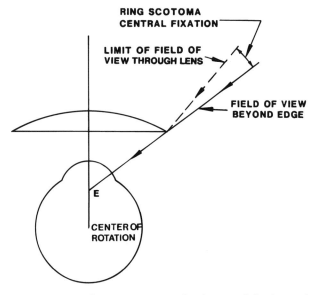

FIGURE 11–7. **Ring scotoma occurring in central fixation (subtended at the center of the entrance pupil) for an aphakic eye.**

a head movement is made. Beyond the scotomatous area the wearer has uncorrected vision, but central to the scotoma the wearer has corrected vision.

The angular size of the gap is equal to the prismatic effect present at the edge of the lens. For example, if an aphakic patient wears a +12.00-D lens, 44 mm wide, centered in front of the center of the pupil, the prismatic effect at the edge of the lens is, according to Prentice's rule,

$$2.2(12) = 26.4 \text{ prism diopters},$$

and the angular extent of the scotoma is approximately 15 degrees.

As the eye rotates, the scotoma moves (hence the term *roving ring scotoma*). As shown in Figure 11–8, the scotoma moves in the direction *opposite* to the direction in which the eyes are moved; as the eye rotates outward, the scotoma moves centrally (inward), and vice versa. The term *jack-in-the-box phenomenon* has been used to describe the way an object seems to jump in and out of the field of view as it moves out of and into the ring scotoma. This event can also occur with a stationary object that can be seen in indirect vision at the periphery of the object field, but the object vanishes into the roving ring scotoma when attempts are made to fixate it directly by rotating the eye. The jack-in-the-box phenomenon also occurs when the eyes are held stationary— an object moving across the field of vision may disappear into the ring scotoma and then appear on the other side of the scotoma, thus apparently popping out of nowhere.

The roving ring scotoma causes little difficulty at a normal reading distance of 40 cm (where it is only 15 degrees wide, extending from 35–50 degrees), and at a distance of 20 feet or beyond (as the range when driving a car); be-

cause the central field is sufficiently wide to allow adequate vision, the scotoma presents no problem. But at *intermediate distances*, especially between about 2 and 10 feet, the ring scotoma often creates a difficult problem. Thus, when the wearer is in an ordinary room, he or she experiences a relatively small area of clear vision enclosed by a wedge of blindness. Moreover, when the eyes move, the wedge-shaped ring of blindness moves also, so that objects or people seem to suddenly appear and disappear. As the eyes move peripherally to fixate an object of attention, the ring scotoma moves in the opposite direction—the wearer does not immediately see the face of another person in the room, clumsily bumps into furniture when moving about, knocks over ashtrays and drinking glasses, stumbles on uneven ground, or misses a step on a flight of stairs with disastrous results. The problems experienced by the spectacle-wearing aphakic are accurately (and amusingly) described in an article by an anonymous aphakic physician.[6]

The following factors have an effect on the size and the position of the ring scotoma:

1. *Lens Power.* The stronger the lens, the larger the ring scotoma.

2. *Vertex Distance.* The farther the lens from the eye, the smaller the ring scotoma. Unfortunately, moving the lens farther out makes the ring scotoma move centrally. Therefore, the closer the vertex distance, the less bothersome the ring scotoma.

3. *Lens Size.* As lens size increases, the ring scotoma increases in size, but it also moves toward the periphery. Increasing the lens size therefore has the same general effect as moving the lens closer to the eye.

4. *Pupil Size.* The smaller the pupil, the larger the ring scotoma.

5. *Lens Thickness.* As the lens thickness increases, so does the magnification and the size of the ring scotoma.

6. *Base Curve.* With increasing steepness of the base curve, both the magnification and the size of the ring scotoma increase.

Increased Ocular Rotations

When a spectacle lens is worn, the angle the eye must turn in changing fixation from one object point to another increases or decreases in comparison with the angle required without the lens (Figure 11–9). The excursions of the eye are increased for plus lenses (A) and decreased for minus lenses (B). The increase or decrease in ocular rotation that occurs with corrective lenses is caused by the presence of *prismatic effects*—the amount of prismatic deviation depending on the power of the lens and the angular separation of the two alternately fixated points.

In plus lenses of the power required for the correction of aphakia, the increase in the amplitude of ocular excursions is significant. Numerically, the increase in ocular rotation exceeds the magnification of the retinal image because the reference point for angular magnification is the entrance pupil of the eye, whereas the reference point for ocular excursions is the center of rotation of the eye.

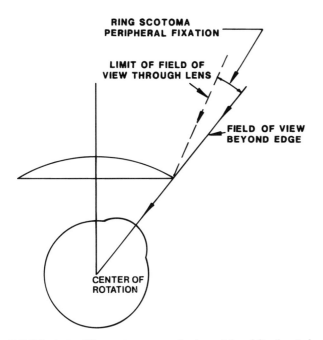

FIGURE 11–8. **Ring scotoma occurring in peripheral fixation (subtended at the center of rotation) for an aphakic eye. Note that the scotoma has moved inward, compared with the scotoma for central fixation shown in Figure 11–7.**

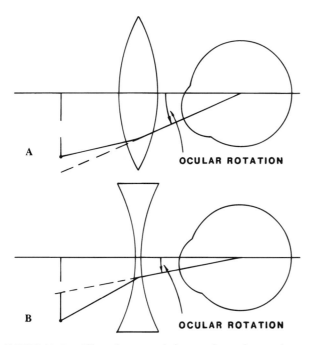

FIGURE 11–9.   **Effect of a spectacle lens on the ocular rotation required to fixate a peripheral object. A, increased for a plus lens; B, decreased for a minus lens.**

Increased Lens Aberrations

As discussed in Chapter 6, any ophthalmic lens is subject to aberrations that degrade the optical image. For plus lenses in the powers needed for the correction of aphakia, the aberrations can be quite severe. These aberrations include:

1. Spherical aberration
2. Coma
3. Oblique astigmatism (or marginal astigmatism)
4. Curvature of image (power error, or mean oblique error)
5. Distortion
6. Chromatic aberration (both axial and transverse)

Some aberrations degrade the image more than others. Spherical aberration and coma occur only for large aperture systems and are ignored by lens designers. Aphakic patients, most of whom have small pupils, are affected very little by these aberrations. However, the off-axis aberrations of oblique astigmatism and curvature of image (mean oblique error) are significant errors that can affect the patient's visual acuity and contrast sensitivity. They are important aberrations, and they are amenable to correction.

As discussed in Chapter 6, to eliminate oblique astigmatism, one may plot a family of *Tscherning ellipses*. For each ellipse, the front or back surface power is plotted as a function of the total refracting power of the lens. The front or back surface required for a particular lens power can be determined by visual inspection of such an ellipse. Similar ellipses can be constructed for zero power error (zero mean oblique error) in which the circle of least confusion of the

image formed by the lens falls on the eye's far-point sphere and, ultimately, on the retina.

The limits of these ellipses are approximately –23.00 D and +8.00 D, depending on a number of factors including (1) whether the lens is designed for zero oblique astigmatism or for zero mean oblique error, (2) the refractive index of the lens, (3) the object distance, and (4) the stop distance (the distance from the lens to the center of rotation of the eye). Outside these limits, neither oblique astigmatism nor mean oblique error can be eliminated if spherical surfaces are used. However, they can be minimized by the judicious selection of spherical surfaces. (See Section 6.10)

For plus lenses above +8.00 D, either oblique astigmatism or power error can be eliminated by making at least one of the surfaces aspheric, but both cannot be eliminated with the same choice of curves. Thus, if oblique astigmatism is eliminated, substantial power error exists; if the power error is eliminated, substantial oblique astigmatism is present. Hence, the lens designer must consider the two aberrations together and attempt to reach a balance between them. The same problem exists when spherical surfaces are used for lens powers falling within the range of Tscherning's ellipse.

As discussed in Chapter 6, Section 6.20, *aspheric surfaces* are rotationally symmetrical surfaces whose cross sections are noncircular. It should be noted that *toric* surfaces form circular cross sections in their principal meridians and, therefore, are not considered as aspheric. Most aspheric surfaces used for ophthalmic lens design are *conicoid* surfaces, obtained by rotating a conic section (ellipse, parabola, or hyperbola) about an axis of symmetry of the conic. The *circle* is considered to be a special case of the ellipse.

Smith and Bailey[7] presented the following mathematical formulation of the conic section:

$$C[Y + (1 + Q)x^2] - 2x = 0$$

where x is the axis of revolution, C is the curvature of the surface at the origin, or vertex $(0,0)$, and Q is a quantity that specifies the type of conicoid, its shape, and degree of asphericity. The type of conicoid can be determined from the value of Q as follows:

$Q < -1$	Hyperboloid
$Q = -1$	Paraboloid
$-1 < Q < 0$	Ellipsoid with the x-axis as the major axis
$Q = 0$	Sphere
$Q > 0$	Ellipsoid with the y-axis as the major axis

For ophthalmic lenses, it is convenient to designate the *x-axis* as the optical axis and C as the curvature in the paraxial region.

Currently, there are two different approaches to the design of aspheric surfaces for ophthalmic lenses. One approach is to manufacture the surface as a *continuous* aspheric surface, as is done with the Signet Armorlite Alfa Full Field lens. The curvature of such a surface reduces continuously from the center toward the edge. The curvature reduction results in a drop in power toward the edge, as shown in Figure 11–10.

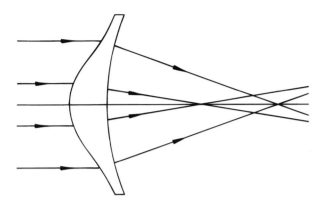

FIGURE 11–10. **The reduced curvature toward the periphery of an aspheric lens results in a drop in refracting power.**

In the other approach, the lens surface is made up of a series of different zones arranged in an annular pattern about the center; each zone is essentially spherical but has progressively decreasing surface power the farther the zone is from the center. To eliminate any obvious dividing lines on the surface, the tangents to the curves of adjacent zones are arranged to coincide to the boundary between adjacent zones, and the junctions between adjacent zones are smoothed by polishing with flexible pads. Such a surface is known as a *zonal* aspheric. The Signet Armorlite Multiple Drop lens, previously known as the Welsh Four-Drop lens, is an example of this design. Zonal aspherics can be ground and finished with tools used for working spherical surfaces. The surfaces of the glass molds used for casting the front surfaces of CR-39 aspheric lenses are formed by a series of spherical generator cuts.

The continuous aspheric surface can be analyzed by conventional third-order aberrational theory if a mathematical description of the surface is available. It is difficult to analyze the zonal aspheric surface unless the zonal surface powers and the outer and inner zonal diameters are known and the radial surface powers of the zones are constant.

Smith and Atchison[8] showed that for a lens having an aspheric front surface in the form of a conicoid, the third-order solution for *oblique astigmatism* is a cubic equation. Therefore, for any front surface asphericity and equivalent lens power, there are one, two, or three solutions for the back surface power for which oblique astigmatism is essentially zero. The results for the elimination of third-order *mean oblique error* (power error) show the same trends as those for the elimination of third-order oblique astigmatism. However, in both cases, the back surface power is often too steep for the solutions to be of practical value.

Distortion, a term frequently misused in describing undesirable optical effects, results from changing magnification across the field of view of a lens. With distortion, the shape, size, or both, of an object is not faithfully reproduced. For an aphakic patient wearing high plus lenses, distortion creates the familiar *pincushion* effect, which causes straight lines to look curved, and the apparent location of an object changes as the observer's eye turns to a different portion of the lens. This happens because of magnification changes. Distortion causes some of the navigational diffi-

culties so vividly described in the literature by aphakic patients. Control of distortion requires steeply curved lenses, which are unsightly and difficult to manufacture. Fortunately, design factors that minimize oblique astigmatism and power error (mean oblique error) also decrease distortion. There is some evidence that newly corrected aphakic patients can adapt quickly to some lens distortion.[9]

Axial and transverse chromatic aberration cannot be eliminated when only a single refractive medium is used. Transverse chromatic aberration is the more bothersome of the two and occurs because the image locations (from axial chromatic aberration) and magnifications differ for different wavelengths. It affects primarily the tangential meridian of oblique astigmatism. Therefore, by controlling the tangential error, the effect of transverse chromatic aberration can be attenuated.

Hence, the aberrations of oblique astigmatism and curvature of image are the most important and have been the main targets of the lens designer. Secondary attention has been directed toward the correction of distortion, which is still a significant aberration in current aspheric lens designs (although considerably less so than in a lens having spherical curves on both the front and back surfaces).[10]

Motion of Objects in the Field of View

When a wearer of high plus lenses holds the eyes steady and moves the head to look at any object not in direct view, a marked reversed motion of the field of view (an "against" motion) is experienced. This motion is often referred to as *swim*. Swim occurs when the field from which the visual axes are moving away is seen in indirect vision, through progressively peripheral portions of the lens with the prismatic base in the direction of the head movement (Figure 11–11).

Swim can be avoided by moving the eyes from one fixation point to another while the head is held stationary; however, this action may produce distortion effects. The best procedure is to turn the head slowly, so that the head and eyes move simultaneously.

Appearance

Among the strong objections to cataract lenses has been the matter of appearance. The appearance of an aphakic spectacle wearer may convey two impressions. The first impression is that of the apparent enlargement of the eyes and their unusual appearance behind bulbous, thick lenses. The second impression is the general awkwardness of the patient's bearing and movements. Both these impressions originate from the magnification and distortion effects of the lenses. The high plus lens required for the aphakic eye causes a large amount of angular magnification, no matter in which direction one looks through the lens. The magnification and distortion of the image experienced by the patient alter the behavior in the environment to the extent that the patient's bearing seems awkward to others.

Aphakic lenses of *lenticular* construction present a particularly bothersome appearance. Such a lens provides the

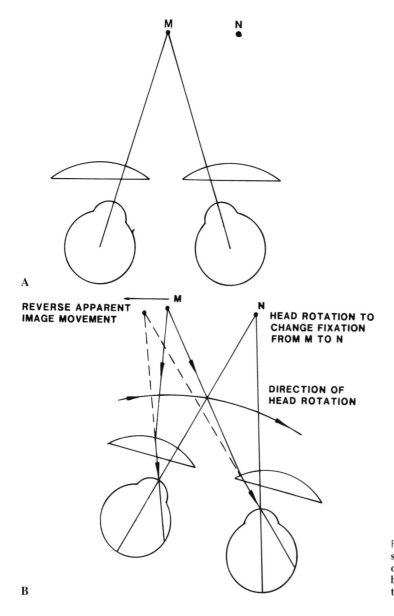

A

REVERSE APPARENT
IMAGE MOVEMENT

HEAD ROTATION TO
CHANGE FIXATION
FROM M TO N

DIRECTION OF
HEAD ROTATION

B

FIGURE 11–11. **Swim, occurring when the eyes are held steady fixating an object, M, and the head moves to look at an object, N, not in direct view. There is a reverse motion, caused by a prismatic effect, with the base of the prism in the direction of the head movement.**

patient's prescription only in the central portion of the lens, as shown in Figure 11–12; the peripheral portion is thin and lightweight and is not optically useful; it serves only as a carrier for the central portion. These lenses provide good optical performance in the central portion, which is usually 30 to 40 mm in diameter, and are lighter in weight than full-field lenses. However, they have a poor cosmetic appearance. Because the magnification is confined to the central portion of the lens, a "bull's eye" or "fried egg" appearance is typically produced. This identifies the wearer as an individual who has a very serious eye defect.

Demands on Convergence

If the distance centers of aphakic lenses are placed in front of the centers of the wearer's pupils, convergence of the visual axes toward a near fixation point creates a *base-out* pris-

matic effect. Because of this base-out effect, the eyes, when reading, must converge considerably more than that for a wearer of lenses of low power. This can place a strain on positive fusional vergence and may lead to discomfort. The effect can be reduced if the distance centers are placed closer together than the patient's distance PD. This change produces a slight base-in effect at distance vision but relieves the load on positive fusional vergence at near vision. This practice is particularly recommended when the patient is exophoric at distance.

11.5. Parameters of Aphakic Lenses

In addition to the unique optical phenomena and effects that occur with aphakic lenses of high power, there are lens specifications (including bend and asphericity) and wearing parameters of spectacles that influence the diop-

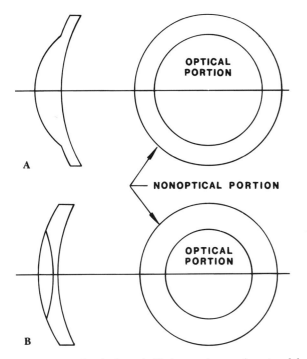

FIGURE 11–12.   **Lenticular aphakic lenses. A, one-piece (used for plastic lenses); B, fused (used for glass lenses).**

tric value and the visual efficacy of the prescription. These factors can alter the prescription by significant amounts, and they demand the same meticulous attention to detail as do those for cataract surgery, refractive technique, and lens design. These critical lens specifications and fitting parameters include vertex distance, pantoscopic tilt, centration, lens weight and thickness, and adjustment of the spectacles.

Vertex Distance

Because most aphakic lenses are of very high plus power, even a small variation in the position of the lens before an aphakic eye produces a substantial change in the optical effect. To correct the ametropia properly, aphakic lenses should be fitted at the vertex distance that was used during the refraction. If the vertex distance must be different because of the structure of the patient's face or because of the style of the frame, compensation in the power must be made by using the effective power formula (see Chapter 3, Section 3.6).

As discussed earlier, if a plus lens is moved toward the eye, the secondary focal length must be shortened by the distance the lens has been moved, which makes the lens stronger. If the plus lens is moved farther from the eye, the secondary focal length must be lengthened by the distance moved, which makes the lens weaker. For example, if a +12.00 D lens is moved 3 mm closer to the eye, the new focal length of the lens is

$$\frac{1}{12} - 0.003 = 0.083 - 0.003 = 0.080 \text{ m},$$

and the power of the lens is

$$\frac{1}{0.08} = +12.50 \text{ D}.$$

For a plus lens, an identical amount of movement closer to the eye causes a greater refractive change than that which occurs when the lens is moved farther from the eye.

Not only does the effective power of the lens change when the position of the lens is changed, but the size of the retinal image changes also, as discussed in Chapter 10, Section 10.9. With a plus lens, the image is made smaller as the vertex distance is decreased, even though the power of the lens must be made stronger. Section 11.4 showed that, in an aphakic eye, the size of the retinal image is 36% larger than that in the normal eye if the correction (+9.34 D) is placed at the anterior focal point of the aphakic eye. However, if the lens is moved to 12 mm from the cornea, the power of the lens must be +10.31 D, but the size of the retinal image is only 22% larger than that for the normal emmetropic phakic eye.

Pantoscopic Tilt

All lenses perform best and provide the widest field of view with minimum aberrations when the optic axis of the correcting lens passes through the center of rotation of the eye. This means that when the visual axis of the eye passes through the optical center of the lens, the visual axis and the optic axis of the lens coincide. All lens designers assume that lenses will be worn so that this occurs.

Usually, spectacle lenses are tilted around a horizontal axis to improve their appearance on the wearer's face. The amount of tilt is typically 8 or 10 degrees (as discussed in Chapter 2, Section 2.20 and illustrated in Figure 2–46); the optical center should be lowered 0.5 mm for every degree of pantoscopic tilt so that the optic axis passes through the center of rotation of the eye. However, in aphakic lenses we must *reverse* this procedure. To minimize thickness and weight, the optical center of the lens should fall at the geometric center, and the optic axis should be made to pass through the center of rotation by altering the vertical position of the frame on the face and by adjusting the pantoscopic tilt. The reversed procedure provides minimum weight and thickness of the lens in addition to proper optical performance.

If the optic axis of the lens does not pass through the center of rotation, then the visual axis is oriented obliquely to the optic axis when the person looks through the optical center, with the result that the effective power of the prescription is changed. With lenses of low power, the induced changes are very small, but with aphakic lenses of high power, the induced changes are significant.

Because the correct prescription is found when the lenses are verified by means of a lensometer, the induced changes are often overlooked as a source of trouble. Formulas for calculating the induced changes when the optic axis of the lens fails to pass through the center of rotation of the eye are given in Chapter 2, Section 2.20.

Positions of Optical Centers

Special care must be taken to determine the distance and near PD accurately. Small errors in PD measurements produce significant effects on aphakic lenses. The monocular PD should be taken, preferably by a method of corneal reflection, to determine the positions of the visual axes. The visual axis does not usually pass through the center of the pupil, even in phakic eyes, and this may be especially true when, as a result of cataract surgery, the pupil is irregular or deformed.

Weight and Thickness

Lenses that correct aphakia are thick and heavy. Weight can be reduced by using CR-39 plastic, but because of its lower index of refraction, lens thickness may increase slightly. Thickness can be reduced by using high-index glass, but the weight remains about the same and the chromatic aberration almost doubles. The use of lenticular aphakic lenses reduces both thickness and weight, but these lenses are not acceptable to some patients because of their unattractive appearance. Lens thickness and weight can be minimized by using frames with symmetrical (and small) eye sizes, placing the optical center at the geometric center of the lens, and ordering the lenses with essentially knife-edge thickness.

Spectacle Adjustments

It is often difficult to maintain aphakic spectacles in the proper position. Because they are heavy, they tend to slip down on the nose. Once the spectacles are removed from the face, the patient has difficulty seeing them, and, in groping for them, they are often knocked to the floor. They rarely break, but are easily bent out of adjustment.

Small changes in position and alignment introduce large errors that greatly reduce the visual efficiency of an already precarious optical system. Frequent office visits should be scheduled so that the frames can be realigned and readjusted to provide the patient with optimal vision and comfort.

11.6. Aphakic Lens Design

The design of spectacle lenses for aphakia has improved during the past decade. Design improvements have occurred as a result of the availability of new lens materials and manufacturing processes and as a result of a better understanding on the part of lens designers of the optimal performance requirements for lenses of high plus power. It is ironic that the important advances in aphakic spectacle lens designs have occurred in tandem with the rapidly increasing popularity of extended-wear contact lenses and intraocular lenses for the correction of aphakia. Advances in aphakic lens design can be considered in terms of the achievement of the following design goals:

1. Reducing lens weight
2. Reducing lens thickness
3. Reducing spectacle magnification
4. Increasing the field of view
5. Minimizing lens aberrations
6. Offering choice of optimum multifocal style and position
7. Providing protection from glare and ultraviolet radiation

Each design goal and methods used to achieve it is discussed below.

Reducing Lens Weight

Reducing lens weight is undoubtedly the easiest goal to achieve, simply by using plastic rather than glass for the manufacture of aphakic lenses. Because CR-39 material has a specific gravity of 1.32 compared with 2.54 for crown glass, the use of this material provides a saving of lens weight close to 50%. Although newer plastic materials (such as polycarbonate, which has a higher index of refraction and a lower specific gravity than those of CR-39) are available, almost all currently available aphakic lenses are made of CR-39 material. An additional method of reducing lens weight involves the restriction of frames to small eye sizes, which makes possible the use of lenses of less weight.

Reducing Lens Thickness

Although lens thickness is to some extent a cosmetic problem, a reduction in lens thickness not only reduces lens weight but, as already noted, reduces the magnification brought about by the lens.

LENTICULAR-APHAKIC LENSES
As described in Section 11.5, an early method of reducing lens thickness was the use of a lenticular form, with the optical zone of the lens having a diameter of 30 to 40 mm, surrounded by a nonoptical carrier lens. For many years, glass aphakic lenses were made in lenticular form, and some plastic lenses are also made in this form. The disadvantage of a lenticular lens is that it gives the wearer's eyes a "bull' eye" or "fried egg" appearance, which calls attention to the visual anomaly.

FULL-DIAMETER ASPHERIC LENSES
Most full-diameter plastic lenses for aphakia are currently made with an aspheric front surface. This construction not only reduces the effects of aberrations but also reduces lens thickness and weight. To keep lens thickness to a minimum, frames with large eye sizes must be avoided. Davis and Torgersen[11] pointed out that more thickness and weight reduction occurs by decreasing the eye size as little as 2 mm than by making a spherical lens aspheric and retaining the same size.

Reducing Spectacle Magnification

As shown by inspection of the spectacle magnification formula (Chapter 10, Equation 10.8), magnification can be reduced by reducing lens thickness or by flattening the front curve of the lens. Atchison and Smith[12] found that aphakic lenses with flat back surfaces and aspheric front surfaces reduce spectacle magnification and look more attractive compared with lenses with steeper forms. However, the amount of asphericity (power drop) seems insufficient to markedly improve peripheral visual performance. Reducing vertex distance also reduces spectacle magnification, and, as already noted, moves the ring scotoma farther out, which makes it less bothersome.

Benton and Welsh[13] recommended *minimal effective diameter* (MED) fitting for aphakic lenses. This term means that the frame size (eye size plus DBL) is chosen to ensure that the frame PD is equal to the patient's distance PD, so that no decentration is required, and so that the lenses can be ground with knife-thin edges. As shown in Figure 11–13, if an aphakic patient is fitted with a modern, large-size frame requiring several millimeters of inward decentration, the center thickness of the lenses must be considerably greater than if no decentration were necessary. In the event that the frame PD cannot be made to exactly match the patient's distance PD, it is usually best to select a frame PD that is slightly *narrower* than the patient's PD and not to decenter the lenses. This creates base-in prism, which helps to reduce the expected exophoria at near.

Increasing the Field of View

The field of view can be increased by fitting the lens at as close a vertex distance as possible. Increasing the lens size also helps (but also adds thickness, weight, and magnification). As already mentioned, reducing vertex distance and increasing lens size both increase the size of the ring scotoma, but this is of little concern because the scotoma

is moved farther out into the periphery. The field of view is also increased by the use of an aspheric front surface, which reduces the power in the periphery of the lens.

Minimizing Lens Aberrations

When discussing the aberrations of oblique astigmatism, curvature of image, and distortion, we are concerned with the aberrations experienced when the eye rotates (using macular vision) to look through a peripheral point in the lens—not with the peripheral field of view of the stationary eye. Varying the form (or bend) of the lens and the use of an aspheric front surface are the designer's principal tools in controlling these aberrations.

As indicated in the discussion of spectacle magnification in Chapter 10, the goals of reducing spectacle magnification and reducing lens aberrations are at odds with one another when it comes to manipulating the form (i.e., the base curve selection) of the lens. Although a base curve of about –20.00 D is effective in minimizing distortion, both the magnification and the appearance of such a lens is unacceptable.

The aberrations encountered on peripheral gaze through lenses with spherical surfaces are large—as large as a few diopters of error at 30 degrees of obliquity, as noted by Whitney.[14] The tangential errors are the largest, with the additive effect of transverse chromatic aberration. A steeper back surface curve (–3.50 D) has the advantage of reducing distortion, lens reflections, and sensitivity to differences in vertex distance. Shallower back surface curves (for example, –1.75 D) reduce both lens thickness and spectacle magnification and help compensate for the power increase as frames slip forward.

The use of an aspheric surface does much more than help control peripheral aberrations. By allowing greater control over the lens periphery, an aspheric surface can provide a greater visual field, reduce lens weight and thickness, reduce magnification, reduce the size of the ring scotoma, and improve the appearance of the lens.

The degree of asphericity (power drop) should be varied with lens power. Ideally, a different aspheric surface should be used for each increment of spherical power. Good lens design requires a wide variety of aspheric lens blanks—the number of aspheric front curves available is one index of the quality of an aphakic lens series.

Important Note. The term *base curve* has taken on a slightly different meaning for aspheric aphakic lenses than the one used for ordinary spherical lenses. Traditionally, the term *base curve* refers to the standardized curvature for a series of lens powers. The same concept applies to aspheric lens design, but the degree of asphericity varies on the basis of base curve. Hence, in aspheric lens design, the number of base curves not only indicates the number of different central curvatures available but also indicates the number of degrees of asphericity.

It is unfortunate that some lens manufacturers have implied that the performance of an aphakic lens depends *solely* on the amount of asphericity, or power drop. Many factors must be considered when one judges the quality of the

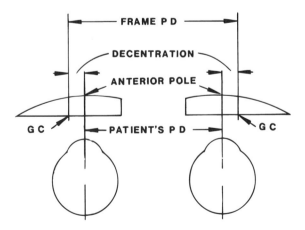

FIGURE 11–13. **If an aphakic patient is fitted with a large-size frame requiring inward decentration, the thickness of each lens (both at the center and at the nasal edge) is greater than if the lenses had not been decentered (GC = geometric center).**

image produced by a strong plus lens. These include errors of sphere (curvature of image), cylinder (oblique astigmatism), and distortion for direct foveal vision and for specified angles of gaze, as well as distortion for indirect peripheral vision.

The choice of aphakic lenses should be based on (1) accurate technical information, with *numerical* detail, and (2) the *number* of base curves, with instructions on how they should be used. Table 11–1 lists some of the current full-field aspheric bifocal aphakic lenses, with the number of base curves and the segment type. All the lenses are CR-39 plastic with an index of refraction of 1.498 to 1.499, an Abbe value of 57.8, and a specific gravity of 1.32.

Choice of Multifocal Style and Position

Most plastic aspheric full-diameter multifocal aphakic lenses are made up in the form of either round or straight-top bifocals (note that although the segment looks very much like a fused segment, it is actually a one-piece segment). Although the front surface of the lens is aspheric, the segment surface is *spherical.* This has important implications for the shape of the segment.

ROUND SEGMENTS

The round segments used in aphakic lenses are usually not perfectly round because the segment shape is modified by the intersection of the spherical segment surface with the aspheric surface of the distance portion of the lens. The result is a pleasant oval shape, which widens more rapidly than a circular segment as the eyes are lowered.

The round segment has several desirable attributes in aphakic lenses. First, there is a reduction in the total prismatic displacement at the reading level because the base-down effect of the segment balances some of the base-up prismatic effect caused by the distance portion of the lens. An aspheric front surface has rotational symmetry because it has a center (pole) of its own. The inside surface should be centered directly behind the pole of the front surface so that the optical center falls at the pole of the aspheric surface. With round-top segments, the bifocal inset may be customized by rotating the lens about the center of the aspheric curve, which moves the segment center laterally to the desired position without changing the segment height significantly. In this manner, the correct bifocal inset can be obtained without altering the distance center and the optics of the aspheric surface.

STRAIGHT-TOP SEGMENTS

The straight-top bifocal segment is relatively wide at the top, has very little image jump as the line of sight enters the segment, and has practically no differential displacement occurring at the reading level. However, unlike round segments, straight-top segments are manufactured with *predetermined* segment inset relative to the center of the aspheric surface. If the prescription is fabricated in such a way as to alter that inset, the distance optical center does not coincide with the center of the aspheric surface, and the patient does not get the full benefit of the aspheric design.

Because of the increasing amount of oblique astigmatism induced as the visual axis moves downward through the lens, bifocal segments for aphakic lenses should be set as high as possible. This applies both to round and to straight-top segments. It is usually a good idea to make the addition as weak as possible, to lessen the demand for convergence and to increase the "arm's length" range through the segment. For vision at closer than the usual reading distance, clear vision may be obtained by pushing the glasses down (only a few millimeters) on the nose.

Segment Inset

For the reading fields for the two eyes to coincide, aphakic lenses may require a larger amount of inset than one would ordinarily provide. American Optical[15] has provided a table, reproduced here as Table 11–2, showing the amount of inset required for the two reading fields to coincide, based on the patient's distance PD, the distance prescription, and the reading distance.

TABLE 11–1
Representative Plastic Full-Field Aphakic Bifocal Lenses

Manufacturer	Lens	Number of Base Curves	Segment Type
Armorlite Signet	Multiple Drop	3	22 round
		3	22 straight-top
	Hyperaspheric	4	22 round
		4	22 straight-top
	Alfa Full Field	3	22 round
		3	22 straight-top
Bristol C&D	Post-Cataract	3	25 straight-top
Bristol	Full Field Post-Cataract	3	22 round
Rodenstock	Perfastar Bifo 22	7	22 round
Silor	Super-Modular Aspheric	5	22 round
Sola	Hi-Drop	4	22 round
		4	22 straight-top
Vision-Ease	High-Base 22mm CFR	7	22 round

TABLE 11–2
Amount of Segment Inset for Each Lens Required for the Two Reading Fields to Coincide, for a Lens Having a –3.00-D Back Surface and a Stop Distance of 27 mm

| Lens Power | | +10.00 D | | +12.00 D | | +14.00 D | | +16.00 D | |
Reading Distance (cm)		33	40	33	40	33	40	33	40
Distance PD (mm)	56	3.5	2.9	3.9	3.3	4.4	3.7	5.0	4.2
	60	3.7	3.1	4.2	3.5	4.7	4.0	5.3	4.5
	64	4.0	3.4	4.4	3.8	5.0	4.2	5.7	4.8
	68	4.2	3.6	4.7	4.0	5.3	4.5	6.0	5.1
	72	4.5	3.8	5.0	4.2	5.6	4.8	6.5	5.4

SOURCE: Adapted from *Optical, Cosmetic and Mechanical Properties of Ophthalmic Lenses*, Lens Information Kit, Table of Seg Insets, American Optical Co., p. 4.201, 1968.

Because an aphakic patient is unable to accommodate, when wearing aphakic bifocals, the patient is limited to the ranges of clear vision provided by the depth of focus surrounding each of the two focal powers. Consequently, it would seem that the aphakic patient would be an ideal candidate for a trifocal. On the contrary, trifocals are almost useless in aphakia and are not recommended. The presence of the intermediate segment requires an excessive downward eye movement to reach the near segment, with the result that the prismatic effects and aberrations at the reading level preclude useful vision. An exception to this general rule is a patient who was myopic before surgery and who requires a distance correction no greater than +8.00 D.

Some older, senile aphakics, who would be in danger of stumbling if bifocals were used, may be fitted with single-vision lenses for distance vision and a separate pair of glasses in the form of bifocals or single-vision glasses for reading. The patient should be instructed that, when the reading glasses are not available, reading may be done for short periods of time by pushing the distance glasses downward on the nose.

Protection from Glare and Ultraviolet Radiation

In answers to a questionnaire presented to 13 spectacle-wearing aphakics by Atchison,[16] *glare* was ranked as the second worst perceptual disturbance (ranking just behind the reduced visual field). When asked in the same questionnaire to identify the factors most important in spectacle lens design, glare again ranked second (again, the reduced visual field ranked first). These findings are understandable; as the eye ages, the crystalline lens becomes increasingly yellow, which causes a significant decrease in the transmission of visible light. After removal of the lens, the eye therefore is more sensitive to visible radiation simply because more of it reaches the retina.

In addition to being a filter for visible light, the crystalline lens contains pigments that act as an ultraviolet radiation filter and prevent much of the radiation from reaching the retina. Removal of the crystalline lens subjects the retina to potential ultraviolet radiation damage for two reasons: (1) In the absence of the lens, the cornea concentrates radiant energy in such a way that the retina receives an increased amount of radiation per unit area; (2) the coefficient of absorption by the retina is greater for ultraviolet radiation than that for visible light. Ham, Muller, and Sliney[17] showed that near ultraviolet radiation and short wavelengths of the visible spectrum can produce retinal damage; Lerman[18] suggested that cystoid macular edema, which has a high incidence in aphakia, may be due to increased ultraviolet radiation reaching the retina.

Although there is disagreement as to the desirable cutoff point for ultraviolet radiation, it would seem that a lens that filters out most ultraviolet radiation below 400 nm and progressively transmits wavelengths between 400 and 500 nm would eliminate most of the near ultraviolet radiation and visible wavelengths that are potentially harmful.

In addition to the ultraviolet-absorbing filter, an aphakic patient may wish to have one of the light tints for general wear. Such a tint has the further advantage of improving the appearance of the lenses. If the patient complains of discomfort when outdoors, a separate pair of prescription sunglasses that contain an ultraviolet absorber should be provided. Ultraviolet-absorbing lenses are discussed in Chapter 7.

11.7. Frames for Aphakic Lenses

A sturdy, lightweight, easily adjustable frame is required for aphakic lenses. Usually the best frame to select is either a metal frame or a combination plastic and metal frame. Frames with thick eyewires should be avoided because an eyewire may increase the width of the ring scotoma. Adjustable pads are a necessity, and for most patients jumbo pads are recommended. The pads should be adjusted so that the lenses fit as close to the eyes as possible (consistent with the wearer's facial features).

To meet the criterion of minimal effective diameter, the patient should be encouraged not only to select a frame with a relatively small eye size, but also to select one having a relatively symmetrical lens shape with no pronounced upsweep and no sharp angles. A useful guide for symmetry is that the effective diameter (ED) of the frame should be no more than 2 mm greater than the marked eye size (the *A* dimension of the box system). A frame so selected ensures that there is little variation in thickness of the lens edge, and if the lens edge is made as thin as possible, the lens has optimal appearance and lightness of weight. To avoid decentration, the frame PD should match the patient's PD.

For a patient with a narrow PD, to keep from making the eye size smaller than necessary, the bridge (DBL) should be kept as narrow as physically possible, which allows the lenses to be as large as possible for the required frame PD. For a patient who has a wide PD, the eye size can be kept relatively small by making the DBL larger than usual.

If a patient insists on a stylish frame, lens thickness can be kept to a minimum only by using lenticular lenses. The practitioner or dispenser should keep on hand an assortment of attractive sample frames that can be used with aphakic lenses.

11.8. The Unilateral Aphakic

The principal problem associated with the correction of unilateral aphakia by spectacles is the difference in the sizes of the retinal images of the two eyes. A second difficulty is the large differential prismatic effects encountered in the peripheral portions of the lenses. As shown in Section 11.4, the spectacle magnification brought about by a typical aphakic spectacle lens is approximately 30%. For the *bilateral* aphakic, this amount of spectacle magnification can be tolerated, after a period of adaptation, because it is essentially the same for both eyes, but for the *unilateral* aphakic, the magnification difference for the two eyes is so great that binocular vision is impossible.

Suppose, for example, that the aphakic eye of a unilateral aphakic patient required the lens described in the example in Section 11.4—a lens with a back vertex power of +13.00 D, a front surface power of +16.00 D, a center thickness of 8.0 mm, an index of refraction of 1.498, and a vertex distance of 10 mm, which created a spectacle magnification of 31.5%. Suppose also that the patient's unoperated eye required a lens having a back vertex power of +2.00 D, a front surface power of +8.00 D, a center thickness of 2.0 mm, an index of refraction of 1.498, and a vertex distance of 10 mm. The spectacle magnification brought about by this lens is

$$SM = \left(\frac{1}{1 - \frac{t}{n} F_1} \right) \left(\frac{1}{1 - hF_V} \right)$$

$$= \left(\frac{1}{1 - \frac{0.002(8)}{1.498}} \right) \left(\frac{1}{1 - 0.013(2)} \right)$$

$$= (1.011)(1.0267) = 1.038$$

$$\%SM = +3.8\%.$$

The difference between the spectacle magnifications for the two lenses is therefore 31.5 − 3.8, or 27.7%. Manipulation of the base curve, thickness, and so forth, of either lens would bring about only an insignificant decrease in this difference. The substantial amount of aniseikonia together with the differential peripheral prismatic effects for the two eyes that occur when a unilateral aphakic wears spectacle lenses are responsible for disturbances in sensory and motor fusion and in stereoscopic spatial projection, which makes binocular vision impossible.

The large magnification difference for the spectacle-wearing unilateral aphakic is manifested by a difference in the *rate of movement* across the visual field of the images of objects seen by the two eyes. The confusing movement of diplopic images is apparently what makes the magnification difference intolerable to the patient. The practitioner, however, has three options—not correct the operated eye, prescribe a "balance" lens or an "occluder" lens for the unoperated eye, or prescribe a *contact lens* for the aphakic eye.

Most patients tend to resist wearing no correcting lens before the operated eye or wearing a balance lens or an occluder lens before the unoperated eye. However, if the visual acuity of the corrected unoperated eye is still reasonably good (e.g., 20/40), the problems of adjusting to an aphakic lens are such that the patient may be much happier to see with the unoperated eye than with the operated eye. Inasmuch as unilateral aphakia is in many cases only temporary because an operation is scheduled for the second eye in the near future, the patient may have to suffer the inconvenience of being monocular for only a relatively short period of time. However, in cases in which the monocular situation is to be relatively permanent, and when an intraocular lens has been ruled out, the best method of achieving binocular vision is to fit a contact lens on the aphakic eye.

In Section 11.4 a +10.31-D spectacle lens was needed at a vertex distance of 12 mm to correct an eye that was the optical equivalent of Gullstrand's schematic eye before surgery. If a contact lens were used to correct such an eye, its power would be

$$\frac{1}{0.097 - 0.012} = \frac{1}{0.085} = +11.76 \text{ D}.$$

The resulting power of this aphakic schematic eye, corrected with a contact lens, would be the sum of the power of the contact lens and the power of the cornea; thus,

$$+11.76 \text{ D} + 43.05 \text{ D} = +54.81 \text{ D}.$$

Since the size of the retinal image is inversely proportional to the refracting power of the eye,

$$\frac{\text{retinal image size corrected by a contact lens}}{\text{retinal image size in emmetropia}} = \frac{+58.64}{+54.81} = 1.07.$$

Hence, there is a retinal image size difference of 7% between the Gullstrand schematic aphakic eye corrected with a contact lens and the Gullstrand emmetropic schematic eye.

Ogle[19] stated that individuals are rarely found who have binocular vision in the presence of aniseikonia greater than 5 or 6%. This figure indicates that, in cases of unilateral aphakia corrected by a contact lens, the amount of residual aniseikonia makes normal binocular vision difficult, if not impossible. Yet, many unilateral aphakic patients corrected with contact lenses appear to have comfortable vision.

The actual amount of residual aniseikonia present in unilateral aphakia corrected with contact lenses depends on the following factors:

1. The refractive error present before the onset of the cataract in the aphakic eye together with the origin of the ametropia (axial or refractive). This is the most important factor.

2. The refractive error in the phakic (unoperated) eye, as well as its origin (axial or refractive) and whether it is corrected by a spectacle lens or a contact lens.

3. Any alteration of the power of the cornea caused by the surgery.

4. The individual variations in the dimensions of the primary refracting components of the eye in question, which often differ greatly from those of the standard schematic eye (and make calculations on the basis of the schematic eye misleading).

5. The shape factor of the spectacle magnification formula. This is often considered to be equal to unity because the lens (either spectacle or contact) is considered as a thin lens. However, the finite thickness of an actual lens, together with the curvatures of the surfaces of the lens, cause the shape factor to vary considerably from unity and from one lens to another.

Each of the above factors obviously may have an effect on the amount of residual aniseikonia present when unilateral aphakia is corrected by contact lenses. The ametropia that was present before the development of the cataract, as well as whether it was axial or refractive, is especially important (although often neglected) in determining the amount of residual aniseikonia in the correction of unilateral aphakia. Ogle, Burian, and Bannon[20] plotted residual aniseikonia on the basis of pre-cataract data, as shown in Figure 11–14, and noted the following:

1. If the ametropia before the onset of the cataract was *axial* in origin and equal in amount for the two eyes:
   (*a*) In high myopia (5 to 6 D), correction of unilateral aphakia with contact lenses for both eyes results in a residual aniseikonia of 15%; the use of a contact lens for the aphakic eye and a spectacle lens for the unoperated eye results in an increase of residual aniseikonia to 26%.
   (*b*) In high hyperopia (again, 5 to 6 D), the correction of unilateral aphakia with contact lenses for both eyes leaves a residual aniseikonia of only 2%; the use of a contact lens for the aphakic eye and a spectacle lens for the unoperated eye

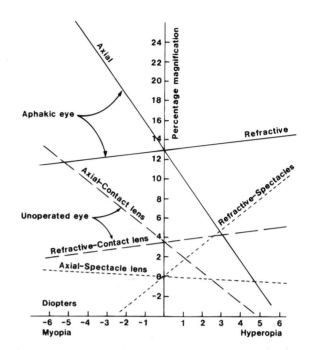

FIGURE 11–14.   **Residual aniseikonia based on pre-cataract data. (Reprinted with permission from K. N. Ogle, H. M. Burian, and R. E. Bannon, *Arch. Ophthalmol.*, Vol. 59, pp. 639–652, © 1958, American Medical Association.)**

reduces the residual aniseikonia to approximately zero.

2. If the ametropia before the onset of the cataract was *refractive* in origin, and of the same magnitude for each eye, the amount of residual aniseikonia if both eyes are fitted with contact lenses is about 10% for both the high myope and the high hyperope. However, if a contact lens is worn on the aphakic eye and a spectacle lens is worn on the unoperated eye, the amount of residual aniseikonia increases to about 24% for the high myope, but decreases to only about 5% for the high hyperope.

3. If both eyes were emmetropic before the cataract onset, and if a contact lens is worn on the aphakic eye and no lens is worn on the unoperated eye, the estimated aniseikonia is about 13%. If contact lenses are worn on both eyes, the residual aniseikonia is about 10%.

The predicted amounts of aniseikonia for each example, with contact lenses worn on both eyes or with a contact lens on the aphakic eye and a spectacle lens on the unoperated eye, are summarized in Table 11–3.

These examples show that, for the high myope before cataract onset (whether axial or refractive), residual aniseikonia can be minimized by fitting contact lenses for both eyes. On the other hand, for the high hyperope before cataract onset (whether axial or refractive), residual aniseikonia can be minimized by fitting a contact lens on the aphakic eye and a spectacle lens on the unoperated (phakic) eye.

Enoch[21] has suggested that binocular vision may be restored in unilateral aphakia by fitting the aphakic eye with a reverse Galilean telescope, which brings about a *minifi-*

TABLE 11–3
Predicted Amounts of Aniseikonia, Depending on the Refractive State of the Aphakic Eye before Cataract Onset*

Pre-cataract Refraction	Origin	Lens for Aphakic Eye	Lens for Phakic Eye	Residual Aniseikonia (%)
–5 to –6 D	Axial	Contact	Contact	15
		Contact	Spectacle	26
–5 to –6 D	Refractive	Contact	Contact	10
		Contact	Spectacle	24
+5 to +6 D	Axial	Contact	Contact	2
		Contact	Spectacle	0
+5 to +6 D	Refractive	Contact	Contact	10
		Contact	Spectacle	5
Emmetropia	—	Contact	Contact	10
		Contact	No lens	13

SOURCE: Adapted from K. N. Ogle, H. M. Burian, and R. E. Bannon, *Arch. Ophthalmol.*, Vol. 59, p. 644, 1958.
*Based on data plotted in Figure 11–14.

cation of the retinal image. The plus power necessary for the eyepiece, or ocular, of the telescope is added to the contact lens prescription for the aphakic eye, and the minus power for the telescope objective is supplied in the form of a spectacle lens. Enoch estimated the residual aniseikonia to be in the range of 6% to 8%, and provided a table (selected values of which are reproduced here as Table 11–4) to indicate the amount of minification available for various vertex distances. If a vertical imbalance occurs at the reading level, Enoch suggested the use of a slab-off prism in the spectacle lens.

Whether the aphakic eye is fitted with a contact lens or a spectacle lens, a bifocal addition or a single-vision lens for reading must be supplied for the aphakic eye. Because most unilateral aphakics are absolute presbyopes, the same bifocal addition or reading lens can usually be supplied for both eyes. If the patient is able to accommodate with the unoperated eye, an add can be given only for the aphakic eye, or unequal adds can be prescribed.

11.9. Determining the Final Aphakic Prescription

Contrary to the usual method of refraction, the frame for an aphakic patient should be selected *before* the refraction is performed. The sample frame should be of the correct eye size and DBL, and should be adjusted to the patient's face so that the vertex distance can be determined. An instrument called the *distometer* has been designed for this purpose. Because the optical center of the lens should be placed at the geometric center, the distance from the geometric center to the level of the center of the pupil determines the amount of pantoscopic tilt to ensure that the optic axis of the lens passes through the center of rotation of the eye. If the pantoscopic tilt exceeds about 8 degrees, the frame may have to be positioned lower on the face than it would ordinarily be fitted, by adjusting the nose pads, to meet the criterion that the optical center should be lowered 1 mm for each 2 degrees of pantoscopic tilt.

There are two methods of refraction that should lead to accurate results. One method is to use the refractor for a careful refraction (sphere, cylinder power, cylinder axis, as usual) and then to refine that result with a trial frame at the correct vertex distance and pantoscopic tilt. After the trial frame refraction, the trial frame with the correcting lenses is carefully placed in a lensometer to determine the final prescription in back vertex power.

The second method involves a technique known as *over-refraction*. Signet Armorlite and Frieder make over-refraction kits, which consist of several frames suitable for aphakic corrections and contain the manufacturer's aphakic lenses in assorted powers and frame PDs. Also included in the kit is a trial lens clip (Figure 11–15) which attaches to the frame

TABLE 11–4
Parameters for the Design of a Reverse Galilean Telescope for the Aphakic Eye in Unilateral Aphakia, Using an Overcorrection for the Contact Lens, F(+), as the Ocular Lens, and a Minus Spectacle Lens, F(–), as the Objective Lens

Aphakic Minification (%)	Vertex Distance (mm)	F(+) (D)	F(–) (D)	Phakic Magnification (%)
12.3	15.4	8.00	9.12	14.1
11.2	13.9	8.00	9.00	12.5
10.0	11.1	9.00	10.00	11.1
9.4	15.8	6.00	6.62	10.4
8.6	10.7	8.00	8.75	9.4
8.0	13.9	5.75	6.25	8.6
7.4	11.9	6.25	6.75	8.0
6.7	9.5	7.00	7.50	7.1
6.0	10.6	5.75	6.12	6.5
5.6	9.1	6.25	6.62	6.0

SOURCE: Adapted from J. M. Enoch, *Am. J. Optom. Arch. Am. Acad. Optom.*, Vol. 45, p. 236, 1968.

FIGURE 11–15. **Trial lens clip, which attaches to the frame for verifying the lens power needed for the frame the patient will be wearing.**

for verifying the power needed with the frame in which the patient's lenses will be ultimately mounted, correctly adjusted for vertex distance and pantoscopic tilt. By utilizing a frame having fitting characteristics similar to the one the patient will be wearing, vertex distance and pantoscopic tilt during refraction will be similar to those during actual wear of the glasses. By using lenses of design and power similar to those that will be dispensed, the optics employed during the final refraction and the final spectacle design will be comparable.

When the finished glasses are received from the laboratory, the frame must be fitted very precisely on the patient's face. The distance optical centers should be "spotted," and the frame should be adjusted so that the optical center of each lens is located 1 mm below the center of the pupil (with the patient's head held erect and the eyes in the primary position) for each 2 degrees of pantoscopic tilt. The reflection method of alignment, as described in Chapter 9, Section 9.17, should be used to verify that the optic axis passes through the center of rotation of the eye.

11.10. The High Hyperope

In general, high hyperopes tend to have the same problems with their glasses as do aphakics: excessive lens weight and thickness, magnified appearance of the wearer's eyes, increased retinal image size, lens aberrations, and decreased field of view. However, very few hyperopes require lenses anywhere near the normal range for aphakic powers—from about +10.00 to +14.00 D. The refractive error distribution curve for unselected subjects shows *very few* hyperopes of more than 5 or 6 D.

With the wide use of plastic lenses, the high hyperope need no longer put up with intolerably *heavy* lenses. *Thickness*, as with aphakic lenses, can be minimized by selecting a frame size that results in little or no decentration so that the lenses can have knife-thin edges. The use of an aspheric front surface helps reduce the weight, thickness, "bulginess," and magnification effects (see Chapter 6,

Section 6.20). Further reduction in thickness may be obtained by using high-index materials.

Contact lenses, if fitted successfully, offer many benefits to the high hyperope. Aside from the generally improved appearance that is usually achieved by moving from spectacles to contact lenses, the weight of the lenses is no longer a factor. The magnification effects of the spectacle lenses are also eliminated; an observer, therefore, sees the eyes as the normal size. Distorted appearances caused by prismatic effects and surface reflections of spectacle lenses are also removed. The field of view is enlarged, and oblique aberrations are essentially absent.

A disadvantage of contact lenses for the high hyperope is the smaller retinal image size with contact lenses as compared with that for glasses. Just as many myopes who change from glasses to contact lenses are aware that "everything looks bigger" with contact lenses, many hyperopes are aware that "everything looks smaller" with contact lenses. For some patients, smaller retinal image size may be sufficient to reduce corrected visual acuity and may cause the patient to reject contact lenses in favor of a return to glasses.

However, for the aphakic patient (who is a refractive hyperope rather than an axial hyperope), the greatly reduced image size with contact lenses is a definite advantage—as are the larger field of view and the absence of peripheral aberrations, the roving ring scotoma, and the jack-in-the-box phenomenon.

Magnification of the retinal image is not as much of a problem for the high hyperope as it is for the aphakic, not only because the lens power is usually much lower than that for an aphakic eye, but also because the hyperope normally has become accustomed to the magnification over a period of years, whereas the aphakic is suddenly presented with extremely high magnification. Nevertheless, as in the case of aphakic lenses, it is possible to minimize both the magnified appearance of the wearer's eyes and the retinal image magnification and to maximize the field of view by placing the lenses as close to the eyes as possible and by choosing base curves that are as shallow as possible to be compatible with good optical performance.

When viewed from the front, the surfaces of a plus meniscus lens act as a pair of reflecting surfaces that form images that have a tendency to hide the wearer's eyes from observers and that also annoy the wearer. The intensity of these images may be greatly reduced by the use of an antireflective coating. In addition, the number of reflected images potentially visible to an observer may be reduced by reducing the object field of view. The size of the object field of view for a spherical surface is directly proportional to the size of the reflecting surface and inversely proportional to its radius of curvature. Thus, the size of the object field of view may be reduced by selecting as small an eye size as possible that is acceptable to the patient and by making the base curve as shallow as possible in terms of optical performance. Of course, a small eye size has the advantage of reducing the lens thickness and weight, and a shallow base curve has the advantage of reducing magnification effects.

LENSES FOR HIGH MYOPIA

11.11. Problems Caused by High Minus Lenses

Lens Weight and Thickness

The problems caused by the lenses required for the correction of high myopia are quite different from those caused by lenses for the correction of aphakia or hyperopia. Lens weight is somewhat less of a problem for the myope than for the hyperope or the aphakic, and is usually not a problem at all if plastic lenses are used. Lens thickness, however, is more of a problem for the myope because thick *edges* are much more obvious to the observer than are thick *centers*.

Minification

High minus lenses obviously bring about a minification of the wearer's eyes, to the observer, as well as minify the retinal image. Both the apparent size of the wearer's eyes and the retinal image size can be increased by fitting the lenses as close to the wearer's eyes as possible. Many myopes have solved this problem for themselves by wearing *contact lenses* rather than glasses. For the high myope, minification of the wearer's eyes is probably at least as great a cosmetic deterrent as are edge thickness and edge reflections. Contact lenses not only allow the eyes to appear normal in size, but bring about an increase in retinal image size that is readily apparent to the high myope.

Field of View

Minus lenses actually *increase* both the peripheral and macular fields of view, as compared with those for an unpowered lens. With an increased macular field of view, rather than having a roving ring scotoma as the aphakic has, the myope may experience a ring-shaped area of overlapping *double-vision*—an area that involves relatively clear vision through the lens but blurred vision outside the lens, as shown in Figure 11–16. However, the *ring of diplopia* is so far in the periphery that it is seldom, if ever, noticed.

Except for the minification caused by the lenses, the problems associated with wearing high minus lenses are almost entirely with the *appearance* of the lenses. These problems include not only the thick edges and the minified appearance of the wearer's eyes, but also the *rings*, caused by reflections from the lens edges, which an observer can see.

11.12. Minimizing Edge Thickness

The relationship between the edge thickness and center thickness of a lens is discussed in Chapter 3, Sections 3.12 through 3.14, and formulas relating power to center and

edge thickness of a lens are given in Equation 3.13, for a spherical lens, and in Equation 3.14, for a sphero-cylindrical lens. In Equation 3.13,

$$t_C - t_P = \frac{F_A h^2}{2(n-1)},$$

where t_C is the center thickness, t_p is the edge thickness, F_A is the approximate power of the lens, h is one-half the diameter (chord length) of the lens, and n is the index of refraction of the lens material.

For a lens of a given power, edge thickness can be minimized (1) by keeping the lens size as small as possible and by using a frame with a PD equal to the patient's distance

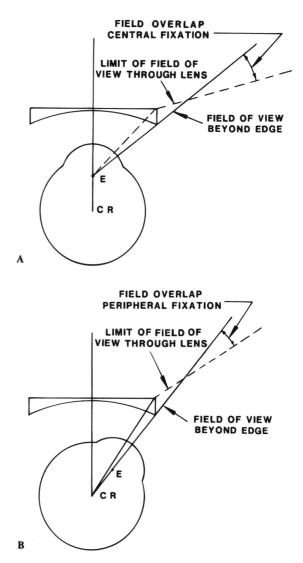

FIGURE 11–16. **The ring-shaped area of diplopia, or field overlap, which may be seen (but is seldom noticed) by the wearer of a high minus lens. A, for central fixation; B, for peripheral fixation (CR = center of rotation).**

PD so that no decentration is required (analogous to the minimal-effective-diameter method of fitting aphakic lenses) and (2) by using a material having as high an index of refraction as possible. However, the current popularity of large lens sizes makes it difficult for the practitioner or dispenser to interest most patients in keeping lens size to a minimum, and the popularity of CR-39 plastic lenses, although they decrease lens weight, has the consequent disadvantage of increasing the edge thickness.

However, *polycarbonate* material is not only lighter in weight than ophthalmic crown glass, but also has a higher index of refraction, with the result that a lens made of this material is both lighter and thinner than one made of glass. Table 11–5 lists the indices of refraction, specific gravities, and Abbe values of CR-39, polycarbonate, and other representative plastic materials.

The edge thickness that can be expected for lenses made of ophthalmic crown glass is compared with that of CR-39 and polycarbonate materials in the following example.

EXAMPLE

Given the prescription –8.00 D sphere, to be mounted in a frame having an eye size of 50 mm, the lens having a center thickness of 2.0 mm. If the patient's PD is equal to the frame PD, which makes decentration unnecessary, what is the edge thickness at the thickest points of the lens edge (assumed to be in the 180° meridian) for (1) an ophthalmic crown glass lens ($n = 1.523$); (2) a CR-39 lens ($n = 1.498$); (3) a polycarbonate lens ($n = 1.586$); and (4) an Optima Hyperindex lens ($n = 1.660$)?

(1) For the ophthalmic crown glass lens:

$$t_C - t_P = \frac{-8(0.025)^2}{2(1.523 - 1)} = \frac{-0.005}{1.046} = -0.0048 \text{ m}.$$

$$t_P = 0.0048 + 0.002 = 0.0068 \text{ m} = 6.8 \text{ mm}.$$

(2) For the CR-39 lens:

$$t_C - t_P = \frac{-0.005}{2(1.498 - 1)} = \frac{-0.005}{0.996} = -0.0050 \text{ m}.$$

$$t_P = 0.0050 + 0.002 = 0.0070 \text{ m} = 7.0 \text{ mm}.$$

(3) For the polycarbonate lens:

$$t_C - t_P = \frac{-0.005}{2(1.586 - 1)} = \frac{-0.005}{1.172} = -0.00427 \text{ m}.$$

$$t_P = 0.00427 + 0.002 = 0.00627 \text{ m}$$
$$= 6.27 \text{ mm}.$$

(4) For the Optima Hyperindex lens:

$$t_C - t_P = \frac{-0.005}{2(1.660 - 1)} = \frac{-0.005}{1.32} = -0.00379 \text{ m},$$

$$t_P = 0.00379 + 0.002 = 0.00579 \text{ m}$$
$$= 5.79 \text{ mm}.$$

Although the edge thickness difference of only 0.2 mm between CR-39 and glass may be considered negligible, the difference of 0.7 mm between CR-39 and polycarbonate is approximately 10% of the edge thickness, and the difference of 1.0 mm between CR-39 and Optima Hyperindex is approximately 15% of the edge thickness. These differences are sufficient to make a noticeable difference in appearance.

An additional alternative is the use of one of the available *high-index* glass or plastic materials. Currently available high-index glasses and plastics, together with their indices of refraction, Abbe numbers, and specific gravities, are listed in Chapter 1, Table 1–2 (glass) and Table 1–3 and in this chapter in Table 11–5 (plastic).

TABLE 11–5
Optical Characteristics of Representative Plastic Lenses

Manufacturer/Supplier	Name	Refractive Index	Abbe No.	Specific Gravity
Pittsburg Plate Glass	CR-39	1.498	58.0	1.32
Transitions Optical	Transitions*	1.500	57.0	1.28
Sola	Spectralite	1.537	47.0	1.21
Signet Armorlite	RLX-Lite	1.555	36.0	1.24
Hoya	Hi-Lux II	1.556	40.0	1.27
Pittsburg Plate Glass	HIP	1.556	37.7	1.22
Seiko	Diacoat Thin	1.556	40.0	1.27
Younger	Younger-Lite	1.556	37.7	1.22
[Numerous]	Polycarbonate	1.586	31.0	1.20
Silor	Thin & Lite	1.595	36.0	1.37
Optima	Hyperindex 160	1.597	37.0	1.34
Signet Armorlite	1.60 High Index	1.600	36.0	1.45
Hoya	Hi-Lux Excellence	1.600	36.0	1.34
Seiko	Super 1.6	1.600	34.0	1.38
Pentax	Superthin 1.6	1.600	36.0	1.34
Zeiss	Claret SL	1.600	36.0	1.34
Optima	Hyperindex 166	1.660	32.0	1.35
Nikon	NL IV HCC	1.660	32.0	1.35

*Photochromic plastic.

The most commonly used high-index glasses are High-Lite, made by Schott, and similar materials made by Chance-Pilkington and by Hoya. Most have an index of refraction of 1.70 and an Abbe value substantially lower than that of ophthalmic crown glass, with the result that the chromatic dispersion is much greater than that for ophthalmic crown glass.

Using the above example, the edge thickness for a high-index (1.70) glass lens is:

$$t_C - t_P = \frac{-0.005}{2(1.70 - 1)} = \frac{-0.005}{1.400} = -0.0036 \text{ m.}$$

$$t_P = 0.0036 + 0.002 = 0.0056 \text{ m} = 5.6 \text{ mm.}$$

The resultant saving in edge thickness compared with that of ophthalmic crown glass is 1.2 mm, or close to 20%.

If one of the recently introduced 1.80 index glasses is used for this lens, an even greater saving in edge thickness results:

$$t_C - t_P = \frac{-0.005}{2(1.80 - 1)} = \frac{-0.005}{1.60} = -0.0031 \text{ m.}$$

$$t_P = 0.0031 + 0.002 = 0.0051 \text{ m} = 5.1 \text{ mm.}$$

The charts shown in Figure 11–17 indicate the expected edge thickness for minus lenses at various distances from the optical center for lenses made of ophthalmic crown glass (A); for 1.70 index glass (B); for 1.80 index glass (C); for CR-39 plastic (D); and for polycarbonate plastic (E). Although the charts are designed to be used for minus lenses having a center thickness of 2.0 mm, they can also be used for predicting the *center* thickness of plus lenses. For example, if it is assumed that the edge thickness of a plus lens should be 1 mm, the predicted center thickness of a given plus lens would be equal to the edge thickness (as found in the chart) minus 1 mm.

In view of the higher specific gravity of high-index glass, the fact that this material produces thinner lenses does not necessarily mean that the lenses weigh less. Tucker[22] compared the weights of CR-39 plastic, ophthalmic crown glass, and high-index glass (1.70) for a 50-mm lens size and for a minimum edge or center thickness of 2 mm. Her results are shown plotted in Figure 11–18. In this diagram, it can be seen that the curves for ophthalmic crown glass and high-index glass cross at back vertex powers of approximately ±8.00 D. Below 8.00 D, lenses made of high-index glass are heavier than lenses made of ophthalmic crown glass, but above 8.00 D they are lighter; so for lenses having a diameter of 50 mm,

A

B

C

D

E

FIGURE 11–17. **Charts showing expected edge thickness for minus lenses at varying distances from the optical center. A, for ophthalmic crown glass, *n* = 1.523; B, for high-index glass, *n* = 1.70; C, for high-index glass, *n* = 1.80; D, for CR-39 plastic, *n* = 1.498; and E, for polycarbonate plastic, *n* = 1.586. (Reprinted with permission from Edge Thickness Comparison Chart, O'Hara Corporation, makers of Index 8, Watchung, New Jersey, and Paul M. Hadley, O.D.)**

if the goal is to reduce *both* thickness and weight, the lenses should be used only for powers in excess of ±8.00 D.

Note, however, that the saving in weight is relatively small, amounting to only 1 or 2 grams for lenses having powers of ±12.00 D. On the other hand, for lenses of relatively low power, the *excess* weight of high-index lenses amounts to only 1 or 2 grams. The crossover values for these curves vary both with lens size and with the criterion for minimum edge or center thickness.

All high-index glass lenses should have an antireflective coating. Because the intensity of the reflections increases with the index according to Fresnel's equation, the reflections from an uncoated high-index lens is quite noticeable. As discussed in Chapter 7, Section 7.30, the ideal antireflective coating has an index of refraction equal to the square root of the index of refraction of the glass to be coated. Magnesium fluoride has an index of refraction of 1.38, which is considerably higher than the square root of the index of ophthalmic crown glass (1.234). However, because the square root of the index of glass having an index of 1.70 is 1.304, an antireflective coating of magnesium fluoride functions more efficiently for a high-index glass than it does for ophthalmic crown glass.

11.13. Minimizing Edge Reflections

As discussed in Chapter 7, Sections 7.27 through 7.33, there are reflections from the surfaces and edges of an opthalmic lens that are not noticed by the wearer but may be annoying or distracting to an observer. The reflections tend to enhance the glassiness of the lenses and to obscure the eyes of the wearer and thus serve as an impediment to communication and present a problem, particularly for an individual who must regularly appear in public.

In addition to the reflections formed by the surfaces of the lenses, the edges of the lenses are responsible for the *multiple rings* seen just inside the edges of high minus lenses. The rings (described in Chapter 7, Section 7.33 and illustrated in Figure 7–43) are images of the edge of the lens, and are caused by internal reflections that begin at the lens edge and reflect their way toward the center of the lens until

they strike the surface at an angle that permits refraction by the lens and into the eye of the observer. The process is then repeated, with the result that multiple rings are seen. The rings are more pronounced for oblique angles of view than for straight-ahead viewing.

Although the use of an *antireflective coating* is helpful in attenuating the intensity of the rings on straight-ahead viewing, for rings seen on oblique viewing, the most effective method of attenuation is the use of one of the available forms of *edge treatment*. Methods of edge treatment include:

1. *Edge Coating*. This helps to reduce the granular appearance of the edge.
2. *Edge Painting*. Using a neutral gray color, painting the edge tends to make the rings less noticeable.
3. *Using a Semitransparent Edge*. For a glass lens, a semitransparent edge can be produced by using an edging wheel that results in a fine, semitransparent grain of the beveled edge rather than the usual coarse white grain.
4. *Buffing the Edge*. For a plastic lens, buffing produces the same effect as a semitransparent edge on a glass lens.
5. *Tinting the Lens*. Another effective procedure for a plastic lens is that of tinting (dyeing) the lens after it has been edged. Even a relatively light tint is effective in reducing the multiple ring effect.
6. *Hide-a-Bevel Technique*. As shown in Chapter 7, Figure 7–44, this procedure results in a flat edge with a small, narrow bevel that protrudes from the edge. Because of the angle between the flat edge and the lens surface, the reflected rays that are responsible for the multiple-ring effect are not apt to enter an observer's eye.

The use of a combination of these methods can be very effective. For example, for a plastic lens one may use the hide-a-bevel technique and buff the edge and tint the lens.

11.14. Lenticular Lenses

In 1933, Obrig[23] introduced a lenticular lens called the Myo-Disc, to correct high myopia. The lens was made by grind-

FIGURE 11–18. **Comparison of the weights of lenses made of CR-39 plastic, ophthalmic crown glass, and high-index glass for a 50-mm lens with a minimum edge or center thickness of 2 mm. (Reprinted with permission from T. Tucker, *Ophthalmic Optician*, Vol. 16, pp. 795–804, 1976.)**

ing a small concave disk on the back surface of a plano lens (Figure 11–19), as shown in (A). This lens was remarkably thin and lightweight. Newer lenticular lenses are generally similar to the original Myo-Disc lens, having a powered portion approximately 30 mm in diameter and surrounded by a carrier lens having either plano or low plus power, as shown in Figure 11–19B. As with plus lenticular lenses, the lenses have the advantage of decreased lens thickness and weight, but the disadvantage of causing a "bull's eye" appearance that calls attention to the fact that the individual is wearing very strong lenses.

Most practitioners consider the use of a minus lenticular lens only for a patient who has *very* high myopia, for example, in excess of 11.00 or 12.00 D. Even for lenses in this power range, the practitioner should consider all options short of using a lenticular lens, as discussed in the preceding paragraphs. Keeping lens size to a minimum and making use of the methods described to minimize edge thickness (including the use of high-index materials) and minimize lens reflections in many cases provides a more cosmetically acceptable pair of glasses than could be provided by the use of minus lenticular lenses. Also, the use of contact lenses should be considered, particularly because, as shown by Gumpelmeyer,[24] with contact lenses instead of glasses, very high myopes tend to have significantly better visual acuity beyond that predicted by the greatly increased spectacle magnification.

The saving in edge thickness by use of a minus lenticular lens for a very high myope is demonstrated by the following example.

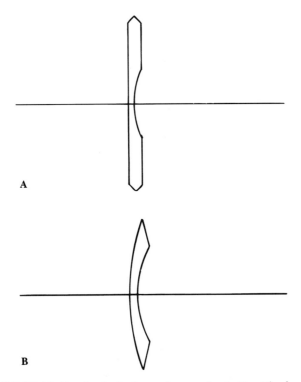

A

B

FIGURE 11–19. **Lenticular lenses for myopia. A, Myo-Disc lens, made by grinding a small concave disk on the back surface of a flat plano lens; B, lens having a powered portion 30 mm in diameter and a plus-powered carrier.**

EXAMPLE
For a patient requiring a lens with a power of –15.00 D sphere, if one uses a lens made of CR-39 material having an index of refraction of 1.498, with a center thickness of 2.0 and if one uses a frame requiring no decentration: (1) What would be the edge thickness at the thickest point if a 50-mm-wide full-diameter lens were to be used? (2) What would be the thickness at the thickest point of the transition between the optical portion and the carrier if a lenticular lens having a 30-mm-wide optical zone is used?

(1) For the full-diameter lens:

$$t_C - t_P = \frac{-15(0.025)^2}{2(1.498 - 1)} = -0.0094 \text{ m.}$$

$$t_P = 0.0094 + 0.002 = 0.0114 \text{ m}$$
$$= 11.4 \text{ mm.}$$

(2) For the minus lenticular lens:

$$t_C - t_P = \frac{-15(0.015)^2}{2(1.498 - 1)} = -0.0034 \text{ m.}$$

$$t_P = 0.0034 + 0.002 = 0.0054 \text{ m}$$
$$= 5.4 \text{ mm.}$$

This example shows that the edge thickness at the thickest point of a full-diameter lens is more than twice the transition thickness for a minus lenticular lens. If the lenticular lens had a *convex* carrier, the edge thickness would be considerably less than the 5.4-mm transition thickness. For very high minus prescriptions for which full-diameter lenses would result in unacceptable edge thicknesses, the "bull's eye" appearance of minus lenticular lenses may be minimized by using lightly tinted lenses having an antireflective coating.

11.15. Fresnel Press-on Lenses

Fresnel press-on lenses are made in much the same manner as Fresnel press-on prisms, described in Chapter 4, Section 4.19; however, the grooves in the material form a concentric pattern on the surface instead of parallel lines (Figure 11–20). Successive concentric grooves cut away from the center have slightly increased apical angles that provide the increased deviating power from the center to the edge. The angle of each groove can be set independently, with the result that any spherical or aspheric surface can be generated. The generation of an aspheric surface is not more expensive nor more difficult than the generation of spherical surfaces.

Fresnel lenses, like Fresnel prisms, provide a thin, lightweight alternative to conventional glass or plastic lenses. Fresnel lenses (in either plus or minus powers) offer unique advantages in many circumstances, including (1) the correction of very high refractive errors, (2) temporary use as a trial or diagnostic lens, (3) additions with high power or

FIGURE 11–20.   **A Fresnel press-on lens.**

eccentric placement of segments, and (4) for use when a lens power or construction is not available or would result in exorbitant costs or long delays.

The grooves cut in the lenses produce scattering of light, which may cause a slight reduction in visual acuity. The most important factor in determining resolution through the lenses is the *width* of the grooves—the smaller the groove width, the more precise the focus and (theoretically) the better the resolution. However, as groove width becomes smaller, diffraction begins to reduce resolution. Therefore, the groove width chosen must represent a balance between precise focus and image deterioration from diffraction. The resolution also depends on the orientation of the object.[25] Components of an object that are parallel to the orientation of the grooves have the poorest resolution; components at right angles to the grooves undergo little deterioration.

The advantages of Fresnel lenses of thinness, light-weight, large aperture, unlimited placement, and in-office application must be weighed against the disadvantages of reduced contrast, a slight reduction in visual acuity, and the visibility of the concentric grooves to observers.

Fresnel lenses in plus powers are available from +0.50 D to +20.00 D; in minus lenses, they are available from –1.00 D to –14.00 D; precut straight-top (D-25) segments are available from +0.50 to +8.00 D. Cylinder powers are not available in Fresnel press-on lenses. If a patient's prescription contains a cylindrical component, the cylinder must be placed on the carrier lens. There appears to be no end to the potential applications of Fresnel lenses—the possibilities seem limited only by the practitioner's imagination.

References

1. Donders, F. C. *On the Anomalies of Accommodation and Refraction of the Eye*, The New Sydenham Society, London, p. 309, 1864.
2. Bettman, J. W. Apparent Accommodation in Aphakic Eyes. *Am. J. Ophthalmol.*, Vol. 33, pp. 921–923, 1950.
3. Laurance, L. *Visual Optics and Sight Testing*, The School of Optics, London, p. 117, 1920.
4. Sanders, D. R., Retzlaff, J., and Kraff, M. C. Comparison of Empirically Derived and Theoretical Aphakic Refraction Formulas. *Arch. Ophthalmol.*, Vol. 101, pp. 965–967, 1983.
5. Ogle, K. N. *Optics: An Introduction for Ophthalmologists*, 2nd edition, Charles C Thomas, Springfield, IL, p. 202, 1968.
6. Anonymous. The Adjustment to Aphakia. *Am. J. Ophthalmol.*, Vol. 35, p. 118, 1952.
7. Smith G., and Bailey I. L. Aspheric Spectacle Lenses—Design and Performance, Part One: Introduction. *The Optician*, Vol. 181, pp. 21–26, 1981.
8. Smith G., and Atchison D. A. Effect of Conicoid Asphericity on the Tscherning Ellipses of Ophthalmic Spectacle Lenses. *J. Opt. Soc. Am.*, Vol. 73, pp. 441–445, 1983.
9. Fowler, C. W. Measurement of Distortion in Single Vision Ophthalmic Lenses. In *Transactions of the First International Congress*, Vol. 1, British College of Ophthalmic Opticians, London, pp. 148–157, 1984.
10. Fowler, C. W. Aspheric Spectacle Lens Design for Aphakia. *Am. J. Optom. Physiol. Opt.*, Vol. 61, pp. 737–740, 1984.
11. Davis, J. K., and Torgersen, D. L. The Properties of Lenses for Correction of Aphakia. *J. Am. Optom. Assoc.*, Vol. 54, pp. 685–693, 1983.
12. Atchison, D. A., and Smith, G. Assessment of Aphakic Spectacle Lenses: High Power Flatback Lenses for the Correction of Aphakia. *Austral. J. Optom.*, Vol. 63, pp. 258–263, 1980.
13. Benton, C. D., and Welsh, R. C. *Spectacles for Aphakia*, Charles C Thomas, Springfield, IL, p. 39, 1966.
14. Whitney, D. B. What Aspheric Design Can and Cannot Do for the Aphakic Patient. *Optom. Wkly.*, pp. 45–52, June 17, 1976.
15. *Optical, Cosmetic and Mechanical Properties of Ophthalmic Lenses*. Lens Information Kit, Lens Development Dept., American Optical Co., Southridge, MA, p. 4.201, March 1968.
16. Atchison, D. A. Problems of Spectacle Wearing Aphakics. *Austral. J. Optom.*, Vol. 66, pp. 216–218, 1983.
17. Ham, W. T., Jr., Muller, H. A., and Sliney, D. H. Retinal Sensitivity to Damage from Short Wavelength Light. *Nature*, Vol. 260, pp. 153–155, 1975.
18. Lerman, S. L. *Radiant Energy and the Eye*, Macmillan, New York, p. 176, 1980.
19. Ogle, K. N. *Researches in Binocular Vision*, W. B. Saunders, Philadelphia, p. 260, 1950.
20. Ogle, K. N., Burian, H. M., and Bannon, R. E. On the Correction of Unilateral Aphakia with Contact Lenses. *Arch. Ophthalmol.*, Vol. 59, pp. 639–652, 1958.
21. Enoch, J. M. A Spectacle-Contact Lens Combination Used as a Reverse Galilean Telescope in Unilateral Aphakia. *Am. J. Optom. Arch. Am. Acad. Optom.*, Vol. 45, pp. 231–240, 1968.
22. Tucker, T. The Use of High Index Glass. *Ophthalmic Optician*, Vol. 16, pp. 795–804, 1976.
23. Obrig, T. E. *Modern Ophthalmic Lenses and Optical Glass*, Chilton Co., New York, p. 106, 1935.
24. Gumpelmeyer, T. F. Special Considerations in the Fitting of Corneal Lenses in High Myopia. *Am. J. Optom. Arch. Am. Acad. Optom.*, Vol. 47, pp. 879–886, 1970.
25. Kapash, R. T., and Barkan, E. Fresnel Optics and Human Visual Performance. Presented at the Annual Meeting of the American Academy of Optometry, Toronto, Canada, December 1971.

Questions

1. According to Laurance, a pre-aphakic eye having 4.00 D of hyperopia needs how much spectacle correction after surgery?

2. According to Sanders et al., an eye that is 24.0 mm long with a pre-aphakic K reading of 44.00 D requires how much spectacle correction after cataract surgery?

3. Where is the far point located for an aphakic eye that has a refractive power of 42.00 D, an axial length of 24.0 mm, and a refractive index of 1.336?

4. If a spectacle lens is to be worn at a distance of 11 mm from the cornea of the patient in Question 3, what must be its power?

5. What is the angular size of the ring scotoma of a +12.50-DS aphakic prescription that is made as a 50-mm round centered lens?

6. If a +12.00-D aphakic spectacle wearer with a vertex distance of 12 mm is fitted with contact lenses, what must be the power of the contact lenses?

7. What is the difference in the edge thickness between a −10.00 D, 50-mm round centered glass lens made of ophthalmic crown glass of refractive index 1.523 (n = 1.523) and one made with an index of refraction of 1.80, if both lenses have a center thickness of 1.5 mm?

8. Why are nuclear and subcapsular cataracts more troublesome outdoors than indoors?

9. Identify the factors affecting the size and position of the ring scotoma and describe the effect of each factor.

10. Discuss how oblique astigmatism and the curvature of the field are addressed in the design of lenses above +8.00 D.

11. Why is it best to place the optical center of aphakic lenses at the geometric center of the lens?

12. Discuss the advantages and disadvantages of trifocals for aphakic spectacle wearers.

13. Why is it important to provide an ultraviolet filter for an aphakic patient?

14. Why should all high-index glasses have an antireflective coating?

15. List methods that can be used to reduce reflections from the edge of high minus lenses.

16. If the optical center is placed at the geometric center of the lens, how can the optic axis of the lens be made to pass through the center of rotation of the eye?

17. Describe the design of aphakic lenses that minimize weight and thickness.

18. Discuss the advantages and disadvantages of lenticular aphakic lenses.

19. What is the meaning of *base curve* when it applies to an aphakic lens with an aspheric surface?

20. Discuss the advantages and disadvantages of contact lenses for aphakia.

21. Discuss the construction and uses of Fresnel press-on lenses.

CHAPTER TWELVE

Optical Principles of Lenses for Low Vision

*L*ow vision, or *partial sight*, has been defined by Mehr and Freid[1] as "reduced central acuity or visual field loss which even with the best optical correction provided by regular lenses still results in visual impairment from the performance standpoint." Most definitions of low vision do not include a visual acuity cutoff point. However, reading ordinary newsprint requires vision of approximately 6/12 to 6/15 (20/40–20/50); thus, a person may be assumed to have low vision if regular spectacle lenses fail to provide vision of this magnitude.

Optical aids designed for patients who have low vision differ from those for other patients in that the main function of the aids is to bring about magnification, with or without changing the vergence of incident light. Many methods of providing magnification are available. For distance vision, telescopic lens systems are used, in the form of professionally prescribed headborne telescopic systems, nonprescription headborne telescopic systems, and handheld telescopes. For near vision, a telescope with a "reading cap" may be used, but more commonly a high plus lens, either in the form of a high add or reading glasses, is prescribed. Many other aids are available for near vision, including hand magnifiers, stand magnifiers, projection magnifiers, and even closed-circuit television.

12.1. Methods of Providing Magnification

Because a patient with low vision, by definition, cannot obtain satisfactory visual acuity in spite of the correction of any existing refractive error, any method of improving visual acuity requires the *enlarging of the retinal image* so that the image of a fixated object (such as a letter on a Snellen chart) stimulates a larger number of photoreceptors. Thus, some form of *magnification* must be provided.

The extent to which magnification actually improves visual acuity depends, to a great extent, upon the *cause* of the low vision. For example, if only a tiny central retinal area is available for vision (as in advanced cases of retinitis pigmentosa), enlarging the retinal image may stimulate only nonfunctioning photoreceptors and either not improve visual acuity, or, possibly, make acuity worse. However, usually any magnification of the retinal image is accompanied by a proportional increase in visual acuity. For example, if the best visual acuity for a given eye when tested at a distance of 3 m (10 ft) is 3/30, or 10/100, a visual aid providing an angular magnification of 2× is expected to result in a visual acuity of 3/15, or 10/50. (Because visual acuity testing for low-vision patients is routinely done at a distance of 3 m (10 ft), this testing distance is used here for all visual acuity examples.)

The intent of magnification is to increase the size of the retinal image of the object of regard. Although the retinal image size may be specified in terms of the angle subtended at any reference point within the eye, a satisfactory point is the center of the eye's exit pupil. Because the centers of the entrance and exit pupils are conjugate points, any alteration of the angular subtense of the object at the center of the entrance pupil produces a proportional change in angular size of the retinal image measured from the center of the exit pupil. The use of the centers of the entrance/exit pupils as reference points has the additional advantage that all equations relating to them are valid for both in-focus and out-of-focus retinal images. Hence, if the angular subtense of the object for the eye's optical system is increased, there is also an increase in the angular size of the retinal image.

To provide magnification for patients having low vision, the methods used increase the angular subtense of the object for the eye's optical system. The methods commonly used can be placed in four basic categories:

1. Relative distance magnification
2. Relative size magnification
3. Projection magnification
4. Angular magnification

When two or more of these methods are used in combination, the *total magnification* is defined as the *product* of each individual magnification.

A brief description of each of the first three methods follows; however, the focus of the discussion in this chapter is on methods of providing *angular magnification*. *Relative distance magnification* is the magnification that results from decreasing the distance of the object from the eye. To specify the amount of magnification, it is necessary to use an initial standard or reference distance, usually 40 cm or 25 cm.

As shown in Figure 12–1, an object (*h* millimeters high) is at a distance *q* millimeters from the entrance pupil of the eye and subtends an angle, α, at the entrance pupil. If the object is moved so that it is at distance *q'* from the entrance pupil, it subtends an angle of α'.

The relative distance magnification, M_D, is found by the relationship

$$M_D = \frac{\tan \alpha'}{\tan \alpha} = \frac{h/q'}{h/q} = \frac{q}{q'}. \qquad (12.1)$$

For example, if an object is moved from the reference distance of 40 cm to 10 cm, the relative distance magnification is

$$M_D = \frac{40}{10} = 4\times.$$

The use of short fixation distances requires large amounts of accommodation. For example, a 10-cm working distance requires 10 D of accommodation. If the patient's accommodation is insufficient, a clear retinal image can be obtained by the use of a plus lens of sufficient power. In this example, the use of a +10.00-D lens requires no accommodation.

Relative size magnification is the magnification obtained by increasing the size of the object at its original position, as shown in Figure 12–2. Large-print books, magazines, and newspapers are examples of this form of magnification. To quantify relative size magnification, the same fixation distance must be used for both object sizes. For example, if at 40 cm an object is 0.5 mm high but is increased to 2.0 mm high, the relative size magnification is

$$M_S = \frac{2.0}{0.5} = 4\times.$$

Projection magnification is the magnification that results from the formation of an enlarged image on a screen, of an opaque or transparent object. The projection system may be optical or electronic—an example of the latter is a closed-circuit television system. Projection magnification makes possible a high level of magnification at a viewing distance that is convenient for the user and has the advantage that

FIGURE 12–1.   **Relative distance magnification.**

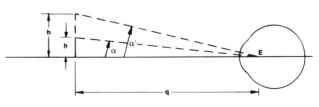

FIGURE 12–2.   **Relative size magnification.**

it may be used in combination with relative distance magnification; that is, a lens that creates relative distance magnification may be used to view the projected image, as shown in Figure 12–3. With such a combination, the aberrations accompanying the use of very strong optical aids are greatly reduced. Projection magnification can be considered as a special form of relative size magnification.

Angular magnification of an optical system (Figure 12–4) is specified by the ratio of the angle subtended by the image of an object formed by the system to the angle subtended by the object when viewed directly; both angles are subtended at the center of the entrance pupil of the eye, or

$$AM=\frac{\text{angle subtended by the image of an object}}{\text{angle subtended by the project when viewed directly}}.$$

Thus, angular magnification compares the apparent increase in the size of the object seen through the optical system with the size of the object seen without the optical system in place.

Although relative size magnification and relative distance magnification can be specified in terms of angular subtense, the term *angular magnification* is usually reserved for the magnification produced by the optical system itself.

FIGURE 12–3. **Projection magnification used in combination with relative distance magnification.**

FIGURE 12–4. **Angular magnification.**

OPTICAL AIDS FOR DISTANCE VISION

12.2. Afocal Telescopes

An *afocal telescope* is defined as an optical system that provides angular magnification without bringing about a change in vergence. Both classical afocal telescope designs—the Galilean and the Keplerian telescopes—are used as aids for low vision. In their simplest construction, afocal telescopes contain two optical elements, the objective lens and the eyepiece. In all telescopes designed to provide angular magnification, the objective lens is positive in power and is placed toward the object to be viewed. The eyepiece, placed close to the eye of the observer, is much stronger in power than the objective lens and may be either a positive or negative lens.

With all afocal telescopes, the basic optical principle is that the secondary focal plane of the objective lens coincides with the primary focal plane of the eyepiece lens. Parallel rays incident on the objective lens form an image at the secondary focal plane, and this image becomes the object for the eyepiece lens. Because the object is located at the primary focal plane of the eyepiece, the rays emerge from the system parallel, but form a greater angle with the optic axis than that formed by the incident rays.

The *Galilean telescope*, shown in Figure 12–5, uses a positive-powered objective lens (O) and a negative-powered eyepiece (E). The objective lens forms an *optically real* image of height *h*, with the chief ray passing through the optical center of the objective lens and forming an angle α with the optical axis. The optically real image of the objective lens

becomes a *virtual object* for the eyepiece lens. The ray passing through the optical center of the eyepiece helps form the tip of the optically real image and emerges undeviated from the eyepiece lens. This ray forms an angle α′ with the optic axis. Thus, parallel rays enter the objective lens at angle α to the optic axis, and a parallel bundle emerges from the eyepiece lens at angle α′ from the optic axis.

The ratio α′/α compares the angular size of the image to the angular size of the object. In Figure 12–5, F_o = power of objective lens; F_e = power of eyepiece lens; f_o' = secondary focal length of objective lens; f_e = primary focal length of eyepiece lens; therefore

$$M = \frac{\alpha'}{\alpha},$$

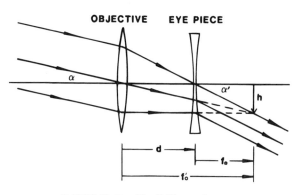

FIGURE 12–5. **The Galilean telescope.**

or, more exactly,

$$M = \frac{\tan \alpha'}{\tan \alpha} = \frac{h/f_e}{h/f_o'} = \frac{f_o'}{f_e},$$

since

$$f_e = -f_e'$$

$$M = -\frac{f_o'}{f_e'}$$

or

$$M = -\frac{F_e}{F_o}. \tag{12.2}$$

The separation, d, of the objective lens and the eyepiece can be determined as follows:

$$d = f_o' - f_e \tag{12.3}$$

or

$$d = \frac{1}{F_o} + \frac{1}{F_e},$$

and

$$F_o = \frac{F_e}{dF_e - 1} \tag{12.4}$$

$$F_e = \frac{F_o}{dF_o - 1}. \tag{12.5}$$

If the value of F_o in Equation 12.4 is substituted in Equation 12.2,

$$M = \frac{-F_e}{\dfrac{F_e}{dF_e - 1}} = -(dF_e - 1),$$

or

$$M = 1 - dF_e. \tag{12.6}$$

If the value of F_e in Equation 12.5 is substituted in Equation 12.2,

$$M = \frac{\dfrac{F_o}{dF_o - 1}}{-F_o} = \frac{1}{-(dF_o - 1)},$$

or

$$M = \frac{1}{1 - dF_o}. \tag{12.7}$$

Galilean telescopes have the following characteristics:

1. Since for a Galilean telescope F_e is always a negative lens and F_o is always a positive lens, in the formula

$$M = \frac{-F_e}{F_o},$$

the magnification has a positive sign, which indicates that the image formed is *erect*.

2. The length, d, of the telescope is the secondary focal length of the objective lens minus the primary focal length of the eyepiece. As discussed later, the Galilean telescope is *shorter* than the Keplerian telescope if both have the same magnification. For constant magnification, increasing the power of both the objective and the eyepiece produces a shorter telescopic unit.

EXAMPLE

An afocal Galilean telescope has a +10.00-D objective lens and a −25.00-D eyepiece lens. What is the magnifying power of the telescope?

$$M = \frac{-F_e}{F_o} = -\frac{-25.00}{10.00} = 2.5\times.$$

What is the separation of the two lenses?

$$d = f_o' - f_e$$
$$= +0.10 - 0.04 = 0.06 \text{ m} = 6 \text{ cm}.$$

The *Keplerian telescope*, shown in Figure 12–6, has a positive-powered objective lens and a stronger positive-powered eyepiece lens. A parallel bundle of rays incident on the objective lens at an angle α to the optic axis forms a real image of height h at the secondary focal plane of the objective lens. Because the primary focal plane of the eyepiece lens coincides with the secondary focal plane of the objective lens, the rays emerge parallel from the eyepiece lens at an angle α' to the optic axis. The magnification brought about by the telescope is

$$M = \frac{\alpha'}{\alpha} = \frac{\tan \alpha'}{\tan \alpha}$$
$$= \frac{h/f_e}{h/f_o'} = \frac{f_o'}{f_e} = \frac{-F_e}{F_o}.$$

Thus, the expression $M = \dfrac{-F_e}{F_o}$ is identical for the Galilean and Keplerian telescopes.

The separation, d, of the objective lens and the eyepiece lens of the Keplerian telescope is given by the relationship

$$d = f_o' - f_e.$$

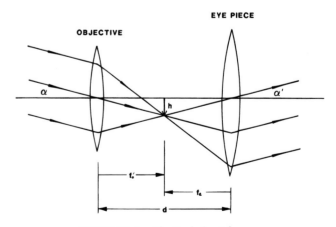

FIGURE 12–6. **The Keplerian telescope.**

Because the secondary focal length of the objective lens is positive and the primary focal length of the eyepiece lens is negative, the separation is the *sum* of the two focal lengths. Hence, as mentioned earlier, a Keplerian telescope is always *longer* than a Galilean telescope of the same magnifying power.

Because F_o and F_e are both positive in power, in the formula

$$M = \frac{-F_e}{F_o},$$

the magnification is negative, which indicates that the image is *inverted*. Therefore, all Keplerian telescopes used as low-vision aids must incorporate an image-erecting lens or prism system; they are referred to as *terrestrial* telescopes. However, when a sense of orientation is not important, an image-erecting system is not incorporated into the Keplerian telescope; such a telescope is described as an *astronomical* telescope.

The basic formulas developed for Galilean telescopes, given below, are valid also for Keplerian telescopes. However, the magnification is positive in sign for the Galilean telescope (image erect) but negative (image inverted) for the Keplerian telescope, unless the telescope is fitted with an erecting system.

$$M = \frac{-F_e}{F_o}$$
$$d = f_o' - f_e$$
$$M = \frac{1}{1 - dF_o}$$
$$= 1 - dF_e.$$

EXAMPLE
An afocal Keplerian telescope has a +10-D objective lens and a +30.00-D eyepiece lens. What is the magnification?

$$M = \frac{-F_e}{F_o} = \frac{-30}{10} = -3\times.$$

What is the separation of the two lenses?

$$d = f_o' - f_e$$
$$= 0.10 - (-0.033) = 0.133 \text{ m} = 13.3 \text{ cm}.$$

Galilean and Keplerian afocal telescopic systems may be compared in the following respects:

1. A Galilean telescope is shorter than a Keplerian telescope of similar magnification.
2. The image formed by a Galilean telescope is erect but that formed by a Keplerian telescope is inverted, which requires an erecting system when the telescope is used as a low-vision aid.
3. The design of a Galilean telescope is usually simpler than that of a Keplerian telescope.
4. Keplerian telescopes are moderately heavy compared with Galilean telescopes.
5. The image quality and brightness across the field of view are usually better in Keplerian telescopes than Galilean telescopes.

6. The magnification available for telescopes of Keplerian design (up to 10×) is higher than that available for those of Galilean design (usually less than 4×).
7. Keplerian telescopes usually have larger fields of view than those of Galilean telescopes. The size and the position of the *exit pupil* of the telescope are important factors in determining the field of view. In the Galilean telescope, the exit pupil is virtual and usually falls inside the telescope between the objective and the eyepiece, at some distance in front of the entrance pupil of the eye. However, in the Keplerian telescope, the exit pupil is *real* and is located a short distance behind the eyepiece, close to the eye's entrance pupil. The position of the exit pupil of the telescope in relation to the eye's entrance pupil increases the field of view of the Keplerian telescope as compared with that of the Galilean telescope.

In discussing afocal telescopes, it is assumed that they are used with emmetropic eyes or those that are made artificially emmetropic, with the distance correction in place. The distance correction can, however, be incorporated into the eyepiece of the telescope.

Some telescopes are adjustable; with such telescopes, it is possible to correct for *spherical* ametropia (for distance vision) by varying the distance between the objective lens and the eyepiece. If the wearer of a telescope is hyperopic with respect to a distant object, the separation of the lenses is *increased* compared with the afocal setting; if the wearer is myopic, the separation is *decreased*. This applies to both Galilean and Keplerian designs.

The tube length required to correct spherical ametropia is illustrated by the following:

EXAMPLE 1
What tube length is required for an uncorrected 5.00-D myope to have clear distance vision through a 4× Galilean telescope having a +5.00-D objective lens?

$$M = +4 = \frac{-F_e}{F_o} = \frac{-F_e}{+5}$$
$$F_e = -20.00 \text{ D}.$$
$$d = f_o' - f_e$$
$$= 0.20 - 0.05 = 0.15 \text{ m}$$
$$= 15 \text{ cm}.$$

Since the telescope is to be used by an uncorrected 5.00-D myope, the vergence leaving the eyepiece must be –5.00 D. The eyepiece lens must therefore be moved a distance, Z, from where the vergence on it is +15.00 D rather than +20.00 D:

$$\frac{+20.00}{1 - Z(+20.00)} = +15.00 \text{ D}$$
$$Z = -\frac{5}{300} = -0.0167 \text{ m} = -1.67 \text{ cm}.$$

Therefore, the value of d, for the 5.00-D myopic eye ($d_{\text{ametropia}}$), compared with its value for the emmetropic eye ($d_{\text{emmetropia}}$), is given by

$$d_{\text{ametropia}} = d_{\text{emmetropia}} + Z$$
$$= 15 + (-1.67)$$
$$= 13.13 \text{ cm}.$$

EXAMPLE 2

What tube length is required for an uncorrected 5.00-D myope to have clear distance vision through a 10× Keplerian telescope having a +5.00 D objective lens?

$$M = -10 = \frac{-F_e}{F_o} = \frac{-F_e}{+5}$$
$$F_e = +50.00 \text{ D}.$$
$$d = f_o' - f_e$$
$$= 0.20 - (-0.02) = 0.22 \text{ m}$$
$$= 22 \text{ cm}.$$

Since the telescope is to be used by an uncorrected 5.00 D myope, the vergence leaving the system must be −5.00 D. The eyepiece lens must therefore be moved a distance of Z, from where the vergence on it is −55.00 D rather than −50.00 D:

$$\frac{-50.00}{1 - Z(-50.00)} = -55.00 \text{ D}$$

$$Z = -\frac{5}{2750} = -0.0018 \text{ m} = -0.18 \text{ cm}.$$

Therefore, the value of d, for the 5.00-D myopic eye ($d_{\text{ametropia}}$), compared with its value for the emmetropic eye ($d_{\text{emmetropia}}$), is given by

$$d_{\text{ametropia}} = d_{\text{emmetropia}} + Z$$
$$= 22 + (-0.18)$$
$$= 21.82 \text{ cm}.$$

When the adjustable feature to correct ametropia for distant objects is used, the effective magnification is changed. For a myope, the angular magnification is reduced with a Galilean telescope and increased with a Keplerian telescope; for a hyperope, the angular magnification is increased with a Galilean telescope and decreased with a Keplerian telescope. Smith[2] developed an expression that provides the effective magnification:

$$M' = M + \frac{d(M)(A)}{M - 1},$$

where M' = the new effective magnification, M = the original magnification, d = the original separation, and A = the refractive correction (a minus sign indicates a myopic correction and a plus sign indicates a hyperopic correction).

EXAMPLE 1

A 2× afocal Galilean telescope has an objective lens of +25.00 D and an eyepiece lens of −50.00 D. If the telescope is adjusted to provide a correction for a 5.00 D myope for distance vision, what is be the effective magnification?

$$d = f_o' - f_e$$
$$= 0.04 - 0.02$$
$$= 0.02 \text{ m} = 2 \text{ cm}.$$
$$M' = M + \frac{d(M)(A)}{M - 1}$$
$$= 2 + \frac{(0.02)(2)(-5)}{2 - 1}$$
$$= 2 + (-0.2)$$
$$= 1.8\times.$$

EXAMPLE 2

If a 2× afocal Keplerian telescope with an objective lens of +25.00 D and a +50.00 D eyepiece lens is adjusted for a 5.00 D myope for distance vision, what is the new effective magnification?

$$d = f_o - f_e$$
$$= 0.04 + 0.02$$
$$= 0.06 \text{ m} = 6 \text{ cm}.$$
$$M' = M + \frac{d(M)(A)}{M - 1}$$
$$= -2 + \frac{(0.06)(-2)(-5)}{-2 - 1} = -2 + \frac{0.6}{-3}$$
$$= -2 + (-0.2)$$
$$= -2.2\times.$$

12.3. Headborne Telescopic Systems

Until recently, most afocal telescopes used as low-vision aids were of Galilean design, but Keplerian telescopes, sometimes referred to as *expanded-field* telescopes, have seen much greater use in recent years. As discussed by Bailey,[3] although these telescopes have the advantage of having a wider field of view than that of Galilean telescopes, they have the disadvantages of being longer, heavier, and about three times more costly. Headborne telescopes, mounted in spectacle frames, are available from many manufacturers as *full-diameter* telescopes, that is, the telescope occupies the entire aperture of the spectacle lens. Also available, from Designs for Vision, is the Bioptic telescope, a small-diameter telescopic unit mounted in the upper part of a carrier lens with the patient's prescription provided in the carrier lens. Keplerian expanded-field telescopes are available in powers ranging from 2× to 8×.

Telescopes of Galilean design are available as full-diameter telescopes in magnifying powers ranging from 1.3× to 2.2× and as Bioptic telescopes in powers ranging from 2.2× to 4×.

Bailey[3] commented that, in his experience, the most useful Galilean Bioptic telescope is the 2.2×; Robert Browning of the University of Houston Low Vision Clinic found that the most useful Keplerian telescopes are the 3× and the 4× (personal communication).

As already stated, the practitioner can usually expect an improvement in the patient's visual acuity proportional to the angular magnification provided by the aid. For example, if, without the telescopic aid, a patient's corrected visual acuity is 3/60 (10/200), a 2× afocal telescope should improve visual acuity to 3/30 (10/100) and a 4× afocal telescope should improve visual acuity to 3/15 (10/50).

Problems Associated with Telescopes for Distance Vision

A telescopic system brings about angular magnification at the expense of making drastic changes in the sizes of perceived objects and in the extent of the visual field. A 2× telescope makes an object appear to be not only twice as *large*, but twice as *near*; it also creates an apparent increase in the rate of motion of moving objects, greatly reduces the visual field, and causes extreme peripheral aberrations. The perceptual problems encountered by a patient wearing a telescopic lens are similar to those experienced by a spectacle-wearing aphakic patient, but they are greatly intensified.

Because of the perceptual problems, full-diameter telescopic spectacles are indicated mainly for relatively sedentary activities rather than for walking and other forms of locomotion. However, some patients can wear a Bioptic telescope for locomotion (and even for driving an automobile).

With such a telescope, the carrier lens, which provides no magnification, is used for routine locomotion, and the head is tilted downward slightly when a magnified view through the telescope is desired.

12.4. Nonprescription Telescopes

Many manufacturers make available nonprescription head-borne telescopic systems, often categorized as *sport-scopes*, which are intended only for occasional use. These aids may also be used by normally sighted individuals in much the same way as prism binoculars are used; therefore, these systems are available at a fraction of the cost of telescopic prescription spectacles.

Other forms of inexpensive telescopic systems include monocular clip-on telescopic units, designed to be clipped to ordinary spectacles, and handheld monocular telescopes. These aids are intended mainly for momentary use, such as identifying a street sign or the route number of a bus, and are available in magnifying powers as high as 6× to 10×. Genensky,[4] a partially sighted researcher for Rand Corporation, recommends the use of ordinary prism binoculars for occasional use for distance vision because they can easily be worn around the neck, are always available when needed, and are more convenient to use than a monocular telescope, even though only one eye may be used with the binoculars.

OPTICAL AIDS FOR NEAR VISION

12.5. Microscopic Lenses

One of the simplest low-vision aids for near vision is the use of high-powered addition in the form of either bifocals or single-vision lenses intended for near vision only. The term *microscopic*, often used to describe such an aid, does not imply a compound lens system as used in a laboratory microscope.

Although microscopic lenses, reading magnifiers, and loupes are often grouped together, a distinction should be made between them. All are basically plus-powered systems that allow the viewing of an object at a short distance with the object located inside the optical system's focal length. *Microscopic lenses* are usually mounted in a conventional frame at a very short vertex distance. A *reading magnifier*, on the other hand, is used at a relatively great distance from the eye; as a result, the diameter of the lens is large to provide an adequate field of view. Increasing the size also increases the weight of the lens, with the result that a reading magnifier is normally handheld or mounted on a stand. *Loupes*, like spectacle lenses, are usually worn on the head with an appropriate device or attached to the spectacle frame. However, the vertex distance is considerably longer

than that ordinarily used for spectacles; hence, the required distance falls between that used for spectacles and that used for reading magnifiers.

To be an effective low-vision aid, the power of the addition of a microscopic lens must be extremely high. Semifinished bifocals kept in stock by ophthalmic laboratories seldom have adds exceeding +4.00 D and, even on special order, additions available for fused bifocals are usually restricted to about +4.50 D because of the increased countersink depth and the resulting increase in lens thickness. However, one-piece bifocals may be obtained with additions as high as +20.00 D on special order.

Wild[5] pointed out that if the segment is placed on the front surface of a high-powered one-piece bifocal, the magnification is increased compared with that obtained by placing the segment on the back surface. Placing the segment on the front surface also has the advantage that if a cylindrical correction is needed, it can be placed on the back surface.

As stated, high additions may be ordered in the form of single-vision lenses intended only for near vision. However, beyond a total power of +10.00 D (in either single-vision lenses or bifocals) ordinary corrected-curve ophthalmic lenses are subject to excessive aberrations, so the use of lenses designed specifically for low-vision patients should be considered.

Many manufacturers have microscopic lenses in both bifocal and single-vision form. For example, Designs for Vision makes a bifocal microscope in magnifying powers from 2× through 10× (+4.00 through +40.00 D) with the distance prescription ground into the carrier lens. The same company also makes full-diameter microscopes in magnifying powers ranging from 2× to 20×.

American Optical has glass microscopic lenses, in bifocal form, in magnifying powers from 2× to 8× (+8.00 to +32.00 D) and plastic aspheric single-vision microscopic lenses in magnifying powers from 6× to 12×. American Optical also markets plastic microscopic lenses in refracting powers from +4.00 to +12.00 D for half-eye frames.

Dioptric Power Notation for Microscopic Lenses

For simplicity in calculation, low-vision lenses are often considered to be single *thin* lenses. For a thin lens, no distinction is made between back vertex power, front vertex power, and equivalent power. In reality, most low-vision magnifiers are *thick* lenses, and the appropriate power notation for such lenses is *equivalent power*. Equivalent power is the negative reciprocal of the distance between the primary principal point and the primary focal point, or the reciprocal of the distance between the secondary principal point and the secondary focal point. In computing the relative sizes of object and image for any thick lens system, object and image distances must be measured from the principal planes. To compare sizes of retinal images accurately for thick low-vision aids, the equivalent powers of the aids must be known. Manufacturers' specifications normally list the equivalent power of low-vision devices.

A disadvantage of using equivalent power (as opposed to back or front vertex power) is that the practitioner cannot easily identify the location of the primary or secondary principal plane of a lens or optical system. However, Bailey[6] described a method of determining equivalent power that can be used in the practitioner's office.

The general formula for angular magnification can be developed from Figure 12–7, in which an object, Y, is placed inside the primary focal point of the lens at a distance l from the lens. The lens rests at a distance h from the center of the entrance pupil of the eye. The object and the image subtend angles α and α', respectively, at the center of the entrance pupil. A formula for the angular magnification may be derived as follows:

$$M = \frac{\tan \alpha'}{\tan \alpha},$$

where

$$\tan \alpha' = \frac{y'}{l' - h} \quad \text{and} \quad \tan \alpha = \frac{y}{l - h}.$$

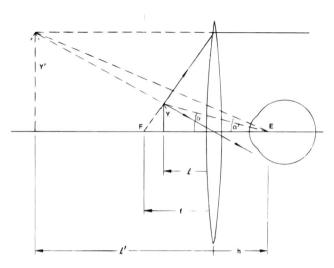

FIGURE 12–7. **Angular magnification of a microscopic lens when the object is placed inside the primary focal plane.**

Substituting,

$$M = \left(\frac{\dfrac{y'}{l' - h}}{\dfrac{y}{l - h}} \right) = \left(\frac{y'}{l' - h} \right) \left(\frac{l - h}{y} \right)$$

$$= \left(\frac{y'}{y} \right) \left(\frac{l - h}{l' - h} \right).$$

Since

$$\frac{y'}{y} = \frac{l'}{l},$$

$$M = \left(\frac{l'}{l} \right) \left(\frac{l - h}{l' - h} \right).$$

Since

$$\frac{1}{l'} = \frac{1}{l} + F,$$

$$l' = \left(\frac{1}{\dfrac{1}{l} + F} \right) = \left(\frac{1}{\dfrac{1 + Fl}{l}} \right).$$

Therefore,

$$M = \left(\frac{l}{1 + Fl} \right) \left(\frac{1}{l} \right) \left(\frac{l - h}{\dfrac{l}{1 + Fl} - h} \right)$$

$$= \left(\frac{l}{1 + Fl} \right) \left(\frac{l - h}{\dfrac{l - h(1 + Fl)}{1 + Fl}} \right),$$

and

$$M = \frac{l - h}{l - h(1 + Fl)}. \qquad (12.8)$$

In this derivation, the distance l is less than the distance f, and the object lies inside the primary focal plane of the lens. Maximum magnification occurs when $l = f$, that is, when the object is located at the primary focal plane of the lens and the image is located at infinity. Therefore, when the object is located at the primary focal plane (Figure 12–8), Equation 12.8 reduces initially to

$$M = \frac{l - h}{l},$$

and, by substituting $-(1/F)$ for l,

$$M = \frac{-\dfrac{1}{F} - h}{-\dfrac{1}{F}} = \frac{\dfrac{1}{F} + h}{\dfrac{1}{F}}$$

$$M = \frac{\dfrac{1 + hF}{F}}{\dfrac{1}{F}} = 1 + hF. \qquad (12.9)$$

This formula gives the amount of *angular magnification* for an object in the primary focal plane of the lens, that is, the ratio of the angular subtense of the object seen through the lens to the angular subtense seen without the lens, with the object at a constant distance from the eye.

The *total magnification* resulting from a microscopic lens is the product of the *angular magnification* and the *relative distance magnification*. Although microscopic lenses provide some angular magnification, the amount is small because of the closeness of the lens to the eye. Most increase in retinal image size originates from relative distance magnification. In situations requiring large amounts of relative distance magnification, the eye is unable to maintain sustained accommodation for such a close distance (in the case of an absolute presbyope, no accommodation is possible).

Therefore, the primary function of a high-powered plus lens is to allow the patient to see near objects clearly with little or no accommodation.

For example, if a +8.00-D lens is placed 15 mm from the eye, the angular magnification for an object in the primary focal plane is

$$\begin{aligned} M &= 1 + hF \\ &= 1 + 0.015(8) \\ &= 1 + 0.12 \\ &= 1.12 \end{aligned}$$

and the percentage magnification is equal to

$$100(M - 1) = 100(1.12 - 1) = 12\%.$$

However, if the reading card was originally held at a distance of 40 cm from the eye, the distance of the card from the eye when viewed through the lens becomes

$$\begin{aligned} 1/8\,\text{m} + 0.015\,\text{m} &= 0.125\,\text{m} + 0.015\,\text{m} \\ &= 0.140\,\text{m} = 14\,\text{cm}. \end{aligned}$$

Therefore, the *relative distance magnification* is

$$40/14 = 2.857\times.$$

Total magnification, also called *effective magnification*, is the product of the angular magnification and the relative distance magnification:

$$1.12(2.857) = 3.2\times.$$

If d in Figure 12–9 is the reference viewing distance, and the quantity $(f - h)$ is the distance of the object from the eye with the lens before the eye, then the angular magnification is equal to

$$\frac{\tan \alpha_3}{\tan \alpha_2} = 1 + hF$$

and the relative distance magnification is

$$\frac{d}{f - h},$$

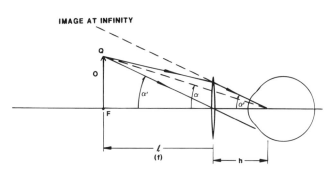

FIGURE 12–8. **Angular magnification of a microscopic lens when the object is placed at the primary focal plane.**

FIGURE 12–9. **Total magnification, or effective magnification. The product of the relative distance magnification and the angular magnification.**

and the total magnification is

$$M = \text{(relative distance magnification}$$
$$\times \text{ angular magnification)}$$

$$= \frac{d}{f - h}(1 + hF)$$

$$= \frac{dF}{fF - hF}(1 + hF)$$

$$= \frac{dF}{\dfrac{f}{-f} - hF}(1 + hF)$$

$$= \frac{dF}{-1 - hF}(1 + hF)$$

$$= \frac{-dF}{1 + hF}(1 + hF)$$

$$M = -dF. \tag{12.10}$$

This formula emphasizes the need for establishing a standard reference viewing distance.

Although arbitrary, this distance historically has been assumed to be 25 cm, a distance known as the *least distance of distinct vision*. Hence, Equation 12.10 is often stated as

$$M = -dF = -(-0.25)F$$

or

$$M = \frac{F}{4}. \tag{12.11}$$

Magnification so stated is called *effective* magnification. Thus, a +4.00-D magnifier designed to view an object at 25 cm has an effective magnifying power of 1×, a +8.00-D magnifier designed to view an object at 12.5 cm has an effective magnifying power of 2×, and so forth. Most optometrists prefer to use 40 cm as the standard reference distance because they are accustomed to testing their patients' near vision at this distance.

Magnifiers are sometimes described in terms of *conventional magnification*, which is defined as the ratio of the angular subtense of the image formed at the standard reference distance from the eye by the optical system to the angular subtense of the object placed at the standard reference distance *without* the optical system in place (Figure 12–10). It is assumed that the ametropia is corrected and that the same amount of accommodation is required with and without the optical system.

From Figure 12–10 it is apparent that

$$M = \frac{O'}{O} = \frac{l'}{l} = \frac{L}{L'}$$

$$= \frac{L' - F}{L'}$$

$$= \frac{L'}{L'} - \frac{F}{L'}$$

$$= 1 - \frac{F}{L'} = 1 - l'F,$$

and since

$$l' = h + d,$$
$$M = 1 - (h + d)F.$$

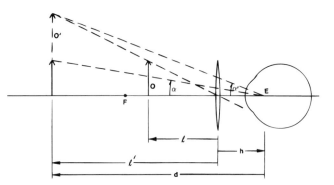

FIGURE 12–10.   **Conventional magnification. The ratio of the angular subtense of the image formed by the optical system at the standard reference distance, *d*, from the eye to the angular subtense of the object placed at the standard reference distance *without* the optical system in place.**

If the magnifying lens is held close to the eye so that the distance h can be ignored and if the standard reference distance, d, is equal to –0.25 m, then the conventional magnification can be stated as

$$M = 1 - (-0.25)F = 1 + \frac{F}{4}. \tag{12.12}$$

When commercially available microscopic low-vision aids are rated only by their magnification, the underlying assumptions used in making such ratings may be impossible to know. It is more reliable, therefore, to simply specify the *equivalent power* instead of the magnifying power.

Specifying magnification in terms of equivalent power has the advantage of not presupposing a standard reference distance and, if the practitioner knows the equivalent power of a given microscopic lens, the magnification and the expected visual acuity that it will provide can be easily determined. For example, if a presbyopic patient's best corrected near acuity with a +2.50-D add as determined by a reduced Snellen chart at a distance of 40 cm is 20/100, a microscopic lens having an equivalent power of +10.00 D will enable the patient to read at 10 cm by providing a magnification of 4×, resulting in an expected visual acuity of 20/25.

Although the use of equivalent power is the most desirable method of specifying the magnifying power of microscopic lenses, most manufacturers still specify magnification on the basis of the standard reference distance of 25 cm. Table 12–1 shows the magnifying power (based on the 25-cm distance) of microscopic lenses of various equivalent powers, with corresponding reading distances for absolute presbyopes.

Problems Associated with Microscopic Lenses

The following problems are associated with the use of microscopic reading aids:

1. *Aberrations.* Lenses of the very high powers required for microscopic aids often produce severe aberrations un-

TABLE 12–1
Magnifying Power of Microscopic Lenses on the Basis of a Standard Reading Distance of 25 cm, Together with the Necessary Reading Distance for an Absolute Presbyope

Equivalent Power (D)	Magnifying Power (times)	Reading Distance (cm)
+4.00	1	25
+6.00	1.5	16.7
+8.00	2	12.5
+10.00	2.5	10
+12.00	3	8.3
+16.00	4	6.25
+20.00	5	5

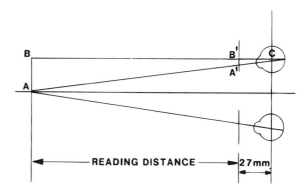

FIGURE 12–11.   Determining the amount of decentration for microscopic lenses.

less they are carefully designed. Aberrations may, however, be controlled by using aspheric surfaces or multiple elements, which adds considerably to the expense.

2. *Illumination.* When reading material is held very close to the eyes, it is difficult to provide adequate illumination for the reading material because much ambient light is blocked by the patient's head.

3. *Centration of Lenses.* Often a patient who requires a microscopic aid for near vision has such a severe visual loss in each eye that an aid is prescribed only for the better eye. For example, if the patient's reduced Snellen acuity at 40 cm is 20/100 with the right eye but less than 20/200 for the left eye, the practitioner may decide to prescribe the aid only for the right eye. On the other hand, if acuity is approximately equal for the two eyes, the patient is very likely able to make use of binocular vision if an aid is prescribed for each eye. In such a case, the practitioner must know where to place the *centers* of the microscopic aids for the two eyes. Because reading will be done at a very close distance, more inward decentration is required than the "2 mm in" normally used for bifocal lenses.

If it is assumed that the *stop distance* (the distance between the back vertex of the lens and the center of rotation of the eye) is 27 cm, inspection of Figure 12–11 (note the similar triangles ABC and A′B′C) shows that the required amount of decentration can be determined by the use of the following formula:

$$\text{total decentration} = \frac{27(\text{distance PD})}{(\text{reading distance}) + 27}. \quad (12.13)$$

For example, for a reading distance of 10 cm and PD of 60 mm, the total decentration is

$$\frac{27(60)}{100 + 27} = 12.8 \text{ mm, rounding to 13 mm,}$$

with the result that each lens should be decentered inward 6.5 mm.

Note that Equation 12.13 does not require the power of the microscope, only the reading distance at which the microscope will be used. Table 12–2 shows the required amount of decentration for typical reading distances, assuming a distance PD of 64 mm and a stop distance of 27 mm.

In discussing decentration of microscopic lenses, Bailey[7] emphasized that when a reading distance closer than 10 cm is necessary, binocularity becomes impractical—only a lens for the better eye should be prescribed. He suggested that when lenses are to be prescribed for both eyes, the amount of decentration may be determined by the following rule: For each diopter of working distance (i.e., add for near vision), give 1.5 mm of total decentration (both eyes), and if the distance PD is greater than 65 mm, add 1 mm of decentration.

4. *Maintenance of the Proper Viewing Distance.* Although a microscopic lens can greatly improve the near acuity of a low-vision patient, many patients have difficulty adapting to the very short reading distance that is necessary. For example, a microscopic lens with an equivalent power of +20.00 D requires a reading distance of 5 cm. Holding the reading material at the correct viewing distance and keeping the facial plane parallel to the page is often a most difficult task.

Because the depth of focus of a strong plus lens is very small, movement of the reading material only a slight distance from the primary focal plane of the lens provides large changes in vergence of the light emerging from the lens. If the reading material falls within the focal point, the emergent light diverges and the retinal image becomes blurred unless accommodation is used. Therefore, for presbyopic or aphakic patients, reading material must be held in the primary focal plane of the lens for the print to be seen clearly. Many elderly patients cannot hold reading material steadily at the required distance for long periods of time.

TABLE 12–2
Decentration Required for Microscopic Lenses, for a Distance PD of 64 mm and a Stop Distance of 27 mm

Reading Distance (cm)	Total Decentration (mm)	Decentration of Each Lens (mm)
40	4	2
33	5	2.5
25	6	3
20	8	4
17	9	4.5
12.5	11	5.5
10	14	7

12.6. Telescopic Lenses for Near Vision

Even if an individual has a high amplitude of accommodation, it is virtually impossible to accommodate for near objects through an afocal telescope because of the *vergence amplification effect;* that is, when diverging rays are incident on a telescope, the emerging rays have considerably more divergence than that of the incident rays (shown in Figure 12–12). Because of this effect, if an attempt is made to accommodate for a near object through an afocal telescope, the amount of accommodation necessary is much greater than that indicated by the object distance.

Bailey[8] proposed an approximate equation for the vergence amplification effect:

$$L'_2 = M^2 L_1, \qquad (12.14)$$

where L'_2 = the emerging vergence, M = the magnifying power of the telescope, and L_1 = the incident vergence.

For a 2× telescope used at a distance of 40 cm, the vergence amplification effect is

$$2^2(-2.50) = 4(-2.50) = -10.00 \text{ D},$$

and therefore the amount of accommodation required at that distance is 10 D. For a 4× telescope used at the same distance, the vergence amplification effect is

$$4^2(-2.50) = 16(-2.50) = -40.00 \text{ D}.$$

The problem of the vergence amplification effect can be solved by placing a plus lens of appropriate power either in front of or behind the telescope. When a plus lens is placed *in front of* a telescope to be used for near vision, parallel rays of light enter the telescope, with the result that the vergence amplification effect does not occur; if a plus lens is placed *behind* the telescope, the vergence amplification effect does occur, and a lens of much higher plus power must be used.

Therefore, a telescopic system to be used for near vision is usually fitted with *reading cap* on the front of the telescope. The reading cap is easily removable and can be carried by the patient and worn when needed for near vision. The reading cap must have the power determined by the desired reading distance; that is, for a reading distance of 40 cm, the reading cap must have a power of +2.50 D, or for a distance of 20 cm, it must have a power of +5.00 D. The combination of an afocal telescope and a reading cap is known as a *telemicroscope.*

For an individual whose ametropia is corrected, the working distance for a telemicroscope is equal to the front focal length of the reading cap lens, which is also the front focal length of the telemicroscope itself because the telescopic unit is afocal. If a lens of front vertex power F_N is placed before the objective lens of an afocal telescope, the resulting telemicroscope has a front vertex power F_N, with a front focal length of f_N (or $1/F_N$). The front focal length of the reading cap determines the working distance of the lens and is inversely proportional to the relative distance magnification created by the reading cap.

As previously discussed, relative distance magnification is based on a standard reference distance for which magnification is considered to be unity; to avoid confusion as to whether the reference distance is 25 or 40 cm, it is appropriate to define or compare low-vision devices in terms of their equivalent power.

The total magnification of a telemicroscope is the product of the angular magnification of the afocal telescope and the relative distance magnification of the reading cap. The total magnification is equal to the relative distance magnification of a single plus lens and is directly proportional to the equivalent power. Hence, different telemicroscopes of the same equivalent power produce the same magnification for the wearer, although the working distances are different.

The equivalent power of a telemicroscope can be found by

$$F_E = F_1 + F_2 - dF_1F_2,$$

where F_E = the equivalent power, F_1 = the sum of powers of the reading cap and the objective lens, F_2 = the power of the eyepiece lens, and d = the separation of the objective and eyepiece lenses.

EXAMPLE

An afocal Galilean telescope has the following specifications:

$$F_1 = +10.00 \text{ D}$$
$$F_2 = -20.00 \text{ D}$$
$$d = 5 \text{ cm}.$$

What is the magnifying power of the telescope?

$$M = \frac{-F_2}{F_1} = -\frac{(-20)}{10} = 2\times.$$

If a +4.00-D reading cap is placed on the objective lens, the equivalent power can be found by use of the formula

$$F_E = F_1 + F_2 - dF_1F_2,$$
$$F_E = +14 + (-20) - 0.05(14)(-20)$$
$$= -6 + 14$$
$$= +8.00 \text{ D}.$$

An alternative method can be developed: The front vertex power of the telemicroscope is equal to the front vertex power of the reading cap and, thus, the front vertex power of the telemicroscope is

$$F_N = \frac{F_2}{1 - dF_2} + F_1,$$

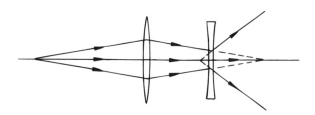

FIGURE 12–12. **The vergence amplification effect. When diverging rays are incident on a telescope, the emerging rays have a greater vergence than that of the incident rays.**

where F_N = the front vertex power of the telemicroscope, F_1 = the sum of the powers of the reading cap and the objective lens, F_2 = the power of the eyepiece lens, and d = the separation of the objective and eyepiece lenses:

$$F_N = \frac{F_2}{1 - dF_2} + \frac{F_1(1 - dF_2)}{1 - dF_2}$$
$$= \frac{F_1 + F_2 - dF_1F_2}{1 - dF_2}$$
$$= \frac{F_E}{1 - dF_2}. \tag{12.15}$$

In Section 12.2 the magnification of an afocal telescope was expressed as

$$M = 1 - dF_2.$$

Thus,

$$F_N = \frac{F_E}{M},$$

or

$$F_E = F_N M. \tag{12.16}$$

Equation 12.16 shows that the equivalent power of a telemicroscope is equal to the *power of the reading cap times the magnifying power of the afocal telescope.*

In the example worked previously, the equivalent power resulting by placing a +4.00 D reading cap on a 2× Galilean telescope was +8.00 D. In the equation

$$F_E = F_N M,$$
$$F_E = +4(2) = +8.00 \text{ D}.$$

In each example, if the standard reference distance is 25 cm, the magnification is

$$M = dF_E = 0.25(8) = 2\times.$$

The magnification of a telemicroscope can also be found by multiplying the magnification of the telescope by the power of the reading cap divided by 4, or

$$M = (\text{magnification of telescope})(F_{RC}/4).$$

This simple relationship—that the equivalent power of a telemicroscope is equal to the power of the reading cap times the angular magnification of the afocal telescope—is useful in selecting the combination of reading cap and afocal telescope to provide the required magnification. For example, each of the following telemicroscopes (Figure 12–13) provides an equivalent power of 24 D and all provide the same magnification: a 4× telescope with a +6.00 D reading cap (A), a 6× telescope with a +4.00 D reading cap (B), and an 8× telescope with a +3.00 D reading cap (C). What varies is the *working distance*, which is 16.67 cm for telemicroscope A, 25 cm for telemicroscope B, and 33.3 cm for telemicroscope C. Each telemicroscope provides the same magnification as a +24.00 D *microscopic* lens with a working distance of 4.17 cm (Figure 12–13D).

When compared to use of a microscopic lens, or high add, a telescope with a reading cap has the following advantages and disadvantages:

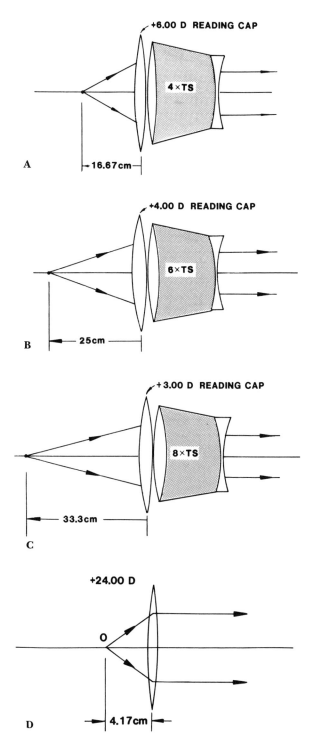

FIGURE 12–13. **Four magnifiers with the same equivalent power (the same magnification) but varying working distances. A, 4× telescope with a +6.00 D reading cap and a reading distance of 16.67 cm; B, 6× telescope with a +4.00 D reading cap and a reading distance of 25.00 cm; C, 8× telescope with a +3.00 D reading cap and a reading distance of 33.30 cm; D, +24.00 D microscopic lens with a working distance of 4.17 cm.**

1. Because of the power of the afocal telescope, the patient can obtain *greater magnification* at the same working distance as that for a microscopic lens. For example, if only a +10.00-D microscopic lens is worn for a working distance of 10 cm, the angular magnification is 2.5× (assuming a reference distance of 25 cm), but with the addition of the 2× afocal telescope, the equivalent power of the resulting telemicroscope, according to Equation 12.16, is 10(2), or +20.00 D, and the total magnification at that reading distance is +20/4, or 5×.
2. Conversely, with the magnifying power provided by the afocal telescope, for a given amount of magnification, a patient wearing a telescope with a reading cap can read at a *greater distance* than that possible if only a microscopic lens is worn. Again using the above example, a patient wearing a 2× afocal telescope and a +10.00 D reading cap is able to read at a distance of 10 cm with a total magnification of 5×, but if only a 5× (+20.00 D) microscopic lens is worn, the patient has to read at a distance of 5 cm, with the same amount of magnification.
3. An afocal lens with a reading cap has the disadvantage of a *smaller field of view* than is present if only a microscopic lens is worn.

All manufacturers of telescopic spectacles have reading caps available in various powers. Designs for Vision makes a low-vision aid called Trioptic, consisting of an afocal telescope (Bioptic) with a reading cap, mounted in the upper part of a carrier lens, and a microscopic lens mounted in the lower part of the carrier lens.

12.7. Hand Magnifiers

Many hand magnifiers are available at relatively low cost, and many patients who have a low-vision problem will have already visited the local drug or variety store and purchased one or more of these aids. The magnifiers are particularly useful for short-term visual tasks such as looking at a telephone number, but they can also be used for prolonged reading.

Although the hand magnifier is a relatively simple device, the optical principles involved in its use are complex because the magnification cannot be represented by a unique number. The magnification depends not only on the equivalent power but also on how the magnifier is used. Both the distance from the lens to the eye and the distance from the object to the lens affect the amount of magnification. Each distance can be altered independently over a wide range, according to the wishes of the user.

Normally, the magnification of a hand magnifier is specified by the manufacturer. The stated magnification is usually based on the formula

$$M = \frac{F_E}{4}.$$

Use of this formula assumes that the standard reference distance for unaided vision is 25 cm and that the object is located at the primary focal point of the lens. In this situation, light from the object emerges parallel from the lens, with the result, as shown in Figure 12–14, that parallel light is incident on the eye, regardless of the distance from the eye to the lens. The fact that parallel light is incident on the eye regardless of the distance from the eye to the lens is responsible for an important property of a hand magnifier: When an object is located in the primary focal plane of the magnifier, the magnification (and therefore the retinal image size) is constant, *regardless of the distance between the magnifier and the eye.*

As shown in Figure 12–14, retinal image size is determined by the angle between the optic axis and the ray from the object point, Q, subtended at the entrance pupil. If the eye is moved from its original position A to position B, farther from the lens, the ray that passes through the entrance pupil creates a retinal image that is equal in linear size to that in the original position. This occurs because all rays leaving the lens are parallel, with the result that any ray passing through the center of the entrance pupil crosses the optic axis at the same angle. However, even though the retinal image size is constant for all magnifier-to-eye distances, the field of view decreases as the distance is increased.

Another explanation may be helpful in accounting for the constancy of the retinal image size. If the object is kept in the focal plane of the magnifier and if the object and the magnifier are moved in unison away from the eye, the *angular magnification* increases. However, the *relative distance magnification* decreases, and the product of the angular magnification and the relative distance magnification is a constant.

If the object is positioned in the primary focal plane of the magnifier, no accommodation need be exerted if the viewer's ametropia is properly corrected. The equivalent power of the system is therefore simply the equivalent power of the magnifier.

When the object is positioned at a distance *closer* to the magnifier than the primary focal length, the image falls behind the magnifier, closer than infinity, as shown in Figure 12–15. To see the image clearly, an emmetropic (or corrected ametropic) observer must resort either to accommodation or to the use of a reading addition. In this situation, the retinal image size is *no longer constant* for all

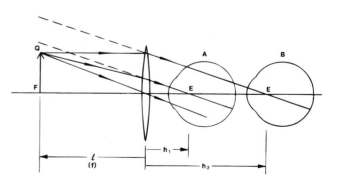

FIGURE 12–14.   **With the object in the primary focal plane of a hand magnifier, the retinal image size is constant and independent of the distance between the magnifier and the eye.**

FIGURE 12–15.   **When an object is positioned closer to a hand magnifier than its primary focal length, the image is located behind the magnifier, closer than infinity.**

viewing distances. In this event, the equivalent power of the system is equal to

$$F_E = F_M + F_A - dF_M F_A,$$

where F_E = the equivalent power, F_M = the power of the magnifier, F_A = the amount of accommodation or power of add, and d = the distance from the magnifier to the spectacle plane.

When the distance from the magnifier to the spectacle plane is equal to the focal length of the magnifier,

$$F_M = \frac{1}{d},$$

and

$$F_E = F_M + F_A - d\left(\frac{1}{d}\right)F_A,$$

therefore

$$F_E = F_M,$$

with the result that the equivalent power of the optical system is equal *solely* to the power of the magnifier; it is independent of the amount of accommodation or of the power of the reading addition. The image of the system is seen clearly if the object is placed so that the image falls at the distance for which the eye is accommodated or at the focal distance of the reading addition.

When the distance from the magnifier to the spectacle plane is *less* than the focal length of the magnifier, the resultant equivalent power is *greater* than the power of the magnifier, reaching a maximum value when the magnifier is placed in the spectacle plane (in which case $d = 0$). In this situation, the equivalent power is equal to the sum of the power of the magnifier and the power of the reading addition. On the other hand, when the distance from the magnifier to the spectacle plane is *greater* than the focal length of the magnifier, the resultant equivalent power is *less* than the power of the magnifier. The greater the separation, the less the resultant equivalent power. These principles are illustrated by the following examples:

EXAMPLE 1
A simple magnifier having a refracting power of +20.00 D is used by a presbyope who wears a +2.50 D add, with the magnifier held 5 cm in front of the spectacle lens (d = 5 cm). What is the equivalent power of the magnifier/reading-add system?

$$F_E = F_M + F_A - dF_M F_A,$$
$$= +20.00 + 2.50 - 0.05(+20.00)(+2.50)$$
$$= +22.50 - 2.50$$
$$= +20.00 \text{ D}.$$

EXAMPLE 2
Using the same magnifier and the same reading add, the magnifier is held in contact with the spectacle lens ($d = 0$). What is the equivalent power of the combination?

$$F_E = F_M + F_A - dF_M F_A,$$
$$= +20.00 + 2.50 - 0(+20.00)(+2.50)$$
$$= +22.50 + 0$$
$$= +22.00 \text{ D}.$$

EXAMPLE 3
Again using the same magnifier and the same reading add, the magnifier is moved to a position 10 cm in front of the spectacle plane. What is the equivalent power of the combination?

$$F_E = F_M + F_A - dF_M F_A,$$
$$= +20.00 + 2.50 - 0.1(+20.00)(+2.50)$$
$$= +22.50 - 5.00$$
$$= +17.00 \text{ D}.$$

To summarize these results, if a magnifier is placed at its focal distance from the spectacle plane, its equivalent power is always equal to the power of the magnifier (regardless of whether a bifocal is used), as shown in Example 1. When a bifocal is used with the hand magnifier, if the magnifier is held at a distance in front of the spectacle plane shorter than its focal length, the equivalent power is greater than that of the magnifier alone (Example 2); if the magnifier is held at a distance in front of the spectacle plane greater than its focal length, the equivalent power is less than that of the magnifier alone (Example 3).

For objects located at arm's length (i.e., beyond the distance for which a bifocal addition is intended) magnification is maximal when the object is placed in the primary focal plane of the magnifier and distance spectacles are used.

Because the magnification of a hand magnifier depends on how it is used, a hand magnifier should not be specified in terms of a fixed magnifying power but by its *equivalent power*.

As described above (Example 2), it is possible for a low-vision patient to use a hand magnifier by placing it in contact with his or her lenses (using it as a high add) and holding the reading material at a suitably close distance. Faye[9] made the point that some patients who resist wearing a high add in the form of a spectacle lens are willing to use a hand magnifier and that, for these patients, the use of a hand magnifier held against the spectacle correction serves as a simple and inexpensive method for the patient to gain experience in using a high addition. After practicing with this combination, some patients actually request to be fitted with a high addition in spectacle form.

When an object is located in the primary focal plane of a hand magnifier, the *linear field of view* is given by the following expression:[10]

$$w = \frac{y}{F_E(d)},$$

where w = the linear width of the field of view, y = the lens diameter in meters, F_E = the equivalent power of the magnifier, and d = the distance of the magnifier to the spectacle plane in meters. For example, if a 50-mm round +20.00-D hand magnifier is held 10 cm from the eye, and the object is located at the primary focal point of the magnifier, the field of view of the magnifier is

$$w = \frac{0.05}{20(0.1)}$$
$$= \frac{0.05}{2}$$
$$= 0.025 \text{ m, or } 25 \text{ mm.}$$

If the object is not located in the primary focal plane of the magnifier, the field of view behaves in the following manner:

1. If the distance from the eye to the magnifier is *greater* than the focal length of the magnifier, the linear field of view *increases* slightly.
2. If the distance from the eye to the magnifier is *less* than the focal length of the magnifier, the linear field of view *decreases* slightly.

12.8. Stand Magnifiers

Although a few focusable stand magnifiers are available, most stand magnifiers are of *the fixed-focus* type, having a fixed object-to-lens distance. The magnifier support is placed directly on the reading material, with the result that both the object distance and the image distance are constant. If the plane of the reading material coincides with the primary focal plane of the magnifier, the image is located at infinity. Usually, the reading material is located just inside the focal plane of the magnifier, with the result that a virtual, erect image is formed behind the magnifier between the plane of the reading material and infinity. For the image to be seen clearly, an emmetrope or a corrected ametrope must accommodate or wear a suitable reading addition.

When a stand magnifier is prescribed for a low-vision patient, the practitioner must locate the image plane to instruct the patient about the proper viewing distance and to estimate the amount of accommodation or the power of the reading addition required to see the image clearly. The location of the image plane can be found by neutralizing the emerging divergence with a plus lens, which causes the image to be formed at infinity (Figure 12–16).

Because a stand magnifier is intended to be used so that the virtual image is located at a standard reading distance, it is possible to calculate the *equivalent power* of the magnifier, which permits such a magnifier to be compared with other magnification systems (such as high add) used close to the eye.

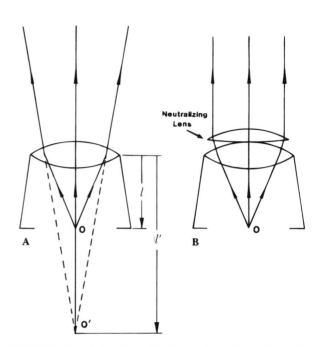

FIGURE 12–16.   **A, Location of the image plane of a stand magnifier; B, the power of the neutralizing lens that renders the emergent light parallel indicates the position of the image plane, *O'*.**

The equivalent power may be found by combining the refractive power of the magnifier and the amount of accommodation in play (or the power of the reading addition) and using the formula used for a hand magnifier,

$$F_E = F_M + F_A - dF_M F_A,$$

where F_E = the equivalent power, F_M = the power of the magnifier, F_A = the amount of accommodation or power of add, and d = the distance from the magnifier to the spectacle plane.

The amount of accommodation or power of the reading addition is

$$F_A = \frac{1}{d - l'}, \tag{12.17}$$

where l' is the negative image distance behind the stand. In the general equivalent power equation,

$$F_E = F_M + F_A - dF_M F_A,$$

or

$$F_E = F_A[F_M/F_A + 1 - dF_M].$$

Substituting the expression for F_A from Equation 12.17 within the brackets,

$$F_E = F_A[F_M(d - l') + 1 - dF_M]$$
$$= F_A[dF_M - F_M l' + 1 - dF_M]$$
$$= F_A(1 - F_M l')$$
$$= F_A\left(1 - \frac{F_M}{L'}\right)$$
$$F_E = F_A\left(\frac{L' - F_M}{L'}\right). \tag{12.18}$$

The expression

$$\left(\frac{L' - F_M}{L'}\right) \qquad (12.19)$$

was coined the MULTACC factor (M_T) by Bailey.[11]

Therefore,

$$F_E = F_A(M_T),$$

where

$$M_T = \left(\frac{L' - F_M}{L'}\right),$$

and since in the simple lens formula,

$$L' - F = L,$$

then

$$M_T = \frac{L}{L'} = \frac{l'}{l}.$$

Therefore, the MULTACC factor is an expression for lateral or transverse magnification.

Bailey recommended that all fixed-focus stand magnifiers be labeled in terms of refracting power, F_M, the image position, l', and the MULTACC factor, M_T, to allow easy calculation of the equivalent power. A stand magnifier creates different equivalent powers depending on the separation of the eye and the magnifier and offers different resolution abilities because resolution ability is directly proportional to equivalent power.

To illustrate how the equivalent power changes with the manner in which a stand magnifier is used, consider a stand magnifier having a refracting power, F_M, of +20.00 D, and an image distance, l', of –20 cm (and, therefore, an image vergence, L', of –5.00 D).

$$M_T = \frac{L' - F}{L'} = \frac{-5 - 20}{-5} = \frac{-25}{-5} = 5.$$

EXAMPLE 1
If the magnifier is located in the spectacle plane and if the distance between the spectacle plane and the image is 20 cm, what is the equivalent power?

$$F_A = \frac{1}{0.2} = +5.00 \text{ D}.$$

Thus,

$$F_E = F_A(M_T) = 5(5) = +25.00 \text{ D}.$$

EXAMPLE 2
If the magnifier is located 20 cm from the spectacle plane and the distance between the spectacle plane and the image is 40 cm (20 cm + 20 cm), what is the equivalent power?

$$F_A = \frac{1}{0.4} = +2.50 \text{ D}.$$

Thus,

$$F_E = F_A(M_T) = 2.50(5) = +12.50 \text{ D}.$$

Hence, changing the distance from the spectacle plane to the magnifier from zero to 20 cm changes the ac-commodation (or power of the required reading addition) from 5.00 to 2.50 D and the equivalent power from +25.00 to +12.50 D. Because resolution ability is directly proportional to equivalent power, the change reduces the observer's resolution ability by one-half.

EXAMPLE 3
If the stand magnifier is used as described in Example 2, by a patient who can barely read 25-point print at 40 cm while wearing a +2.50-D add, what size print can the patient resolve?

With the stand magnifier specified in Example 2, the equivalent power of the combination of the +20.00-D stand magnifier and the +2.50-D addition is

$$F_E = F_A(M_T) = 2.50(5) = +12.50 \text{ D}.$$

The +12.50-D system should improve resolution by a factor of 5 compared with that obtained with the +2.50-D add, so that the patient can be expected to resolve 5-point print.

12.9. The Paperweight Magnifier

The "paperweight magnifier" is a very popular reading aid. It is a thick, plano-convex lens that is held in contact with the reading material and is moved along the page as the person reads; it is therefore a modification of the stand magnifier with a magnifier-to-print distance of zero.

Although the magnifying power of a paperweight magnifier is relatively low, it has the advantage of very good light-gathering properties and is very easy to use, particularly for an older person with unsteady hands. When given a choice of a large number of commercially available aids, many low-vision patients choose such a magnifier.

The magnifying power of a paperweight magnifier can be determined by finding the image position and applying the linear magnification formula for a single spherical refracting surface; thus,

$$M = \frac{h'}{h} = \frac{nl'}{n'l} = \frac{L}{L'}.$$

EXAMPLE 1
A paperweight magnifier has a spherical surface with a radius of curvature of 5 cm, a thickness of 3 cm, and an index of refraction of 1.53. (1) What is the position of its image? (2) What is its magnification?

(1) Using the single spherical refracting surface formula (Figure 12–17),

$$\frac{n'}{l'} - \frac{n}{l} = \frac{n' - n}{r}$$

$$\frac{1}{l'} - \frac{1.53}{-0.03} = \frac{1 - 1.53}{-0.05}$$

$$\frac{1}{l'} + 51 = +10.6$$

$$\frac{1}{l'} = -40.4$$

$$l' = -0.0248 \text{ m} = -2.48 \text{ cm}.$$

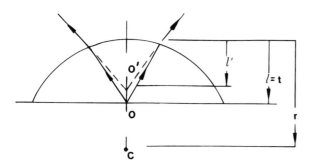

FIGURE 12–17.   **Location of the image position and magnification for a paperweight magnifier (see Section 12.9, Example 1).**

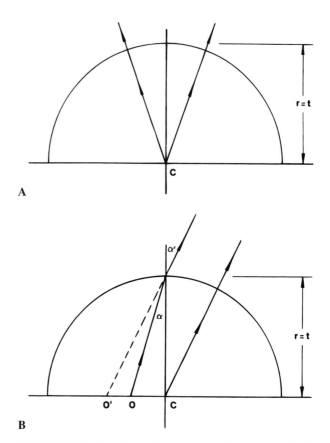

A

B

FIGURE 12–18.   **Location of the image position and magnification for a paperweight magnifier whose thickness is equal to its radius of curvature, being hemispherical in shape (see Section 12.9, Example 2).**

(2) The magnification can be determined by use of the expression

$$M = \frac{nl'}{n'l}$$
$$= \frac{1.53(-0.0248)}{1(-0.03)} = \frac{0.0379}{0.03}$$
$$M = 1.26\times.$$

An interesting form of the paperweight magnifier occurs when the radius of curvature is equal to the center thickness, that is, when the magnifier is in the form of a *hemisphere*, as shown by the following example.

EXAMPLE 2

A paperweight magnifier has a spherical surface with a radius of curvature of 5 cm, a thickness of 5 cm, and an index of refraction of 1.53. (1) What is the position of its image? (2) What is its magnification?

(1) Referring to Figure 12–18 and using the formula for a spherical refracting surface,

$$\frac{n'}{l'} - \frac{n}{l} = \frac{n' - n}{r}$$
$$\frac{1}{l'} - \frac{1.53}{-0.05} = \frac{1 - 1.53}{-0.05}$$
$$\frac{1}{l'} + 30.6 = +10.6$$
$$\frac{1}{l'} = -20$$
$$l' = -0.05 \text{ m} = -5 \text{ cm}.$$

The image of this paperweight magnifier is therefore located *in the plane of the object* (A).

(2) Referring again to Figure 12–18, the magnification is

$$M = \frac{nl'}{n'l}$$
$$= \frac{1.53(-0.05)}{1(-0.05)} = \frac{0.0379}{0.05}$$
$$M = 1.53\times.$$

Hence, for a paperweight magnifier in the form of a hemisphere, the *magnification is equal to the index of refraction* (B).

References

1. Mehr, E. B., and Freid, A. M. *Low Vision Care.* Professional Press, Chicago, 1975.
2. Smith, G. Magnification of Afocal Telescopes When Used Focally. *Austr. J. Optom.,* Vol. 64, No. 5, pp. 202–205, 1964.
3. Bailey, I. L. New "Expanded Field" Bioptic Systems. *Optom. Monthly,* Vol. 69, pp. 895–898, 1978.
4. Genensky, S. M. Binoculars: A Long-Ignored Aid for the Partially Sighted. *Am. J. Optom. Physiol. Opt.,* Vol. 51, pp. 648–673, 1974.
5. Wild, B. W. A Low-Vision Aid Design for Reading. *Optom. Weekly,* Vol. 59, pp. 36–37, 1968.
6. Bailey, I. L. Traditional Methods for Measuring the Magnification of Telescopes. *Optom. Monthly,* Vol. 70, pp. 128–131, 1979.
7. Bailey, I. L. Centering High Addition Spectacle Lenses. *Optom. Monthly,* Vol. 69, pp. 981–984, 1978.
8. Bailey, I. L. Telescopes: Their Use in Low Vision. *Optom. Monthly,* Vol. 69, pp. 634–638, 1978.
9. Faye, E. *Clinical Low Vision.* Little, Brown, Boston, 1976.
10. Johnston, A. W. Technical Note: The Relationship between the Magnification and Field of View for Simple Magnifiers. *Austr. J. Optom.,* Vol. 65, No. 2, pp. 74–77, 1982.
11. Bailey, I. L. The Use of Fixed Focus Stand Magnifiers. *Optom. Monthly,* Vol. 72, pp. 37–39, 1981.

Questions

1. A patient with a best-corrected acuity of 10/80 must read 20/40 on the job. What approximate magnification is needed?

2. If an object is moved from 40 to 15 cm, what is the relative distance magnification?

3. An afocal Keplerian telescope has an objective lens of +5.00 D and an eyepiece lens of +12.50 D.

    (a) What is the magnifying power for a distant object?
    (b) What is the length of the telescope?

4. An afocal 4× Galilean telescope has a telescopic length of 7.5 cm. What is the power of the objective lens and the eyepiece lens?

5. An afocal 4× Galilean telescope has an objective lens of +5.00 D. What telescopic length is required for an uncorrected 5.00 D hyperope to have clear distance vision?

6. If a 4× afocal Keplerian telescope with an objective lens of +10.00 D and a +40.00 D eyepiece lens is adjusted to allow an uncorrected 5.00 D hyperope to see clearly at distance, what is the new effective magnification?

7. A microscopic lens has an equivalent power of +20.00 D. If the lens is used 15 mm from the eye, what is the angular magnification for an object placed at its primary focal point?

8. If the object in Question 7 was originally placed at a distance of 40 cm from the eye, what is the total magnification of the lens described in Question 7?

9. If a 2× afocal telescope is used for an object at 50 cm without a reading cap, what is the approximate amount of accommodation required to see the object clearly?

10. If a 4× afocal telescope is fitted with a +4.00 D reading cap, what is the equivalent power of the combination?

11. What is the working distance of the telemicroscope described in Question 10?

12. What is the total magnification relative to a reference distance of 25 cm of a 2× afocal Galilean telescope with a +10.00-D cap?

13. A printer needs 4× magnification to perform his duties. However, the working distance must be 20 cm. What combination of afocal telescope and reading cap provides the desired magnification?

14. A +12.00 D hand magnifier is used in conjunction with a +3.00 D spectacle addition at a distance of 20 cm from the spectacle plane. What is the equivalent power of the magnifier/reading-add system?

15. What is the linear field of view for a 60-mm round +15.00 D hand magnifier held 10 cm from the eye, with the object at the primary focal plane of the magnifier?

16. A +25.00 D stand magnifier is 20 cm from the spectacle plane. The virtual image formed by the stand magnifier is located 20 cm from the stand magnifier. What is the equivalent power of the stand magnifier/reading add when used by a presbyopic patient wearing a +2.50 D add?

17. What is the magnification of a plastic paperweight magnifier with an index of refraction of 1.49, a curved surface with a radius of curvature of 5 cm, and a thickness of 4 cm?

18. What is the magnification of a glass hemispheric paperweight magnifier with an index of refraction of 1.60 and a curved surface whose radius of curvature is 6 cm?

19. The image formed by a stand magnifier is viewed clearly by a presbyope with an add power of +2.00. If the legs of the magnifier are 5 cm long, and the patient's eye is 25 cm from the magnifier, what is the power of the lens in the stand magnifier?

20. A stand magnifier has a lens power of +10.00 D and an emerging vergence of −5.00 D. The distance from the spectacle plane to the magnifier is 30 cm for a presbyope wearing a +2.00 D add.

    (a) What is the MULTACC factor?
    (b) What is the equivalent power?

CHAPTER THIRTEEN

Optics of Contact Lenses

Contact lenses differ from spectacle lenses in many respects. Some of the differences are obvious, but others are not.

The Contact Lens as a Thick Lens. Without doubt, the least obvious difference is that although a spectacle lens can often be considered a *thin lens*, a contact lens must always be considered a *thick lens*. Although a contact lens is much thinner than a spectacle lens, because it is so steeply curved means that use of the approximate power formula results in serious errors.

Effective Power. One of the more obvious ways in which contact lenses differ from glasses is that contact lenses *touch the eyes*. One result of the proximity of the contact lens to the eye is that the *effective power* of a correcting lens changes as it is brought toward the eye. Thus, for a myope, a contact lens must be *weaker* than a spectacle lens for the same eye and, for a hyperope, a contact lens must be *stronger* than a spectacle lens for the same eye.

The Contact-Lens/Eye System. Because contact lenses touch the eyes, a contact lens (particularly if it is a hard lens) can alter the refractive state of the eye. Conversely, the eye can alter the refractive power of the contact lens (particularly if the lens is a soft contact lens). The effects are of particular importance in dealing with *astigmatism.* A spherical hard contact lens tends to mask (eliminate) corneal astigmatism, but a spherical soft lens tends to conform to the toricity of the cornea and thus has little or no effect on astigmatism. If astigmatism is to be corrected with soft contact lenses, *toric* lenses must be used.

Magnification Effects. Another effect of the proximity of a contact lens to the eye is the change in *magnification* that occurs when one changes from glasses to contact lenses. Because the power factor of the spectacle magnification formula includes the distance h (the distance from the correcting lens to the center of the entrance pupil of the eye), moving a correcting lens closer to the eye brings about a change in magnification. For a myope, a contact lens provides a *larger* retinal image than that of a spectacle lens; for a hyperope, a contact lens provides a *smaller* retinal image. Thus, a high myope who switches from glasses to contact lenses often is delighted because "everything looks bigger," and a hyperope (particularly an aphakic) may be relieved to find that objects appear to be more nearly their normal sizes with contact lenses than they were with glasses.

Changes in Accommodative Demand. A myope who wears spectacles has the advantage that the minus lenses reduce the amount of accommodative demand compared with that for an emmetropic eye; but if contact lenses are worn, the myope loses this advantage. On the other hand, when a hyperope wears spectacles, the plus lenses increase the accommodative demand compared with that for the emmetropic eye, with the result that the hyperope needs to accommodate less when switching to contact lenses. The change in accommodative demand has an important implication for the correction of *presbyopia.* It often happens that a myope who is on the verge of becoming presbyopic needs an add for near work *earlier* if the person wears contact lenses, whereas a hyperope who switches from glasses to contact lenses may not need an add for near vision as soon as if glasses were worn.

Changes in Accommodative Convergence. The increased accommodative demand while contact lenses are worn means that the myope uses *more* accommodative convergence while wearing contact lenses than while wearing glasses, but the hyperope uses *less.* Therefore, an esophoric myope has to use more *negative fusional vergence* while wearing contact lenses than while wearing glasses, and an exophoric hyperope has to use more *positive fusional vergence* while wearing contact lenses than while wearing glasses.

The effects on the demand for accommodation and fusional vergence are negligible for small refractive errors but may be of importance for larger refractive errors, particularly if the *AC/A* ratio (the ratio between accommodative convergence and accommodation) is also large.

Changes in Prismatic Effects. Correctly fitted contact lenses remain *centered* on the eyes in spite of convergence or divergence of the visual axes, and this situation is responsible for an additional change in fusional vergence demand. If spectacle lenses are centered for the wearer's distance PD—the usual situation—the lenses induce prismatic power when worn for near vision—Minus lenses induce *base-in* prism, and plus lenses induce *base-out* prism. Therefore, an exophoric myope, when switching from glasses to contact lenses, is at a disadvantage because of the lack of base-in prismatic effect for near work, and an esophoric hyperope switching to contact lenses is at a similar disadvantage because of the lack of base-out prismatic effect for close work.

Fortunately, the effects on fusional vergence demand caused by the lack of decentration tend to cancel the effects caused by changes in accommodative demand. However, for some patients, one effect can outweigh the other to the extent that it causes an adaptation problem.

The absence of induced prismatic effects caused by contact lenses provides a decided advantage for an anisometrope wearing contact lenses. When an anisometrope wears spectacles, a vertical prismatic imbalance is induced at the reading level, but when contact lenses are worn, no vertical imbalance is present if the contact lenses remain centered on the eyes during downward gaze.

Aberrations and Field of View. The fact that well-fitted contact lenses are centered on the eyes and remain so when the eyes are moved, is responsible for two additional optical differences between contact lenses and glasses.

These are the difference in the *aberrations* experienced by the wearer and the difference in the wearer's *field of view.*

The aberrations of most importance in the design of spectacle lenses are oblique astigmatism, curvature of image, and distortion. Oblique astigmatism and curvature of image occur only when the wearer rotates the eyes to look through the periphery of the lens—this occurs when spectacles are worn, but a contact lens wearer is unable to fixate an object through the periphery of the lens. Distortion, on the other hand, occurs partially as a result of the distance between the aperture of the lens and the aperture (pupil) of the eye. Because this distance is at a minimum when a contact lens is worn, distortion, too, is at a minimum.

Most contact lens wearers are pleased to find that they have a larger *field of view* when they wear contact lenses than when they wear glasses. Although the *peripheral field of view* of the stationary eye may be no larger when wearing a contact lens than when wearing a spectacle lens—in many cases it is actually *smaller*—a contact lens wearer has the advantage that there is no limit to the *macular field of view* for the moving eye because, in the absence of a spectacle rim, the macular field is limited only by the wearer's field of fixation (i.e., ability to move the eye to maintain macular vision).

BASIC OPTICS OF CONTACT LENSES

13.1. The Contact Lens as a Thick Lens

Any lens may be considered "thin" if its radii of curvature are large compared with its thickness. For such a lens, the *approximate power formula* may be used:

$$F_A = F_1 + F_2$$

However, the surfaces of a contact lens are so highly curved that the sagitta of the lens cannot be considered to be small in terms of the chord length; thus, in spite of its obvious thinness, a contact lens must be considered a thick lens. The necessity for treating a contact lens as a thick lens is shown by an example.

EXAMPLE

Given a contact lens having both the front and back radii of curvature (r_1 and r_2) equal to 7.5 mm, a center thickness (t) equal to 0.20 mm, and made of a material having an index of refraction of 1.490, find the approximate power and the back vertex power of the lens.

Approximate Power. The values of F_1 and F_2 are

$$F_1 = \frac{1.490 - 1}{0.0075} = +65.33 \text{ D.}$$

$$F_2 = \frac{1 - 1.490}{0.0075} = -65.33 \text{ D.}$$

Therefore, the approximate power of this lens is

$$F_1 + F_2 = +65.33 \text{ D} + (-65.33 \text{ D}) = 0.00 \text{ D.}$$

Back Vertex Power. Using the back vertex power formula,

$$F_V = \frac{F_1}{1 - \frac{t}{n} F_1} + F_2$$

$$= \frac{+65.33}{1 - \frac{0.0002}{1.490}(65.33)} + (-65.33)$$

$$= +65.91 - 65.33 = +0.58 \text{ D.}$$

This example shows that the use of the approximate power formula instead of the back vertex power formula results in an error of more than 0.50 D. For a thicker lens (such as an aphakic lens) the error would be much greater.

Because contact lenses, like spectacle lenses, are specified in terms of back vertex power, the power of a contact lens is measured in the same way the power of a spectacle lens is measured—by using a lensometer and mounting the lens so that the concave side of the lens rests against the lensometer aperture. However, because of the steepness of the contact lens, the lensometer should be fitted with a smaller stop than that ordinarily used for a spectacle lens (Figure 13–1). Most modern lensometers are supplied with such a stop.

The Base Curve of a Contact Lens

The concave side of a contact lens is designated as the *base curve* of the lens. The base curve radius is selected mainly to meet the criteria for a comfortable and physiologically

FIGURE 13–1. **The use of a small lensometer stop for measuring the back vertex power of a contact lens.**

acceptable fit on the wearer's eye, with good centration and adequate movement. However (particularly for a hard contact lens), the base curve radius also has important *optical* significance.

In the fitting of hard contact lenses, the base curve radius is usually selected to be equal (or nearly so) to the radius of curvature of the front surface of the cornea, as measured by the keratometer. This method of fitting a contact lens is known as the *parallel fit* or *on K* method. In a laboratory order for a contact lens, the practitioner specifies the base curve radius, r_2, the back vertex power, F_v, and the center thickness, t; on the basis of this information, the laboratory selects the necessary front curve radius, r_1.

When the finished lens is received from the laboratory, the practitioner verifies the base curve radius by means of an instrument known as a *radiuscope*. The radiuscope measures the actual (physical) distance between the back surface of the lens and its center of curvature (see Section 13.18).

EXAMPLE

A practitioner orders a contact lens having a base curve radius of 8.0 mm, a back vertex power of –3.00 D, and a center thickness of 0.20 mm. If the lens is made from a material having an index of refraction of 1.490, what is the power (F_1) and the radius of curvature (r_1) of the front curve?

$$F_2 = \frac{1 - 1.490}{0.008} = -61.25 \text{ D.}$$

To find F_1, we begin with the back vertex formula,

$$F_V = \frac{F_1}{1 - \dfrac{t}{n}F_1} + F_2$$

and solve for F_1.

$$F_V - F_2 = \frac{F_1}{\left(1 - \dfrac{t}{n}F_1\right)}$$

$$(F_V - F_2)\left(1 - \frac{t}{n}F_1\right) = F_1.$$

Expanding the left-hand side of the equation and rearranging, we have

$$F_V - F_2 = F_1\left(1 + F_V\frac{t}{n} - F_2\frac{t}{n}\right).$$

Therefore,

$$F_1 = \frac{F_V - F_2}{1 + \dfrac{t}{n}(F_V - F_2)}$$

$$= \frac{-3.00 - (-61.25)}{1 + \dfrac{0.0002}{1.490}[-3.00 - (-61.25)]}$$

$$= +57.80 \text{ D.}$$

$$r_1 = \frac{1.490 - 1}{57.80} = 8.48 \text{ mm.}$$

13.2. The Effective Power of a Contact Lens

As discussed in Chapter 3, Section 3.6, the term *effective power* is used to indicate the change in lens power required when a lens is moved from one position to another in front of the eye. For example, a plus lens is more effective (has more effectivity) when it is moved farther from the eye, and a minus lens is more effective when moved closer to the eye. In Equation 3.16, in which the letters A and B refer to the original and altered positions of the lens,

$$F_B = \frac{F_A}{1 - dF_A},$$

the letter d, indicating the distance the lens has been moved, is given a plus sign if the lens is moved toward the eye and a minus sign if the lens is moved away from the eye.

EXAMPLE 1
A 4.00-D myope, refracted at a vertex distance of 12 mm, is to be fitted with contact lenses (Figure 13–2). Assuming that the contact lens does not change the refractive power of the eye (that is, its back surface is parallel to the air/tear interface), what is the required power of the contact lenses?

$$F_B = \frac{-4.00}{1 - 0.012(-4.00)} = -3.82 \text{ D.}$$

EXAMPLE 2
An aphakic is refracted at a distance of 15 mm and is found to require a +13.00-D lens (Figure 13–3). Assuming, again, that the contact lens does not change the refraction of the eye, what is the required power of a contact lens for this eye?

$$F_B = \frac{+13.00}{1 - 0.015(13.00)} = +16.15 \text{ D.}$$

These examples show that, for a myopic eye, the required power of a contact lens is *less* than the power of a spectacle lens but, for a hyperopic eye, the required power of a con-

FIGURE 13–2. **For a 4.00-D myope, effective power of a contact lens refracted at a vertex distance of 12 mm.**

tact lens is *greater* than that for a spectacle lens. For refractive errors of less than ±3.00 D, the difference in the power of a contact lens and a spectacle lens is approximately no more than 0.12 D, which is considered negligible. For an aphakic eye, the second example shows that the difference between the power of a spectacle lens and a contact lens for the same eye is about 3.00 D.

13.3. The Keratometer: Notation and Calibration

The cornea is both a convex refracting surface and a *convex* mirror. The *keratometer* employs the relationship between the object size and image size formed by a convex mirror to measure the radius of curvature of the anterior surface of the cornea. With a given radius of curvature, the power of the corneal surface is determined by assigning an index of refraction to the cornea and applying Equation 2.3 in Chapter 2, that is,

$$F = \frac{n' - n}{r}.$$

Although keratometers that provide readings either in radii of curvature or corneal surface powers are available, most provide the reading in surface power.

The power along the horizontal meridian is usually recorded first, followed by the vertical meridian. The notation @ is used for *at, along,* or *in* before the designated meridian. Typical findings are recorded as follows:

OD 42.50 @ 180; 43.50 @ 90
OS 42.25 @ 10; 43.75 @ 100

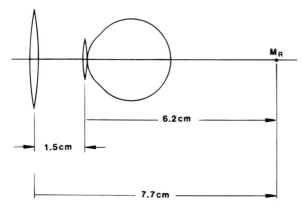

FIGURE 13–3. **Effective power of a contact lens for an aphakic patient requiring a +13.00-D lens, refracted at a vertex distance of 15 mm.**

The findings for the right eye indicate that the corneal refractive power at (along or in) the 180° meridian is 42.50 D and the refractive power along the 90° meridian is 43.50 D. To prevent misunderstanding, the meridian along which the power is measured should not be recorded as the axis (x) position.

Although the index of refraction of the cornea is considered to be 1.376, most keratometers (including the Bausch & Lomb and American Optical instruments) are calibrated for an index of refraction of 1.3375. This value, originally used by Helmholtz, was selected because it considers the refraction at the *back* surface of the cornea (because of the small index change, which amounts to 1.336–1.376, the refraction taking place at this interface is only about 5.00 D). Because measuring the radius of curvature of the back surface of the cornea is difficult in routine clinical practice, the assumption is made that the back surface radius of curvature is equal to that of the front surface of the cornea.

It is an interesting coincidence that the index of refraction used for the calibration of the keratometer is very close to the actual index of refraction of the *tear layer* (1.336). Thus, the keratometer comes very close to measuring the refraction taking place at the *air/tear interface*. The initial refraction that we usually think of as taking place between air and the cornea actually takes place at the interface between air and the *tear layer*. When a hard contact lens is placed on the cornea, the front surface of the tear layer tends to conform to the back surface curvature of the contact lens, with the result that the contact lens may alter the radius of curvature of the front surface of the tear layer. However, the contact lens would not be expected to alter the radius of curvature of the tear/cornea interface or the refraction taking place at that interface. Hence, the radius of curvature of the tear/cornea interface can be considered as a constant.

Using the actual values for the indices of the tears and the cornea, let us calculate the sum of the refracting power of the air/tear interface and the tear/cornea interface for a tear layer having a radius of curvature of 7.5 mm (Figure 13–4). At the air/tear interface,

$$F_{A/T} = \frac{1.336 - 1}{0.0075} = +44.80 \text{ D},$$

and at the tear/cornea interface,

$$F_{T/C} = \frac{1.376 - 1.336}{0.0075} = +5.33 \text{ D}.$$

$$F_{total} = +44.80 + 5.33 = +50.13 \text{ D}.$$

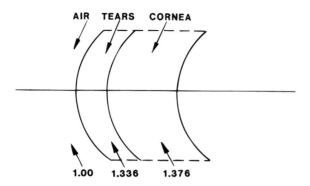

FIGURE 13-4.   **Calculation of the refracting power at the air/tear interface and the tear/cornea interface, using actual values for indices of the tears and cornea.**

If these two interfaces are treated as a single surface, having a radius of curvature of 7.5 mm, the index of refraction of that surface may be found as follows:

$$\frac{n-1}{0.0075} = +50.13$$

$$n - 1 = 0.376$$

$$n = 1.376.$$

Thus, from a practical point of view, in measuring the radius of curvature of the cornea we can ignore the tear layer. If we assume it is infinitely thin, it has zero power and therefore acts as a plano lens. We can, therefore, consider that all refraction takes place at the air/cornea interface:

$$F = \frac{n' - n}{r} = \frac{1.376 - 1}{0.0075} = +50.13 \text{ D.}$$

For the same reason, the tear layer *on the front surface of a contact lens* can also be ignored. However, because the keratometer is calibrated for an index of refraction of 1.3375, the keratometer reading for a cornea having a radius of curvature of 7.5 mm is

$$F_{\text{K}} = \frac{1.3375 - 1}{0.0075} = +45.00 \text{ D.}$$

As mentioned earlier, this discrepancy in the apparent power of the cornea, as determined by the keratometer, takes into consideration the power of the back surface of the cornea. The front surface power of the cornea is actually

$$F_{\text{A/C}} = \frac{+1.376 - 1}{0.0075} = +50.13 \text{ D,}$$

and the back surface power of the cornea is

$$F_{\text{C/aq}} = \frac{1.336 - 1.376}{0.0075} = -5.33 \text{ D.}$$

The resultant refracting power of the cornea is therefore

$$+50.13 + (-5.33) = +44.80 \text{ D,}$$

or 0.20 D less than the keratometer reading of 45.00 D.

The keratometer underestimates the front surface power of the cornea by a factor of

$$\frac{5.33}{50.13} = 0.106, \text{ or approximately } 10\%.$$

The keratometer finding, therefore, measures approximately 9/10 of the total front surface power of the cornea. If corneal astigmatism is present, the keratometer measures only 9/10 of the actual amount, underestimating it by 1/10. However, this does not produce a 10% error, because the back surface of the cornea has a negative power (in each principal meridian) of approximately 1/9 of the total front surface power. In marked corneal astigmatism, the negative back surface is likely to be responsible for reducing a similar percentage of front surface astigmatism. On this basis, the refractive index for which the keratometer is calibrated works very well in practice.

The calibration index of 1.3375 not only provides keratometric readings that consider the back corneal surface, but also provides, through an averaging process, an approximate power of the entire cornea, as if the cornea were a homogeneous medium having an index of refraction of 1.3375. This index is so close to the actual index of the tears (1.336) that one can assume that the corneal astigmatism indicated by the keratometer is essentially neutralized when a hard contact lens having a spherical back surface is placed on the eye and, thereby, renders the front surface of the tear layer spherical. However, as discussed later, complications arise if the contact lens has a *toroidal*, rather than spherical, back surface.

For convenience in problem solving, the index of refraction of the tears is assumed to be equal to the index for which the keratometer has been calibrated—that is, the front surface power of the cornea is equal to the back surface power of the tear layer, but opposite in sign. This assumption involves only a very small constant error (0.20 D as shown in the above example) and greatly simplifies calculations.

In solving contact lens problems, it is helpful to make use of an important general principle of optics: If an optical system is composed of two media on either side of a spherical surface, the power of the system will be the same (1) if the two surfaces are considered to be in contact with each other, or (2) if the two surfaces are considered to be separated by a thin layer of air. This principle is illustrated by an example:

EXAMPLE

If two media, the first having an index of 1.60 and the second having an index of 1.50, with adjacent surfaces with radii of curvature of 20 cm are in contact with each other (Figure 13-5), the power at the interface is

$$F_1 = \frac{1.50 - 1.60}{0.2} = -0.50 \text{ D.}$$

If the two surfaces are considered to be separated by an infinitely thin layer of air (Figure 13-6), the sum of the two surface powers is

$$F_1 = \frac{1 - 1.60}{0.2} = -3.00 \text{ D.}$$

$$F_2 = \frac{1.50 - 1}{0.2} = +2.50 \text{ D.}$$

$$F_1 + F_2 = -3.00 \text{ D} + 2.50 \text{ D} = -0.50 \text{ D.}$$

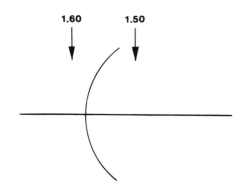

FIGURE 13–5.   **Calculation of refracting power at the interface between media having indices of 1.60 and 1.50, with the two surfaces in contact.**

FIGURE 13–6.   **Calculation of refracting power at the interface between media having indices of 1.60 and 1.50, with the two surfaces considered to be separated by an infinitely thin layer of air.**

THE CONTACT LENS/EYE OPTICAL SYSTEM

13.4. The Contact Lens on the Eye

The optical system consisting of the contact lens and the eye can be considered by the use of either of two methods, based on the methods just described: the *in situ* method, or the *exploded* method. Using either method, the contact lens is assumed to be infinitely thin.

1. Using the *in situ* method, the lens is treated as if it were in place on the cornea (Figure 13–7). Using this method, we are concerned with two refractions: one taking place at the air/contact-lens interface and the other taking place at the contact-lens/tear interface. Therefore, if the contact lens perfectly corrects the eye,

(power at air/lens interface) + (power at lens/tear interface)
= (corneal refracting power) + (ocular refraction)

or

$$F_{A/C} + F_{C/T} = K + R_x. \qquad (13.1)$$

Important Note. With the in situ method, power can be transferred back and forth between the air/contact-lens interface and the contact-lens/tear interface, as long as the power at the two interfaces adds up to the sum of the corneal refracting power (as determined by the keratometer) and the ocular refraction. With use of this method, it is assumed that the tear/cornea interface is not affected by the presence of the contact lens. Also, the term R_x in Equation 13.1 indicates the *ocular* refraction, that is, refraction determined at the plane of the cornea. This is equal to the power of the contact lens in air only if the back surface of the contact lens has the same radius of curvature as the front surface of the cornea (fit on K).

2. Using the *exploded* method, we assume that there is a layer of air between the contact lens and the tear layer

FIGURE 13–7.   **The in situ method of determining the power of a contact lens on the eye. This method considers two refractions, one taking place at the air/contact-lens interface and the other at the contact-lens/tear interface.**

and also between the tear layer and the cornea (Figure 13–8). Using this method, we are concerned with the refraction by the contact lens in air and the refraction by the tear lens in air. Therefore, if the contact lens perfectly corrects the eye,

(power of contact lens in air) + (power of tear lens in air) = ocular refraction

or

$$F_C + F_T = R_x. \qquad (13.2)$$

Important Note. With the exploded method, power can be transferred back and forth between the tear lens and the contact lens, as long as the two add up to the ocular refraction. With use of this method, the back surface curvature of the tear layer is assumed to match that of the front surface of the cornea.

The two methods can be compared by the use of some examples. The examples assume that the patient is being fitted with a hard contact lens (a hard lens is one consid-

FIGURE 13–8.   **The exploded method of determining the power of a contact lens on the eye. This method considers refractions by the contact lens and by the tear lens, with an infinitely thin layer of air considered to be between the contact lens and the tear layer and between the tear layer and the cornea.**

ered as a lens that is sufficiently rigid so that it maintains its curvature while on the eye, but does not change the curvature of the tear/cornea interface).

EXAMPLE 1

Assume that we are providing a perfect optical correction for a patient by using a contact lens having an index of refraction of 1.490 and having both front and back surface radii of curvature of 7.5 mm, to be fitted on a cornea having an apical radius of curvature (i.e., keratometer finding) of 7.5 mm. Neglecting the thickness of the contact lens, find the ocular refraction, using (1) the in situ method and (2) the exploded method.

(1) Using the in situ method (Figure 13–9),

$$F_{A/C} + F_{C/T} = K + R_x,$$

or

$$R_x = F_{A/C} + F_{C/T} - K$$

$$= \frac{1.490 - 1}{0.0075} + \frac{1.3375 - 1.490}{0.0075} - \frac{1.3375 - 1}{0.0075}$$

$$= +65.33 + (-20.33) + (-45.00) = +45.00 - 45.00$$

$$= 0.00 \text{ D}.$$

(2) Using the exploded method (Figure 13–10),

$$R_x = F_C + F_T$$

$$= F_{C1} + F_{C2} + F_{T1} + F_{T2}$$

$$= \frac{1.490 - 1}{0.0075} + \frac{1 - 1.490}{0.0075} + \frac{1.3375 - 1}{0.0075} + \frac{1 - 1.3375}{0.0075}$$

$$= +65.33 + (-65.33) + 45.00 - 45.00$$

$$= 0.00 \text{ D}.$$

EXAMPLE 2

An eye has an apical radius of curvature of 7.5 mm and the refraction in the plane of the corneal apex is –3.00 D. If the back surface (base curve) of the contact lens is to have the same radius of curvature of the corneal apex, what is the power of the front surface of the required contact lens, using (1) the in situ method and (2) the exploded method?

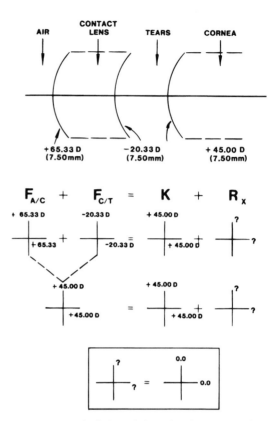

FIGURE 13–9.   **Calculation of the refracting power of a contact lens on the eye, by using the in situ method, for a contact lens having an index of refraction of 1.490, front and back radii of curvature of 7.5 mm, and fitted on a cornea having an apical radius of curvature of 7.5 mm.**

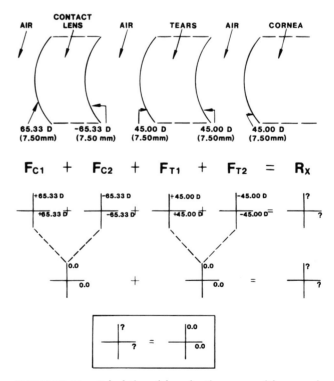

FIGURE 13–10.   **Calculation of the refracting power of the example shown in Figure 13–9, with use of the exploded method.**

(1) Using the in situ method (Figure 13–11),

$$F_{A/C} + F_{C/T} = K + R_x$$
$$F_{A/C} = K + R_x - F_{C/T}$$
$$= \frac{1.3375 - 1}{0.0075} + (-3.00) - \frac{1.3375 - 1.490}{0.0075}$$
$$= 45.00 + (-3.00) - (-20.33)$$
$$= +62.33 \text{ D.}$$

(2) Using the exploded method (Figure 13–12),

$$R_x = F_C + F_T$$
$$= F_{C1} + F_{C2} + F_{C1} + F_{T2}$$
$$F_{C1} = R_x - F_{C2} - F_{T1} - F_{T2}$$
$$= -3.00 - \frac{1 - 1.490}{0.0075} - \frac{1.3375 - 1}{0.0075} - \frac{1 - 1.3375}{0.0075}$$
$$= -3.00 - (-65.33) + 45.00 - 45.00$$
$$= +62.33 \text{ D.}$$

A Soft Contact Lens on the Eye

A soft contact lens behaves on the eye quite differently than a hard contact lens. Whereas a hard lens, as already stated, is assumed to maintain its shape while on the eye, a soft lens is assumed to conform completely to the corneal surface, with the result that there is no tear lens, as such.

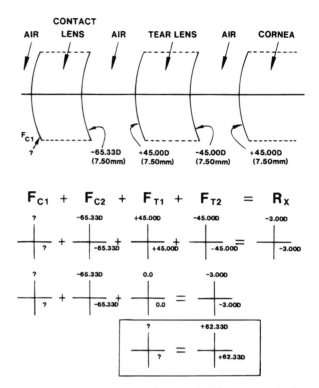

FIGURE 13–12.   **Use of the exploded method for the example shown in Figure 13–11.**

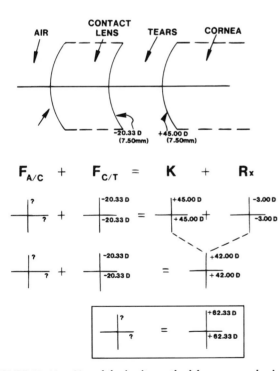

FIGURE 13–11.   **Use of the in situ method for a cornea having an apical radius of curvature of 7.5 mm, fitted with a contact lens having a back surface radius (base curve) of 7.5 mm and a refracting power of –3.00 D.**

There is, of course, an extremely thin layer of tears between the soft lens and the cornea, but, except in an extreme case such as a very thick plus lens in aphakia, the contact lens is sufficiently flexible so that the tear lens has no power.

In spite of the fact that a soft lens tends to conform to the cornea, a soft lens can be considered to behave in the same way as a hard lens as long as:

1. The lens is fitted on a *spherical* cornea.
2. The back surface of the lens has the same radius of curvature as the front surface of the cornea.

Thus, for the two examples just discussed, the results would have been the same if a soft lens had been fitted because the cornea was assumed to be spherical and the lens was fitted so that its back surface had the same radius of curvature as that found by the keratometer. However, in Sections 13.6 and 13.7, which deal with contact lenses fitted on astigmatic corneas and contact lenses fitted "steeper than K" and "flatter than K," the tear lens concept applies only to the *hard lens*; a soft lens will fit very differently than a hard lens on an astigmatic cornea or if it is fitted steeper or flatter than the corneal radius. Parenthetically, in actual practice, a soft contact lens is normally fitted somewhat *flatter* than the corneal apex, parallel to the corneal periphery, with the result that the lens is considered to "drape" the corneal apex.

13.5. Over-Refraction

In the routine fitting of contact lenses, the optometrist often does an *over-refraction*—a refraction with the patient wearing either a pair of trial contact lenses or his or her own contact lenses. Over-refraction (OR) through trial contact lenses has the advantage that, rather than depending on the *prediction* that a given contact lens will correct the eye's ametropia, the practitioner determines the actual refractive state while the patient wears the lens.

For calculating the results of a contact lens in situ, for an eye whose refractive error is perfectly corrected by the contact lens, we can use Equation 13.1:

$$F_{A/C} + F_{C/T} = K + R_x.$$

If the OR demonstrates that the contact lens does not provide a complete correction, the formula must read

$$F_{A/C} + F_{C/T} + F_{OR} = K + R_x. \qquad (13.3)$$

If the eye is perfectly corrected by the contact lens, the exploded system may be used in the following manner (using Equation 13.2):

$$F_C + F_T = R_x.$$

However, if the contact lens does not provide a complete correction, the equation for the exploded system changes to

$$F_C + F_T + F_{OR} = R_x. \qquad (13.4)$$

EXAMPLE
Given the following information, what is the ocular refraction?
Keratometer: 44.00 @ 180/44.00 @ 90
Trial lens: base curve = 7.58 mm
power = plano
OR: −1.00 DS.

Using the in situ method (Figure 13–13),

$$F_{A/C} + F_{C/T} + F_{OR} = K + R_x$$

$$\frac{1.49 - 1}{0.00758} + \frac{1.3375 - 1.49}{0.00758} + (-1) = 44.00 + R_x$$

$$64.64 + (-20.12) + (-1) = 44.00 + R_x$$

$$R_x = 64.64 - 21.12 - 44.00$$

$$= -0.48 \text{ D.}$$

Using the exploded method (Figure 13–14),

$$F_C + F_T = F_{OR} = R_x, \text{ but } F_C = \text{plano.}$$

The power of the front surface of the tear lens is equal to

$$F_{T1} = \frac{1.3375 - 1}{0.00758} = \frac{0.3375}{0.00758} = +44.52 \text{ D.}$$

The power of the back surface of the tear lens is equal to the power of the cornea but opposite in sign, or,

$$F_{T2} = -44.00 \text{ D,}$$

and

$$F_{T1} + F_{T2} = +44.52 + (-44.00) = +0.52 \text{ D.}$$

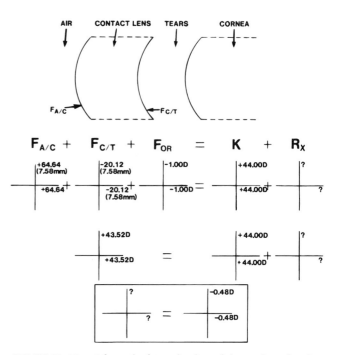

FIGURE 13–13. **Schematic determination of the ocular refraction when the keratometer reading, base curve, contact lens power, and OR are known, by using the in situ method.**

Since

$$F_C + F_T + F_{OR} = R_x,$$

therefore,

$$0 + 0.52 + (-1) = R_x,$$

or

$$R_x = -0.48 \text{ D.}$$

13.6. Contact Lenses and Corneal Astigmatism

To understand the effect of a hard contact lens on corneal astigmatism, it must be realized, as already pointed out, that a contact lens interfaces with (or fits on) the *tear layer*, rather than on the cornea. Because a contact lens, unless fitted very badly, has no effect on the curvature of the cornea itself, we need be concerned only with the relationship between the contact lens and the tear layer. Thus, when a spherical hard contact lens is fitted on a spherical cornea, the lens has no effect on the tear layer if its back surface is parallel to the front surface of the cornea.

Although in fitting spectacles a cylindrical or toric lens is routinely used for an astigmatic eye, in fitting hard contact lenses, toric lenses are seldom used. The reason is that, as long as the hard lens maintains its curvature while on the eye, the interface between the lens and the tear layer is *spherical*, no matter how much corneal astigmatism existed before the lens was put on. A spherical hard lens, in effect, *eliminates* corneal astigmatism. *Internal astigmatism* (astigmatism caused by ocular factors *other* than the toricity of the

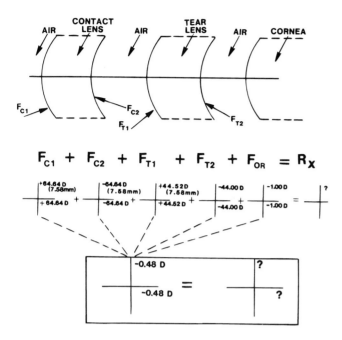

$$F_{C1} + F_{C2} + F_{T1} + F_{T2} + F_{OR} = R_x$$

$$\begin{vmatrix} +64.64\,D \\ (7.58mm) \\ +64.64\,D \end{vmatrix} + \begin{vmatrix} -64.64\,D \\ (7.58mm) \\ -64.64\,D \end{vmatrix} + \begin{vmatrix} +44.52D \\ (7.58mm) \\ +44.52D \end{vmatrix} + \begin{vmatrix} -44.00\,D \\ -44.00\,D \end{vmatrix} + \begin{vmatrix} -1.00\,D \\ -1.00\,D \end{vmatrix} = \begin{vmatrix} ? \\ ? \end{vmatrix}$$

$$\begin{vmatrix} -0.48\ D \\ -0.48\ D \end{vmatrix} = \begin{vmatrix} ? \\ ? \end{vmatrix}$$

FIGURE 13–14.   **Schematic determination of the ocular refraction when the keratometer reading, base curve, contact lens power, and OR are known, by using the exploded method.**

front surface of the cornea) is obviously *not* corrected by the spherical contact lens. Internal astigmatism averages about –0.50 D axis 90, and, using a retinoscope or subjective refraction, the practitioner almost always finds a small amount of against-the-rule astigmatism when doing an over-refraction on a patient wearing a hard contact lens.

EXAMPLE
Given an eye having the following subjective refraction and keratometer readings:
Subjective refraction: plano –1.00 DC x 180
Keratometer reading: 44.00 @ 180/45.00 @ 90.

If the back surface radius of a spherical hard contact lens is fitted parallel to the flattest corneal meridian (on K fitting), what is the required front surface radius of curvature, using (1) the in situ system and (2) the exploded system?

(1) Using the in situ method (Figure 13–15), one finds the radius of curvature of the back surface of the contact lens by using the index of refraction for which the keratometer is calibrated and the keratometer reading in the horizontal meridian,

$$r_2 = \frac{1.3375 - 1}{44.00} = 0.00767 \text{ m}$$

(normally, this would be done by the use of a table). The refraction taking place at the interface between the contact lens and the tear layer is the same in both the horizontal and vertical meridians because the contact lens renders the front surface of the tear layer spherical,

$$F_{C/T} = \frac{1.3375 - 1.490}{0.00767} = -19.88 \text{ D},$$

and at the front surface of the contact lens,

$$F_{A/C} + F_{C/T} = R_x + K$$
$$F_{A/C} = R_x + K - F_{C/T}$$
$$= 0.00 + 44.00 - (-19.88)$$
$$= +63.88 \text{ D}.$$

Therefore,

$$r_1 = \frac{1.490 - 1}{63.88} = 0.00767 \text{ m} = 7.67 \text{ mm}.$$

(2) Using the exploded system (Figure 13–16), one finds the refracting power of the *tear lens*, first for the horizontal meridian and then for the vertical meridian, by using the subscripts T1 and T2 for the front and back tear layer surfaces.

In the *horizontal meridian*,

$$F_{T2} = \frac{1 - 1.3375}{0.00767} = -44.00 \text{ D}.$$
$$F_{T1} = \frac{1.3375 - 1}{0.00767} = +44.00 \text{ D}.$$
$$F_T = F_{T1} + F_{T2} = 44.00 + (-44.00) = 0.00 \text{ D}.$$

In the *vertical meridian*,

$$r_2 = \frac{1 - 1.3375}{-45.00} = 0.0075 \text{ m}.$$

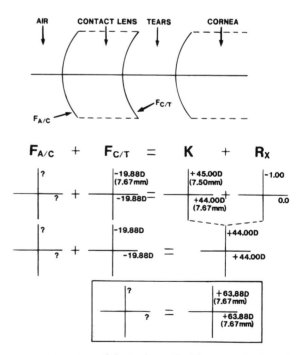

FIGURE 13–15.   **Use of the in situ method for an eye having a keratometer reading of 44.00 @ 180/45.00 @ 90 and a refraction of plano –1.00 DC x 180, fitted with a hard contact lens whose back surface radius is parallel to the flattest meridian of the cornea.**

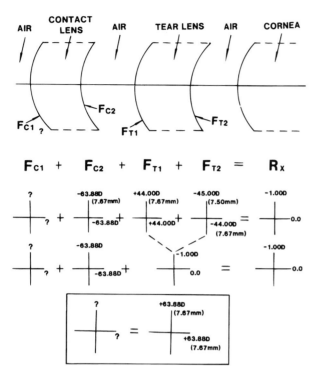

FIGURE 13–16.   **Use of the exploded method for the example shown in Figure 13–15.**

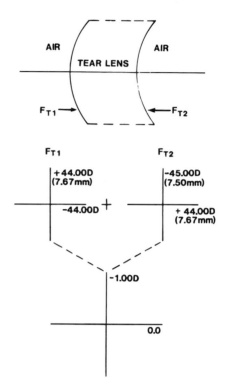

PLANO -1.00 DC X 180

FIGURE 13–17.   **Power diagram used for determining the power of the contact lens illustrated in Figure 13–16.**

Therefore,

$$F_{T2} = \frac{1 - 1.3375}{0.0075} = -45.00 \text{ D.}$$

$$F_{T1} = \frac{1.3375 - 1}{0.00767} = +44.00 \text{ D.}$$

$$F_T = F_{T1} + F_{T2} = +44.00 + (-45.00) = -1.00 \text{ D.}$$

Considering both meridians, the power of the tear lens (as shown in the power diagram in Figure 13–17) is

$$F_T = \text{plano} - 1.00 \text{ DC axis } 180.$$

As for the *contact lens,* in the horizontal meridian,

$$F_{CL} + F_T = R_x = 0.00,$$

and since

$$F_T = 0.00 \text{ D,}$$
$$F_{CL} + 0.00 = 0.00$$
$$F_{CL} = 0.00 \text{ D,}$$

and in the vertical meridian,

$$F_{CL} + F_T = R_x = -1.00,$$

and since

$$F_T = -1.00 \text{ D,}$$
$$F_{CL} + (-1.00) = -1.00$$
$$F_{CL} = 0.00 \text{ D.}$$

Because the back surface of the contact lens is spherical, having a radius of 7.67 mm, the back surface power of the contact lens *in both meridians* is

$$F_{CL2} = \frac{1 - 1.490}{0.00767} = -63.88 \text{ D.}$$

Since the contact lens has zero refracting power in both meridians,

$$F_{CL1} + F_{CL2} = 0.00$$
$$F_{CL1} + (-63.88 \text{ D}) = 0$$
$$F_{CL1} = +63.88 \text{ D,}$$

and therefore

$$r_1 = \frac{1.490 - 1}{+63.88} = 0.00767 \text{ m} = 7.67 \text{ mm.}$$

Therefore, the contact lens is spherical on both surfaces with zero power. The example illustrates that corneal astigmatism is neutralized with a hard contact lens that has a spherical back surface.

Soft Contact Lenses and Corneal Astigmatism

Unlike a hard contact lens, a soft lens is not fitted parallel to the cornea but, as already described, is normally fitted considerably *flatter* than the optical zone of the cornea. Because the radius of curvature of the peripheral portion of the cornea is typically much flatter than the corneal optical zone, a soft contact lens roughly parallels the corneal periphery and "drapes" over the corneal apex.

Moreover, although diagnostic lens sets for hard contact lenses are available in any desired radii of curvature (usually in steps of 0.05-mm radius), a diagnostic set for soft contact lenses may include no more than two or three radii (such as 8.0, 8.3, and 8.6 mm), which are expected to fit all corneas.

For the eye having a subjective refraction of plano –1.00 DC X 180 and a keratometer finding of 44.00 @ 180/45.00 @ 90, Figure 13–18 shows that the lens parallels the cornea in both principal meridians, with the result that it does not correct astigmatism. Thus, the refractive power of this lens system while on the eye, instead of plano –1.00 X 180, is simply *plano*. This example shows that if a lens parallels a toric cornea in both principal meridians (Figure 13–18), no corneal astigmatism is corrected.

13.7. Fitting Steeper or Flatter Than the Cornea

Some philosophies of fitting hard contact lenses require that the lens be fitted either steeper or flatter than the flattest corneal meridian, rather than with the more conventional on K fit. When this is done, the effect of the contact lens on the curvature of the tear layer must be taken into consideration for the contact-lens/tear interface in the in situ system and for the air/tear interface in the exploded system.

EXAMPLE
An emmetropic eye having a spherical keratometer reading of 45.00 D (therefore having a corneal radius of 7.5 mm) is fitted with a hard contact lens having a radius of curvature of 7.3 mm (0.2 mm steeper than the cornea).

What is the required radius of the front surface of the contact lens?

(1) Using the in situ method (Figure 13–19), for the refraction at the interface between the contact lens and the tear layer,

$$F_{C/T} = \frac{1.3375 - 1.490}{0.0073} = -20.89 \text{ D},$$

$$F_{A/C} = R_x + K - F_{C/T}$$

$$= 0.00 + 45.00 - (-20.89)$$

$$= +65.89 \text{ D}.$$

$$r_1 = \frac{1.490 - 1}{65.89} = 0.00744 \text{ m}.$$

Is there something wrong here? Even though the wearer of this contact lens is emmetropic, the two radii of curvature, r_1 and r_2, are not equal, which indicates that the lens is not a plano lens. The required power of the lens can be found by use of the exploded system.

(2) Using the exploded system (Figure 13–20), we first determine the refraction occurring at each surface of the tear lens:

$$F_{T2} = \frac{1 - 1.3375}{0.0075} = -45.00 \text{ D}.$$

$$F_{T1} = \frac{1.3375 - 1}{0.0073} = +46.23 \text{ D}.$$

$$F_T = +46.23 - (-45.00) = +1.23 \text{ D},$$

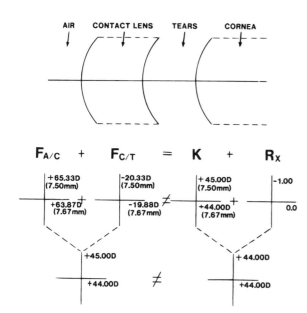

FIGURE 13–18. **The refracting power of a soft contact lens on the eye used in the example illustrated in Figure 13–15, by using the in situ method.**

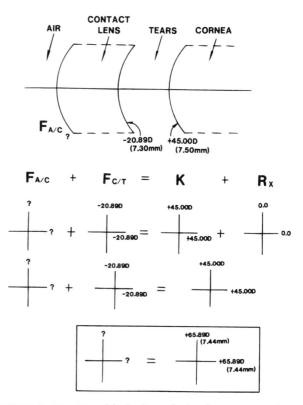

FIGURE 13–19. **Use of the in situ method to fit an emmetropic eye with a hard contact lens 0.2 mm steeper than the cornea with a radius of curvature of 7.5 mm. The front surface of the contact lens must have a radius of curvature of 7.44 mm.**

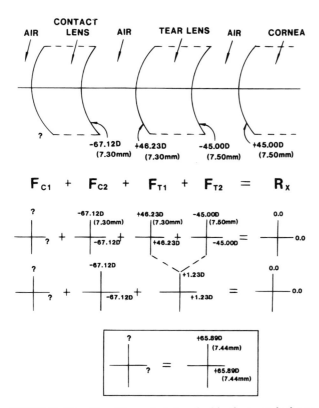

FIGURE 13–20.   **Use of the exploded method for the example shown in Figure 13–19.**

and for the contact lens,

$$F_{CL} + F_T = R_x$$
$$F_{CL} = R_x - F_T = 0.00 - 1.23 = -1.23 \text{ D.}$$
$$F_{CL2} = \frac{1 - 1.490}{0.0073} = -67.12 \text{ D.}$$
$$F_{CL1} = F_{CL} - F_{CL2}$$
$$= -1.23 - (-67.12) = +65.89 \text{ D.}$$
$$r_{CL1} = \frac{1.490 - 1}{+65.89} = 0.00744 \text{ m.}$$

These results show (1) when a lens is fitted steeper than the flattest corneal meridian, the front surface must be made *flatter* to maintain the same refracting power while on the eye (which means that *more minus* power must be added to the lens), and (2) the amount of added minus power is approximately 0.50 D per 0.1 mm of lens steepening.

Clinical Note. Many optometrists think of steepening or flattening in terms of diopters of change in the keratometer finding. In the example just given, instead of steepening the back surface of the lens from 7.50 to 7.30 mm, the optometrist could think of steepening the curve from 45.00 to 46.23 D. This has the advantage that the optometrist knows immediately the change that must be made in the *back vertex power* of the contact lens, as compared with that required for an on K fit. In the example, the back vertex power of the lens must be –1.23 D rather than plano as re-

quired if the lens were fitted on K. If the base curve were to be fitted *flatter* than the flattest corneal meridian, it would be necessary to *steepen* the front surface of the lens, thus adding *plus power* to the lens.

We therefore have the following general rules:

1. If a hard contact lens is to be fitted steeper than the flattest corneal meridian, add more minus power to the lens.
2. If a hard contact lens is to be fitted flatter than the flattest corneal meridian, add plus power to the lens.
3. The amount of minus or plus power to be added is approximately 0.50 D for each 0.1 mm of steepening or flattening of the radius of the back surface of the lens. If the base curve is specified in diopters (that is, in diopters as determined by the keratometer), a straight diopter-for-diopter relationship exists, in which minus power is added to the lens when the back surface is steepened, and plus power is added when the back surface is flattened.

Important Note. Some practitioners (and even some textbooks), when explaining the need for altering the power of a contact lens when the base curve is steepened or flattened, make the mistake of attributing changes in power to the *tear lens*. A steep contact lens is said to result in a "plus tear lens" and a flat contact lens is said to result in a "minus tear lens." Even a casual inspection of the two tear lenses in Figure 13–21 shows why this mistake is repeatedly made: The front surfaces of the two tear lenses cause them to *look like* plus and minus lenses, respectively. However, *when the lens is on the eye*, in both cases the tear lens acts as a *minus lens* because there is a greater index change at the contact-lens/tear interface (a *minus* refraction) than there is at the tear/cornea interface (a *plus* refraction). The refracting power of the tear lens—and its

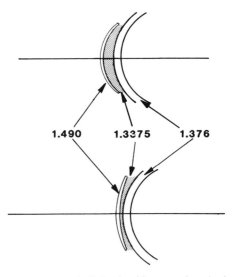

FIGURE 13–21.   **A steeply fitting hard lens may be mistakenly considered to result in a tear lens having plus power, and a flat-fitting hard lens may be mistakenly considered to result in a tear lens having minus power. However, in both cases, the tear layer acts as a *minus lens* (see text for explanation).**

change when the base curve is steepened—is shown by an example.

EXAMPLE

A cornea has a keratometer reading of 45.00 D. Assuming that the tear layer is infinitely thin, what is the refracting power of the tear lens if the lens is fitted (1) parallel to the cornea or (2) 0.2 mm steeper than the cornea. This, of course, is the problem we just considered, but now we will calculate the in situ power of the lens.

(1) The refraction taking place at the contact lens/tear interface is

$$\frac{1.3375 - 1.490}{0.0075} = -20.33 \text{ D},$$

and the refraction taking place at the tear/cornea interface is

$$\frac{1.376 - 1.3375}{0.0075} = +5.13 \text{ D}.$$

The total refraction by the tear lens is therefore

$$-20.33 + 5.33 = -15.20 \text{ D}.$$

(2) With the lens fitted 0.2 mm steeper than the cornea, the refraction taking place at the contact-lens/tear interface will be

$$\frac{1.3375 - 1.490}{0.0073} = -20.89 \text{ D},$$

and since the refraction at the tear/cornea interface is still +5.13 D, the total refraction by the tear layer is

$$-20.89 + 5.13 = -15.76 \text{ D}.$$

We see, therefore, that by fitting the lens 0.2 mm steeper than the corneal radius, the refraction by the tear lens is now 0.56 D *more minus* than it would have been for an on K fit. If a tear lens that looks like a plus lens is actually a *minus* (diverging) lens, and if fitting the contact lens steeper than the cornea *increases* the minus power of the tear lens, why do we have to add minus power to the contact lens to properly correct the eye?

When we steepen the base curve of the contact lens *while keeping the same back vertex power*, we are steepening *both* the front and back surfaces of the lens, and, as shown in part (1) of the solution to the original example, steepening of the front surface results in the front surface power increasing from its original value of

$$\frac{1.490 - 1}{0.0075} = +65.33 \text{ D}$$

to the value

$$\frac{1.490 - 1}{0.0073} = +67.12 \text{ D},$$

or an increase in refracting power of +1.79 D.

Therefore, by steepening the lens 0.2 mm (both front and back surfaces), we bring about an increase in plus

power at the air/contact-lens interface of 1.79 D and an increase in the minus power at the contact-lens/tear interface of –0.56 D (from –20.33 to –20.89 D), so the *net* change is equal to

$$+1.79 \text{ D} - .56 \text{ D} = +1.23 \text{ D},$$

which is the same as the original +1.23 D that we found would have to be compensated by reducing the plus power of the front surface.

The ratio between the power change at the front surface and the change at the back surface brought about by steepening or flattening the lens is

$$\frac{1.79}{0.56}, \quad \text{or approximately} \quad \frac{3.2}{1},$$

which is the same ratio as the index change at the front surface of the contact lens to the index change at its back surface, or

$$\frac{1.490 - 1}{1.3375 - 1.49} = \frac{3.2}{1}.$$

Fitting Soft Contact Lenses Steeper or Flatter Than the Cornea

As stated in Section 13.5, soft contact lenses are routinely fitted much flatter than the optical zone of the cornea and because a soft lens conforms to the corneal surface so completely, not only is there no tear lens, but a flattening or steepening of the lens has no clinically significant effect on the ability of the lens to correct the eye's refractive error. An exception to this rule is a very *thick* lens designed for an aphakic eye, which may fail to completely conform to the corneal curvature. In addition, a *badly fitting* soft contact lens sometimes flexes or bends on the cornea in such a way that the refractive error is not adequately corrected by the lens.

13.8. The Optics of Bifocal Contact Lenses

As with spectacle lenses, a bifocal contact lens may be made either by using two materials having different indices of refraction (a fused bifocal) or by using a lens made of a single material but having two different radii of curvature on either the front or the back surface (a one-piece bifocal). Although both methods are used in the manufacture of bifocal contact lenses, we first consider one-piece hard bifocals, having two radii of curvature on the back surface.

One-Piece Back Surface Hard Bifocals

Referring to Figure 13–22, the power of the addition (on the eye) is equal to the difference in the back surface interface powers of the two portions of the lens:

$$F_{add} = F_{near} - F_{distance}$$

where F_{near} = the back surface interface power of the near portion of the lens, and $F_{distance}$ = the back surface interface power of the distance portion of the lens.

For a material having an index of refraction of 1.490, a distance portion radius of curvature of 7.50 mm, and an addition of +2.00 D, we can find the radius of curvature of the back surface of the near portion r_n of the lens as follows:

$$+2.00 = \frac{1.3375 - 1.490}{r_n} - \frac{1.3375 - 1.490}{0.0075}$$

$$+2.00 = \frac{0.1525}{r_n} - \left(\frac{-0.1525}{0.0075}\right)$$

$$+2.00 = \frac{0.1525}{r_n} - (-20.33)$$

$$-18.33 = \frac{0.1525}{r_n}$$

$$r_n = 0.00832.$$

What is the power of the add if we verified the finished lens (above) by means of a lensometer? The refracting power of the distance and near portions of the back surface of the lens, *in air*, are

$$F_{distance} = \frac{1 - 1.490}{0.0075} = -65.33 \text{ D.}$$

$$F_{near} = \frac{1 - 1.490}{0.00832} = -58.89 \text{ D.}$$

Because the refraction at the front surface of the lens is the same for the distance and near portions, the power of the add when measured on the lensometer is

$$F_{near} - F_{distance} = -58.89 - (-65.33) = +6.44 \text{ D.}$$

Thus, the ratio of the power of the add as found by the lensometer (in air) compared with the power of the add on the eye (the contact-lens/tear refraction) is

$$\frac{6.44}{2.00} = \frac{3.2}{1},$$

or the familiar 3.2/1 ratio discussed in Section 13.7.

One-Piece Front Surface Hard Bifocals

Both hard and soft contact lens bifocals may be made in one-piece form, with the segment on the front surface. Because

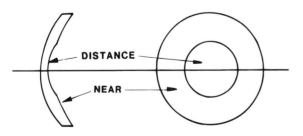

FIGURE 13–22.   **For a one-piece back surface hard bifocal, the power of the addition is equal to the difference in the back surface interface powers in the two portions of the lens. With use of a lensometer, the power of the addition is equal to the difference in back vertex powers in air (3.2 times the power of the addition on the eye).**

the power of the add is the difference between the powers of the distance and near portions of the front surface, when a front surface segment is verified on the lensometer, we expect to find the exact power of the add that was ordered.

Fused Front Surface Hard Bifocals

The optical principles of fused front surface bifocal contact lenses (available for hard lenses only) are similar to the principles of fused bifocal spectacle lenses, as discussed in Chapter 8, Section 8.14. The basic formula Equation (8.11) is

$$\text{power of add} = \frac{F_1 - F_C}{\text{ratio}},$$

where F_1 = the front surface power of the major lens and F_C = the surface power of the countersink surface. In this expression, the term *ratio* is equal to

$$\frac{n' - n}{n'' - n'},$$

where n = the index of refraction of air, n' = the index of the major lens, and n'' = the index of the segment.

When a fused front surface bifocal contact lens is verified by means of the lensometer, the power of the add is equal to the difference between the powers of the distance and near portions of the lens.

Fused Back Surface Hard Bifocals

This lens is made by fusing a higher index material into a countersink curve on the back surface of the lens. The curvature of the back surface of the segment is the same as that of the base curve (i.e., the back surface of the major lens). Because of the strong concave curvature of the back surface of the lens, there is an increase in *minus* power at the back surface of the segment compared with that of the back surface of the major lens. Therefore, the radius of curvature of the countersink surface must be much shorter for a fused back surface bifocal than for a fused front surface bifocal.

Suppose, for example, that we wish to make a fused back surface bifocal, using a major lens having an index of refraction of 1.490, a segment having an index of refraction of 1.570, with the lens having a base curve radius of 7.5 mm and an addition of +2.00 D. What is the radius of curvature of the countersink surface (Figure 13–23)?

With use of the in situ method, the power of the contact-lens/tear interface in the distance portion is

$$F_{C/T} = \frac{n_T - n_{C'}}{r_2} = \frac{1.3375 - 1.490}{0.0075} = -20.33 \text{ D.}$$

The power of the contact-lens/tear interface in the near portion is

$$F_{C/T} = \frac{n_T - n_{C''}}{r} = \frac{1.3375 - 1.570}{0.0075} = -31.00 \text{ D.}$$

Therefore, the near contact-lens/tear interface is more minus in power than the distance contact-lens/tear interface by

$$-31.00 - (-20.33) = -10.67 \text{ D.}$$

FIGURE 13–23. **For a fused back surface hard bifocal, the in situ method is used to find the curvature of the countersink curve for a lens having a base curve radius of 7.5 mm and an addition of +2.00 D, for a major lens having an index of 1.490 and a segment having an index of 1.570.**

To determine the radius of curvature of the countersink curve, we use the following relationship: The power of the addition is equal to the power of the front surface of the segment plus the power change between the distance and near contact-lens/tear interfaces, or

$$\text{power of add} = \frac{n_{C''} - n_{C'}}{r_C} + (-10.67)$$

$$+2.00 = \frac{1.570 - 1.490}{r_C} + (-10.67)$$

$$\begin{matrix}\text{power of} \\ \text{countersink} \\ \text{interface}\end{matrix} = +12.67 \text{ D} = \frac{1.570 - 1.490}{r_C}$$

$$+12.67 = \frac{0.08}{r_C}$$

$$r_C = \frac{0.08}{12.67} = 0.00631 \text{ m} = 6.31 \text{ mm}.$$

If the back surface of the contact lens were in air, the power of the contact-lens/tear interface for the distance portion of the lens would be

$$F_{C/A} = \frac{n - n_{C'}}{r_2} = \frac{1.00 - 1.490}{0.0075} = -65.33 \text{ D},$$

and the power of the contact-lens/tear interface for the segment portion of the lens would be

$$F_{C/A} = \frac{n - n_{C''}}{r_2} = \frac{1.00 - 1.57}{0.0750} = -76.00.$$

The change in power between the distance and near contact-lens/air interfaces is therefore

$$-76.00 - (-65.00) = -10.67 \text{ D},$$

which is the same as we found when the back surface of the lens was placed against the tear layer. Thus, the effective power of the addition on the eye will be the same as the power of the add as determined by the use of a lensometer.

13.9. Residual Astigmatism and Its Correction

Residual astigmatism is the astigmatism that is present when a contact lens with spherical surfaces is placed on the cornea to correct the eye's ametropia. Residual astigmatism may be caused by any of a number of optical and anatomical components of the contact-lens/eye system. An anatomical factor that may cause residual astigmatism is the displacement of the fovea from the posterior pole of the eye, with the result that the visual axis and the optic axis fail to coincide—astigmatism caused by obliquity of incidence. Other sources of residual astigmatism include the back surface of the cornea, toroidal crystalline lens surfaces, and the tilting of these surfaces.

The relationship between the total astigmatism of the eye (also called *refractive* astigmatism), corneal astigmatism, and residual astigmatism is given by the relationship

$$\begin{aligned}\text{total astigmatism} &= \text{corneal astigmatism} \\ &+ \text{residual astigmatism.}\end{aligned} \quad (13.5)$$

According to *Javal's rule*, which attempts to predict the total astigmatic correction on the basis of keratometric findings,

$$\begin{aligned}\text{total astigmatism} &= (1.25)(\text{corneal astigmatism}) \\ &+ (-0.50 \text{ DC x } 90).\end{aligned}$$

Although Javal's rule was determined strictly on an empirical (rather than a theoretical) basis, residual astigmatism can be thought of as averaging about –0.50 DC x 90. (Note that Javal's rule is in the form $y = mx + b$, with the result that b represents residual astigmatism.) Residual astigmatism has a rather narrow distribution, normally ranging from zero to about 1.50 DC x 90, and very seldom has its axis at or near 180.

Because a hard contact lens (unless it is very thin and flexible) eliminates corneal astigmatism, a spherical hard lens is expected to leave only *residual* astigmatism uncorrected. For this reason, if retinoscopy or subjective testing is done while a patient wears spherical hard contact lenses, the expected finding is –0.50 D of astigmatism with the axis at or near 90°. To predict the amount of uncorrected astigmatism a patient will have when fitted with hard contact lenses, we compare total astigmatism (as determined by retinoscopy or by subjective testing) to keratometric astigmatism. This process is illustrated by three examples.

EXAMPLE 1
A given eye has the following keratometric finding and subjective refraction:
Keratometer: 42.50 @ 180/45.00 @ 90
Subjective: plano –2.00 DC x 180.

What is the amount of astigmatism that is not corrected by a spherical hard contact lens (i.e., the residual astigmatism)?

$$\begin{aligned}\text{Residual astigmatism} &= \text{refractive astigmatism} \\ &- \text{corneal astigmatism} \\ &= (-2.00 \text{ DC x } 180) - (-2.50 \text{ x } 180) \\ &= +0.50 \text{ DC x } 180, \text{ or } -0.50 \text{ DC x } 90.\end{aligned}$$

If retinoscopy or subjective refraction is done while a spherical hard contact lens is worn on this eye, the astigmatic portion of the refractive finding should be –0.50 DC x 90.

EXAMPLE 2
A given eye has the following keratometric finding and subjective refraction:
Keratometer: 44.00 @ 180/43.50 @ 90
Subjective: plano –1.50 DC x 90.

What is the amount of astigmatism that is not corrected by a spherical hard contact lens?

Residual astigmatism = (–1.50 DC x 90) – (–0.50 DC x 90)

= –1.00 DC x 90.

EXAMPLE 3
Given the keratometric findings and subjective refraction:
Keratometer: 42.50 @ 180/42.50 @ 90
Subjective: plano –0.75 DC x 90.

What is the amount of astigmatism that is not corrected by a spherical hard contact lens?

Residual astigmatism = (–0.75 DC x 90) – 0.00

= –0.75 DC x 90.

In this case, because there is no corneal astigmatism, *all* the refractive astigmatism is accounted for by residual astigmatism.

In routine hard contact lens fitting, once the lens has been placed on the eye and has been allowed to settle down, the predicted residual astigmatism is verified by performing an over-refraction.

Correction of Residual Astigmatism

As a general rule, a contact-lens wearer can tolerate, without asthenopia or blurred vision, as much as 0.50 D of against-the-rule or oblique astigmatism, or as much as 0.75 D (or even 1.00 D) of with-the-rule astigmatism. Therefore, when it is estimated (by comparing keratometer readings and subjective findings) or found by direct measurement (i.e., by OR) that a spherical contact lens results in more than these amounts of uncorrected astigmatism, the use of a toric contact lens should be seriously considered.

Because both hard and soft spherical contact lenses tend to *rotate* while on the wearer's eye, some method must be found to *stabilize* a toric lens to prevent it from rotating on the eye. The most common method of stabilizing a contact lens on the eye is *prism ballast* (Figure 13–24)—base-down prism is placed on the lens, in the lathe cutting process, so that the bottom of the lens is thicker than the top. The increased thickness of the lower part of the lens keeps the lens from rotating on the eye.

For either a hard or soft contact lens, a toric surface may be put on either the front or the back of the lens. In most cases, a *front* toric surface is used. However, both possibilities are examined here.

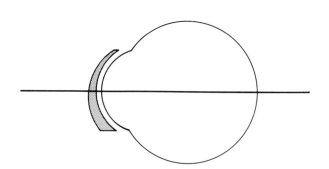

FIGURE 13–24.   **A prism-ballasted lens used for the correction of astigmatism, having base-down prism so that the bottom of the lens is thicker than the top.**

EXAMPLE 1
Given the keratometer readings and subjective refraction findings:
Keratometer: 44.00 @ 180/43.00 @ 90
Subjective: plano –2.00 DC x 90.

(1) What is the amount of uncorrected astigmatism if a *spherical* hard contact lens is fitted with its back surface radius parallel to the flattest corneal meridian? (2) What are the required parameters of a *front surface toric* lens, fitted so that the astigmatism is corrected in both principal meridians? (3) What is the back vertex power of the contact lens in (2) above?

(1) Since the corneal astigmatism can be corrected by a –1.00 D cylinder axis 90 and the refractive astigmatism can be corrected by a –2.00 D cylinder axis 90, the residual astigmatism with a spherical hard contact lens is

(–2.00 DC x 90) – (–1.00 DC x 90) = –1.00 DC x 90.

The parameters of a spherical hard lens for this eye can be determined with the aid of Figure 13–25, by the in situ method. For the 43.00-D keratometer reading in the *vertical meridian*, the use of a table (or calculation) results in a back surface radius of 7.85 mm. Therefore, for the refraction at the back surface of the contact lens (contact-lens/tear interface),

$$F_{C/T} = \frac{1.3375 - 1.490}{0.00785} = -19.43 \text{ D},$$

and, for the refraction at the front surface of the contact lens if the lens is ordered in plano power (because the spherical portion of the spectacle refraction is plano) and if the lens is assumed to be infinitely thin,

$$F_{A/C} = \frac{1.490 - 1}{0.00785} = +62.43 \text{ D}.$$

To be perfectly corrected in each principal meridian, the power of the air/contact-lens interface ($F_{A/C}$) plus the power of the contact-lens/tear interface ($F_{C/T}$) must be equal to the keratometer reading plus the ocular refraction. For the horizontal meridian, the keratometer

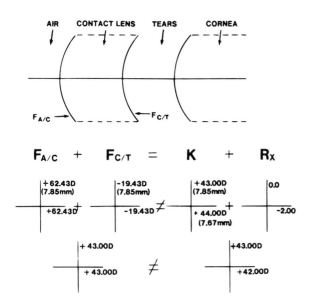

$$F_{A/C} + F_{C/T} = K + R_X$$

FIGURE 13–25. Diagram used for determining the parameters of a spherical hard contact lens for an eye having a keratometer reading of 44.00 @ 180/43.00 @ 90 and a subjective refraction of plano –2.00 DC x 90. Note that the horizontal meridian is overcorrected by +1.00 D.

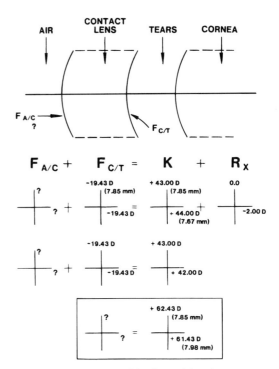

FIGURE 13–26. Diagram used for determining the parameters of a front surface toric hard contact lens for the eye considered in Figure 13–25.

reading plus the ocular refraction is

$$44.00 + (-2.00) = 42.00 \text{ D},$$

and for the vertical meridian the sum of the keratometer reading and the ocular refraction is

$$43.00 + 0.00 = 43.00 \text{ D}.$$

We now determine how well this lens corrects the refractive error of the eye in each of the principal meridians:

Horizontal: $\qquad F_{A/C} + F_{C/T} = K + R_x$

$$+62.43 + (-19.43) = +44.00$$

$$+(-2.00) + 43.00 \neq +42.00 \text{ D}.$$

Vertical: $\qquad +62.43 + (-19.43) = 43.00 + 0.00$

$$+43.00 \text{ D} = +43.00 \text{ D}.$$

The result shows that although the refractive error is corrected in the vertical meridian, the horizontal meridian is overcorrected by +1.00 D (Figure 13–25). This, of course, is what we found by comparing the keratometric and refractive astigmatism.

(2) Referring to Figure 13–26, the parameters of a *front surface toric* hard lens for this eye are determined with use of the in situ method. Because the correction in the vertical meridian is plano, the radius of curvature of the front surface in the vertical meridian is the same as the radius of the back surface, that is, 7.85 mm. Therefore, we are concerned only with the horizontal meridian. We first determine the refracting power of the front surface, $F_{A/C}$, in the horizontal meridian and then the radius of curvature, r_{1H}:

Horizontal: $F_{A/C} + F_{CT} = K + R_x$

or

$$F_{A/C} = K + R_x - F_{C/T}$$

$$= -2.00 + 44.00 - (-19.43)$$

$$= +61.43 \text{ D},$$

and

$$r_{1H} = \frac{1.490 - 1}{61.43} = +0.00798 \text{ m}.$$

Hence, the radii of this lens is

Back surface: 7.85 mm

Front surface:

vertical meridian = 7.85 mm

horizontal meridian = 7.98 mm.

(3) The back vertex power is more easily seen if the exploded method is used. This method is more easily visualized if schematic power crosses are used (Figure 13–27). The use of these power crosses shows that the radii of curvature of this lens are

Front surface:
    vertical meridian = 7.85 mm,
    therefore $F_{A/C}$ = +62.43 D.
    horizontal meridian = 7.98 mm,
    therefore $F_{A/C}$ = +61.43 D.

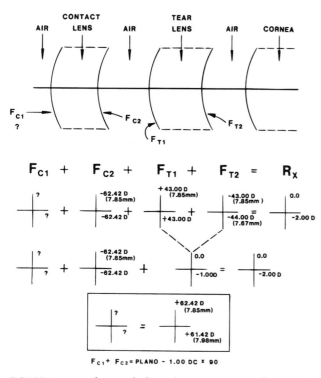

FIGURE 13–27.   **The use of schematic power crosses to illustrate the exploded method of determining the back vertex power of the front toric hard contact lens referred to in Figure 13–25.**

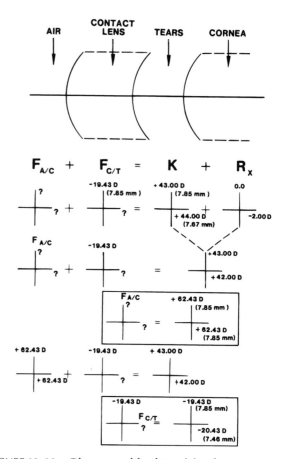

FIGURE 13–28.   **Diagram used for determining the parameters of a back surface toric hard contact lens, by using the in situ method, for the eye referred to in Figure 13–25.**

Back surface = 7.85 mm,
therefore $F_{C/A}$ = –62.43 D.

Hence the back vertex power of this contact lens is plano –1.00 DC x 90.

EXAMPLE 2

For the same eye, what are the required parameters of a *back surface* toric hard lens, with one principal meridian of the back surface of the lens parallel to the flattest corneal meridian? What is the back vertex power of the contact lens?

Referring to Figure 13–28, and again by using the in situ method, the radius of curvature in the *vertical meridian* of the back surface parallels the cornea and, hence, is 7.85 mm. This contact-lens/tear interface, therefore, generates the following power:

$$F_{C/T} = \frac{1.3375 - 1.490}{0.00785} = -19.43 \text{ D.}$$

Since the correction in the vertical meridian is plano, the power in the *vertical meridian* of the front surface is

$$F_{A/C} + F_{C/T} = K + R_x$$
$$F_{A/C} = K + R_x - F_{C/T}$$
$$= +43.00 + 0.00 - (-19.43)$$
$$= +62.43 \text{ D.}$$

Hence, the radius of curvature in the vertical meridian of the front surface is found by the relationship

$$r_{IV} = \frac{1.490 - 1}{62.43} = 0.00785 \text{ m.}$$

Since the front surface is spherical, the radius of curvature in the horizontal meridian of the front surface is also 7.85 mm.
In the horizontal meridian,

$$F_{A/C} + F_{C/T} = K + R_x$$
$$F_{C/T} = K + R_x - F_{A/C}$$
$$= +44.00 + (-2.00) - 62.43$$
$$F_{C/T} = -20.43 \text{ D}$$
$$r_{2H} = \frac{1.3375 - 1.490}{-20.43}.$$

Therefore, in the horizontal meridian,

$$r_{2H} = 0.00746 \text{ m, or } 7.46 \text{ mm.}$$

A schematic diagram of the power of this contact lens, in air, is given in Figure 13–29. The diagram shows that the radii of curvature of this lens are:

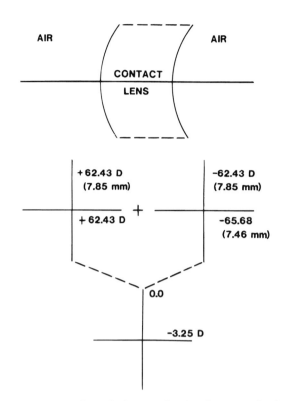

FIGURE 13–29. **Schematic diagram showing the power, in air, of the back surface toric hard contact lens illustrated in Figure 13–28.**

Front surface = 7.85 mm,

therefore

$$F_{A/C} = +62.43 \text{ D}.$$

Back surface:

vertical meridian = 7.85 mm,

therefore $F_{C/A} = -62.43$ D.

horizontal meridian = 7.46 mm,

therefore $F_{C/A} = -65.68$ D.

Hence, the back vertex power of this lens is plano –3.25 DC x 90.

Note that a comparison of the power of the back surface cylinder to that of the front surface cylinder gives us the familiar ratio,

$$\frac{3.25}{1.00}, \text{ or approximately } 3.2/1.$$

The Effect of Lens Flexure on Residual Astigmatism

The preceding discussion assumed that a hard contact lens maintains its spherical curvature when fitted on a toric cornea. However, when a spherical polymethyl methacrylate (PMMA) contact lens is made with a center thickness of less than about 0.13 mm, the lens has a tendency to *flex* or bend on a toric cornea in such a manner that it assumes a part of the corneal toricity. Gas-permeable hard lenses (e.g., those made of silicone acrylate) are even more flexible than PMMA lenses and must be made somewhat thicker to prevent excessive flexure. The amount of flexure may be measured by taking a keratometer reading while the spherical lens is worn—if the front surface of the lens is spherical, no flexure is present; if astigmatism is found, it is the result of flexure.

Flexure can be an advantage or a disadvantage in terms of its effect on residual astigmatism. If a lens flexes on a cornea having with-the-rule toricity in such a manner that it fails to eliminate 0.50 to 0.75 D of the corneal astigmatism, the uncorrected astigmatism may be just sufficient to compensate for 0.50 to 0.75 D of against-the-rule *internal* astigmatism, with the result that little or no residual astigmatism is found when an OR is done. However, if a lens flexes *more* than 0.50 to 0.75 D (which may occur with a thin lens on a highly toric cornea), a large amount of astigmatism may remain uncorrected. In such a case, a thicker lens (or one made of a less flexible material) may be used, or a toric contact lens may be fitted.

Residual Astigmatism and Soft Contact Lenses

When the term *residual astigmatism* is used in connection with soft contact lenses, it has a different meaning than that used in connection with hard lenses. Rather than being used as a synonym for internal astigmatism, the term is used to denote any astigmatism not corrected by the contact lens in question, which may better be termed *uncorrected astigmatism.*

As stated earlier, a well-fitting soft contact lens completely conforms to the corneal surface, with the result that it fails to correct any corneal astigmatism; because a contact lens cannot correct internal astigmatism, it follows that a spherical soft contact lens *does not correct astigmatism.* Thus, the astigmatism that is not corrected by a spherical soft contact lens (the "uncorrected" astigmatism) is the *refractive,* or *total,* astigmatism. To illustrate this principle, each of the above examples for a spherical soft lens is recalculated.

EXAMPLE 1
What is the amount of uncorrected astigmatism for a spherical soft contact lens, given the following findings?
Keratometer: 42.50 @ 180/45.00 @ 90
Subjective: plano –2.00 DC x 180.

Since a spherical soft contact lens corrects no corneal astigmatism, the answer is
–2.00 DC x 180.

EXAMPLE 2
What is the amount of uncorrected astigmatism for a spherical soft contact lens, for the following findings?

Keratometer: 44.00 @ 180/43.50 @ 90
Subjective: plano −1.50 DC x 90.

The uncorrected astigmatism is the refractive astigmatism, or −1.50 DC x 90.

EXAMPLE 3
Given the following findings, what is the amount of uncorrected astigmatism for a spherical soft contact lens?
Keratometer: 42.50 @ 180/42.50 @ 90
Subjective: plano −0.75 DC x 90.

The answer is, again, the refractive astigmatism, or −0.75 DC x 90.

On the basis of these examples, if a prospective contact lens wearer has any amount of astigmatism, he or she is likely to have *less* uncorrected astigmatism if a *hard* contact lens is worn than if a *soft* lens is worn. Furthermore, because internal astigmatism is almost always against-the-rule and because corneal astigmatism and refractive astigmatism are more commonly with-the-rule, it follows that:

1. When a spherical hard lens is worn, any uncorrected astigmatism is most likely to be *against-the-rule* astigmatism.
2. When a spherical soft lens is worn, any uncorrected astigmatism is very likely to be *with-the-rule* astigmatism.

Correction of Astigmatism with Soft Contact Lenses

When a patient is to be fitted with soft contact lenses, the use of a toric soft lens is normally considered whenever the total astigmatism of the eye exceeds 0.50 or 0.75 D of against-the-rule or oblique astigmatism or 0.75 or 1.00 D of with-the-rule astigmatism. A toric soft contact lens can be made in either front toric or back toric form; the discussion here is limited to the front toric form. Because a well-fitting soft lens conforms completely to the corneal surface, it is assumed that a front surface toric lens fits in such a way that the back surface radii of curvature of the lens are equal, in each of the principal meridians, to the radii of curvature of the cornea. Because soft contact lenses contain a high percentage of water, they have a lower index of refraction than hard contact lenses, usually considered to be approximately 1.430.

EXAMPLE
Given the following keratometric and subjective findings:
Keratometer: 44.00 @ 180/43.00 @ 90
Subjective: plano −2.00 DC x 90.

Using the index of refraction of 1.430, find the necessary front and back radii of curvature in each of the principal meridians of the contact lens.

We first calculate the radii of curvature of the cornea in each meridian:

$$r_{\text{H}} = \frac{1.3375 - 1}{44.00} = 0.00767 \text{ m.}$$

$$r_v = \frac{1.3375 - 1}{43.00} = 0.00785 \text{ m.}$$

Thus, the radii of curvature of the back surface of the lens is 7.67 mm in the horizontal meridian and 7.85 mm in the vertical meridian.
The power of the contact-lens/tear interface in the *horizontal* meridian is

$$F_{\text{C/T}} = \frac{1.3375 - 1.430}{0.00767} = \frac{-0.0925}{0.00767} = -12.06 \text{ D,}$$

and the power of the contact-lens/tear interface in the *vertical* meridian is

$$F_{\text{C/T}} = \frac{1.3375 - 1.430}{0.00785} = -11.78 \text{ D.}$$

With use of the in situ method for the refraction in the horizontal meridian at the *front surface* of the contact lens,

$$F_{\text{A/C}} + F_{\text{C/T}} = K + R_x$$
$$F_{\text{A/C}} = K + R_x - F_{\text{C/T}}$$
$$= +44.00 + (-2.00) - (-12.06)$$
$$= +54.06 \text{ D.}$$

The radius of curvature of the front surface of the lens in the horizontal meridian is

$$r_{\text{1H}} = \frac{1.430 - 1}{54.06} = 0.00795 \text{ m,}$$

and for the refraction in the vertical meridian of the front surface,

$$F_{\text{A/C}} = K + R_x - F_{\text{C/T}}$$
$$= +43.00 + 0.00 - (-11.78)$$
$$= +54.78 \text{ D.}$$

Hence, the radius of curvature of the front surface in the vertical meridian is

$$r_{\text{1V}} = \frac{1.430 - 1}{54.78} = 0.00785 \text{ m.}$$

The radii of curvature of this soft contact lens on the eye is therefore:

Front surface:
   horizontal = 7.95 mm
   vertical   = 7.85 mm.

Back surface:
   horizontal = 7.67 mm
   vertical   = 7.85 mm.

with the flattest curvature of the lens parallel to a spherical cornea that measures 45 D on a keratometer?

15. A front surface toric contact lens has a power of plano −3.00 DC x 020. The contact lens is placed on a patient's eye, but it is suspected that the lens is not oriented properly on the eye. An OR of +0.50 DS −1.00 DC x 60 gives the best acuity. Assume the orientation is the only reason for the nonzero over-refraction. What is the approximate minus axis cylinder orientation on the eye?

16. A patient is fitted with the following rigid contact lens: base curve radius = 7.67 mm, power = −2.00 D. At the time of the fitting, the OR was plano and the patient's K readings were 44.00 D at 180° and 44.50 D at 90°. Three months later, the K readings were found to be 44.75 D at 180° and 45.25 D at 90°. The patient wishes to wear spectacle lenses immediately after removal of the contact lenses. What is the spectacle prescription found immediately on removal of the contact lenses?

17. A patient's refractive error is fully corrected with a spherical corneal contact lens. The base curve of the lens is 43.00 D and the power is −3.00 D. The patient is refitted with a bi-toric lens having a base curve of 43.50 D at 180° and 45.50 D at 90°. What is the power ordered for this lens?

18. A fused bifocal is made on the back surface of a hard contact lens with the back surface of the segment having the same radius of curvature as the base curve, that is, 8.0 mm. The refractive index of the segment is 1.57 and the radius of the countersink surface is 6.67 mm. What is the power of the add on the eye?

19. A fused bifocal is made on the back surface of a hard contact lens (of refractive index 1.49) with the back surface of the segment having the same radius of curvature as the base curve, that is, 8.0 mm. The index of the segment is 1.56 and the power of the add on a lensometer is +3.00 D. What is the radius of curvature of the countersink surface?

20. A rigid one-piece back surface bifocal contact lens is ordered with a distance power of −3.00 D with a +2.50 D add. When verified on a lensometer, what is the difference in the readings between the near and distance portions of the lens?

21. A front surface spherical/back surface toric rigid contact lens (index 1.49) is ordered to match a cornea with 2.00 D of corneal toricity. How much cylinder power is measured with a lensometer?

22. An add of +2.00 D is generated by changing the curvature of the peripheral portion of the back surface. The central back portion has a radius of curvature of 7.50 mm.
    (a) What is the radius of curvature of the peripheral portion?
    (b) What is the power of the add read on a lensometer?

23. A patient is wearing a spherical rigid corneal contact lens with a base curve of 43.00 D (7.85 mm) and a back vertex power of −3.00 D. This lens fully corrects his refractive error. He is refitted with a bi-toric lens having a base curve of 45.00 D (7.50 mm) in the vertical meridian and 42.00 D (8.05 mm) in the horizontal meridian, which are the principal meridians. What lens power in the contact lens completely corrects the patient?

Answers to Questions

No answers are provided for essay or discussion questions.

Chapter 2

1. 2.99 mm
2. 1.698
3. +5.07 D
4. F_1 of major portion = +12.83 D
   F_1 of segment = +16.92 D
5. +2.65 D
6. 1.625
7. 1.70
8. 1.60
9. +70.00 D
10. +3.50 DS +2.50 DC x 90
11. (a) −1.50 D
    (b) −4.50 D
12. (a) +1.00, +2.00, +1.73, +1.00, −1.00, −2.00, −1.00, +1.00 D
    (b) −1.50, +0.50, +1.87, +3.00, +3.50, +1.50, −1.00, −1.50 D
13. +1.31 D
14. Horizontal line

(a)	(b)	(c)
+10 cm	+20 cm	+20 cm
(d)	(e)	
−20 cm	+33.3 cm	

Vertical line

(a)	(b)	(c)
+20	−20	∞
(d)	(e)	
−10	−33.3	

Circle

(a)	(b)	(c)
+13.3	∞	+40
(d)	(e)	
−13.3	∞	

15. +2.00 DS +1.00 DC x 90
16. 1 − 7
17. −2.00 DS +8.00 DC x 180
18. (a) −1.80 DS +4.85 DC x 2°45′ or
        +3.05 DS −4.85 DC x 92°45′
    (b) +0.85 DS +3.30 DC x 51°42′ or
        +4.15 DS −3.30 DC x 141°42′
    (c) −0.71 DS +0.91 DC x 8°26′ or
        +0.21 DS −0.91 DC x 98°26′
    (d) −1.52 DS +5.05 DC x 69°4′ or
        +3.52 DS −5.05 DC x 159°4′
    (e) −3.90 DS +6.05 DC x 30°21′ or
        +2.15 DS −6.05 DC x 120°21′
19. +3.00 DC x 180/+1.00 DC x 90
20. +10.00 D
21. 1.622
22. −10.10 DS −0.31 DC x 180
23. +3.50 D
24. +0.75 DS
25. +0.25 DS −2.00 DC x 120
26. +4.00 D
27. 13.9 cm

Chapter 3

1. −5.00 D
2. +11.27 D
3. +9.80 D
4. (a) −12.00 D
   (b) −13.03 D
   (c) −13.03 D
   (d) −3.03 D
5. −9.26 D
6. +13.90 DS −3.38 DC x 180
7. 1.33 cm
8. −2.25 DS +1.75 DC x 15
9. +9.14 D
10. +16.67 D
11. +25.00 D
12. +2.00 DS −6.00 DC x 180
13. −4.00 D
14. +2.00 DS +1.25 DC x 15, add +2.00 D
15. +2.50 DS −7.50 DC x 30
16. 2.3 mm
17. 4.4 mm
18. −10.46 D
19. +0.39 D increase
20. 4.5 mm
21. +12.5 D
22. −12.60 D

Chapter 4

1. (a) 1°22′
   (b) 1°5′
2. 2.6 prism diopters
3. 2 prism diopters base-up
4. (a) 4.47 prism diopters, base at 243°29′
   (b) 2.2 prism diopters, base at 116°34′
5. (a) 2.59 prism diopters, base-in/1.5 prism diopters, base-up
   (b) 1 prism diopter, base-in/1.73 prism diopters, base-down
6. 12 prism diopters
7. 4.4 degrees
8. 11.39 prism diopters
9. (a) 0.6 prism diopter, base-out/3.6 prism diopters, base-up
   (b) 0.4 prism diopter, base-in/none vertical
   (c) none horizontal/2.4 prism diopters, base-up

10. (a) 3.8 BU
        0.2 BI
    (b) 4.5 BU
        3.0 BI
    (c) 2.68 BU
        2.18 BI
11. 1.40 prism diopters BD in the OD
    1.64 prism diopters BO in the OS
12. +3.00 DS +7.00 DC x 180
13. −5.00 DS +8.33 DC x 180
14. 13.33 prism diopters
15. 3 mm in from the geometric center
16. 2.688 mm
17. 2 prism diopters
18. 3 mm temporally
19. 65 mm
20. 5.0 mm in; 1 mm out
21. 2.4 mm
22. 1.2 mm less
23. 1.25
24. 2 prism diopters, base-out
25. 7 prism diopters

Chapter 5

1. 0.77 D
2. OD +1.55 D
   OS + 1.36 D
3. (a) +2.36 D add
   (b) 0.62 D
4. 3.29 D
5. 2.01 D
6. +2.97 DS −7.97 DC x 90
7. +2.40 DS +5.60 DC x 180
8. 0.33 m in front of the eye
9. 10 cm
10. 10.00 D
11. 20 cm
12. 2.00 D hyperopia
13. 1.50 D
14. 1.00 D myopia
15. 6.00 D

Chapter 6

1. 0.1
2. 10.0
3. 0.092 D
4. 0.7 prism diopter
5. +0.19 D
6. +11.66 D and −6.67 D
7. Crown = 8.18 prism diopters
   Flint = 5.18 prism diopters
8. −72.00 cm
9. +4.00 D
10. 0.18 D

11. 0.26 D
12. −508 mm
13. +360 mm
14. −20.00 D

Chapter 7

1. 1.3
2. 116 nm
3. 5.6%
4. 87.0%
5. 95.6%
6. 6.25%
7. 2.1
8. 25
9. 1.4
10. 10.0%
11. 30 mm
12. 20.17%
13. 4.74%
14. 68.1%
15. 10
16. 0.1%
17. 4.48 mm
18. –
19. 3.94%
20. 12.00 D
21. −6.00 D
22. 82.7%

Chapter 8

1. 3.3 prism diopters, base-down
2. 1.1 cm
3. 1.2 prism diopters, base-down
4. 4.0 prism diopters, base-up
5. 4.4 prism diopters, base-down
6. 30 mm
7. 7 mm below the top of the segment
8. −6.00 D
9. plano
10. +3.00 D
11. +15.00
12. Near segment = 1.60
    Intermediate segment = 1.54
13. 0.756 mm
14. F_1 = +22.00 D
    F_2 = −31.00 D
15. 1.58 mm
16. 10 mm
17. +1.00 DS −1.50 DC x 90; add = +2.25 D.
18. −4.50 D horizontal
    +6.00 D vertical
19. 1.18 D
20. 0.21 D
21. 41.76%
22. 0.30 D too weak

Chapter 9

1. 5.0%
2. 63.2 mm
3. 62.05 mm
4. 2 mm in; 2 mm in
5. 4 mm in; 4 mm in
6. 3.5 mm each
7. 3 mm below the geometric center
8. +2.00 D
9. 18.0 mm

Chapter 10

1. 2.5 prism diopters OD
2. 9 prism diopters BU
3. OD R-5; OS R-9 or OD R-6; OS R-10
4. (e) OD Executive; OS Kryptok
5. 1.08 mm
6. +11.50 D
7. 2.5 mm above the reading level
8. 1.0 prism diopter left hyperphoria
9. orthophoria
10. 2.0%
11. −14.00 D
12. 6.75 mm
13. +11.00 D
14. 20.2% increase
15. 12.0% decrease
16. Increase by 3%
17. 1.0% decrease
18. 2.0% increase
19. +26.15%
20. 16.28%
21. −9.37 D
22. 12.8 mm
23. (a) 12.5 mm
    (b) +5.71 D

Chapter 11

1. +13.00 D
2. +10.00 D
3. 73.15 mm behind the corneal apex
4. +11.88 D
5. 31.25 prism diopters
6. +14.02 D
7. 2.07 mm

Chapter 12

1. 4×
2. 2.67×
3. (a) −2.5×
   (b) 28 cm

4. Objective lens = +10.00 D
Eyepiece lens = −40.00 D

5. 16 cm

6. −3.5×

7. 1.30 or 30%

8. 8×

9. 8 D

10. 16 D

11. 25 cm

12. 5×

13. 3.2× telescope with a +5.0 D reading cap

14. +7.8 D

15. 40 mm

16. +15.00 D

17. 1.36×

18. 1.60×

19. +16.00 D

20. (a) 3
(b) 6 D

Chapter 13

1. +18.25 D

2. −2.50 DC x 90

3. 7.70 mm

4. −0.50 DS −0.75 DC x 90

5. −3.00 D

6. 43.75 D at 180; 45.00 D at 90

7. +7.75 D

8. −3.00 DS −0.50 DC x 90

9. 44.50 D at 180; 45.50 D at 90

10. −2.00 D

11. 42.25 D

12. 7.258 mm

13. 7.89 mm

14. +1.00 DS −1.00 DC x 90

15. 10 degrees

16. −2.75 DS −0.50 DC x 180

17. −3.50 DS −2.00 DC x 180

18. +2.00 D

19. 5.96 mm

20. 8.03 D

21. 2.90 D

22. (a) 8.31 mm
(b) 6.43 D

23. −2.00 DS − 3.00 DC x 180

Index

The Use of a Toric Back Surface Hard Lens for a Highly Toric Cornea

For a highly toric cornea, a spherical hard contact lens tends to fit very badly, "rocking" on the flat meridian of the cornea and causing discomfort because of pressure on the lid margins. In such a case, the use of a toric back surface lens often provides a comfortable physical fit. The lens is fitted *only* for the purpose of providing a comfortable fit—from the *optical* point of view, such a lens fails to mask corneal astigmatism (as does a spherical lens), with the result that uncorrected astigmatism may be a problem unless a toric *front* surface is also used.

EXAMPLE

Given the following findings:
Keratometer: 43.50 @ 180/46.50 @ 90
Subjective: plano –2.00 DC x 180.

If a back surface toric lens is fitted so that it is parallel to the cornea in each principal meridian, what are the parameters of the resulting lens, designed in such a way as to completely correct the eye's astigmatism?
With use of the in situ method, the problem can be solved by reference to the optical crosses shown in Figure 13–30. As shown in the figure, the lens radii are:

Back surface interface:
    horizontal   = 7.76 mm ($F_{C/T}$ = –19.65 D).
    vertical = 7.26 mm ($F_{C/T}$ = –21.00 D).
Front surface:
    horizontal   = 7.76 mm ($F_{A/C}$ = +63.15 D).
    vertical = 7.48 mm ($F_{A/C}$ = +65.15 D).

The back vertex power of the contact lens, in air (Figure 13–31), is plano –2.00 DC x 180.
It is obvious that this lens is *bi-toric.* When a toric back surface matching the toricity of the cornea is used, a front toric curve usually must be used to provide adequate correction of the eye's astigmatism.

13.10. Magnification Effects of Contact Lenses

As stated in Chapter 10, Section 10.9, if we assume a correcting lens to be infinitely thin (so that the shape magnification factor is equal to unity), the size of the retinal image formed by a lens is inversely proportional to the power of the lens; when this relationship is applied to the fitting of a contact lens as opposed to a spectacle lens on the same

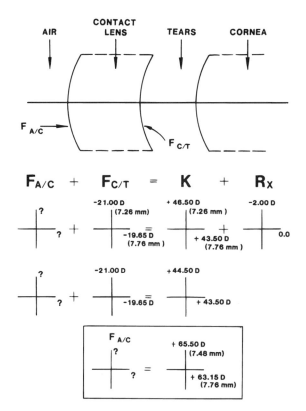

FIGURE 13–30.   **Diagram used for determining the parameters of a back surface toric hard lens used to provide a comfortable physical fit on a highly toric cornea.**

Figure 13–31.   **Diagram showing the power, in air, of the back surface toric lens illustrated in Figure 13–30.**

eye, the equation is

$$\frac{\text{retinal image size with a contact lens}}{\text{retinal image size with a spectacle lens}} = \frac{F_S}{F_C},$$

and fitting a spectacle lens as opposed to a contact lens, the equation is

$$\frac{\text{retinal image size with a spectacle lens}}{\text{retinal image size with a contact lens}} = \frac{F_C}{F_S},$$

where F_S is the back vertex power of the spectacle lens and F_C is the back vertex power of the contact lens. For a myopic eye, a contact lens has a lower back vertex power than does a spectacle lens for the same eye, with the result that the retinal image is *larger* with a contact lens than with a spectacle lens. For a hyperopic eye, a contact lens has a higher power than a spectacle lens, with the result that the retinal image is *smaller* with a contact lens than with a spectacle lens. These relationships are illustrated in two ways in the following example.

EXAMPLE
Assuming the correcting lens to be infinitely thin in each case, what is the change in retinal image size when switching from a spectacle lens to a contact lens for each of the following eyes: (1) an eye requiring a −5.00-D spectacle lens at a vertex distance of 12 mm, and (2) an eye requiring a +13.00-D spectacle lens at a vertex distance of 10 mm.

(1) The required power of a contact lens for this eye is

$$\frac{-5.00}{1 - 0.012(-5.00)} = -4.72 \text{ D}.$$

$$\text{Magnification ratio} = \frac{F_S}{F_C} = \frac{-5.00}{-4.72} = 1.06,$$

and

%SM change = (1.06 − 1.00)100 = +6%. (The spectacle magnification is 6% *larger* with contact lenses than that for spectacle lenses.)

(2) The required power of a contact lens for this eye is

$$\frac{+13.00}{1 - 0.010(+13.00)} = +14.94 \text{ D}.$$

$$\text{Magnification ratio} = \frac{F_S}{F_C} = \frac{+13.00}{+14.94} = 0.87,$$

and

%SM change = (0.87 − 1.00)100 = −13%. (The spectacle magnification is 13% *smaller* for contact lenses than that for spectacle lenses.)

A more exact comparison can be made by using the entire spectacle magnification formula, which takes into

consideration the shape factor as well as the power factor. This is calculated below for the +13.00-D spectacle lens with a front curve of +16.00 D and a center thickness of 8.0 mm, and made of a plastic having an index of refraction of 1.498, and for the contact lens with a front curve of +77.00 D and a center thickness of 0.4 mm, made of a plastic having an index of 1.490.

For the spectacle lens,

$$\text{SM}_S = \left(\frac{1}{1 - \frac{0.008}{1.498}(+16)}\right)\left(\frac{1}{1 - 0.013(+13)}\right)$$
$$= (1.094)(1.203) = 1.316,$$

and for the contact lens,

$$\text{SM}_C = \left(\frac{1}{1 - \frac{0.0004}{1.490}(+77)}\right)\left(\frac{1}{1 - 0.003(+14.94)}\right)$$
$$= (1.021)(1.047) = 1.069.$$

$$\text{Magnification ratio} = \frac{\text{SM}_C}{\text{SM}_S} = \frac{1.069}{1.316} = 0.81.$$

%SM change = (0.81 − 1.00)100 = −19%. (The spectacle magnification is 19% *smaller* for contact lenses than that for spectacle lenses.)

The error of 6% (i.e., 19% − 13%) caused by considering an aphakic lens as an infinitely thin lens, shows that this is an invalid assumption, and that an aphakic lens (whether a spectacle lens or a contact lens) must be treated, for purposes of determining spectacle magnification, as a thick lens.

Relative Spectacle Magnification

The discussions in Chapter 10, Sections 10.12, 10.13, and 10.20 showed that when a patient has anisometropia, if the difference in the spherical ametropia for the two eyes is assumed to be caused by a difference in axial length, a minimum of aniseikonia is induced if spectacles are prescribed; if the difference in the spherical ametropia is assumed to be caused by a difference in the refractive power of the two eyes (i.e., cornea, anterior chamber, or lens), a minimum of aniseikonia is induced if contact lenses are prescribed. Because astigmatism is always refractive in origin, when a patient has significant astigmatism (particularly if the axes are oblique and symmetrical), a minimum of meridional aniseikonia is induced if contact lenses are prescribed.

Nevertheless, because most instances of spherical anisometropia tend to have both axial and refractive components, the above statements should not be interpreted as incontrovertible. For example, if an anisometropic patient desires contact lenses, he or she should not be told that contact lenses cannot be worn—the patient should be allowed to wear contact lenses for a trial period before the final decision is made.

EFFECTS OF CONTACT LENSES ON BINOCULAR VISION

13.11. Accommodative Demand

Because accommodation, like refraction, takes place at the first principal plane of the eye (which is only slightly more than 1 millimeter behind the corneal apex), the accommodative demand can be significantly different for a contact lens wearer than for a spectacle wearer. The difference increases with increasing ametropia, and reaches significance in the pre-presbyopic and presbyopic years. As shown in Chapter 5, Section 5.7, a spectacle-wearing 10.00 D hyperope must accommodate 3.29 D for a 40 cm reading distance, but a spectacle-wearing 10.00 D myope needs to accommodate only 1.83 D for the same distance.

Because the amount of accommodation while wearing contact lenses is very close to 2.50 D, no matter what the refractive error, the examples show that the 10.00 D hyperope has to accommodate about 0.75 D *less* while wearing contact lenses than while wearing glasses, but the 10.00 D myope has to accommodate about 0.75 D *more* while wearing contact lenses than while wearing glasses. Even for patients who have far less than 10.00 D of myopia, the increased accommodative demand required for contact lenses may constitute a problem. For example, if a 42-year-old 5.00-D myope who has had no problem with near work while wearing glasses is fitted with contact lenses, he or she may immediately find that close work is difficult because this myopic patient has lost the advantage of having to accommodate less than an emmetrope or a spectacle-wearing hyperope. On the other hand, sometimes a spectacle-wearing hyperope who has just begun to need an add while wearing spectacles finds that switching to contact lenses allows reading and other near work to be done comfortably without the need for an add.

13.12. Accommodative Convergence

The change in accommodative demand that occurs when a patient switches from glasses to contact lenses means that there is also a change in the amount of accommodative convergence present for reading and other close work, which causes a change in the amount of fusional convergence required for fusion. The amount of change in accommodative convergence depends on the AC/A ratio.

For example, if a 10.00 D myope changes from glasses to contact lenses, the increased accommodative demand of almost 0.75 D is accompanied by an increase in accommodative convergence. For a 6/1 AC/A ratio, the increased amount of accommodative convergence at 40 cm is 6(0.75), or 4 prism diopters. Thus, if the patient is exophoric at 40 cm, the exophoria is reduced by 4 prism diopters, but if the patient is esophoric at 40 cm, the esophoria is increased by 4 prism diopters. In the former case, the patient uses 4 prism diopters less positive fusional vergence; in the latter case, the person has to use 4 prism diopters more negative fusional vergence.

Similarly, the decrease in accommodative demand for the high hyperope results in a decreased amount of accommodative convergence, the change in accommodative convergence again depending on the value of the AC/A ratio. For the 10.00 D hyperope having a 6/1 AC/A ratio, switching from glasses to contact lenses increases any exophoria at 40 cm and decreases any esophoria at 40 cm by 4 prism diopters.

Fortunately, most contact lens wearers have refractive errors in the range of ±1.00 to ±4.00 or ±5.00 D, with the result that the change in accommodative convergence required with contact lenses is not often a problem.

13.13. Prismatic Effects

When spectacles are worn, whether primarily for distance vision or for both distance and near vision, they are normally centered in front of the wearer's pupils, which avoids prismatic effects during distance vision but allows prismatic effects to be induced for near vision or for viewing through the lens periphery. When spectacle lenses of minus power are centered for the distance PD, *base-in* prism is induced for near vision; when plus-powered spectacle lenses are centered for the distance PD, *base-out* prism is induced for near vision.

The induced prism power may be an advantage or a disadvantage to the wearer, depending on the near phoria. As shown in Figure 13–32, if a myope has a significant exophoria at near, the presence of the induced base-in prism at the near point is an advantage (by reducing the amount of positive fusional vergence that must be used to compensate for the phoria), but a myope having esophoria at near is at a disadvantage because the prismatic effect at near increases the amount of negative fusional vergence needed to compensate for the esophoria. On the other hand, for a hyperopic patient (Figure 13–33), a *base-out* prismatic effect is present at near, which is an advantage

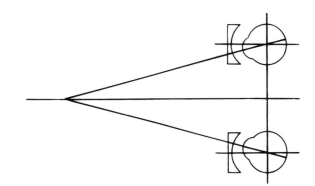

FIGURE 13–32.   **If a myope's spectacle lenses are centered for distance vision, induced base-in prism is encountered for near work.**

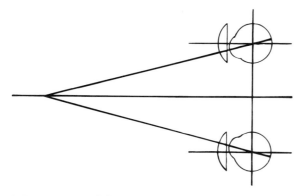

FIGURE 13–33.   **If a hyperope's spectacle lenses are centered for distance vision, induced base-out prism is encountered for near work.**

if the wearer is esophoric at near but a disadvantage if the person is exophoric at near.

When contact lenses are worn rather than glasses, the contact lenses (if fitting correctly) are centered before the pupils for both distance and near vision, with the result that the induced prismatic effects for near vision are no longer present. For relatively small refractive errors, the change in the near phoria does not often present a problem. However, it is possible that many symptoms reported by contact lens wearers that are considered by practitioners to be caused by adaptation to the contact lenses are actually caused by the change in prismatic effects for near vision.

For myopic patients, changing from spectacles to contact lenses causes *an increase* in both the accommodative and convergence stimuli for near vision. The general effect is *as if* the near-vision task has been moved a little closer because the patient must now accommodate and converge more than previously. For the hyperopic patient, changing from spectacles to contact lenses causes *a decrease* in both the accommodative and convergence stimuli for near vision. It is *as if* the near-vision work has moved farther away because the patient must now accommodate and converge less than previously.

If a patient has normal linkage between accommodation and convergence (average AC/A ratio) and has no trouble with spectacles, the person should not experience difficulties in changing from spectacles to contact lenses. The exception is the pre-presbyopic myope who, newly introduced to contact lenses, may immediately become presbyopic. Because a myopic patient must accommodate and converge more with contact lenses than with spectacles, and because both functions must increase in about the same proportion, a new, higher level of accommodation–convergence activity is established, but no imbalance in the accommodation–convergence relationship occurs.

Changes for the hyperopic patient are the opposite, that is, both accommodation and convergence are less, but the same conclusions regarding the stability of the accommodation–convergence relationship apply as discussed for the myopic patient.

When ametropia is significant and when there is an anomalous relationship between accommodation and con-

vergence—too much convergence (high AC/A ratio) or too little convergence (low AC/A ratio) associated with each diopter of accommodation, the patient may develop visual problems. These problems, however, may be studied and possibly resolved through one of the standard methods of case analysis and treatment.

The clinical ramifications of changing from spectacles to contact lenses are listed as follows:

1. For a patient with high myopia and a significant near exophoria (low AC/A ratio), an *increase* in the near exophoria with contacts is more likely to occur—because of the absence of induced base-in prismatic effects of the spectacles—than is a *decrease* because of the greater amount of accommodative convergence in play.

2. For a patient with high myopia and a significant near esophoria (high AC/A ratio), an *increase* in the near esophoria is more likely to occur—because of increased accommodative convergence—than is a *decrease* because of the absence of the induced base-in prismatic effects of the spectacles.

3. For a patient with high hyperopia and a significant near exophoria (low AC/A ratio), the near exophoria is likely to *decrease* more because of the removal of the induced base-out prismatic effects of the spectacles than to an increase because of a reduction in the accommodative convergence. The net effect is a *decrease* in the near exophoria.

4. For a patient with high hyperopia and a significant near esophoria (high AC/A ratio), the near esophoria is likely to *decrease* more to a reduction in accommodative convergence than to increase because of the absence of induced base-out prismatic effects of the spectacles. The net change is a *decrease* in the near esophoria.

The binocular vision ramifications of changing from spectacles to contact lenses are summarized in Table 13–1.

13.14. Prescribing Prism in a Contact Lens

As already discussed, a contact lens may be provided with base-down prism (prism ballast) to eliminate rotation of the lens on the eye. Vertical prism may also be prescribed to compensate for a vertical heterophoria. Articles in professional literature have stated that when a contact-lens-containing prism is placed in contact with tear fluid, the lens retains only about one-fourth its deviating power in air.[1,2] However, both Bailey[3] and Mandell[4] showed that placing a contact lens on the eye has no effect on the prism power; that is, for a given amount of prism power for *distance vision*, the deviation is the same for a contact lens as for a spectacle lens. However, for *near vision*, a given amount of prism in a contact lens produces somewhat *more* deviation than a prism in a spectacle lens because (as stated in Chapter 4, Section 4.17) when a prism is used for near objects, its deviating power is greater as the prism is moved closer to the center of rotation of the eye; that is, for a given amount of prism, the effective power of the prism for near objects is greater for a contact lens than for a spectacle lens.

Regardless of whether a contact lens contains prism, the presence of *refractive power* in a contact lens brings about a vertical prismatic effect whenever the lens moves upward or downward on the eye with respect to the center of the pupil. The induced vertical prismatic effect adds to (or subtracts from) the prismatic effect caused by any vertical prism present in the lens.

TABLE 13–1
Some Binocular Vision Ramifications of Changing from Spectacles to Contact Lenses

Patient	Changes in Accommodative Demand	Changes in Accommodative Convergence and Phoria (at near vision)	Changes in Prismatic Effects and Phoria[a] (at near vision)
High myopia with exophoria at near (low AC/A ratio)	Increase	Increase; decreased exophoria	Lack of BI effect; increased exophoria[b]
High myopia with esophoria at near (high AC/A ratio)	Increase	Increase; increased esophoria[c]	Lack of BI effect; decreased esophoria
High hyperopia with exophoria at near (low AC/A)	Decrease	Decrease; increased exophoria	Lack of BO effect; decreased exophoria[d]
High hyperopia with esophoria at near (high AC/A)	Decrease	Decrease; decreased esophoria[e]	Lack of BO effect; increased esophoria

[a] Assuming that spectacle lenses were centered for distance vision.
[b] Increased exophoria at near caused by lack of BI prismatic effect is likely to be greater than the decreased exophoria caused by the greater amount of accommodative convergence.
[c] Increased esophoria at near caused by a greater amount of accommodative convergence is likely to be greater than decreased esophoria at near caused by a lack of BI prismatic effect.
[d] Decreased exophoria at near caused by lack of BO prism is likely to be greater than an increased exophoria caused by a reduction in accommodative convergence.
[e] Decreased esophoria at near caused by a reduction in accommodative convergence is likely to be greater than an increase because of the lack of a BO prismatic effect.

ABERRATIONS AND FIELD OF VIEW

13.15. Aberrations

All lenses are subject, in varying degrees, to chromatic aberration and to the five monochromatic aberrations. The effects of each aberration on contact lenses is briefly described.

Chromatic Aberration

As discussed in Chapter 6, Section 6.2, chromatic aberration may be considered as either (1) *longitudinal* chromatic aberration, defined as the separation along the optic axis of the focus for rays of light originating from a single axial point, or (2) *transverse* chromatic aberration, considered in terms of (1) the chromatic difference in magnification produced by a thick lens, which occurs in the image plane for rays from an extended object, or (2) the angular dispersion caused by the presence of prismatic effects. The eye tolerates longitudinal chromatic aberration very well, probably because the eye itself is subject to about 1 D of longitudi-

nal chromatic aberration. As for transverse chromatic aberration, the angular dispersion caused by prismatic effects is present only when the eye turns to look through a point in or near the periphery of a high-powered lens. Because a contact lens wearer always looks through a point at or near the optical center of the lens, the aberration does not present a problem.

Monochromatic Aberrations

The aberrations of *spherical aberration* and *coma* occur only for large-aperture optical systems. As with spectacle lenses, the aberrations do not present a problem for contact lenses of moderate power because the eye looks through only a small portion of the lens (the apical portion, in the case of a contact lens) at any time.

The aberrations of *oblique astigmatism* and *curvature of image* occur when a narrow pencil of light from an object passes obliquely through a spherical surface. For a spectacle lens, the aberrations occur only when the eye rotates away from the primary position so that the foveal line of sight passes through a peripheral point in the lens. Because a contact lens fits the eye in such a way that the foveal line of sight always passes through a point at or near the optical center of the lens, the aberrations do not present a problem for the contact lens wearer.

The aberration of *distortion*, although a problem for wearers of spectacle lenses of high power, applies only to extended objects and occurs as a result of the gradual change in magnification brought about by a lens from the center toward the periphery. The aberration increases in magnitude with the distance between the correcting lens and the pupil of the eye. Because the eye always fixates through the center of a contact lens and because the distance between the contact lens and the pupil of the eye is very small, distortion is not apt to be a problem for wearers of contact lenses. In summary, neither chromatic aberration nor any of the five monochromatic aberrations is likely to present a problem to the contact lens wearer.

13.16. Field of View

As discussed in Chapter 11, Section 11.4, field of view may be considered either in terms of the *peripheral* field of view, subtended at the entrance pupil of a steadily fixating eye, or in terms of the *macular* field of view of the moving eye (also known as field of fixation), subtended at the center of rotation of the eye.

As given in Equations 11.4 and 11.5 and illustrated in Figures 11–5 and 11–6, the extent of the peripheral field of view can be determined by the relationship

$$\tan \phi = y(E - F),$$

and the extent of the macular field of view can be determined by the relationship

$$\tan \theta = y(S - F),$$

where ϕ = one-half the peripheral field of view, θ = one-half the macular field of view, y = one-half the lens aperture, in meters, E = the vergence of light at the entrance pupil of the eye, S = the vergence of light at the center of rotation of the eye, and F = the power of the correcting lens.

The difference between the peripheral fields of view for a spectacle lens and for a contact lens is illustrated by the following examples.

EXAMPLE 1

How does the size of the peripheral field of view compare for a 3.00-D myope (1) for a spectacle lens having an aperture of 50 mm, located 15 mm from the entrance pupil of the eye, and (2) for a contact lens having an aperture of 7 mm, located 3 mm from the entrance pupil?

For the spectacle lens (1),

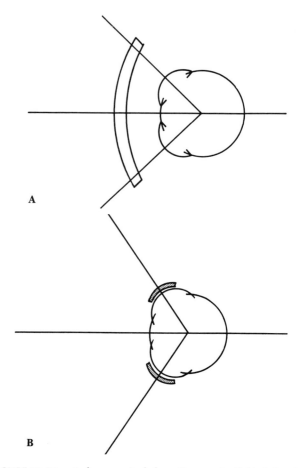

FIGURE 13–34.   **A, for a spectacle lens, the macular field of view is limited by the rim, or edge, of the lens; B, for a contact lens, the macular field of view is limited only by the ability of the eye to make rotational movements.**

$$\tan \phi = 0.025(66.67 + 3) = 1.742$$
$$\phi = 60.14°$$
$$2\phi = 120.28°,$$

and for the contact lens (2),

$$\tan \phi = 0.0035(333.33 + 3) = 1.1777$$
$$\phi = 49.65°$$
$$2\phi = 99.31°.$$

EXAMPLE 2

How does the size of the peripheral field of view compare for an aphakic patient (1) wearing a +12.50-D spectacle lens having an aperture of 50 mm, located 15 mm from the entrance pupil of the eye, and (2) wearing (for the same eye) a +14.50-D contact lens having an aperture of 7 mm, located 3 mm from the entrance pupil?

For the spectacle lens (1),

$$\tan \phi = 0.025(66.67 - 12.50) = 1.3543$$
$$\phi = 53.56°$$
$$2\phi = 107.12°,$$

and for the contact lens (2),

$$\tan \phi = 0.0035(333.33 - 14.50) = 1.116$$
$$\phi = 48.135°$$
$$2\phi = 96.27°.$$

Because many people (including many vision practitioners) believe that "the field of view is bigger" with a contact lens than with a spectacle lens, it is of interest that, in both examples above, the peripheral field of view is about 20 degrees *smaller* with a contact lens than with a spectacle lens. Although these results could vary somewhat, depending on the vertex distance of the spectacle lens and the aperture sizes of the spectacle lens and the contact lens, it is apparent that a contact lens does not necessarily provide a *larger* peripheral field of view than a spectacle lens. Why, then, does the idea persist that a contact lens provides a larger field of view?

The answer is that the field of view that is larger for a contact lens wearer is not the peripheral field of view, but the *macular* field of view. The macular field of view can be shown to be larger for a minus lens than for a plus lens (as in the case of the peripheral field of view). However, the important consideration is that, for a spectacle wearer, the macular field of view (as shown in Figure 13–34) is limited by the presence of the rim, or edge, of the lens; for a contact lens, the lens moves with the eye, with the result that the macular field of view is limited only by the eye's ability to make rotational movements.

Therefore, when the statement is made that "a contact lens provides a larger field of view than a spectacle lens," the statement is true if it is applied to the *macular* field of view, but not if it is applied to the *peripheral* field of view.

APHAKIA

13.17. Aphakic Contact Lenses

As discussed in Chapter 11, Section 11.4, aphakic spectacle lenses present a number of inherent problems. Although most problems can be controlled to a great extent by careful selection of aphakic lenses and frames, it is fortunate that the problems can, for all practical purposes, be *eliminated* by prescribing contact lenses rather than glasses and thereby allow the aphakic patient to function in very much the same manner as in the pre-aphakic condition. Problems caused by aphakic spectacles include the following:

1. Increased retinal image size
2. Decreased field of view
3. Presence of a ring scotoma
4. Increased ocular rotations
5. Increased lens aberrations
6. Motion of objects in the field of view
7. Demands on convergence
8. Appearance of the wearer

Increased Retinal Image Size

In Chapter 11, Section 11.4, it was found that for the aphakic schematic eye, corrected by a +10.34-D lens at a vertex distance of 12 mm, spectacle magnification (including both the shape factor and the power factor) was 28%. What is the contact lens magnification if the aphakic schematic eye is fitted with a contact lens rather than a spectacle lens?

First, the power of the aphakic contact lens differs from that of the spectacle lens because of the change in vertex distance. With use of the effective power formula,

$$F_{CL} = \frac{F_S}{1 - dF_S}$$
$$= \frac{+10.34}{1 - .012(+10.34)}$$
$$= +11.80 \text{ D.}$$

To apply the spectacle magnification formula, we must supply values for the index of refraction, the center thickness, and the front surface power of the contact lens. Assuming that these values are 1.490, 0.50 mm, and +74.00 D, respectively, the magnification brought about by the contact lens is

$$SM = \left(\frac{1}{1 - \frac{0.0005}{1.490}74}\right)\left(\frac{1}{1 - 0.003(11.80)}\right)$$
$$= (1.025)(1.037) = 1.063$$
$$\%SM = (1.063 - 1.00)100 = 6.3\%.$$

Although 6.3% is a large amount of magnification, it is sufficiently small (when compared with the 28% magnification brought about by spectacle lenses) that the bilateral aphakic is able to adapt relatively easily to the aphakic world. Even this amount of magnification can be a problem for the *unilateral* aphakic (see Chapter 11, Section 11.8, for a discussion of unilateral aphakia).

Decreased Field of View and Presence of a Ring Scotoma

As shown in Chapter 11, Section 11.4, when the pre-aphakic and aphakic fields of view are compared for a typical spectacle-wearing aphakic patient, the peripheral field of view decreases by about 7 degrees, but the macular field of view decreases by about 17 degrees. The decreases in both the peripheral and macular fields of view are responsible for the *ring scotoma* that is encountered when the eye rotates toward the periphery of the lens. However, because the macular field of view is virtually *unlimited* when a contact lens is worn (as shown in the previous section), an aphakic wearing contact lenses is not aware of any limitation in the field of view.

As for the problem of the ring scotoma and the accompanying jack-in-the-box phenomenon, the ring scotoma occurs because the spectacle-wearing aphakic has peripheral vision *beyond* the edge of the correcting lens. This, obviously, is not possible with a contact lens, with the result that the ring scotoma and the jack-in-the-box phenomenon are not present.

Increased Ocular Rotations

The increase in magnitude of ocular rotation when viewing an object in the periphery, for the spectacle-wearing aphakic eye as compared with the pre-aphakic state, is caused by the *prismatic effect* that is present when the visual axis passes through a peripheral point in the lens. Because a contact lens rotates with the eye, the visual axis of an aphakic wearing contact lenses always passes through the center of the lens, with the result that increased ocular rotations are not required.

Increased Lens Aberrations

As concluded in Section 13.14, neither chromatic aberration nor the five monochromatic aberrations are likely to present problems for the contact lens wearer. This statement applies equally well to the *aphakic* contact lens wearer.

Motion of Objects in the Field of View

This problem, sometimes referred to as swim, is an "against motion" of the field of view that occurs when a wearer of aphakic spectacles moves the head to look at a peripheral object while the eyes are held stationary (but move with the movement of the head). Swim occurs because as the head is moved, the visual axes pass through progressively more peripheral portions of the spectacles lenses, and thus bring about progressively increasing prismatic effects (with the prism base corresponding to the direction of the head movement). When an aphakic wearing contact lenses moves his or her head (and eyes) to look at a peripheral object, all objects in the field of view are seen (as the head moves) through the central or para-central portion of each contact lens, with the result that swim does not occur.

Demands on Convergence

As discussed in Section 13.13, when spectacle lenses are centered for the wearer's distance PD, a horizontal prismatic effect is encountered during reading and other close work and requires either an increase or a decrease in the demand on fusional vergence. For an aphakic lens, the base-out effect occurring with any plus lens is exaggerated and can be easily determined by the use of Prentice's rule. Because a contact lens wearer looks through the centers of his or her lenses for reading as well as for distance vision, no base-out prismatic effect is present at near vision, with the result that the demand on fusional vergence is only that required by the patient's near phoria.

Appearance

Even before the patient has undergone surgery (and is therefore relatively unaware of the perceptual problems brought about by aphakic spectacles), many patients choose contact lenses strictly because they consider aphakic spectacles to be unsightly.

INSTRUMENTATION

Just as the optics of a spectacle lens can be assessed by the use of the lensometer, the lens measure, and the thickness calipers, the optics of a contact lens can be assessed by means of the lensometer, the radiuscope, and the thickness gauge.

The optical principles of the *lensometer* were described in Chapter 3. The back vertex power of a contact lens is measured by placing the back surface of the lens against the lensometer stop. As described in Section 13.1 and illustrated in Figure 13–1, modern lensometers are equipped with a smaller stop than that used for a spectacle lens to provide for the steeper back surface curvature of a contact

lens. A *thickness gauge* is a mechanical instrument (similar to that used by a machinist) having a stage on which the contact lens is placed and having a gear assembly that supplies a direct reading to the nearest 0.01 mm.

The radiuscope, whose optical principles are described below, was developed by American Optical Corporation specifically for the measurement of the back surface radius of curvature of a hard contact lens (as with other instrumentation such as the refractor, the keratometer and the lensometer, the term *radiuscope* is now used in a generic sense).

13.18. The Radiuscope

The radiuscope is an instrument designed to measure the radius of curvature of the back surface (the base curve) of a contact lens. The instrument is based on a principle described by Drysdale[5] in 1900. The Drysdale principle is incorporated in all radiuscopes, although these instruments differ from one another in design and in the method of displaying the reading.

If a collimated beam of light is focused on a concave reflecting surface, the light is reflected along the same path as the incident light; if the focus of the collimated beam is then moved to the center of curvature of the concave surface, it is again reflected back along the same path as the incident light. Because the center of a concave reflecting surface and the center of curvature of the surface both cause incident light to be reflected back along its original path, these points are sometimes referred to as *self-reflecting points.*

The radiuscope incorporates a compound microscope in which an internally illuminated target (a radial-line target similar to a clock dial) is projected along the axis of the instrument. An image of the target is seen clearly by an observer, through the eyepiece, when the microscope objective focuses the image of the target either on the concave reflecting surface or at its center of curvature. The instrument is fitted with a half-silvered mirror, set at an angle of 45°, above the microscope objective (Figure 13–35).

The measurement consists of placing a contact lens (with its concave surface upward) on the stage of the instrument, with the convex surface in contact with a small pool of water. The water reduces the intensity of the image reflected from the lower (convex) surface of the contact lens so that it cannot be readily seen when the reflection from the upper (concave) surface is scrutinized. The stage of the instrument is then adjusted so that the illuminated target is aligned with the mirror, with the result that light from the mirror is reflected through the objective lens and forms a real image in the working plane of the objective lens.

Once the instrument has been aligned, the microscope objective is moved downward, toward the surface of the contact lens, until the working plane of the objective lens coincides with the plane of the back surface of the contact lens. When this occurs, the light is reflected back along its incident path and passes through the half-silvered mirror to form an image in the focal plane of the eyepiece, where it can be seen clearly by the observer, as shown in Figure 13–35A. This is the zero reading, and the operator places a fiduciary line on the zero point on the instrument's scale.

The microscope objective is then raised until a second position is found where the image of the target is in opti-

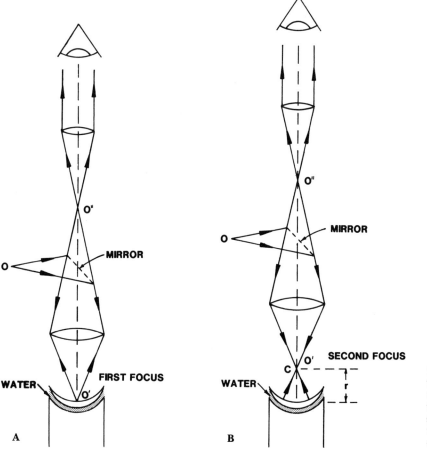

FIGURE 13–35. **The radiuscope. A,** the zero position (first focus) in which the working plane of the microscope objective coincides with the plane of the back surface of the contact lens; **B,** the final position (second focus), in which the working plane of the microscope objective coincides with the center of curvature of the back surface of the contact lens.

mal focus. This occurs when the working plane of the objective lens is positioned at the center of curvature of the back surface of the contact lens, as shown in Figure 13–35B. In this position, the concave surface again returns the light along its own path, which is normal to the back surface of the contact lens.

The distance through which the microscope has been moved between the first and second clearly focused images is the actual (physical) length of the radius of curvature of the concave surface (the base curve radius) of the contact lens.

References

1. Girard, L. J., Soper, J. W., and Sampson, W. G. *Corneal Contact Lenses*, C. V. Mosby, St. Louis, p. 290, 1964.
2. Filderman, I. P., and White, P. F. The Effect of Surrounding Media on Prismatic Contact Lenses. *Optom. Weekly*, Vol. 56, No. 26, pp. 19–24, July 1, 1965.
3. Bailey, N. J. Prism in a Contact Lens. *J. Am. Optom. Assoc.*, Vol. 37, pp. 44–45, 1966.
4. Mandell, R. B. The Prism Controversy. *J. Am. Optom. Assoc.*, Vol. 38, pp. 188–189, 1967.
5. Drysdale, C. V. On a Simple and Direct Method of Obtaining the Curvature of Small Lenses. *Trans. Ophthalmol. Soc. UK*, Vol. 2, pp. 1–12, 1900.

Questions

In working these problems, it is assumed that the keratometer is calibrated for an index of refraction of 1.3375 and that both the cornea and tears have an index of refraction of 1.3375. The index of refraction of rigid contact materials is assumed to be 1.49.

1. A patient's refraction using a phoropter at a vertex distance of 13 mm is +14.75 DS OU. If hard contact lenses are prescribed, what is the approximate power of the contact lenses for this patient?

2. Given:

    K readings: 43.00 D @ 180/44.25 D @ 090
    Spectacle R_x: –1.00 DS –1.25 DC x 090
    Base curve of contact lens: 43.00 D

    What is the residual astigmatism predicted with a hard contact lens in place?

3. A hard contact lens with a refractive index of 1.49 has a center thickness of 0.19 mm and a vertex power of –2.00 D. If the radius of curvature of the back surface is 7.4 mm, what is the radius of curvature of the front surface?

4. A 7.50-mm (45.00 D) base curve, –3.00 D hard contact lens is placed on a patient with a refraction of –3.50 DS –0.25 DC x 090, central K readings of 44.50 D in the 180° meridian and 45.00 D in the 90° meridian. What is the probable OR?

5. A patient had K readings of 42.50 D at 180° and 44.00 D at 90° and a spectacle refraction of –1.50 DS –1.50 DC x 180. What standard rigid contact lens power is needed if a 7.67 mm base curve (44.00-D) lens is fitted on this patient?

6. Given the following data:

    Spectacle refraction: –1.00 DS –1.00 DC x 180
    Hard contact lens specifications:
    Base curve = 7.80 mm
    Power = plano DS
    Refraction, contact lens, in situ = –0.25 DS –0.25 DC x 090

    What are the corneal curvatures?

7. A +6.50 D hyperopic patient who wears her spectacle prescription at a 16-mm vertex distance is to be fitted with a hard contact lens (of refractive index 1.49). Her cornea is spherical and measures 44.25 D. If the contact lens is fitted 0.50 D flatter than K, what is the expected contact lens prescription with consideration given to lens effectivity changes?

8. Consider the following clinical information:

    Spectacle Rx: –3.00 DS –0.50 DC x 180
    K readings: 44.00 @ 180/45.00 @ 090
    Base curve of the contact lens: 7.58 mm

    What is the contact lens power necessary for complete correction?

9. If a patient has a spectacle prescription of –1.50 DS –1.00 DC x 180 with a 7.50 mm base curve radius, –2.00 D rigid diagnostic lens on the eye, and the refractive error completely corrected, what is the patient's keratometer reading?

10. A patient with a spectacle correction in one eye of –1.00 DS –0.50 DC x 180 is to be fitted with a rigid contact lens. A diagnostic lens with a radius of curvature of 8.04 mm and power –3.00 D is placed on the eye. OR to best acuity is +1.50 DS. The decision is to order a lens with a base curve radius of 7.94 mm for the patient. What power should be ordered for the contact lens?

11. A patient having a spectacle correction of –3.00 DS –0.50 DC x 180 is fitted with a –3.50 DS contact lens. If keratometer readings are 42.75 D at 180° and 43.25 D at 90°, and the OR is +1.00 DS, what is the power of the base curve of the contact lens measured on a keratometer?

12. A patient has K readings of 43.50 D at 180° and 46.50 D at 90°. The spectacle prescription is plano. The patient is fit with a toric back surface that matches perfectly with the cornea. What is the radius of curvature of the vertical meridian of the front surface of the contact lens?

13. A hard contact lens with a spherical front curve is analyzed on a lensometer to be –0.50 DS –4.37 DC x 180. The radius of curvature is 8.49 mm in the horizontal meridian on the back surface.

    What is the radius of curvature in the vertical meridian on the back side?

14. The power of a toric-base spherical front surface contact lens is measured with a lensometer and is found to be plano –3.25 DC x 180. What is the approximate OR when the lens is properly placed on an emmetropic eye